ATHLETIC INJURIES of the SHOULDER

ATHLETIC INJURIES of the SHOULDER

Editor

FRANK A. PETTRONE, M.D.

Associate Clinical Professor
Department of Orthopaedics
Georgetown University Medical School
Washington, D.C.

McGraw-Hill, Inc.
HEALTH PROFESSIONS DIVISION

New York St. Louis San Francisco Auckland Bogotá
Caracas Lisbon London Madrid Mexico City Milan Montreal
New Delhi San Juan Singapore Sydney Tokyo Toronto

ATHLETIC INJURIES OF THE SHOULDER

1 2 3 4 5 6 7 8 9 0   KGPKGP   9 8 7 6 5 4

ISBN 0-07-049742-7

This book was set in Melior by Compset, Inc. The editors were Jane E. Pennington and Lester A. Sheinis. The production supervisor was Clare Stanley. The cover designer was Marsha Cohen/Parallelogram. The indexer was Tony Greenberg, M.D.
Arcata Graphics/Kingsport was printer and binder.

The book is printed on acid-free paper.

Library of Congress Cataloging-in-Publication Data

Athletic injuries of the shoulder / [edited by] Frank A. Pettrone.
    p.   cm.
  Includes bibliographical references and index.
  ISBN 0-07-049742-7
  1. Shoulder—Wounds and injuries. 2. Sports injuries.
I. Pettrone, Frank A.
  [DNLM: 1. Shoulder—injuries. 2. Rotator Cuff—injuries.
3. Athletic Injuries. WE 810 A8715 1995]
RD557.5.A833 1995
617.5'72044—dc20
DNLM/DLC
for Library of Congress   93-44977

CONTENTS

v

CONTRIBUTORS

NOTE: Numbers in brackets refer to the chapters written or co-written by the contributor.

David W. Altchek, M.D.
Assistant Attending Surgeon at the Hospital for
    Special Surgery
Assistant Professor of Surgery at Cornell University
    Medical College
Team Physician, New York Mets
Medical Director Association of Tennis
    Professionals
New York, NY   [6]

James R. Andrews, M.D.
Clinical Professor of Orthopedics and Sports
    Medicine at the University of Virginia Medical
    School
Clinical Professor University of Kentucky Medical
    School
Orthopedic Department
Orthopedic Surgeon
Alabama Sports Medicine and Orthopedic Center
Birmingham, Alabama   [24]

James P. Bradley, M.D.
Board Certified Orthopedic Surgeon
Clinical Assistant Professor University of
    Pittsburgh
Team Physician for Pittsburgh Steelers Football
    Club
Pittsburgh, Pennsylvania   [2]

Robert S. Burnham, M.D., M.S., F.R.C.P.C.
Assistant Professor
Division of Physical Medicine and Rehabilitation
Faculty of Medicine
University of Alberta
Medical Consultant
Rick Hansen Centre
Faculty of Physical Education and Sports Studies
University of Alberta
Edmonton, Alberta, Canada   [28]

Richard B. Caspari, M.D.
Clinical Professor
Department of Orthopedic Surgery
Medical College of Virginia
Director Orthopedic Research of Virginia
Glen Allen, Virginia   [14]

Edward V. Craig, M.D.
Associate Professor
Department of Orthopedic Surgery
University of Minnesota
Minneapolis, Minnesota   [15]

Kathleen A. Curtis, Ph.D., P.T.
Assistant Professor
Division of Physical Therapy
Department of Orthopedics and Rehabilitation
University of Miami School of Medicine
Miami, Florida   [28]

Wilson Del Pizzo, M.D.
Attending Orthopaedic Surgeon
Southern California Orthopaedic Institute
Van Nuys, California   [11]

Nick M. DiGiovine, M.D.
Reconstructive Surgery of the Shoulder, Elbow, and
    Knee
Oakland Orthopaedic Associates
Brackenridge, Pennsylvania   [2]

Perry S. Esterson, M.S., P.T., S.C.S., A.T.C.
Director
Center for Orthopaedic and Sports Physical
    Therapy
Vienna, Virginia   [20]

Gregory C. Fannelli, M.D.
Department of Orthopaedic Surgery
Sports Injury Clinic
Geisinger Medical Center
Danville, Pennsylvania   [16]

Susan Foreman, M.E.D., A.T.C., M.P.T.
Assistant Athletic Trainer
McCue Center
University of Virginia
Charlottesville, Virginia   [27]

Peter J. Fowler, M.D., F.R.C.S.(C)
Professor
Orthopaedic Surgery
Head, Sports Medicine Section
University Hospital of West Ontario
London, Ontario, Canada   [22]

Joe Gieck, Ed.D., A.T.C., P.T.
Head Athletic Trainer
Professor
Curry School of Education
Associate Professor
McCue Center
University of Virginia
Charlottesville, Virginia   [27]

Bruce J. Goldberg, M.D.
Orthopedic Surgeon
Park Ridge Orthopedic Surgeons, S.C.
Park Ridge, Illinois   [7]

Richard J. Hawkins, M.D., F.R.C.S.(C)
Clinical Professor
Department of Orthopaedics
University of Colorado
Orthopaedic Consultant
The Steadman-Hawkins Clinic
Vail, Colorado   [8]

Charles Jackson, M.D.
Team Physician
Washington Redskins Football Team
Arlington, Virginia   [25]

Ronald P. Karzel, M.D.
Attending Orthopaedic Surgeon
Southern California Orthopaedic Institute
Van Nuys, California   [9,11]

John J. Kelly, M.D.
Professor and Chairman
Department of Neurology
George Washington University Medical Center
Washington, D.C.   [17]

William Benjamin Kibler, M.D.
Medical Director
Lexington Clinic
Sports Medicine Center
Lexington, Kentucky   [3]

Donald Knowlan, M.D.
Professor of Medicine
Georgetown University School of Medicine
Team Physician
Washington Redskins
Director of Medical Education
Arlington Hospital
Arlington, Virginia   [18]

Robert E. Leach, M.D.
Professor of Orthopaedic Surgery
Boston University Medical School
Waltham, Massachusetts   [23]

John R. McCarroll, M.D.
Methodist Sports Medicine Center
Indianapolis, Indiana   [21]

Frank C. McCue III, M.D.
Alfred R. Shands
Professor of Orthopaedic Surgery and Plastic
* Surgery of the Hand*
Director
Division of Sports Medicine and Hand Surgery
Team Physician
University of Virginia
Department of Athletics
Charlottesville, Virginia   [13,27]

Mehrdad M. Malek, M.D.
Associate Professor
Department of Orthopaedics
Howard University
Washington, D.C.
Director
Washington Orthopaedic and Knee Clinic, Inc.
Oxon Hill, Maryland   [16]

Leslie S. Matthews, M.D.
Chief
Orthopaedic Surgery
Union Memorial Hospital
Baltimore, Maryland   [1]

William D. Morin, M.D.
Director, Sports Medicine Service
Department of Orthopaedic Surgery
Naval Hospital of San Diego
San Diego, California   [8]

Martha C. Nelson, M.D.
Associate Professor
Director of Musculoskeletal Radiology
Georgetown University Medical Center
Washington, D.C.   [4]

William E. Nelson, M.D.
Fellow
Division of Sports Medicine and Hand Surgery
Department of Orthopaedics
University of Virginia School of Medicine
Charlottesville, Virginia   [13]

Robert P. Nirschl, M.D., M.S., P.C.
Attending Orthopedic Surgeon
Arlington Hospital
Arlington, Virginia
Director
Orthopedic Sports Medicine Fellowship Program
Nirschl Orthopedic Sports Medicine Clinic
Arlington Hospital and Georgetown Hospital
Arlington, Virginia   [7,12]

Jeffrey S. Noble
Crystal Clinic
Akron, Ohio   [8]

Francis G. O'Connor, M.D.
Director of Primary Care–Sports Medicine
Dewitt Army Community Hospital
Fort Belvoir, Virginia   [26]

Michael J. Pagnani, M.D.
Attending Orthopedic Surgeon
The Lipscomb Clinic
St. Thomas Hospital
Nashville, Tennessee   [6,10]

Frank A. Pettrone, M.D.
Associate Clinical Professor
Department of Orthopaedics
Georgetown University Medical School
Team Physician
George Mason University
Arlington, Virginia   [5,7,26]

David C. Reid, M.D., M.C.H. (ortho), F.R.C.S.(C)
Professor
Division of Orthopedic Surgery
Faculty of Medicine
University of Alberta
Director
Glen Sather University of Alberta
Sports Medicine Center
Edmonton, Alberta, Canada   [28]

Louis J. Ruland, M.D.
Fellow in Sports Medicine
Union Memorial Hospital
Baltimore, Maryland   [1]

Ethan Saliba, Ph.D., A.T.C., P.T., S.C.S.
Associate Athletic Trainer
McCue Center
University of Virginia
Charlottesville, Virginia   [27]

Stephen J. Snyder, M.D.
Orthopedic Surgeon (specializing in arthroscopic
and reconstructive surgery limited to the
shoulder)
Southern California Orthopedic Institute (SCOI)
Van Nuys, California   [9]

Janet Sobel, R.P.T.
Clinical Director
Orthopedic and Sports Rehabilitation Center
Chevy Chase, Maryland   [19]

Raymond Thal, M.D.
Town Center Orthopaedic Associates
Reston, Virginia
Assistant Clinical Professor of Orthopaedic Surgery
George Washington School of Medicine
Washington, D.C.   [14]

James E. Tibone, M.D.
Associate Clinical Professor
University of Southern California
Inglewood, California   [2]

Laura A. Timmerman, M.D.
Assistant Professor
Orthopaedic Surgery and Sports Medicine
University of California Davis School of Medicine
Sacramento, California   [24]

Bubba Tyer
Head Trainer
Washington Redskins Football Team
Ashburn, Virginia   [25]

Dana R. Verch, M.D.
Fellow
Washington Orthopaedic and Knee Clinic, Inc.
Oxon Hill, Maryland   [16]

Russell F. Warren, M.D.
Chief, Sports Medicine
Hospital for Special Surgery
Professor of Orthopedic Surgery
Cornell Medical College
New York, New York   [10]

Kevin E. Wilk, P.T.
National Director of Research and Clinical
Education
Associate Clinical Director
HealthSouth Sports Medicine and Rehabilitation
Corporation
Director
Rehabilitative Research American Sports Medicine
Institute
Birmingham, Alabama   [24]

PREFACE

In the past decade, we have witnessed an explosion in knowledge concerning the shoulder. Physicians as well as athletes and the general public are keenly aware of the frequency and impact of sports-related injuries of the shoulder. Advances in biomechanics and the advent of arthroscopy and magnetic resonance imaging have broadened our knowledge of this unique and complex joint.

In contrast to other texts of shoulder pathology and disorders, this book focuses solely on shoulder disorders sustained as a result of sports participation. This has been accomplished with contributions from many acknowledged authorities in the field. It has been our objective to create a basic clinical reference for the orthopedist and sports medicine physician. In each chapter, the authors discuss techniques of diagnosis and treatment thoroughly. The text is significantly enhanced by the abundant use of illustrations to amplify critical points. Each chapter also provides a historical review of its subject and a comprehensive list of references.

I recognize that knowledge of the shoulder is changing nearly daily. Each author's approach recognizes this evolution in the field. This text may be one still-frame in a moving picture, but I hope we have produced a clear image of the current state of our knowledge and practice. It is my hope that this book will be of benefit not only to practitioners but ultimately to the individual athlete.

CHAPTER 1

Gross Arthroscopic Anatomy

Louis J. Ruland
Leslie S. Matthews

Over the past 20 years, arthroscopy has become established as a both diagnostic and therapeutic modality.[1-12] Recently shoulder arthroscopy has gained acceptance as a valuable tool in the evaluation and treatment of impingement syndrome,[13-17] rotator cuff disease,[18] shoulder instability,[19-21] acromioclavicular joint arthritis,[22] and other miscellaneous disorders.[23,24] The popularity of shoulder arthroscopy stems from the detailed visualization of intraarticular anatomy not provided by open surgical procedures and the increasing number of procedures performed with less morbidity using arthroscopic techniques. Because of the importance of arthroscopy in the diagnosis and treatment of various shoulder pathology, the orthopedic surgeon must be intimately familiar with normal shoulder anatomy and its variations as visualized through the arthroscope.

SURFACE ANATOMY

Arthroscopy of the shoulder is performed in the lateral decubitus, or beach chair, position. A patient who is undergoing shoulder arthroscopy in the lateral decubitus position will be oriented with the involved side up. With a slight posterior tilt in the shoulder position, the glenoid articular surface will be parallel to the floor.[25] The involved forearm is secured in a device with the application of traction at an angle of approximately 45 to 60° of abduction and 20° of forward flexion.[26] In this position, the following surface anatomy is identified: spine of the scapula, the acromion, the clavicle, the acromioclavicular joint, the coracoid process, the posterior humeral head, and the glenohumeral joint (Fig. 1-1). The spine of the scapula, the clavicle, and the acromion are generally easy to palpate and are the key to the surface anatomy of the shoulder. With palpation of the clavicle one can identify the retroclavicular space, or the "soft spot" just posterior to the acromioclavicular joint, and provide some guidance to locating the acromioclavicular joint. Anterior and posterior translation of the humeral head often allows the surgeon to palpate the glenohumeral joint. The superior glenohumeral joint is usually palpated at a point approximately 1 cm medial and 2 cm inferior to the posterolateral angle of the acromion, and is the location of posterior portal placement for arthroscopy. A low entry site may injure the axillary nerve with the arm abducted.[27] The coracoid process anteriorly provides a guide for the introduction of the arthroscope as its position roughly approximates the orientation of the joint. Palpation of the coracoid may also serve as a key for placing anterior portals. The coracoid process lies deep to pectoralis major muscle and helps protect the underlying brachial plexus and axillary vessels. Because of the neurovascular structure relationship to the coracoid, the entry point for anterior portals should be lateral to the tip of the coracoid to avoid injury to the musculocutaneous nerve or other axillary structures beneath the coracoid process. Once the glenohumeral joint has been entered by the arthroscope, a systematic diagnostic arthroscopy should be performed.[26,28] The biceps tendon is the best intraarticular landmark for initial orientation in the glenohumeral joint and should be identified before adoption of a seven-area approach to diagnostic arthroscopy of the shoulder. The seven-area approach includes 14 specific structures: (1) biceps tendon and bicipital groove, (2) rotator cuff, (3) glenoid articular surface and posterior glenoid labrum, (4) inferior recess and posterior recess, (5) humeral articular surface, (6) anterior glenoid labrum, (7) glenohumeral ligaments, subscapularis tendon, subscapularis recess, synovium, and coracoid process.

BICEPS TENDON AND BICIPITAL GROOVE

The tendon of the long head of the biceps muscle is the most prominent soft tissue structure seen upon entering the shoulder joint from the posterior portal. The biceps tendon attaches to the superior margin of the glenoid labrum at the supraglenoid tubercle. It takes an angular course approximately 10 to 15° away from an imaginary vertical line to the glenoid over the humeral head and through the superior anterior capsule as it enters the bicipital groove of the humerus (Fig. 1-2). The capsular exit of the biceps tendon through the intertubercular groove separates the insertion of the supraspinatus and subscapularis.

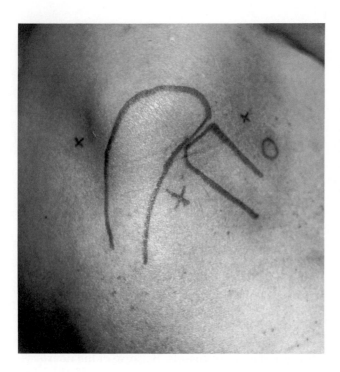

FIGURE 1-1
Outline of bony landmarks and portal sites, left shoulder.

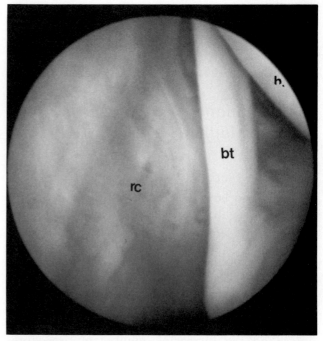

FIGURE 1-2
Initial orienting view of the right shoulder. The biceps tendon (bt) attaches to the glenoid and takes an angular course superiorly to the humeral head (h). The synovium and capsule cover the undersurface of the rotator cuff (rc), making it difficult to define the various muscles and tendons. The biceps tendon courses superiorly to the humeral head and the insertion of the rotator cuff.

The insertion is usually a very smooth, tendinous structure that seems to consistently blend with the fibers of the glenoid labrum. In fact, the long head of the biceps has a four-part attachment to the scapula including anterior and posterior labrum, supraglenoid tubercle, and base of coracoid. Recent arthroscopic descriptions of the superior labral-biceps complex emphasize a role in anterior stability and depression of the humeral head in the glenoid.[29] There is a normal free edge of labrum overlying the glenoid in this area with a potential space normally present between the labrum and the underlying glenoid articular surface (Fig. 1-3). Multiple synovial bands surround the tendon at its exit, and rarely a large synovial mesentery that attaches to the supraspinatus tendon is observed.[29] Elbow flexion introduces additional tendon into the glenohumeral joint for inspection. Some variations in the normal anatomy of the biceps have been noted ranging from total absence of a biceps tendon to the presence of a double structure.[30a]

Disorders of the superior complex, or "SLAP" lesions (superior labrum anterior posterior lesions), are disruptions of the biceps anchor to the superior labrum. Snyder et al. classified the SLAP lesion into four specific types.[36] The type I SLAP lesion demonstrates fraying of the superior labrum with an intact biceps tendon. The type II SLAP lesion shows stripping of the biceps anchor attachment from the

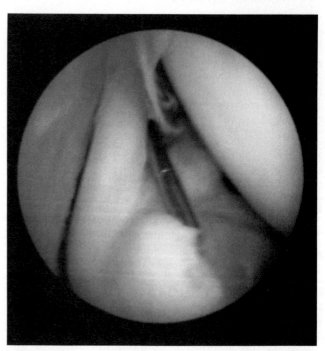

FIGURE 1-3
Arthroscopic view of right shoulder, the probe demonstrating mobility and free edge of biceps tendon attachment to the labrum.

2

supraglenoid tubercle. Type III SLAP lesions are bucket handle tears of the superior labrum with both an intact biceps tendon and biceps attachment to the glenoid. Type IV SLAP lesions are bucket handle tears of the superior labrum with extension of the tear into the biceps tendon. In both type III and IV SLAP lesions the central portion of the labrum commonly displaces into the joint.

Degenerative changes and fraying, narrowing, and adhesions between biceps tendon and surrounding capsule may be observed in patients with chronic tenosynovitis or impingement syndrome. Fragmentation, synovitis, and even complete ruptures of the tendon are noted, often accompanied by degenerative lesions of the supraspinatus tendon.[30–34]

It is important to note the majority of pathology associated with the proximal biceps tendon is actually extraarticular at the transverse humeral ligament or coracohumeral ligament and not well visualized arthroscopically.[35,36] Patients with partial tears or dislocations in the bicipital groove are better differentiated clinically with a history of acute trauma, tenderness over the bicipital groove, pain with resisted flexion and supination, and failure to respond to conservative treatment for bicipital tendinitis and impingement.[35–36]

The rotator interval is an area between the supraspinatus and subscapularis tendon including the exit of the biceps tendon, the subscapularis recess, and the upper tendinous portion of the subscapularis tendon.[37] Because of the extraarticular nature of the rotator interval lesions, arthroscopic findings are subtle. Partial rupture of the subscapularis tendon together with fraying of the biceps tendon is pathognomonic for a rotator interval lesion.[35] Biceps tendon dislocation not only can occur because of a disrupted transverse humeral ligament but can be classified as a rotator interval lesion.[38] Dislocations of the bicipital tendon can occur anterior to an intact subscapularis muscle or posterior to a partially avulsed subscapularis tendon. Evidence of fraying or partial rupture of the tendon as it enters the groove without other findings associated with impingement helps to differentiate rotator interval lesions from impingement syndrome.

ROTATOR CUFF

The rotator cuff consists of tendons from the supraspinatus, infraspinatus, teres minor, and subscapularis muscles. The intraarticular aspect of the rotator cuff tendons, particularly those of the supraspinatus

and subscapularis, can be well visualized arthroscopically. After inspection of the supraglenoid attachment of the biceps tendon, rotation of the scope upward allows one to visualize the supraspinatus tendon just superior to the biceps tendon. The supraspinatus muscle originates in the supraspinatus fossa and blends with the infraspinatus and teres minor at the level of the glenoid. Continuing laterally to their insertion on the greater tuberosity the supraspinatus becomes tendinous about 1 cm medial to the lateral edge of the acromion and then inserts on the superior facet of the greater tuberosity. The most anterior portion of the supraspinatus may be determined by locating the exit site of the tendon of the long head of the biceps. Arthroscopically, it is often difficult to define the various muscles that make up the rotator cuff, as the tendon is normally covered with capsule and synovium (Fig. 1-2). The infraspinatus portion of the rotator cuff can be visualized from the anterior portal. The infraspinatus muscle originates in the infraspinatus fossa and it inserts on the middle facet of the greater tuberosity. The infraspinatus portion of the rotator cuff tendon can be visualized arthroscopically and extends from the capsular insertion on the posterior glenoid to its insertion on the greater tuberosity. The teres minor originates from the lateral border of the scapula and inserts on the lowest facet of the greater tuberosity. The lowest fibers of the infraspinatus muscle blend with the narrow and elongated teres minor muscle which is rarely visualized arthroscopically. Partial and complete tears of the rotator cuff are most commonly seen on the undersurface of the supraspinatus near their insertion on the greater tuberosity. Synovitis in the superior foramen of the subscapularis bursa or at the exit of a biceps tendon may be associated with tears of the rotator cuff.

GLENOID SURFACE

Rotation of the scope posteriorly will allow visualization of the articular surface of the glenoid. The glenoid fossa articulates with the humeral head (Fig. 1-4). Distraction and rotation of the humeral head allows complete visualization of the glenoid, a kidney-shaped cavity with a midanterior sulcus, approximately one-fourth the size of the humeral head. DePalma has noted a thinning of the articular surface slightly inferior to the center of the glenoid that occurs normally with aging. This area is bluish and 3 to 5 mm in diameter. In contrast, degenerative changes of the glenoid are more diffuse, with fraying

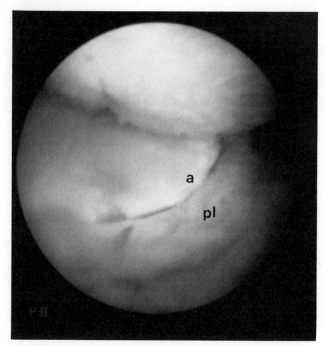

FIGURE 1-4
The posterior labrum (pl) attaches to the glenoid near the articular surface (a).

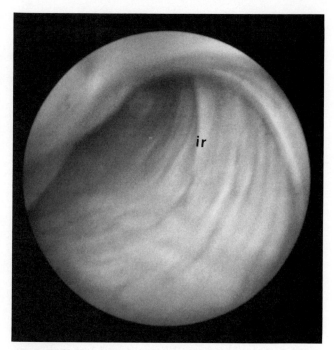

FIGURE 1-5
The inferior recess (ir) attaches to the inferior glenoid and the anatomic neck of the humerus, right shoulder.

and fragmentation of the articular surface and eventually exposure of the subchondral bone. Osteochondritis and impaction injuries can occur as a result of trauma. Snyder recently coined the term GARD (glenoid articular rim divot) lesions, which includes osteochondritis and impaction injuries. The defect observed involves the peripheral glenoid rim articular cartilage (type I), a wafer of subchondral bone (type II), or a large deeper "divot" of bone (type III). The GARD lesion, unlike the Bankart lesion, has no association with instability. Neviaser recently described another source of anterior shoulder pain termed a GLAD lesion (gleno labral articular disruption). The lesion consists of a superficial anterior inferior labral tear associated with an anterior inferior articular cartilage injury.[39] There is no demonstrable shoulder instability. The lesion is similar to the GARD lesion.

INFERIOR RECESS

Continued rotation of the scope inferiorly reveals the inferior capsular reflection onto the humeral head. The inferior recess is a reflection of the synovial and capsular lining of the shoulder joint. The inferior recess corresponds to the axillary pouch of the inferior glenohumeral joint and is a common location for loose bodies (Fig. 1-5). It is also contiguous with the posterior capsular recess, which is the reflection of the posterior capsule prior to its attachment to the

posterior glenoid labrum. The posterior recess is a large cavity in most patients.

HUMERAL HEAD

Only the anterior aspect of the humeral head cannot be examined from the posterior portal. The remaining humeral head examination is facilitated by rotating the humeral head into internal and external rotation. The articular cartilage of the humeral head may not cover the entire intracapsular humerus (Fig. 1-6). It is important to recognize the "bald spot," or normal sulcus, between the posterior extent of the articular surface and the insertion of the teres minor muscle (Fig. 1-7). The normal sulcus should not be mistaken for a Hill-Sachs lesion[40] since (1) the bony sulcus is located more inferiorly; (2) it allows the entry of several interosseous vessels that cause pitting on its surface; and (3) unlike a Hill-Sachs lesion, the bald area is sharply delineated from the surrounding articular surface (Fig. 1-8). Osteochondritis of the humeral head involves the articular surface but is more central on the head and has a wider irregular depression.

GLENOID LABRUM

By advancing the arthroscopy anteriorly, one can visualize the glenoid labrum, a triangular fibrous

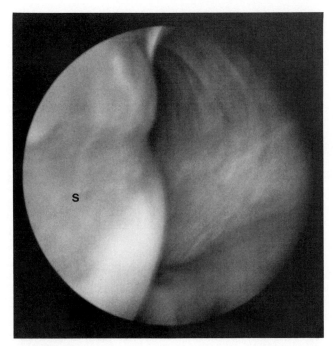

FIGURE 1-6
The normal sulcus (s) or "bald spot" on the posterior aspect of the right humeral head.

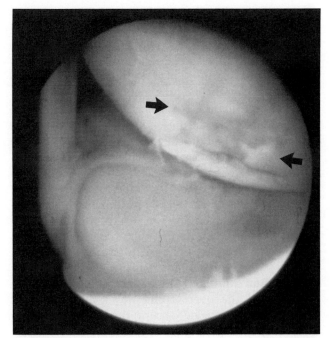

FIGURE 1-8
Hill-Sachs lesion (arrow).

structure surrounding and contiguous with the glenoid articular surface (Fig. 1-9). This wedge-shaped structure that borders the glenoid cavity provides inherent stability to the glenohumeral joint and restricts anterior and posterior excursion of the humerus.[29,41–44] The labrum adds to stability of the glenohumeral joint by increasing the depth of the glenoid cavity and contributing to the suction effect on the humeral head to enhance stability. The structure of the labrum in the lower half of the glenoid fossa is felt to contribute 50 percent to the total concavity or depth of the glenoid fossa. The glenoid surface of the labrum via a fibrocartilaginous transition zone is continuous with the hyaline cartilage of the glenoid cavity while the capsular surface blends with the periosteum of the scapular neck and joint capsule.[42,45] The glenoid labrum is usually made up of the same fibrous material as the surrounding joint capsule and constitutes a thickening of the capsule that provides attachment of synovial and capsular structures, most importantly the glenohumeral ligaments.

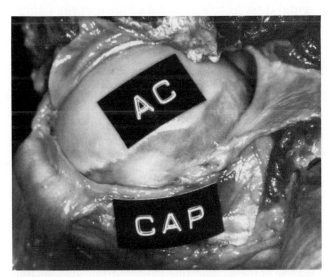

FIGURE 1-7
Posterior view of the left humeral head demonstrating normal sulcus between articular cartilage (AC) and capsule (CAP).

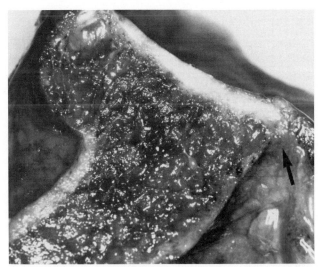

FIGURE 1-9
Horizontal section through cadaveric specimen demonstrating points of attachments of the anterior labrum in the glenoid.

Detrisac and Johnson described the five variations in labral anatomy.[29] The classification is based on the location of a detached central portion of the labrum resulting in separation from the articular cartilage and overlapping of the glenoid articular surface. Type A refers to labral specimens where the superior labrum is not attached to the articular surface of the glenoid and a probe can be passed between the articular surface of the glenoid and the undersurface of the superior labrum. The labrum, located inferiorly, posteriorly, and anteriorly, is firmly attached to the articular surface of the glenoid, unlike the superior labrum which is attached peripherally to the superior scapular neck. In type B (posterior wedge labrum) the posterior labrum is wedge-shaped and thus is attached only at its periphery. Separation extends only a variable distance toward the superior glenoid, and a probe will pass between the articular surface and the overlapping posterior labrum. In type C (anterior wedge labrum) the labrum is firmly attached inferiorly, posteriorly, and superiorly; however, anteriorly the superior band of the inferior glenohumeral ligament is large and covers the labrum. The articular surface is overlapped by the large superior band and relatively small labrum. The type D labrum is a combination of types A and C. In the type E labrum a free central margin is noted around the circumference of the glenoid and a probe can be passed between the labrum and the glenoid articular surface in any position around the glenoid. This classification has been simplified and contains two type of labra: Type I demonstrates a detached central labrum and type II refers to an attached central labrum. Cooper et al. confirmed that the superior and anterosuperior portion of the labrum attaches loosely to the glenoid, while the inferior portion of the labrum is firmly attached to the glenoid rim.[46] They

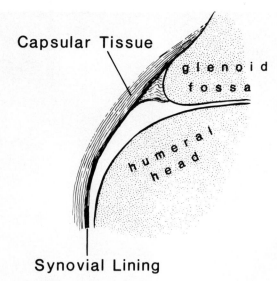

FIGURE 1-11
Illustration of the anterior labrum with external rotation of the shoulder.

also noted in 4 of the 11 specimens the anterosuperior portion of the labrum did not attach to the glenoid or scapular neck and communicated with the subscapularis recess beneath the free edge of the labrum.[46] It is not uncommon to have some synovial fronding or minor labral fraying at the midglenoid notch that is of no clinical significance.

The configuration of the glenoid labrum will vary with changes in arm position.[28] With internal rotation of the arm the capsule folds upon itself, producing a larger labral structure that may overlap the glenoid rim (Fig. 1-10). With external rotation of the arm, the capsule tightens and flattening of the labrum occurs (Fig. 1-11). A variety of tears can be visualized, ranging from the previously described SLAP lesions, degenerative fraying lesions, and bucket handle tears to complete detachment of the labrum from its bony anterior inferior glenoid attachment. The relationship of the individual capsular ligaments to the labrum is also important to understand and is discussed in the next section.

GLENOHUMERAL LIGAMENTOUS-LABRAL COMPLEX

Considerable controversy surrounds the normal anatomy and variants of the glenohumeral ligaments and their relationship to the labrum.[43,44,48–50] Recent arthroscopic and anatomical studies have further increased our understanding of the intimate relationship that exists between these capsular ligaments and the capsular labrum. The superior, middle, and inferior glenohumeral ligaments are thickened regions of the anterior shoulder capsule that stabilizes

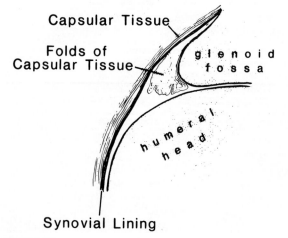

FIGURE 1-10
Illustration of the anterior labrum with internal rotation of the shoulder.

6

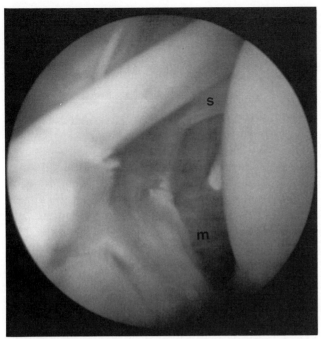

FIGURE 1-12
Arthroscopic view of the right shoulder demonstrating normal appearance of the anterior capsule. Note superior glenohumeral ligament (s) and middle glenohumeral ligament (m).

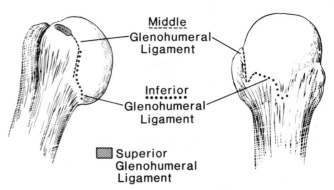

FIGURE 1-13
Illustration of the normal humeral attachments of the glenohumeral ligaments.

the anterior and inferior portions of the joint capsule. Normally they lie close to the glenoid rim; however, these ligaments are anteriorly displaced when the joint is distended with fluid for arthroscopy (Fig. 1-12).[28] Disruptions of these structures result in loss of the stabilizing force of the glenohumeral joint in particular to forward subluxation of the humeral head on the glenoid. The size and den-

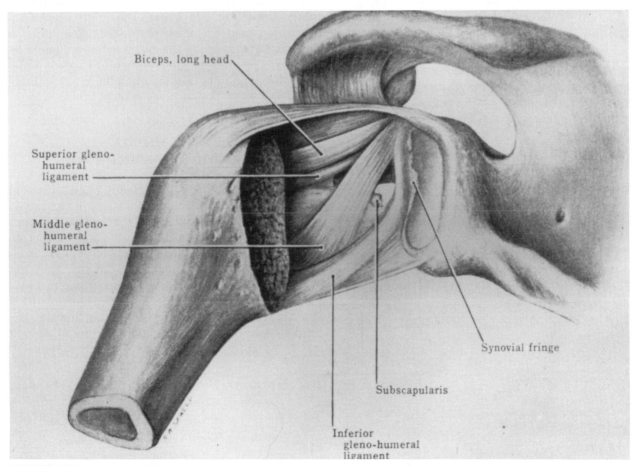

FIGURE 1-14
Illustration of the normal glenoid attachments of the glenohumeral ligament. (*Reprinted from Grant's Atlas of Anatomy.*)

7

sity of the glenohumeral ligaments are variable. All three usually originate from the anterior and inferior humeral head (Fig. 1-13) at the anatomic neck and insert on the glenoid at the glenoid labrum (Fig. 1-14). The major glenohumeral ligaments are named for their attachment on the humeral head.

SUPERIOR GLENOHUMERAL LIGAMENT

The superior glenohumeral ligament is diminutive but consistent, having two proximal attachments: one to the superior aspect of the labrum at that point of attachment of the long head of the biceps tendon and one to the base of the coracoid. The ligament crosses the floor of the rotator interval deep to the coracohumeral ligament and inserts into the fovea capitis of the proximal part of the humerus which is located at the superior aspect of the lesser tuberosity. Arthroscopically, the superior glenohumeral ligament is poorly visualized because of its synovial covering as well as its anterior position relative to the biceps tendon. The superior glenohumeral ligament and the rotator interval capsule, of which the extraarticular coracohumeral ligament is a compo-

nent, may be important for preventing inferior and posterior instability of the glenohumeral joint.[37]

MIDDLE GLENOHUMERAL LIGAMENT

The middle glenohumeral ligament originates from the midportion of the anatomic neck of the humerus, courses superiorly, and inserts into the midportion of the anterior glenoid labrum. Although the attachments of the ligament are wide, they are often difficult to visualize arthroscopically. The middle portion of the ligament can be seen just posterior to the subscapularis tendon, with which it sometimes fuses (Fig. 1-15). This ligament extends from just beneath the superior glenohumeral ligament along the anterior border of the glenoid to the junction of the middle and inferior third of the glenoid rim. It then blends with the capsule of the anteroinferior aspect of the shoulder joint and inserts near the lesser tuberosity over the anterior aspect of the anatomic neck of the humerus. Occasionally the middle glenohumeral ligament will insert medially to the glenoid labrum, in which case the inferior glenohumeral ligament will cross the middle glenohumeral ligament and attach to the entire anterior glenoid labrum.[28] The middle glenohumeral ligament stabilizes the glenohumeral joint when the shoulder is abducted to 45°.

VARIATIONS IN THE MIDDLE GLENOHUMERAL LIGAMENT

Four variations of the middle glenohumeral ligament were identified in an anatomical study in 182 cadaveric specimens without Hill-Sach or labral lesions (Table 1-1).[51] Type I, the classic arrangement, was observed in 66 percent of the specimens. Type II, a confluent middle glenohumeral and inferior glenohumeral ligament described in Grant's Atlas in 1947, comprised 7 percent of these specimens. Type III, a cordlike middle glenohumeral ligament that attaches to the superior glenoid, was observed in 19 percent

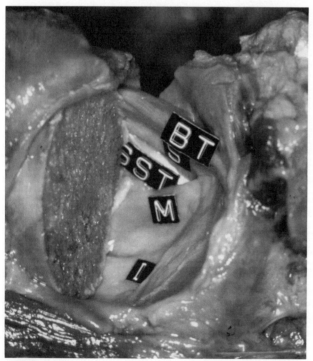

FIGURE 1-15
Posterior view of the left shoulder joint after resection of the humeral head, (BT) biceps tendon, (S) superior glenohumeral ligament, (SST) subscapularis tendon, (M) middle glenohumeral ligament, (I) inferior glenohumeral ligaments.

TABLE 1-1

Type I	Classic appearance
Type II	Confluence of MGHL* and IGHL[†]
Type III	Cordlike MGHL
Type IV	No discernible ligaments

*Middle glenohumeral ligament.

[†]Inferior glenohumeral ligament.

of the specimens. Type IV, no discernible ligaments observed in the anterior capsular sheath, comprised 8 percent of the specimens. Shoulders with the type II variation of the middle glenohumeral ligament were unlikely to demonstrate anterior instability. Shoulders with type IV variation of the middle glenohumeral were predisposed to anterior instability.

Another normal variant described by Snyder et al. is the "Buford complex," which consists of a cordlike middle glenohumeral ligament contiguous with the anterior superior labrum at the base of the biceps tendon and no other labral tissues in the area.[52]

INFERIOR GLENOHUMERAL LIGAMENT

The inferior glenohumeral ligament is often larger than the other glenohumeral ligaments, occasionally demonstrating a separate thickened band along its upper border, and is best visualized when the arm is in abduction in the lateral decubitus position. This triangular ligament arises primarily from the antero-inferior margin of the labrum and inserts into the inferior aspect of the surgical neck of the humerus. The thickest aspect of the inferior glenohumeral ligament along its superior edge is defined as the superior band of the inferior glenohumeral ligament.[54] The size and density of the superior band are variable.[29] A small posterior insertion to the posterior labrum and capsule exists with an axillary insertion directly into bone.[29] In shoulders in which the middle glenohumeral ligament originates medial to the labrum along the scapular neck, the inferior glenohumeral ligament origin extends more superiorly, eventually attaching to the middle and upper glenoid labrum after crossing the middle glenohumeral ligament.[28]

Instability lesions result when a failure of the capsuloligamentous complex occurs. Failure can occur at the glenoid attachment, intracapsular or at the humeral attachment. Detachment of the anterior glenoid labrum will compromise the integrity of the glenohumeral ligaments. Turkel et al. has described the importance of the normal inferior glenohumeral ligament for anterior stability, defining the classic Bankart lesion that involves avulsion of the anterior inferior glenohumeral ligament and labral complex from the anterior rim of the glenoid with an associated rupture of the anterior scapular periosteum.[47] This allows the labral complex to float anterior to the glenoid with an obvious space between it and the rim.

Neviaser has described the anterior labroligamentous periosteal sleeve avulsion lesion (ALPSA) observed in subacute anterior shoulder dislocations.[53] Arthroscopically, there appear to be no ligaments or labrum arteroinferiorly because the labro-ligamentous complex displaces in a sleevelike fashion medially and inferiorly.[53] This lesion differs from the classic Bankart lesion because the anterior scapular periosteum does not rupture but is stripped from the anterior neck of the glenoid. In chronic cases where the lesion heals below the glenoid rim, a crease between the glenoid rim and complex identifies the ALPSA lesion.[53] Other glenoid attachment lesions of the capsuloligamentous-labral complex include the bony Bankart lesion and Perthes lesion. The bony Bankart is an avulsion fracture of the anterior glenoid rim with bone and capsuloligamentous-labral complex displaced from the scapular neck. In the Perthes lesion, capsular stripping from the scapular neck results in an incomplete avulsion of labrum from the glenoid margin. Acute intracapsular lesions uncommonly occur. A tear in the capsule just anterior to the labrum exposes the subscapularis muscle. When no specific lesion is visible but instability has been demonstrated, the diagnosis of exclusion is intrasubstance laxity. In the HAGL lesion (humeral avulsion of glenohumeral ligaments) described by Nicola[54] the deep portion of the subscapularis muscle can sometimes be recognized in the depth of the defect because of avulsion of the glenohumeral ligaments from the humerus.

SUBSCAPULARIS TENDON AND SUBSCAPULARIS RECESS

The well-defined subscapularis tendon is seen anterior to the humeral head. After advancing the arthroscope through the intraarticular triangle, which is bounded by the humeral head, the biceps tendon, and the anterior glenoid rim, one sees the anterior capsule (Fig. 1-16).[55] The posterosuperior edge of the subscapularis tendon can be seen in the anterior aspect of the shoulder between the superior and middle glenohumeral ligaments after they pass over the subscapularis tendon to insert into the anterior glenoid labrum (Fig. 1-17). Only the upper border of the subscapularis is actually visualized with the arthroscope, since most of the broad tendon is extracapsular and covered by the synovium and middle glenohumeral ligament. The fibers of the intraarticular portion of the tendon are more white and compact than the other anterior capsular structures that course across it. These fibers are parallel to the long head of the biceps and perpendicular to the surface of the glenoid. Arthroscopically, one normally sees a

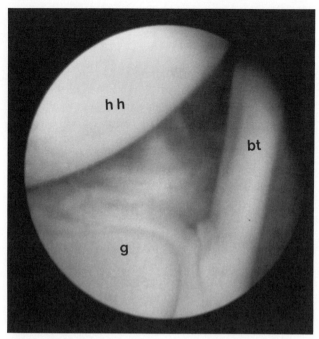

FIGURE 1-16
The intraarticular triangle is bounded by the humeral head (hh), the biceps tendon (bt), and the glenoid (g). The floor of the triangle is the anterior capsule in this right shoulder.

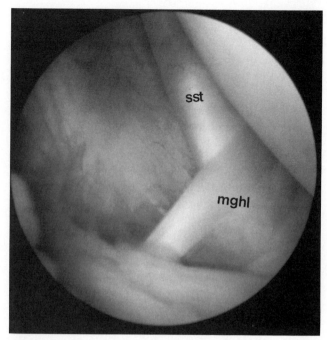

FIGURE 1-17
Arthroscopic view of the anterior aspect of the right shoulder with the perpendicular course of the middle glenohumeral ligament (mghl) to the subscapularis tendon (sst) and its attachment to the anterior labrum and glenoid.

single slip of the subscapularis tendon inserting on the humeral head; however, normal variations include exposure of a larger portion of the musculotendinosis attachment that consists of multiple slips of tendon superiorly and primarily muscle inferiorly.[29] Pathologic findings in this region are unusual but can include ruptures and tears of the subscapularis tendon associated with rotator interval lesions and subluxation of the biceps tendon.

SUBSCAPULARIS RECESS

The subscapularis tendon and muscle are partially separated from the anterior capsular ligaments by the subscapularis bursa. The bursa is located primarily between the subscapularis muscle and the scapula from the level of the glenoid to the coracoid process. Openings of this bursa into the glenohumeral joint are found within the anterior glenohumeral capsular ligaments and are referred to as recesses[30] or foramina.[29] The subscapularis recess opens into the joint just superior to the subscapularis tendon. The synovial space extends anteriorly and is best visualized using one of the higher-angle arthroscopes. The entrance to the space lies between the subscapularis tendon and the superior glenohumeral ligament. This recess is a gap between the superior glenohumeral ligament and the middle glenohu-

meral ligament. This void in the capsule allows one to visualize the superior portion of the subscapularis tendon since it is now intraarticular. Normal variations have been noted by DePalma and include recesses above and below the middle glenohumeral ligament (46 to 89 percent), one recess alone above the middle glenohumeral ligament (6 to 30 percent), one recess only below the middle glenohumeral ligament (25 percent), one large recess above the inferior glenohumeral ligament (9 percent), and two small folds (0 to 11 percent). The second recess, or inferior foramina to the subscapularis bursa, is a void in the middle glenohumeral ligament. This hiatus is located in the inferior portion of the middle glenohumeral ligament, always lateral to the plane of the glenoid.[29,30] In this situation, the width of the middle glenohumeral ligament may be reduced, producing a less substantial middle glenohumeral ligament than seen in cases where one recess is visualized.

CORACOID PROCESS AND SYNOVIUM

The base of the coracoid process can be visualized with the arthroscope from the subacromial space and palpated anteriorly. It is located superior to the subscapularis tendon and medial to the surface of the superior third of the articular surface of the glenoid. The coracoid is an important landmark for localizing

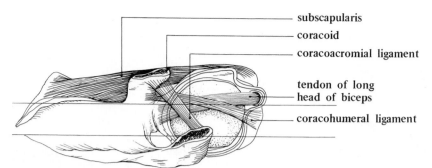

subscapularis
coracoid
coracoacromial ligament
tendon of long
head of biceps
coracohumeral ligament

FIGURE 1-18
Illustration of the anterior zone of the subacromial space.

the vital neurovascular structures that lie inferior and medial to it. The synovium surrounds the shoulder joint and invests all the bony and soft tissue structures. It is important to note the composition of the synovial structure while examining the shoulder joint, since hypertrophy and inflammation of the synovium are associated with pathologic entities including pigmented villonodular synovitis, rheumatoid arthritis, synovial osteochondromatosis, and traumatic etiologies of synovitis.[56–58]

SUBACROMIAL ANATOMY

Arthroscopic subacromial decompression is becoming a standard procedure. If the standard portal is used for introducing the arthroscope posteriorly, visualization of the subacromial space is relatively simple. From the posterior portal the following subacromial structures are appreciated: rotator cuff, acromioclavicular joint, acromion, and the coracoacromial ligament. Dissections and clinical correlation have resulted in the following concept of the subacromial space as it pertains to arthroscopic evaluation and treatment.[59] The roof is composed of the undersurface of the distal clavicle (distal to the coracoclavicular ligaments), the acromioclavicular joint, acromion, and overlying coracoacromial ligament. The insertion of the musculotendinous units of the supraspinatus and the superior 20 percent of the sub-

scapularis and infraspinatus constitute the floor. The coracoid process marks the anterior extent of the subacromial space. Posteriorly, the deltoid muscle limits the subacromial space; medially, the base of the coracoid process and the vertical fibrous bands to the supraspinatus epimysium mark the medial wall. The lateral extent is limited by the deltoid muscle.

Adopting a three-zone concept of the subacromial space is useful for understanding subacromial pathology as it pertains to arthroscopy.[59] The subacromial space is divided into three coronal zones, anterior, middle, and posterior. The anterior or ventral zones contain the structures that lie deep to or to which the coracoacromial ligament attaches and include: the intraarticular portion of the long head of the biceps, the coracoid process, the coracoacromial ligament, and the superior 20 percent of the subscapularis tendon (Fig. 1-18). The middle zone contains the acromioclavicular joint, the anterior two-thirds of the supraspinatus tendon, the anterior one-third of the acromion, and the insertion of the coracoacromial ligament on the acromion (Fig. 1-19). The structures in the anterior and middle zone all may play a role in the impingement syndrome.[60–64] The posterior or dorsal zone contains the remaining portion of the supraspinatus tendon as well as the superior 20 percent of the infraspinatus tendon (Fig. 1-20). The subacromial bursa exists to a variable extent throughout all three zones.

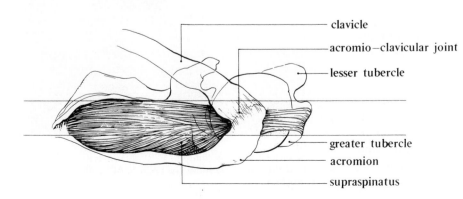

clavicle
acromio–clavicular joint
lesser tubercle
greater tubercle
acromion
supraspinatus

FIGURE 1-19
Illustration of the middle zone of the subacromial space.

11

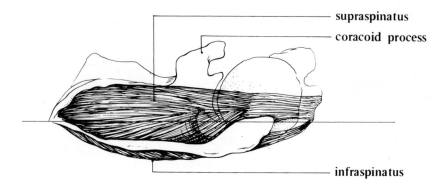

supraspinatus

coracoid process

infraspinatus

FIGURE 1-20
Illustration of the posterior zone of the sub-acromial space.

BURSAS

The bursal cavity is located beneath the anterior half of the acromion, making the bursa a relatively anterior structure. It is therefore possible to enter the subacromial space and yet not enter the bursal space. Subacromial bursa has two spaces, the subacromial space and the subdeltoid space. In addition, the subacromial bursal sac has two layers; one is adherent to the bone above and the other is adherent to the rotator cuff below. Entry into the subacromial space from the standard posterior portal often reveals the bursa to consist of normal filmy, spiderweblike strands of adventitial material.[65] The subacromial space in patients with chronic impingement may contain extensive scarring of the subacromial bursa and one may see hypertrophic tissue consisting of thick fibrous strands.[29,65] Preliminary debridement of the bursa allows visualization of the subacromial space and the structures contained within.

ROTATOR CUFF

The intraarticular surface of the cuff is largely tendinous, but the bursal surface of the rotator cuff is largely muscular. The fibers of the supraspinatus, infraspinatus, and part of the subscapularis are visible. The insertion of the cuff into the greater and lesser tuberosities is also directly visualized. The level of the rotator cuff musculotendinous junction is highly dependent upon the arm's position. In neutral position the musculotendinous junction is approximately at the level of the medial border of the acromion and acromioclavicular joint. All three zones previously described should be visualized to adequately evaluate the rotator cuff. The region of the rotator cuff that is hypovascular lies 1 cm medial to the attachment of supraspinatus tendon and can be evaluated for cuff tear or fraying.[66] The anterior zone should be visualized, especially for patients without rotator cuff disease but with symptoms of impinge-

ment. The rotator cuff underlying the coracoacromial ligament and anterior acromion should be scrutinized for early pathology.

ACROMION

The undersurface of the acromion is usually covered with thick periosteum and a layer of the coracoacromial ligament (Fig. 1-21). The fibers of the coracoacromial ligament insertion blend with the thick inferior capsule of the acromioclavicular joint (Fig. 1-22).[67] The deltoid muscle, the undersurface of which is largely tendinous, attaches to the entire lateral extent of the acromion. One can visualize posteriorly the lateral extent of the scapular spine which is the neck of the acromion.

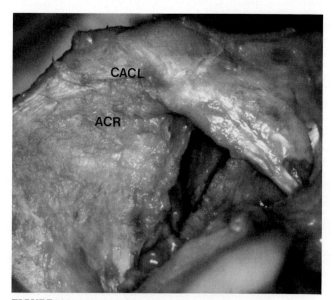

FIGURE 1-21
Inferior surface of the acromion (ACR) demonstrating thick insertion of the coracoacromial ligament (CACL) blending with the periosteum.

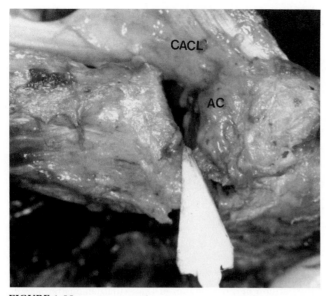

FIGURE 1-22
Fibers of the coracoacromial ligaments (CACL) seen to blend with the inferior capsule of the acromioclavicular joint (AC).

ACROMIOCLAVICULAR JOINT

The acromioclavicular joint is a true synovial articulation. The inclination of the joint is variable. The joint is enveloped by a capsule that attaches to the edges of the articular cartilaginous surface. These surfaces of the acromion and clavicle are separated by an articular disk that is composed of fibrocartilage. The acromioclavicular joint is reinforced both superiorly and inferiorly with the acromioclavicular ligaments.[67]

The acromioclavicular joint is an important landmark lying at the anterior extent of the arthroscopic field. The undersurface can be identified with a needle placed percutaneously into the joint. The acromioclavicular joint is enclosed with a thick fibrous capsule inferiorly that must be opened to visualize inferior osteophytes adequately (Fig. 1-23).

CORACOACROMIAL LIGAMENT

The coracoacromial ligament is the soft tissue extension of the bony acromion. It averages almost 3 cm in width at its origin on the coracoid process, narrowing to 1 cm at its insertion. No functional significance has been attributed to this ligament. The ligament consists of two major bands originating on the coracoid process and joining to form a single insertion. The superiormost insertion on the acromion is in close proximity to the deltoid origin. Fibers of the coracoacromial ligament contribute to the inferior capsule of the acromioclavicular joint. This strong ligament can be easily palpated by the probing finger through the skin and by the arthroscopic probe during surgery. Beneath the coracoacromial ligament lies the anterior portion of the rotator cuff at rest and the long head of the biceps tendon (Fig. 1-24). With forward elevation and abduction of the glenohumeral joint this portion of the rotator cuff comes into contact with the coracoacromial ligament.

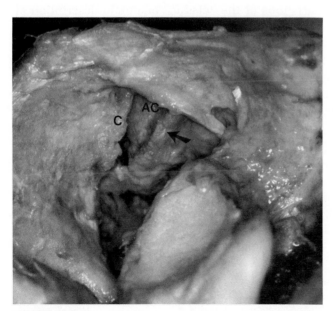

FIGURE 1-23
Inferior view of the acromioclavicular joint (AC) with thick inferior capsules (C) open to reveal inferior osteophyte (arrow).

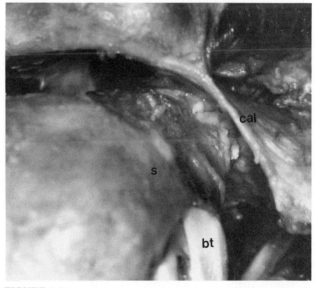

FIGURE 1-24
Biceps tendon (bt) and upper 20 percent of the subscapularis (s) shown to lie under the coracoacromial ligament (cal).

13

SUBSCAPULAR ANATOMY

Cuillo recently introduced endoscopic management of painful subscapular snapping.[68] The scapulothoracic articulation is congruent and consists of the concave scapula gliding over the convex chest wall. The serratus anterior and subscapularis muscle contribute to the normal smooth articulation by cushioning the scapula from the undulating surface of the ribs. Snapping scapula usually is secondary to a compensatory overuse of the scapulothoracic articulation because of primary pathology involving the glenohumeral joint (i.e., SLAP lesion, multidirectional instability, posterior capsulitis), the subacromial space (i.e., subdeltoid adhesions, impingement), or fractures of the scapula or ribs. Anatomic dissections show the scapulothoracic articulation has two spaces: the serratus anterior space and the subscapularis space.[69] (Fig. 1-25) These two spaces are divided by the serratus anterior muscle that courses obliquely from the anteromedial border of the scapula to the anterior lateral chest wall. The boundaries of the serratus anterior space are the rhomboids medially, the serratus anterior posterolaterally, and the chest wall anterolaterally. The subscapularis space boundaries include the subscapularis muscle posteriorly, the serratus anterior muscle anteriorly, and the axilla laterally. A well-defined bursa occupies the serratus anterior space. Portals for arthroscopy should avoid the transverse cervical artery and accessory nerve at the superomedial angle of the scapula and the dorsal scapular nerve and artery that course parallel to the vertebral border of the scapula. Knowledge of the depth of penetration and orientation of instruments is essential to prevent pneumothorax and injury to the contents of the axilla. Normally a dendritic-appearing bursa similar to the subacromial space is observed. Thickened bands, avulsed bone or muscle, healing fractures, and osteo-

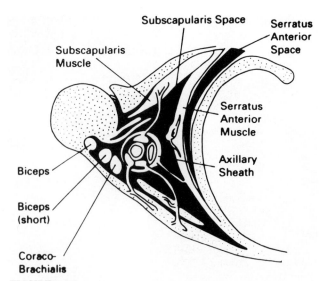

FIGURE 1-25
Illustratiuon of cross section of the axilla demonstrating subscapular spaces.

chondromas are lesions encountered in the subscapular space.

SUMMARY

Knowledge of the normal relationships of various anatomic structures provides the necessary information to understand the normal arthroscopic anatomy of the shoulder. A systematic approach to arthroscopy of the shoulder yields a reproducible method to evaluate the normal anatomy and recognize the abnormal anatomy. Familiarity with normal variations of the "classic" anatomic description allow the surgeon to delineate true pathology from variations of the normal shoulder. This information clarifies the decision-making process for treatment of anatomic abnormalities of the shoulder.

REFERENCES

1. Johnson LL (ed): *Arthroscopic Surgery,* 3d ed. St Louis, Mosby, 1986.
2. Andrews JR, Carson WG Jr, McLeod WD: Glenoid labrum tears related to the long head of the biceps. *Am J Sports Med* 13:337–341, 1985.
3. Andrews JR, Carson WB: Shoulder joint arthroscopy. *Orthopedics* 6:1157–62, 1983.
4. Johnson LL: Arthroscopy of the shoulder. *Orthop Clin North Am* 11:197–204, 1980.
5. Matthews LS, Oweida SJ: Glenohumeral instability in athletes: Spectrum, diagnosis, and treatment. *Adv Orthop Surg* 8:236–249, 1985.
6. Ha'eri GB, Maitland A: Arthroscopic findings in the frozen shoulder. *J Rheumatol* 8:149–152, 1981.
7. McMaster WC: Anterior glenoid labrum damage: A painful lesion in swimmers. *Am J Sports Med* 14:383–387, 1986.
8. Ogilvie-Harris DJ, Wiley AM: Arthroscopic surgery of the shoulder: A general appraisal. *J Bone Joint Surg (Am)* 68B:201–207, 1986.
9. Dolk T, Gremark O: Arthroscopy and stability testing of the shoulder joint. *Arthroscopy* 2:35–40, 1986.

10. Caspari RB: Shoulder arthroscopy: A review of the present state of the art. *Contemp Orthop* 4:523–530, 1982.

11. Lloyd GJJ, Older MW, McIntyre JC: Distention arthroscopy of the shoulder joint. *Can J Surg* 19:203–207, 1976.

12. Johnson LL: The shoulder joint. An arthroscopist's perspective of anatomy and pathology. *Clin Orthop* 223:113–125, 1987.

13. Ellman H: Arthroscopic subacromial decompression: Analysis of one to three years' result. *Arthroscopy* 3:173–181, 1987.

14. Paulos AE, Chamberlain S, Murray S: Arthroscopic shoulder decompression: Technique and preliminary results. *Orthop Trans* 10:22, 1986.

15. Gartsman GH: Arthroscopic subacromial decompression: A clinical study. Presented at the Fourth Open Meeting of the American Shoulder and Elbow Surgeons, Atlanta, Feb 7, 1988.

16. Mendoza FX, Nicholas JA, Rubinstein MP: The arthroscopic treatment of subacromial impingement. *Clin Sports Med* 6:573–579, 1987.

17. Ellman H: Arthroscopic subacromial decompression, in Parisien JS (ed): *Arthroscopic Surgery*. New York: McGraw-Hill, 1988, pp 243–248.

18. Andrews JR, Broussard TS, Carson WG: Arthroscopy of the shoulder in management of partial tears of the rotator cuff: A preliminary report. *Arthroscopy* 1:117–122, 1985.

19. Johnson LL: Arthroscopic management for shoulder instability: Stapling. Presented at the meeting of the Arthroscopy Association of North America, Atlanta, Feb 7, 1988.

20. Wiley AM: Arthroscopy for shoulder instability and a technique for arthroscopic repair. *Arthroscopy* 4:25–30, 1988.

21. Morgan CD, Bodenstab AB: Arthroscopic Bankhart suture repair: Technique and early results. *Arthroscopy* 3:111–122, 1987.

22. Flatow EL, Cordasco FS, Bigliani LU: Arthroscopic resection of the outer end of the clavicle from a superior approach: A critical, quantitative radiographic assessment of bone removal. *Arthroscopy* 8(1):55–64, 1992.

23. Ellman H, Kay SP: Arthroscopic treatment of calcific tendonitis. *Ortho Trans* 13:240, 1989.

24. Ark JW, Flock TJ, Flaton EL, Bigliani LU: Arthroscopic treatment of calcific tendonitis of the shoulder. *Arthroscopy* 8(2):183–188, 1992.

25. Gross RM, Fitzgibbons TC: Shoulder arthroscopy: A modified approach. *Arthroscopy* 1:156–159, 1985.

26. Matthews LS, Fadale PD: Technique and instrumentation for shoulder arthroscopy. *Instr Course Lect* 38:169–176, 1989.

27. Bryan WJ, Schauder K, Tullos HS: The axillary nerve and its relationship to common sports medicine shoulder procedures. *Am J Sports Med* 14:113–116, 1986.

28. Matthews LS, Terry G, Vetter WL: Shoulder anatomy for the arthroscopist. *Arthroscopy* 1:83–91, 1985.

29. Detrisac DA, Johnson LL: *Arthroscopic Shoulder Anatomy: Pathologic and Surgical Implications*, Thorofare, NJ, Slack, 1986.

30. DePalma AF: *Surgery of the Shoulder*, 2d ed. Philadelphia, Lippincott, 1973.

30a. Neer CS: Anterior acromioplasty for the chronic impingement syndrome in the shoulder: a preliminary report. *J Bone Joint Surg (Am)* 54:41–50, 1972.

31. Neviaser TJ, Neviaser RJ, Neviaser JS: Four in one arthroplasty for the painful arc syndrome. *Clin Orthop* 163:107, 1982.

32. Johansson JE, Barrington TW: Coracoacromial ligament division. *Am J Sports Med* 12:138–141, 1984.

33. Warren RF: Lesions of the longhead of the biceps tendon. *Instr Course Lect* 34:204–209, 1985.

34. Neviaser TJ: The role of the biceps tendon in the impingememt syndrome. *Orthop Clin North Am* 18:383–386, 1987.

35. Grauer JD, Paulos LE, Smutz WP: Biceps tendon and superior labral injuries. *Arthroscopy* 8(4):488–497, 1992.

36. Curtis AS, Snyder SJ: Evaluation and treatment of biceps tendon pathology. *Orthop Clin North Am* 24(1):33–43, 1992.

37. Harryman DJ, Sidles JA, Harris SL, et al: The role of the rotator interval capsule in passive motion and stability of the shoulder. *J Bone Joint Surg (Am)* 74(A):53, 1992.

38. Nobuhara K, Ikeda H: Rotator interval lesion. *Clin Orthop* 223:44–50, 1987.

39. Neviaser TJ: The GLAD lesion: Another cause of anterior shoulder pain. *Arthroscopy* 9(1):22–23, 1993.

40. Hill SA, Sachs MD: The grooved defect of the humeral head. A frequently unrecognized complication of dislocations of the shoulder joint. *Radiology* 35:690–700, 1940.

41. Bankart ASB: The pathology and treatment of recurrent dislocation of the shoulder joint. *Br J Surg* 26:23, 1938.

42. DePalma AF, Callert G, Bennett GA: Variational anatomy and degenerative lesions of the shoulder joint. *Instr Course Lect* 6:255, 1949.

43. Townley CO: The capsular mechanism in recurrent dislocation of the shoulder. *J Bone Joint Surg (Am)* 32:370–380, 1950.

44. Moseley HF, Overgaard B: The anterior capsular mechanism in recurrent dislocation of the shoulder. Morphological and clinical studies with special references to the glenoid labrum and the gleno-humeral ligaments. *J Bone Joint Surg (Br)* 44:913–927, 1962.

45. Pappas AR, Gross IP, Kleinman PK: Symptomatic shoulder instability due to lesions of the glenoid labrum. *Am J Sports Med* 11:279–288, 1983.

46. Cooper DE, Arnaczky SP, O'Brien SJ, et al: Anatomy, history, and vascularity of the glenoid labrum. *J Bone Joint Surg (Am)* 74-A:46–52, 1992.

47. Turkel SJ, Panio MW, Marshall J, Girgis FG: Stabilizing mechanisms preventing anterior dislocation of the gleno-humeral joint. *J Bone Joint Surg (Am)* 63:1208–1217, 1981.

48. Fick R: *Handbuch der Anatomie und Mechanik der Gelenke unter Berucksichtingung der bewegenden Muskeln.* Jena, Fisher, 1904.

49. Delorme D: Die Hemmungsbander des Schultergelenks und Ihre Bedeutung für die Schulterluxationen. *Arch Klin Chir* 92:79–101, 1910.

50. Williams PL, Warwick R: *Gray's Anatomy,* Philadelphia, Saunders, 1980.

51. Morgan CD, Rames RD, Snyder SJ: Anatomical variation of the glenohumeral ligaments. Presented at the 10th Annual Meeting of the Arthroscopy Association of North America. San Diego, CA, Apr. 25, 1991.

52. Snyder S, Wu H, Buford D Jr: The Buford complex, loose anterior superior labrum, middle glenohumeral ligament complex: A normal anatomical variant. Unpublished paper.

53. Neviaser TJ: The anterior labroligamentous periosteal sleeve avulsion lesion: A cause of anterior instability of the shoulder. *Arthroscopy* 9(1):17–21, 1993.

54. O'Brien SJ, Neves MC, Arnoczky SP, et al: The anatomy and histology of the inferior glenohumeral ligament complex of the shoulder. *Am J Sports Med* 18:449–456, 1990.

55. Matthews LS, Zarins B, Michael RM, et al: Anterior portal selection for shoulder arthroscopy. *Arthroscopy* 1:33–39, 1987.

56. Curran JF, Ellman MH, Brown NL: Rheumatologic aspects of painful conditions affecting the shoulder. *Clin Orthop* 173:27–37, 1983.

57. Epps CH Jr: Painful hematologic conditions affecting the shoulder. *Clin Orthop* 173:38–43, 1983.

58. Bateman JE: Neurologic painful conditions affecting the shoulder. *Clin Orthop* 173:44–54, 1983.

59. Matthews LS, Ladazo P: Subacromial anatomy for the arthroscopist. *Arthoscopy* 5:36–40, 1989.

60. Salter EG, Nasia RJ, Shelley BS: Anatomical observations on the acromioclavicular joint and supporting ligaments. *Am J Sports Med* 15:199–206, 1987.

61. Neer GS: Impingement lesions. *Clin Orthop* 173:70–77, 1983.

62. Hawkins RJ, Abrams JS: Impingement syndrome in the absence of rotator cuff tear. *Orthop Clin North Am* 18:373–382, 1987.

63. Tibone JE, Jobe FM, Kerlan RK, et al: Shoulder impingement syndrome in athletes treated by anterior acromioplasty. *Clin Orthop* 198:134–140, 1985.

64. Laumann V: Decompression of the subacromial space: An anatomical study, in Bayley, Kessell (eds): *Shoulder Surgery.* Berlin, Springer-Verlag, 1982, pp 14–21.

65. Richardson AB: Arthroscopic anatomy of the shoulder, in Paulos L, Tibone J (eds): *Operative Techniques in Shoulder Surgery.* Rockville, MD, Aspen, 1991, pp 1–7.

66. Rathbun JB, Macnab I: The microvascular pattern of the rotator cuff. *J Bone Joint Surg (Br)* 52:540, 1970.

67. Gerber G, Terrier T, Ganz R: The role of the coracoid process in the chronic impingement syndrome. *J Bone Joint Surg (Br)* 67:703–708, 1985.

68. Cuillo JV: Subscapular bursitis: Treatment of "Snapping Scapula" or "Washboard Syndrome." *Arthroscopy* 8(3):412–413, 1992.

69. Ruland LJ III, Ruland CM, Matthews LS: Scapulothoracic anatomy for the arthroscopist. Presented at the 12th Annual Meeting of Arthroscopy Association of North America. Palm Desert, CA, Apr 2, 1993.

CHAPTER 2

Shoulder Biomechanics in the Athlete

James P. Bradley
Nick M. DiGiovine
James E. Tibone

INTRODUCTION

The shoulder intrinsically enjoys a global three-dimensional mobility by virtue of its skeletal and muscular characteristics. During activity, it is capable of highly mobile, dynamic, and coordinated forceful motion. While most activities of daily living require the shoulder to elevate and position the arm in space, athletic endeavors demand exact and precise motions associated with repetitive propulsive movements. These intricate shoulder movements mandate the maintenance of a delicate balance between functional mobility and stability. The problem is that stability may be jeopardized by accentuated rotation, velocity, force, and repetitiveness inherent to sports activities. An elaborate interaction between dynamic neuromuscular units and static restraints allows the versatile motion, precise positioning, and repetitive forces that are mandatory in effective athletic performance. Unfortunately, minor aberrations (usually secondary to microtrauma) in the mechanisms controlling stability have a significant and cumulative effect on shoulder biomechanics and increase the risk of injury. Clinically, impingement syndrome, eccentric tendon overload, and glenohumeral instability are the most predominant injuries affecting the athletic shoulder. Recently, basic science research has shown that each entity produces individual abnormal variances in the muscle firing and amplitude patterns of the shoulder, thereby reducing overall shoulder function.

In 1944, Inman and associates presented the first comprehensive biomechanical analysis of the shoulder.[1] The shoulder was studied as a dynamic model utilizing anatomic, roentgenographic, and electromyographic (EMG) systems of analysis. Examination of the muscle activity in relation to motion was a revolutionary new approach. The capacity to examine dynamic shoulder motion in standard single planes, as well as during athletic activities with motion analysis and EMGs, produced several axioms of shoulder biomechanics that are now accepted. Recent and ongoing investigations have expanded our understanding of single plane movements, as well as normal athletic shoulder motion. New studies have isolated and studied specific clinical pathologies and correlated them with known normal movements in order to demonstrate anomalous variations in muscle firing and motion biomechanics of the injured shoulder.

This chapter presents a fundamental biomechanical foundation of the shoulder complex including glenohumeral and scapulothoracic motion, static and dynamic restraints, and muscle and joint forces; subsequently, examination of recent concepts in the mechanics of athletic overhead motion illustrated with EMGs and motion analysis; and finally, the effect of specific injuries on athletic shoulder biomechanics.

THE SHOULDER JOINT

The function of the shoulder requires coordinated motion of four articulations, the glenohumeral, scapulothoracic, acromioclavicular, and sternoclavicular joints (Fig. 2-1). In order to achieve coordinated, precise, and many times forceful motion, a synchronous interaction must occur between the articulations and the muscles that control the shoulder system to maintain the delicate balance between mobility and stability.

The Glenohumeral Joint

The skeletal characteristics of the glenohumeral joint permit its global three-dimensional mobility. The articular surface of the humerus is a superomedially oriented hemisphere with a diameter from 35 to 55 mm.[2,3] It forms approximately one-third of the surface of a sphere with an arc of about 120°.[8] The average radius of curvature of the coronal plane is 24 ± 2.1 mm.[9] The surface is retroverted approximately 30° with an upward tilt of 45° (Fig. 2-2).[4–6]

The glenoid, in relation to the humeral head, is small and shallow with half the contour and one-third the surface area.[7] It has an arc of approximately 75° in the coronal plane.[8] The shape is described as an "inverted comma" or "pear-shaped." The dimensions are 39 ± 3.5 mm in the long axis, by 29 ± 3.2

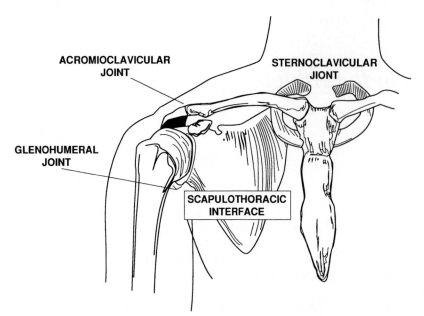

ACROMIOCLAVICULAR JOINT

STERNOCLAVICULAR JIONT

GLENOHUMERAL JOINT

SCAPULOTHORACIC INTERFACE

FIGURE 2-1
The four articulations of the shoulder.

mm in the transverse plane. The radius of curvature of the glenoid in the coronal plane averages 2.3 ± 0.2 mm greater than the humeral head.[9] In the resting position, the glenoid has an upward tilt of 5° and is retroverted approximately 7° (Fig. 2-3).[10] The area and depth of the glenoid is enhanced by the fibrocartilaginous labrum. It has been estimated that the labrum increases the humeral contact area to 75 percent coronally and 56 percent transversely.[11] It ap-

pears, however, that only one-third of the humeral head is in contact with the glenoid at any one time.[6]

The movement of the glenohumeral joint is classified by three patterns of motion: arm elevation, external-internal rotation, and horizontal flexion and extension. Arm elevation is believed to be the most important function of the shoulder. Elevating the arm from the resting position should approach 180°; however, the mean range in men is 167° and 171° in women.[12,13] Extension or posterior elevation is about 60°.[14]

In order to elevate the arm, three planes of motion are possible; they include neutral (scapular), flexion, or abduction. Neutral elevation occurs in the scapular plane (Fig. 2-4). The angle of the arm is approximately 30° anterior to the coronal plane of the body.[15] Basically, the glenohumeral joint is designed to follow the plane of the scapula, because in this position, the path of the humerus is perpendicular to the face of the glenoid and thus in neutral alignment. Also, the inferior capsule has no torsional component when the arm is elevated in the scapular plane.[16] Sagittal plane elevation or flexion aligns the humerus in an oblique orientation to the glenoid and the inferior capsule twists to accommodate.[16] Elevation in abduction requires horizontal extension and external rotation so that the greater tuberosity clears the acromion. Clinically, elevation in the scapular plane is the simplest path of motion and patients with limited strength spontaneously will choose this plane when asked to raise their arms.[17]

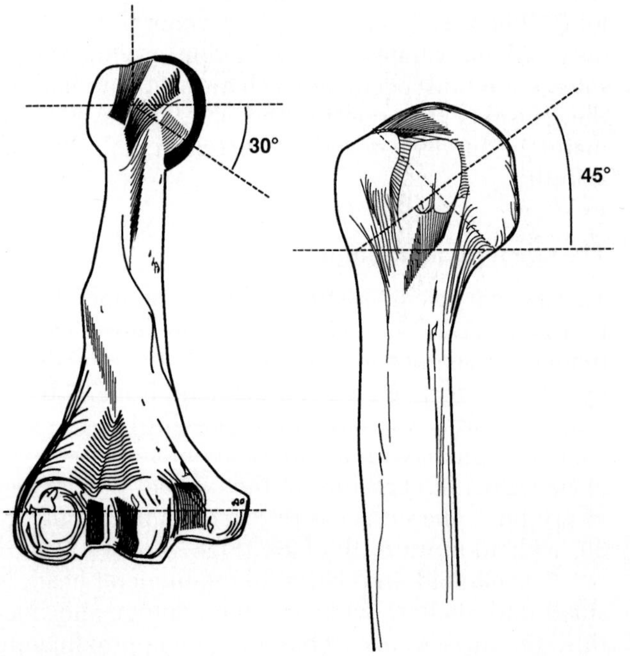

SCAPULOHUMERAL RHYTHM

Total arm elevation requires the contribution of two motion segments: the glenohumeral joint and the

FIGURE 2-2
The humeral head has an upward tilt of 45° and is retroverted approximately 30 to 40° compared with the transverse axis of the elbow.

30°

45°

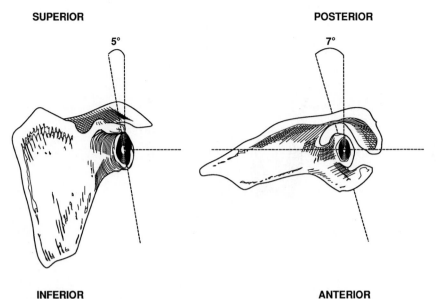

SUPERIOR

5°

INFERIOR

POSTERIOR

7°

ANTERIOR

FIGURE 2-3
In its position, the scapula has an upward tilt of 5° and is retroverted approximately 7°.

gliding of the scapula on the thorax. Scapulohumeral rhythm is the synchronous interaction of both segments to produce fluid arm elevation. During total arm elevation, there is a lag in the scapular motion. The amount depends on the plane (scapular, forward flexion, or abduction) in which the arm is raised. Scapular lag may be as much as 60° in flexion while only 30° in abduction. Scapular participation may be absent, minimal, or even reversed.[17,18] The contribution, in terms of total motion of the humerus vs. the scapula, is controversial. Inman noted a 2:1 ratio of relative humeral to scapular motion.[18] Subsequent investigators have reported both higher (2.5:1) and lower (1.25:1) ratios.[3,11–13] Poppen and Walker noted a 4:1 ratio during the first 25° of elevation, after which a ratio of 5:4 was apparent. Their overall average was 2:1.[19] Bergmann summarized multiple investigations concerning scapulohumeral rhythm.[20]

Generally, during the first 30° of arm elevation, greater motion occurs at the glenohumeral joint, while during the last 60° an equal contribution occurs between the glenohumeral and scapulothoracic segments. The overall ratio throughout the entire arc of motion is approximately 2:1 (Fig. 2-5).

AXIAL ROTATION

The glenohumeral joint controls external and internal rotation. The amount is determined by the relative changes in the capsular length, which is dependent on arm position. Approximately 180° of motion is present with the arm at the side, of which 60 percent is provided by external rotation.[21,22] Abduction of the arm to 90° decreases the rotation arc to 120° with the greater component being internal rotation. In professional pitchers, the external rotation com-

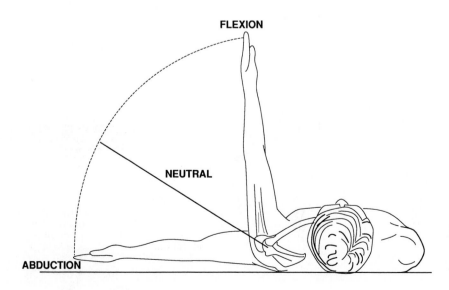

FLEXION

NEUTRAL

ABDUCTION

FIGURE 2-4
Elevation of the arm in the plane of the scapula is neutral. This plane is approximately 30° anterior to the coronal plane of the body.

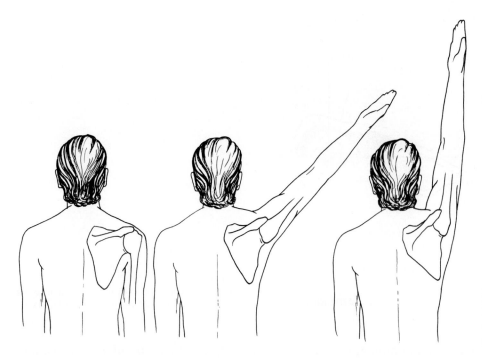

FIGURE 2-5
Complete arm elevation requires the contributions of both glenohumeral and scapulothoracic motion segments.

ponent may be relatively greater secondary to the demands of the sport.[21] At total elevation of the arm, only slight rotation is noted (Fig. 2-6).

Maximal elevation of the arm requires obligatory external rotation.[23] Theoretically, two elements necessitate this external rotation. External rotation allows the greater tuberosity to clear the coracoacromial arch. Also, external rotation of the humeral head, which is retroverted with respect to the glenoid, is rotated anteriorly to enhance its articulation with the glenoid. Morrey and An observed that external rotation also loosens the inferior ligament of the glenohumeral joint, thereby releasing the inferior checkrein effect.[8]

CENTER OF ROTATION

Defining the true instant center of rotation of the humeral head is fraught with technical problems concerning accurate measurement techniques. This complex problem is simplified when limited to glenohumeral motion in a single plane.[24,25] Poppen and Walker defined the center of rotation of the glenohumeral joint as a locus of points situated within 6.0 ± 2.0 mm of the geometric center of the humeral head.[19] Walker found that initial elevation of the arm (0 to 30°) causes a 3-mm upward shift that seems to correct for arm sag in the dependent position. As elevation continued, the point of glenohumeral con-

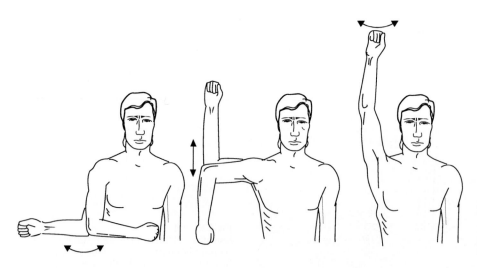

FIGURE 2-6
The relative amount of attainable internal and external rotation at zero, 90°, and terminal shoulder elevation.

tact remained within 1 mm of the center of the fossa.[15] Therefore, it is felt that rolling is not a significant component of shoulder motion. The dominant type of mechanism appears to be gliding of the humeral surface on the glenoid controlled by the intact labrum and the dynamic stabilizers of the shoulder.[17]

Pathologic conditions of the glenohumeral joint alter the center of rotation and allow translation to become a larger component of the motion.[8] Evaluation of patients with painful shoulders illustrated that one-half of them had abnormal mechanics.[17]

CONSTRAINTS

Constraints of the glenohumeral joint are divided into dynamic and static. The static stabilizers are further subdivided into articular (bony) and capsular-ligamentous. Most investigators have focused on the glenoid and labrum when describing the articular stability contribution of the glenohumeral joint. Recent literature depicts the glenoid as having minimal effect on the stability of the joint, and clinically significant variations of the articular orientation are uncommon.[34] The contribution of the labrum in glenohumeral stability has vacillated throughout recent literature. Early literature established the labrum as significantly increasing glenohumeral stability. In 1962, the pendulum swung back by describing the labrum as a specialized portion of the anterior capsule that flattens with external rotation and serves only as an attachment of the inferior glenohumeral ligament.[35] In 1987, data suggested that the labrum effectively increases the depth of the glenoid and therefore has a role in static stability.[36] At present, the precise role of the glenoid labrum regarding static stability is unresolved and further study is warranted.

Bony geometry and negative intraarticular pressure have also been presented as increasing articular static stability.[37,38] However, contemporary literature establishes that the articular geometry minimally aids in the static stability of the shoulder. Static shoulder stability is also enhanced by contributions from the anterior capsuloligamentous complex. This complex consists of the superior, middle, and inferior glenohumeral ligaments, as well as the coracohumeral ligament (Plate 1).

The superior glenohumeral ligament (SGHL) originates at the tubercle of the glenoid anterior to the biceps tendon and progresses inferior and lateral to insert on the humerus close to the superior tip of the lesser tuberosity. It appears that the SGHL func-

tions to passively resist inferior translation of the humerus.[39] Schwartz et al. demonstrated that the humeral head will not translate inferiorly or posteriorly even when the inferior ligament and capsule are released. Therefore, translation in the inferior direction increases the tension in the SGHL and superior capsule.

The middle glenohumeral ligament (MGHL) arises from the supraglenoid tubercle and anterior superior aspect of the labrum and progresses inferiorly to insert on the humerus 2.0 cm medial to the lesser tuberosity. When the MGHL is cut in selective sectioning studies, an increase in anterior translation is noted; however, this does not generally result in instability.[41] Functionally, the ligament tightens as the shoulder is abducted and externally rotated.[40]

The inferior glenohumeral ligament (IGHL) consists of three well-described components: anterior-inferior, inferior, and posterior-inferior.[40] The complex originates along the entire anterior labrum and then progresses inferiorly and laterally to insert on the inferior margin of the humeral articular surface and continues around the anatomic neck of the humerus. The IGHL functions in controlling anterior as well as anterior-inferior instability of the shoulder. Attenuation or detachment of the IGHL appears to be the essential lesion in recurrent anterior subluxation dislocations.[42–44]

The coracohumeral ligament arises from the anterolateral base of the coracoid process and progresses as two bands laterally to blend with the anterior capsule at the rotator interval, finally inserting on both the greater and lesser tuberosities.[45] Although research has been limited, this ligament tightens with external rotation and appears to resist inferior subluxation of the joint.[37]

In conclusion, the primary static stabilizer of the glenohumeral joint is the capsuloligamentous complex. The IGHL appears to be the most important structure in this complex. Morrey and An noted that although the IGHL is the major component of the complex, the other components must not be overlooked and presented a "load-sharing" concept of the soft tissue constraints.[8] This concept postulates that the ligaments function in a coordinated fashion to resist joint translation, chiefly by resisting displacement through their presence and secondarily by transmitting increased joint contact pressure opposite the direction of displacement, thereby increasing joint stability.[8]

The dynamic constraints of the glenohumeral joint primarily consist of the four rotator cuff muscles. The mechanisms utilized by the rotator cuff to increase joint stability include (1) passive muscle tension from the bulk effect of the muscle itself; (2) contraction-producing compression of the articular surfaces; (3) joint motion that secondarily tightens the passive ligament constraints; and (4) the barrier effect of the contracted muscle.[8,38,39,46] Recently, more emphasis is being placed on the scapular rotators (serratus anterior, levator scapulae, trapezius, and rhomboids) in their ability to position the glenoid beneath the humeral head to provide a stable bony platform and thereby assist in dynamic stabilization.[17,43]

The passive stability function demonstrated by muscle bulk in joint stability is illustrated by the increased passive arc of motion when the muscle is removed.[46,47] Many investigators have established increases in anterior, superior, posterior, and inferior translations when the muscles were removed or released.[36,38,46–48]

When the rotator cuff contracts, a centering of the humeral head on the glenoid occurs; this is the so-called centering phenomenon.[8,36] It appears this centering increases joint stability by maximizing contact area and compression; it is thought to be mediated by secondary tightening of the glenohumeral ligaments.[8]

Active joint motion secondarily tightens the glenohumeral ligaments in the direction opposite the rotation.[5,49] As the glenohumeral ligaments become taut, an increase in stability is appreciated.

The barrier effect is the dampening effect of the shoulder musculature during active motion with the ensuing restriction of the active arc of motion.[49] Jobe has described the subscapularis as an important anterior barrier to resist anterior-inferior humeral head displacement in the throwing athlete.[9] Incompetence or stretching of the subscapularis may lead to anterior instability; therefore, many anterior instability rehabilitation protocols try to maximize the muscular function. The subscapularis and the external rotators of the shoulder (infraspinatus and teres minor) represent a force couple that applies approximate equal torques to the humeral head, thereby resisting both anterior and posterior humeral head translation and increasing this barrier effect.[8]

In summary, the glenohumeral joint possesses a vast degree of global mobility; however, there exists a delicate balance between mobility and stability. Stability is monitored by a complex system of static (articular, capsuloligamentous) constraints and dynamic stabilizers. The articular static component supplies a minimal contribution to overall shoulder stability. The majority of the inherent stability of the shoulder is provided by the static capsuloligamentous complex and the dynamic muscular stabilizers.

The Sternoclavicular Joint

The sternoclavicular joint is a saddle-shaped joint. The long axis of the joint is from superior to inferior and the short axis from anterior to posterior.[26] The orientation of the joint is minimally posterolateral, and upward.[5] Motion of the joint appears to be (1) anterior to posterior and (2) superior and inferior translation in addition to axial rotation.[8] An intraarticular meniscus is present, similar to the acromial clavicular joint.

The joint is stabilized by a four-ligament complex arrayed about the joint anteriorly, posteriorly, superiorly, and inferiorly. The intraarticular disk also enhances stability.[27] The interclavicular ligament is the superior constraint that attaches to the superomedial aspect of each clavicle and the middle of the manubrium. Arm depression tightens the ligament while elevation causes it to become lax.[28] Anterior stability is provided by the anterior sternoclavicular ligament which originates from the medial epiphysis of the clavicle and inserts on the sternal articulation border. The anterior sternoclavicular ligament is stronger than the posterior sternoclavicular ligament.[29] Inferior stability is furnished by the costoclavicular ligament which consists of two elements, anterior and posterior. This ligament originates on the undersurface of the medial clavicle and attaches on the first rib. The anterior fibers resist upward displacement while the posterior portion inhibits downward rotation of the medial clavicle.[29]

Six motions occur at the sternoclavicular articulation: elevation, depression, retraction, protrusion, and upward and downward rotation.[5] The joint is capable of about 35° of upward rotation, 35° of anterior and posterior rotation, and up to 50° of axial rotation.[8,18,30] The ligamentous complex controls the amount of motion at the joint, with the costoclavicular ligament being the most important single constraint in limiting motion.[26]

The Acromioclavicular Joint

The acromioclavicular joint is a plane-type joint most commonly oriented anteriorly, medially, and superiorly.[8] The articular surface of the acromion is flat or slightly convex, whereas the accompanying surface of the clavicle is sloped inferiorly and is flat or slightly convex. Because the adjoining articular surfaces are not perfectly matched, an interarticular meniscus is present to aid in force transmission. Stability of the joint is provided by two well-known ligament complexes: the acromioclavicular and costo-clavicular (conoid and trapezoid) ligaments. Many studies have addressed clavicular motion, and at present the subject remains controversial.[18,28,31,32] The potential motion at both the acromioclavicular and sternoclavicular joints surpasses what is actually achieved during active arm elevation.[8] Inman et al. demonstrated during the elevation of the arm that 30° of clavicular elevation occurs. This is accompanied by forward rotation of 10° during the first 40° of elevation, no change in the next 80°, and then an additional 20° during terminal elevation.[18] Rockwood, however, noted only 10° of clavicular forward rotation, placing pins in the clavicle.[28] Rockwood's position is supported by the fact that fixation of the clavicle with a screw to the coracoid does not significantly limit shoulder elevation.[33]

THROWING BIOMECHANICS

Biomechanical comparison of many overhead activities illustrates that the throwing motion is common to many sports, particularly the tennis serve, javelin throw, and football pass. However, the prototype in terms of abundance of biomechanical data is the baseball pitch. Many investigators have studied this complex motion, in both the normal and the pathologic state.[43,44,50–53] These studies detail an elaborate pattern of synchrony of muscular, capsuloligamentous, and bony interactions. Recent studies evaluating electromyographic and motion analysis data have provided new information in the biomechanics and possible mechanisms of injuries sustained by the throwing athlete.[43,50,53]

The glenohumeral joint is the primary site of pathology because it is particularly sensitive to alterations in throwing mechanics. Owing to its vast three-dimensional motion, this joint is constantly trying to maintain an equilibrium between functional mobility and adequate stability.[54] Biomechanical investigations have delineated that throwing transmits tremendous stresses on the shoulder's stabilizing mechanisms, which include the articular contact area, the capsuloligamentous complex, the rotator cuff, and the scapular rotators. During the acceleration phase of throwing, angular velocities of 6100° per second produce a humeral internal rotation torque of 14,000 in-lb.[55,56] A shoulder joint compressive force of 860 newton-meters was observed also during acceleration.[55]

Basically, the stresses generated from throwing

must be dissipated and absorbed by the static and dynamic stabilizers of the shoulder. The articular contact area (humeral and glenoid articular cartilage) provides two primary functions: (1) it disseminates joint loading over a broad area, thus decreasing the compressive force; and (2) it allows movement of opposing joint surfaces with minimal friction and wear.[43] Aberrations in the normal joint compressive pattern resulting from anterior instability produce deleterious changes in the articular cartilage that may lead to osteoarthritis.[43]

The static stabilizers comprised of the anterior capsule (anterior, middle, inferior glenohumeral ligaments), posterior capsule, and labrum provide a restraining effect at the margin of the glenoid. Synchronous firing of the rotator cuff muscles centers the humeral head in the most stable position in the glenoid while providing the maximum available leverage. The scapular rotators contribute by positioning the scapula for optimum bony stability in any overhead position. The scapula moves swiftly, almost simultaneously with the humerus, to maintain the balance and thus the stability of the shoulder.[43]

The act of throwing subjects the shoulder stabilizers to stresses that are sometimes at or near their physiologic limit. If these stresses are applied at a rate that is faster than the rate of tissue repair, progressive stabilizer damage is produced. Small deficiencies in any of the stabilizing mechanisms will have a significant and cumulative effect on shoulder function.

Therefore, if a shoulder is performing at or near its physiologic limitation, any anomalies in throwing mechanics, conditioning, or warm-up will eventually cause stabilizer damage and subsequent decreased function.[53,57]

ELECTROMYOGRAPHY OF THE BASEBALL PITCH

The shoulder muscles provide two salient functions during the throwing motion: activation and stabilization. Activation involves concentric muscle contraction and energy production, which ultimately results in ball velocity. Stabilization embodies eccentric or isometric muscular contractions that function to provide protection dynamically to the skeletal linkage complex during the transfer of energy.[50] As the energy is transferred from proximal to distal, the body parts energized become smaller. Thus the velocity of these parts must proportionally increase to conserve energy. Therefore, the timing of the muscular contractions in the upper extremity is just as important as the absolute force generated. This synchronization of muscular activation is imperative to the smooth and safe transfer of energy through the shoulder during the pitching sequence.[50] The baseball pitch is divided into five phases for the EMG and motion analysis (Fig. 2-7).[54,58]

Stage I   The windup or preparation phase, ending when the ball leaves the gloved hand.

Stage II   Termed early cocking, a period of shoulder abduction and external rotation that starts as the ball is released from the nondominant hand and terminates with contact of the strike foot on the ground.

Stage III   The late-cocking phase that continues until maximum external rotation at the shoulder is obtained.

Stage IV   The short-acceleration phase that starts with internal rotation of the humerus and concludes with ball release.

Stage V   The follow-through phase that starts with ball release and ends when all motion is complete.

Dynamic EMGs and high-speed film analysis of muscles responsible for glenohumeral motion (10 muscles) and scapular rotation (7 muscles) have been investigated.[43,50,54,58] These studies have augmented the understanding of the biomechanics of the shoulder during pitching.

Deltoid

The deltoid muscle is the major motor responsible for arm elevation with active forward flexion and abduction of the humerus.[17,18] All three divisions of the deltoid attain peak EMG activity in early cocking when the arm is elevated 90°.[17] The activity of the deltoid decreases during late cocking as the rotator cuff muscles become more dominant. This sequen-

tial pattern of muscular activity, starting with the deltoid and terminating with the rotator cuff, contradicts the obligatory "force couple" proposed by Inman et al.[18]

Biceps Brachii

The biceps muscle acts predominantly at the elbow, particularly during late cocking and while decelerating the elbow during follow-through.[43,53] However, both the biceps and rotator cuff muscles were utilized to a greater extent during acceleration by amateur pitchers when compared with professionals.[62]

Rotator Cuff

The rotator cuff muscles illustrate an elaborate firing pattern to achieve both activation and stabilization. The supraspinatus muscle during routine elevation helps to initiate humeral abduction.[3,60,61] However, during pitching, its peak activity presents in late cocking when the shoulder is already abducted and most prone to anterior subluxation.[60] The supraspinatus high activity during late cocking is believed to contribute to stability by compressing the humeral head toward the glenoid.[3] The significantly higher activity of the supraspinatus by amateur pitchers in comparison with professionals demonstrates that as expertise increases, so does muscle selectivity.[43,59] Since amateur pitchers fire the supraspinatus to a greater extent, fatigue may precipitate aberrations of dynamic stability, thus jeopardizing the joint. Professional pitchers are much more selective, economical, and proficient in their use of both the supraspinatus and remaining cuff muscles.[59]

The infraspinatus and teres minor function primarily as external rotators. They provide dynamic stability by compressing the humeral toward the glenoid fossa, as well as by external rotation. Both mus-

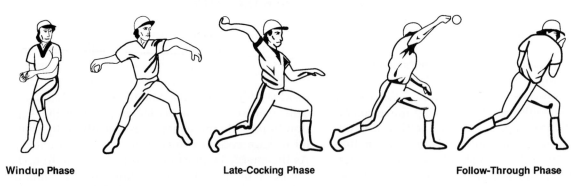

Windup Phase   **Late-Cocking Phase**   **Follow-Through Phase**

    Early-Cocking Phase   **Acceleration Phase**

FIGURE 2-7
Phases of the baseball pitch.

cles have peak EMG activity during late cocking and follow-through; their activation temporarily lags behind the supraspinatus.[62]

The subscapularis demonstrates peak EMG activity in late cocking when it is eccentrically contracting. Theoretically, it functions to decelerate the shoulder's external rotation and therefore presumably stabilize the anterior joint. The subscapularis functions as an internal rotator during acceleration and follow-through.[62]

Professional pitchers demonstrate selective use of the rotator cuff. The activity patterns of the rotator cuff during windup, cocking, and follow-through stages are similar for both amateur and professional throwers. However, the patterns are dissimilar during the acceleration phase when professional pitchers fire the subscapularis selectively over the other cuff muscles.[63]

Rotator cuff injuries may occur during throwing even in advanced pitchers. The thrower who utilizes the rotator cuff muscles inappropriately is predisposed to overuse injuries; this applies to the firing patterns not only of the shoulder but also of the trunk and lower extremities.[17,65] Effective, efficient rotator cuff, trunk, and lower extremity synchrony, acquired through repetitive training and preventive programs, may preclude injuries secondary to overuse.[44,53,54,57,64]

Pectoralis Major and Latissimus Dorsi

The pectoralis major and latissimus dorsi functionally provide internal rotation of the humerus. During late cocking, these muscles, along with the subscapularis, contract eccentrically to dynamically stabilize the anterior glenohumeral joint.[50,66] As the late cocking phase ends, these muscles are already cocked in a prestretched mode; they start the acceleration phase by contracting concentrically, propelling the humerus into rapid internal rotation. The pectoralis and latissimus are the main muscles that actively impart velocity to the ball. The subscapularis is primarily a steering muscle to position the humeral head precisely in the glenoid and protect the head from levering out of the joint.[17,50]

Scapular Rotators

Scapular rotation is controlled by six muscle units: the serratus anterior; upper, middle, and lower trapezius; rhomboids; and levator scapulae. Synergistic action of the muscles varies with the desired scapular motion, which is divided into four basic movements: upward rotation, retraction, protraction, and depression.

The principal concern during throwing is upward rotation with concomitant arm elevation. The primary upward rotators are the serratus and trapezius.[51] Inman et al.[18] noted that only the upper trapezial segment produced consistent activity in both abduction and flexion. Therefore, the serratus is probably responsible for the major burden of scapular elevation; however, both muscles must be available to achieve maximal scapular rotation.[43,51]

EMG analysis has heightened our understanding of the magnitude of serratus muscular contribution during throwing. During routine arm elevation (to 90°), testing showed serratus activity averaged 41 percent of maximum, continuing to full elevation, which required 66 percent of maximum.[17] However, serratus activity during pitching demonstrated a short period that exceeded 100 percent of maximum.[17] The activity of the serratus was consistently greater than that of the trapezius, which showed only 34 to 42 percent of maximum. Interestingly, the two muscles are of equivalent size (12.8 and 12.6 cm²) and therefore should produce similar force potentials.[61] This greater demand placed on the serratus muscle during pitching has led investigators to advise selective serratus training to enable it to withstand the added burden while throwing.[43,51]

Basically, the serratus muscle primarily controls the scapula to provide a stable glenoid to serve as a secure platform for the humeral head. This is particularly important during late cocking, when the serratus controls upward rotation and protraction, thus allowing the scapula to accompany the humerus, which is horizontally flexing and externally rotating. Trapezius activity is relatively low during both cocking and acceleration, indicating that this muscle predominantly provides supplemental scapular stabilization to improve the rotational action of the serratus. Trapezial peak activity is demonstrated during follow-through, where its adduction action aids in deceleration of scapular protraction.[17]

Early throwing studies concentrated on the roles of the deltoid and rotator cuff. Recently, more attention has been directed toward the role of the scapular rotators in providing a stable platform for the actions of the humerus. Impairment of the scapular rotators (specifically the serratus), exhibited by early fatigue, may generate additional stress on the anterior shoulder stabilizers and thus become a harbinger of injury.[52,57]

In summary, the muscles of the shoulder during the baseball pitch fire in a highly coordinated manner, balancing the requirements of stabilization with rapid motion. Every muscle has a unique role in this process. It is now apparent that the scapular rotators contribute by first functioning to optimally position the glenoid against the humeral head, then provide a stable base for the rapid humeral motion, and finally control the deceleration of the scapula after ball release. The supraspinatus functions with the deltoid as it fine-tunes the position of the humeral head against the glenoid. The subscapularis, pectoralis major, and latissimus dorsi are part of the components of the "anterior wall" that provide stability during the period of maximum humeral external rotation; the pectoralis and latissimus are the primary "power driver" muscles to impart velocity to the ball.

Clinical Impingement and the Throwing Shoulder

EMG analysis of throwers with clinical pure impingement demonstrated aberrations in the muscle firing patterns between normals and impingers. Specifically noted is a lower level of supraspinatus activity during late cocking, with a concomitant prolongation of deltoid activity. Presumably this impedes the ability of the supraspinatus to assist the deltoid in cocking and alters its ability to draw the humeral head into the glenoid. Theoretically this reduction in supraspinatus activity is an attempt to reduce tension in the injured tendon, thus setting up the shoulder for a dynamic muscle imbalance.[51]

The most significant differences occurred in the internal rotators (subscapularis, pectoralis major, and latissimus muscles) and serratus anterior. This lower activity may allow increased external rotation, superior humeral head migration, and impaired scapular rotation, all of which could predispose or magnify the impingement process.[17] These findings may provide evidence that neuromuscular anomalies account for the initial and persistent impingement symptoms experienced by throwing athletes.[17]

Clinical Instability and the Throwing Athlete

EMG analysis of pitchers with clinical anterior glenohumeral instability revealed anomalies in the muscle firing patterns between normals and subluxators.[53] In contrast to the firing activity in impingers, the supraspinatus demonstrated enhanced activity through late cocking and acceleration. Presumably this increased activity may help in compensating for lax anterior restraints. The infraspinatus firing pattern was also increased during early cocking and acceleration. Theoretically this increased activity may hold the humeral head posteriorly, thus resisting anterior humeral translation.[53] Similar to the activity in impingers, the internal rotators (subscapularis, pectoralis major, and latissimus) in subluxators illustrated a marked decrease in activity compared with

normals. Inhibition of the synergistic activity of these muscles could allow accentuated external rotation of the humerus and nullifies their ability as dynamic stabilizers of the anterior shoulder. These findings may be associated in producing or perpetuating chronic anterior instability in the throwing athlete.[17,53]

In normal throwers, the biceps brachii appears to play a minimal role and acts primarily at the elbow. However, in subluxators, biceps activity is notably increased during acceleration when the shoulder is prone to instability. Hypothetically the biceps may contribute as a compensatory mechanism to assist in dynamic stabilization.[53] What remains obscure is whether the neuromuscular imbalance presented in subluxators is the primary etiology of instability or a secondary phenomenon.

EMG AND MOTION ANALYSIS OF SWIMMING

Freestyle swimming has many of the same shoulder biomechanical characteristics as overhead throwing. In competitive swimming, the shoulder is subjected to multiple stresses that lead to a high rate of injury very similar to that of the throwing shoulder.[51] Utilizing EMG and motion analysis, the freestyle was broken down into four distinct stages similar to the five stages of throwing.[67] The examination specifically documented that the supraspinatus and serratus anterior muscles produced constant firing activity during the stroke cycle.[67] Presumably this constant activity may lead to fatigue, which may progress to a muscular imbalance and hamper dynamic stabilization. Conditioning and rehabilitation programs currently being constructed address these muscle groups and hopefully will prevent their overuse.[51]

Painful shoulders during freestyle swimming were also analyzed in comparison with normals.[68] Significant differences were recorded in the activity amplitude levels of 7 of the 12 muscles tested. The lack of a specific clinical diagnosis limits the ability to draw definite biomechanical conclusions. However, the data confirm that no differences in the firing pattern were appreciated, while significant amplitude differences were noted in several muscles. Further studies are planned to segregate swimmers with painful shoulders into clinical diagnostic categories.[51]

Multiple other strokes, including butterfly, backstroke, and breaststroke, have already been examined, concentrating on both normal and painful shoulders.[51] Integration and assimilation of those data are presently being completed and compared. Similar investigations studying the tennis stroke and golf swing have also been completed.[17]

SUMMARY

The shoulder complex biomechanically demonstrates an intricate interaction between skeletal and muscular components permitting vast three-dimensional motion. However, a delicate balance exists between functional mobility and adequate stability. Static and dynamic stabilizers allow versatile motion, precise positioning, and forceful propulsion. During athletic activity (especially throwing), tremendous stresses are placed on these stabilizers, which may be at or near their physiologic limit. Even a small deficiency, either skeletal or muscular, has a significant and cumulative effect on shoulder function and may be a harbinger of injury. Thus it is helpful to have a good biomechanical foundation and understand the demands placed on the upper extremity during athletic activities to allow thoughtful treatment and rehabilitation.

REFERENCES

1. Bankart ASB: The pathology and treatment of recurrent dislocation of the shoulder joint. *Br J Surg* 26:23, 1938.
2. Maki S, Gruen T: Anthropometric study of the glenohumeral joint. *Transactions, 22nd Annual Meeting of American Orthopedic Research Society* 1:173, 1976.
3. Poppen NK, Walker PS: Normal and abnormal motion of the shoulder. *J Bone Joint Surg (Am)* 58A:195, 1976.
4. Codman EA: *The Shoulder.* Boston, Thomas Todd, 1934.
5. Dempster WT: Mechanisms of shoulder movement. *Arch Phys Med Rehabil* 46A:49, 1965.
6. Steindler A: *Kinesiology of the Human Body under Normal and Pathological Conditions.* Springfield, IL, Charles C Thomas, 1955.
7. Kent BE: Functional anatomy of the shoulder complex. *Phys Ther* 51:867, 1971.
8. Morrey BF, An K-N: Biomechanics of the shoulder, in Rockwood CA, Matsen FA III (eds): *The Shoulder,* vol 1. Philadelphia, Saunders, 1990, chap 6, pp 208–245.
9. Iannotti JP, Gabriel JP, Schneck SL, et al: The normal glenohumeral relationships. *J Bone Joint Surg (Am)* 74A:491, 1992.
10. Saha AK: Dynamic stability of the glenohumeral joint. *Acta Orthop Scand* 42:491, 1971.
11. Saha AK: Mechanics of evaluation of the glenohumeral joint: Its application in rehabilitation of flail shoulder in upper brachial plexus injuries and poliomyelitis and in replacement of upper humerus by prosthesis. *Acta Orthop Scand* 44:668, 1973.
12. Doody SG, Freedman L, Waterland JC: Shoulder movements during abduction in the scapular plane. *Arch Phys Med Rehabil* 51:595, 1970.
13. Freedman L, Munro RR: Abduction of the arm in the scapular plane: Scapular and glenohumeral movements. *J Bone Joint Surg* 48A:1503, 1966.
14. Matsen FA III: Biomechanics of the shoulder, in Frankel VH, Nordin M (eds): *Basic Biomechanics of the Skeletal System.* Philadelphia, Lea & Febiger, 1980, p 221.
15. Walker PS: *Human Joints and Their Artificial Replacements.* Springfield, IL, Charles C Thomas, 1977.
16. Johnston TB: The movements of the shoulder joint. *Br J Surg* 25:252, 1937.
17. Perry J, Glousman R: Biomechanics of throwing, in Nicholas JA, Hershman EB, Posner MA (eds): *The Upper Extremity in Sports Medicine.* St Louis, Mosby, 1990, chap 32, pp 725–750.
18. Inman VT, Saunders JB de CM, Abbott LC: Observations on the function of the shoulder joint. *J Bone Joint Surg* 26:1, 1944.
19. Poppen NK, Walker PS: Normal and abnormal motion of the shoulder. *J Bone Joint Surg (Am)* 58A:195, 1976.
20. Bergmann G: Biomechanics and pathomechanics of the shoulder joint with reference to prosthetic joint replacement, in Kibel R et al (eds): *Shoulder Replacement.* Berlin, Springer-Verlag, 1987.
21. Bechtol CO: Biomechanics of the shoulder. *Clin Orthop* 146:37, 1980.
22. Boone DC, Azen SP: Normal range of motion in joints in male subjects. *J Bone Joint Surg (Am)* 61A:756, 1979.
23. Johnston TB: The movements of the shoulder joint. A plea for the use of the "plane of the scapula" as the plane of reference for movements occurring at the humero-scapular joint. *Br J Surg* 25:252, 1937.
24. Sigholm G, Herberts P, Almstrom C, Kodifors R: Electromyographic analysis of shoulder muscle load. *J Orthop Res* 1:379, 1984.

25. Taylor CL, Blaschke AC: Method for kinetic analysis of motions of the shoulder, arm and hand complex. *Ann NY Acad Sci* 1251:19, 1970.

26. Kapandji I: *The Physiology of Joints.* Baltimore, Williams & Wilkins, 1970, vol 1.

27. Grant JCB: *Method of Anatomy,* 7th ed. Baltimore, Williams & Wilkins, 1965.

28. Rockwood CA Jr, Green DP (eds): *Fractures in Adults,* 2d ed. Philadelphia, Lippincott, 1984.

29. Bearm JG: Direct observation on the function of the capsule of the sternoclavicular joint in clavicular support. *J Anat* 101:159, 1967.

30. Lucas DB: Biomechanics of the shoulder joint. *Arch Surg* 107(3):425, 1973.

31. Landon GC, Chao EY, Cofield RH: Three dimensional analysis of angular motion of the shoulder complex. *Trans Orthop Res Soc* 3:297, 1978.

32. Fukuda K, Craig EV, An K-N, et al: Biomechanical study of the ligamentous system of the acromioclavicular joint. *J Bone Joint Surg* 68A:434, 1986.

33. Kennedy JC, Cameron H: Complete dislocation of the acromioclavicular joint. *J Bone Joint Surg* 36B:202, 1954.

34. Bergman RA, Thompson SA, Afifi A: *Catalog of Human Variation.* Baltimore, Urban & Schwarzenberg, 1984.

35. Moseley HE, Overgaard B: The anterior capsular mechanism in recurrent anterior dislocation of the shoulder. *J Bone Joint Surg (Am)* 44B:913, 1962.

36. Howell SM, Galinat BJ: The containment mechanism: The primary stabilizer of the glenohumeral joint. Paper presented at the annual meeting of the AAOS, San Francisco, Jan. 23, 1987.

37. Basmajian JV, Bazant FJ: Factors preventing downward dislocation of the adducted shoulder joint. *J Bone Joint Surg (Am)* 41A:1182, 1959.

38. Kumar VP, Balasubramaniam P: The role of atmospheric pressure in stabilizing the shoulder: An experimental study. *J Bone Joint Surg (Am)* 67B:719, 1985.

39. Terry GC, Hammon D, France P: Stabilizing function of passive shoulder restraints, unpublished data from the Hughston Orthopaedic Clinic, Columbus, GA, 1988.

40. Turkel SJ, Panio MW, Marshall JL, Girgis FG: Stabilizing mechanisms preventing anterior dislocation of the glenohumeral joint. *J Bone Joint Surg (Am)* 63A:1208, 1981.

41. Schwartz E, Warren RF, O'Brien SJ, Fronek J: Posterior shoulder instability. *Orthop Clin North Am* 18(3):409, 1987.

42. Neer CS II, Foster CR: Inferior capsular shift for involuntary inferior and multidirectional instability of the shoulder. *J Bone Joint Surg* 62A:897, 1980.

43. Bradley JP, Perry J, Jobe FW: The biomechanics of the throwing shoulder. *Perspect Orthop Surg* 1(2):50, 1990.

44. Jobe FW, Bradley JP: The diagnosis and nonoperative treatment of shoulder injuries in athletes. *Clin Sports Med* 8(3):419, 1989.

45. DePalma AF, Callery G, Bennett GA: Variational anatomy and degenerative lesions of the shoulder bone. *Instr Course Lect* 16:255, 1949.

46. Browne A, Morrey BF, An K-N: Elevation of the arm in the scapula. Submitted for publication.

47. Partridge MJ: Joints. The limitation of their range of movement, and an explanation of certain surgical conditions. *J Anat* 108:346, 1923.

48. Ovesan J, Nielsen S: Anterior and posterior shoulder instability. *Acta Orthop Scand* 57:324, 1986.

49. Cleland D: Notes on raising the arm. *J Anat Physiol* 18:275, 1884.

50. DiGiovine NM, Jobe FW, Pink M, Perry J: An electromyographic analysis of the upper extremity in pitching. *J Shoulder Elbow Surg* 1(1):15, 1992.

51. Bradley JB, Tibone JE: Electromyographic analysis of muscle action about the shoulder. *Clin Sports Med* 10(4):789, 1991.

52. Jobe FW, Bradley J: Rotator cuff injuries in baseball. Prevention and rehabilitation. *Sports Med* 6:378, 1988.

53. Glousman R, Jobe FW, Tibone JE, et al: Dynamic electromyographic analysis of the throwing shoulder with glenohumeral instability. *J Bone Joint Surg* 70A:220–226, 1988.

54. Jobe FW, Tibone JE, Moynes DR, et al: An EMG analysis of the shoulder in pitching and throwing: A preliminary report. *Am J Sports Med* 11:3, 1983.

55. Feltner M, Dapena J: Dynamics of the shoulder and elbow joints of the throwing arm during a baseball pitch. *Int J Sports Biomech* 2:235, 1986.

56. Pappas AM, Zawacki RM, Sullivan TJ: Biomechanics of baseball pitching: A preliminary report. *Am J Sports Med* 13:216, 1985.

57. Jobe FW, Bradley JB, Pink M: Treatment of impingement syndrome in overhand athletes: A philosophical basis, vol I. *Surg Rounds Orthop* 4:19, 1990.

58. Jobe FW, Moynes DR, Tibone JE, et al: An EMG analysis of the shoulder in pitching: A second report. *Am J Sports Med* 12:218, 1984.

59. Perry J: Anatomy and biomechanics of the shoulder in throwing, swimming, gymnastics and tennis: Symposium on injuries to the shoulder in the athlete. *Clin Sports Med* 2:247, 1983.

60. Colachis SC, Strohm BR: Effects of suprascapular and axillary nerve blocks in muscle force in the upper extremity. *Arch Phys Med Rehabil* 52:22, 1971.

61. VanLinge B, Mulder JD: Function of the supraspinatus muscle and its relationship to the supraspinatus syndrome. *J Bone Joint Surg (Am)* 45B:750, 1963.

62. Nuber GW, Gowan ID, Perry J, et al: EMG analysis of classical shoulder motion. *Trans Orthop Res Soc* 11:20, 1986.

63. Poppen NK, Walker PS: Forces at the glenohumeral joint in abduction. *Clin Orthop* 136:165, 1978.

64. Jobe FW, Perry J, Pink M: Electromyographic shoulder activity in men and women professional golfers. *Am J Sports Med* 17:782, 1989.

65. Watkins RG, Dennis S, Dillin WH, et al: Dynamic EMG analysis of torque transfer in professional baseball pitchers. *Spine* 14:404, 1989.

66. Jobe FW, Bradley JP, Pink M: Treatment of impingement syndrome in overhand athletes, vol II. *Surg Rounds Orthop* 4:39, 1990.

67. Pink M, Perry J, Jobe FW, et al: The normal shoulder during freestyle swimming: An EMG and cinematographic analysis of twelve muscles. *Am J Sports Med*. Submitted for publication.

68. Scovazzo ML, Brown A, Pink M, et al: The painful shoulder during freestyle swimming: An EMG and cinematographic analysis of twelve muscles. *Am J Sports Med*. Submitted for publication.

CHAPTER 3

Clinical Examination of the Shoulder

William Benjamin Kibler

The purpose of the clinical exam of the shoulder is to allow the clinician to understand the entire spectrum of abnormalities in bones, muscles, ligaments, and mechanics that cause decreased performance and clinical symptoms at the shoulder joint. Because the "shoulder joint" is quite complex, consisting of several joints on one end of a kinetic chain, a systematic approach utilizing both a detailed, sport-specific history and a comprehensive physical exam should be employed. Specific shoulder forms can aid in the orderly and complete collection of these data. An example of such a form is illustrated in Table 3-1.

HISTORY AS PART OF THE CLINICAL EXAM

The taking of an accurate history is one of the most crucial parts of the clinical exam of the shoulder. Without this as a basis, much time will be wasted in trying to arrive at the proper diagnosis. The history provides background about previous injuries, provides keys and guides for the physical exam, provides directions and types of tests to employ in the exam, and may give information about some of the more unusual presentations of shoulder problems. The clinician should come to the exam prepared to obtain the maximum amount of information. It is very important that the examiner tries to understand the mechanism of injury, asks questions about how the injury or presenting problem affects performance of the shoulder and where the location of the shoulder dysfunction is, and understands the role of sport-specific demands in the production of symptoms. The history questionnaire may be filled out by the patient and reviewed by the examiner at the start of the exam.

Mechanism of Injury

Three types of mechanism of injury are most common in shoulder problems—acute macrotrauma, chronic repetitive microtrauma, and acute exacerbation of chronic injury.

Acute macrotrauma is characterized by one single event. In most of these cases, the shoulder is basically normal before the event and is then abnormal after the event. Most often this results from a fall or other direct trauma, although it may be a tear or a pop with a certain athletic or throwing movement. The patient can usually date the onset of symptoms precisely to that particular moment. There is almost always alteration or cessation of athletic activity as a result of that particular incident. In shoulder pathology, however, the acute macrotrauma mechanism of injury is one of the least common methods of presentation. Examples of acute macrotrauma include a fall with anterior dislocation of the shoulder, a fall with acromioclavicular (AC) joint separation, or a fractured clavicle.

Chronic repetitive microtrauma results from repeated small insults to the supporting structures of the shoulder, culminating in a series of events that eventually lead to clinical symptoms. The pathophysiology of this mechanism means that it is a process of gradual worsening. Recent studies have shown that this process involves a failure of the cells to adequately repair the damage from use, thereby leading to cell degeneration and failure of matrix integrity which eventually causes failure of the structures in a tensile fashion.[1] During this process, adaptations occur in anatomy and physiology that then render the athlete more susceptible to further insults.[2,3] The point at which symptoms occur is usually distant in time from the point where the pathologic condition first started. As a result, the structures usually are not normal just before the onset of symptoms, and there are usually adaptations in flexibility, strength, and mechanics that need to be evaluated and treated at the same time the symptoms are being treated. This particular type of process is very common in the shoulder and occurs for a large majority of the cases of shoulder problems. Examples of this include rotator cuff tendinitis of the shoulder, subtle instabilities of the anterior or posterior aspects of the glenohumeral joint, and superior glenoid labral tears.

Acute exacerbation of a chronic problem differs slightly from the second mechanism of injury in that there may be one event that gets the attention of the athlete, but the real problem lies in the chronic nature of the underlying problems. Once again, the athlete can usually pinpoint the time at which symptoms occurred, and this is usually associated with some type of throwing or overhead motion incident.

TABLE 3-1
Shoulder Evaluation Form

Name _____ Age _____ Date_____

Sex _____ Years of Play _____ Sport_____

Dominant hand   R   L   Height _____ Weight_____

Fill out the following history form to the best of your ability.
The physician will ask you questions only about your "yes" answers.

Section I	Injury and Medical History	Comments

   1. Neck injury   Yes _____ No _____

   2. Back injury   Yes _____ No _____

   3. Arm injury   Yes _____ No _____

   4. Hand injury   Yes _____ No _____

   5. Elbow injury   Yes _____ No _____

   6. Shoulder injury   Yes _____ No _____

   7. Rib injury   Yes _____ No _____

   8. Hip injury   Yes _____ No _____

   9. Leg injury   Yes _____ No _____

  10. Knee injury   Yes _____ No _____

  11. Ankle injury   Yes _____ No _____

  12. Foot injury   Yes _____ No _____

  13. Other (including medical problems) _____

  _____

  14. Operations (list)   Yes _____ No _____

  15. Medications (list)   Yes _____ No _____

Section II	Present Injury

  1. Where in shoulder are most of symptoms?
  2. When did injury occur?
         First symptoms
         Disabling symptoms
  3. Mechanism of injury
         Acute onset
         Chronic onset
         Acute or chronic onset
  4. When in playing do symptoms occur?
  5. Modifications in serving or hitting
  6. Performance changes
         Before symptoms were severe
         Since severe symptoms are present
  7. Changes in play (new strokes, extra play, etc.)

TABLE 3-1 (*continued*)

Section III	Physical Evaluation					

1. General posture
   a. Shoulder sloping   Y   N
   b. Thoracic kyphosis   Y   N
   c. Cervical lordosis   Y   N

2. Range of motion   DOM   NDOM
   a. SHD INT ROT   _____   _____
   b. SHD EXT ROT   _____   _____
   c. SHD ABD   _____   _____
   d. SHD ADD   _____   _____
   e. SHD FLEX   _____   _____
   f. SHD EXT   _____   _____
   g. H-ABD   _____   _____
   h. H-ADD   _____   _____
   i. Hamstring   _____   _____
   j. GASTROC   _____   _____
   k. Quadriceps   _____   _____
   l. I T band   _____   _____
   m. Hip flexion   _____   _____
   n. Hip IR   _____   _____
   o. Hip ER   _____   _____
   p. Forearm pronation   _____   _____
   q. Forearm supination   _____   _____
   r. Wrist flexion   _____   _____
   s. Wrist extension   _____   _____
   t. Sit and reach   _____ cm

3. Strength
   a. Muscle atrophy   DOM   Y   N   NDOM   Y   N

   Manual muscle testing
   b. Pectoralis   DOM   1   2   3   4   5
       NDOM   1   2   3   4   5
   c. Latissimus   DOM   1   2   3   4   5
       NDOM   1   2   3   4   5
   d. Deltoid   DOM   1   2   3   4   5
       NDOM   1   2   3   4   5
   e. Biceps   DOM   1   2   3   4   5
       NDOM   1   2   3   4   5
   f. Triceps   DOM   1   2   3   4   5
       NDOM   1   2   3   4   5
   g. Supraspinatus   DOM   1   2   3   4   5
       NDOM   1   2   3   4   5
   h. Infraspinatus   DOM   1   2   3   4   5
       NDOM   1   2   3   4   5
   i. Subscapularis   DOM   1   2   3   4   5
       NDOM   1   2   3   4   5
   j. Sit-ups (1 min)   _____
   k. Push-ups (1 min)   _____
   l. Grip strength   DOM _____   NDOM _____
   m. Medicine ball push   _____ in
   n. Cybex—attach copy of results

4. Scapula
   a. Winging or prominence   DOM   Y   N   NDOM   Y   N
   b. Abnormal rhythm   DOM   Y   N   NDOM   Y   N
   c. Shoulder shrugs   DOM   1   2   3   4   5
       NDOM   1   2   3   4   5

TABLE 3-1 (continued)

Section III		Physical Evaluation				

d. Scapular pinch	DOM	1	2	3	4	5
	NDOM	1	2	3	4	5
e. Scapular winging	DOM	1	2	3	4	5
	NDOM	1	2	3	4	5

f. Lateral slide position

	DOM	NDOM
Position 1	_____	_____
Position 2	_____	_____
Position 3	_____	_____

g. Scapular motion

DOM Retract/Protract	NDOM Retract/Protract
_____	_____

5. Provocative testing
   a. Impingement (injection)
   b. Apprehension
   c. Anterior drawer   0   45   90   Neutral
                       0   45   90   EXT ROT
   d. Relocation
   e. Posterior inferior
   f. Direct posterior
   g. Sulcus
   h. Clunk
   i. Anterior slide
   j. AC joint
   k. Biceps
6. Neurovascular
   a. Sensation
   b. Reflexes
   c. Pulses
   d. Bruits
   e. Adson's
7. Imaging
   Plain x-ray
   CT (arthro CT)
   Arthrogram
   MRI

Section IV	Working Diagnosis

1. Anatomic alterations
2. Functional alterations

If this is taken as an acute macrotrauma injury, the surrounding adaptations and alterations may be missed. Failure to recognize these on the history will lead to incomplete clinical exam and will hamper rehabilitation and performance. Examples of this include the sudden pop and pain in throwing athletes when the process of anterior instability finally gets bad enough that the shoulder subluxes or in the sudden exacerbation of rotator cuff tendinitis when the athlete resumes play after resting a mildly symptomatic shoulder for a couple of weeks. During that time, the symptoms have decreased but the underlying conditions have not changed and, therefore, when athletic effort is exerted the symptoms are exacerbated.

Questions about Symptoms and Performance

The questions that are asked on the history are very important in elucidating which mechanism of injury exists. Questions need to be asked about the timing of the symptoms, the mechanism of production of the symptoms, any prior history of pain or soreness in the shoulder, or any problems that may exist in other parts of the kinetic chain, such as the back or legs, that may preexist and predispose to injuries around the shoulder.

Questions should also reflect how the injury affects performance. Does this hurt all the time, or just at certain times during athletic activity? What aspects of performance are involved: endurance, velocity, location, etc.? Finally, questions should be directed toward any substitute actions that the athlete may employ to maintain performance. These actions could include change in arm position on the throw, change of stroke pattern in swimming, or serving with a different motion in tennis.

If possible, the location of the dysfunction should be pinpointed. This includes both the anatomic site (AC joint, anterior deltoid, scapular border) and the biomechanical phase (cocking, acceleration, follow-through, pull-through, recovery) of the athletic activity. The location helps guide the physical exam, and the biomechanical phase helps the clinician to know how the different sports' demands put stress on the shoulder joint.

Biomechanical Demands

The information gained from the history can be made more accurate and relevant for the individual athlete if it is gathered and interpreted in the context of the biomechanical demands of the sport. Every sport imposes certain demands on the athlete. Biomechanical motions and forces, loads, and frequency and duration of activities are specific to certain sports. The results of the clinical exam should be evaluated with respect to their effect on sport-specific athletic activity. For example, the motion of shoulder external rotation is more biomechanically necessary in pitching than in serving; 100° of external rotation would be acceptable and probably normal in tennis players but may be unacceptable and potentially pathologic in baseball players. Similarly, baseball throwing produces higher rotational velocities and distraction forces on the shoulder,[4,5] and higher levels of strength and balance, especially in force couples, should be expected and tested for in baseball players.

Finally, the information from the history should be gathered in the context of the shoulder as a link in a kinetic chain. The velocities and forces that occur at the shoulder cannot be generated at the shoulder. They are generated in the legs, trunk, and back, and are funneled through the shoulder to the arm and hand. Alterations in these other areas, whether by injury, muscle imbalance, or poor mechanics,

may place abnormal demands on the shoulder, leading to or exacerbating shoulder symptoms. Questions should be asked about preexisting or coexisting problems in these areas.

Summary

The history is the cornerstone of the clinical exam of the shoulder. The physical exam is much more difficult in the absence of guidelines that may be elucidated by the history. However, the clinician must be prepared for the history by understanding the mechanisms of shoulder injury, how the clinical symptoms of shoulder may present, how the injury may affect athletic performance, and how biomechanical demands affect the shoulder.

THE PHYSICAL AS PART OF THE CLINICAL EXAM

Based on clues and guidelines from the history, the physical exam can be used to assemble the rest of the information to make a complete and accurate diagnosis of the structural and mechanical alterations occurring in shoulder pathology. After completion of the history and physical, a fairly complete diagnosis should be possible in a large majority of cases. The physical should also be done systematically, and can be aided by the use of forms.

Inspection

Visual inspection should start the exam. This should be done with clothes off for males. Alternatives for women include the use of swimsuits or tank tops. Inspection should be from both the front and the back. Posture, or the resting position of the athlete, should be checked for the shoulder, neck, back, and arm. Abnormal sloping of the shoulders, neck lordosis or thoracic kyphosis, or abnormal positioning of the arm should be noted. Muscle atrophy around the shoulder is significant. Scapular winging or lateral displacement may be subtle but is usually fairly obvious.

Palpation

All bony landmarks around the shoulder girdle should be palpated for prominence, tenderness, excessive motion, or crepitus. This includes the clavicle, the acromioclavicular and sternoclavicular joints at both ends of the clavicle, the acromion, the scapular spine, and the neck.

Muscular palpation can be done to detect tears, as in the biceps or pectoralis tendons, or to elicit areas of point tenderness, which are common in the trapezius, deltoid, or infraspinatus, or along the medial scapular border.

Thoracoscapulohumeral Rhythm

Passive but especially active motion of the scapula and humerus with respect to the thorax should be checked in both abduction-adduction and flexion-extension. Smooth motion of all three links is essential for shoulder function, and abnormalities in motion may indicate clinical symptoms, mechanical substitutions, or imbalance in the force couples that govern the coordinated movements. Motion should be watched in the "force generation" phase, either abduction or flexion (Fig. 3-1), but most commonly abnormal motion may be seen in the "force regulation" phase of adduction or extension (Fig. 3-2). This phase requires eccentric work, which often is the weak component of the muscular force couple.

Motion

Passive motion of all the relevant joints contributing to the shoulder should be measured using standard physical therapy techniques. If the neck has been identified on the history as an area of importance, range of motion in all planes should be measured.

Glenohumeral motion is a sensitive measure of early shoulder pathology and is often abnormal before the onset of clinical symptoms. Therefore, accurate measurement is important. Measurements should be done from standardized positions that are agreed upon by all examiners at the sports medicine

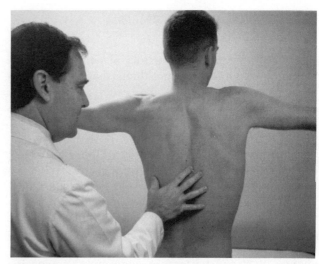

FIGURE 3-2
Abnormal thoracoscapulohumeral motion in eccentric position. The right shoulder is high, the right trapezius is contracting abnormally, and the right scapula is prominent, with loss of smooth motion.

facility. The most optimum position for external-internal rotation is supine, with measurements made in the plane of the scapula (Fig. 3-3). For flexion-extension, abduction-adduction, and horizontal abduction-adduction, the standing or seated position is optimum, with measurements in the plane of the scapula. Measurements are made by goniometers centered on the axis of joint motion. Results can be compared with standard physical therapy or preparticipation exam manuals, and also should be compared with the opposite side. Active motion should be compared with passive motion. There should be

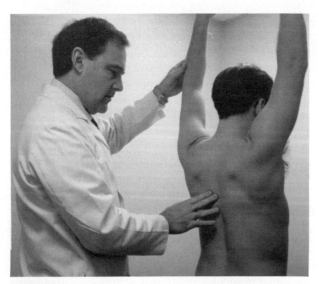

FIGURE 3-1
Thoracoscapulohumeral motion in normal abduction. Muscle tone is equal, scapular movement is symmetrical, and there are no substitute motions.

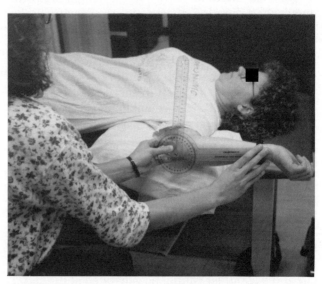

FIGURE 3-3
Glenohumeral external rotation. Arm has been positioned in scapular plane by placing it on pillow. Neutral position for initiation of test indicated by goniometer arm.

36

only slight differences. Larger differences may reflect strength deficits or imbalances.

Other joints and their motion affect shoulder pathology. Tight hip flexors or rotators, or tight trunk muscles, may affect smooth mechanical motion. Restricted motion of forearm, elbow, or wrist may place more strain on the shoulder. These areas should be included in the range of motion evaluations. Scapular motion from full retraction to full protraction can be measured by using the closest spinous process as a reference point and bilaterally measuring the distance from that point to the tip of the scapula in full retraction and full protraction. Any major differences may reflect inability to position the scapula for optimal glenohumeral function.

Strength

On the clinical exam, strength should be estimated by means of manual muscle testing, in addition to more objective testing by isokinetic devices. Manual muscle testing requires some precision and experience to maintain high test-retest reliability, but there are general advantages to learning and doing the evaluation. In many offices and in "on the field" situations, isokinetic equipment or physical therapists will not be available. Also, individual muscles are more easily evaluated by manual muscle testing than by isokinetics, which really evaluates force couples and motions.

The technique of manual muscle testing involves placing the muscle in the position that most isolates it, and then applying a set amount of resistance. These positions are described in most physical therapy or preparticipation manuals. Smoothness of muscle contraction, length of muscle contraction against resistance, and substitute muscle contraction patterns are parameters to check. If the muscle contracts quickly and smoothly, resists pressure without "breaking" or giving way, "springs back" after resistance ceases, and does not require assistance from other muscles, the muscle receives a rating of 5 (Table 3-1), muscle weakness without the use of assisted muscles rates a 4+, while the need for assistive muscles receives a 4. Weakness even with assistive muscles receives a 4−. Grades of weakness below this level, which require positioning to eliminate gravity or are accompanied by atrophy, receive lower ratings, shown in Table 3-2. Key points to emphasize are the consistent use of the same applied resistance by the examiner and strict adherence to the rating criteria.

Neck musculature should be manually checked if there is any suggestion of neck pathology or stiff-

TABLE 3-2
Manual Muscle Grading Criteria

5	Quick contraction, no giving way, no assistive muscles
4+	Slight weakness, no assistive muscles
4	Weakness, assistive muscles
4−	Weakness with assistive muscles
3	Atrophy, substitute activities
2	Atrophy, gravity elimination

ness. Scapular muscles can be checked by shrugging the shoulders upward to check upper trapezius, pinching the scapula posteriorly to check rhomboids and lower trapezius, and a wall push-up (Fig. 3-4) to check serratus anterior. Sometimes these motions need to be held for 10 to 15 s, or the motions repeated, to bring out mild weakness or endurance deficits.

Extrinsic shoulder musculature, including the deltoid (anterior, middle, and posterior), latissimus dorsi, pectoralis, biceps, and triceps, can be easily isolated and tested. Both the absolute rating and the rating compared with the opposite side are important measurements.

The intrinsic shoulder musculature of the rotator cuff is very important, in terms of both absolute strength and strength balance, and cannot be measured by isokinetic devices. Therefore, manual muscle testing is very important for these muscles. There is some variation of opinion about the best position for isolating the supraspinatus, whether in the "empty can" position (Fig. 3-5) or the prone position (Fig. 3-6). Both seem to be effective but must be stipulated in the evaluation. The subscapularis and the infraspinatus–teres minor are best tested with the arm at the side.[5] Resistive force should be applied to rotational movements, and substitute muscular activities like abduction should be eliminated.

Strength in other muscles affects shoulder effectiveness and should be tested. Grip strength can be measured with a hand-held dynamometer. Push-ups and sit-ups, done to a specific protocol, measure overall arm and trunk strength. A medicine ball push, using a 4-lb ball, measures overall upper body power. If available, isokinetic testing can also provide more evidence of muscle strength and balance.

Provocative Testing

In this section of the clinical exam, the examiner deliberately tries to reproduce pathologic positions and

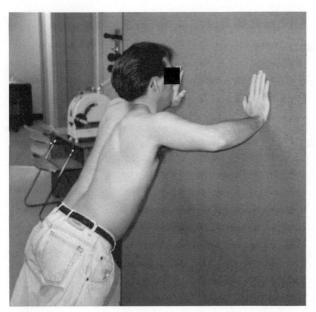

FIGURE 3-4
Wall push-up to check serratus anterior strength.

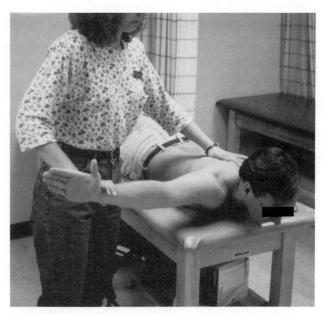

FIGURE 3-6
Prone position for testing supraspinatus strength.

forces, and to elicit symptoms from these positions. Obviously, care must be taken so that overt problems, such as frank shoulder dislocations, are not created by the testing.

Stability of the scapula on the thorax is measured by progressively increasing the load that the scapular-stabilizing musculature must oppose and bilaterally measuring the distance from the spinous process to the scapular tip as the loads increase (Fig. 3-7). These bony landmarks are palpable even in heavily muscled individuals. The loads increase,

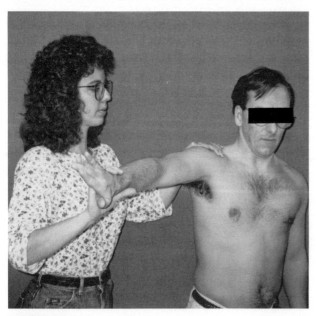

FIGURE 3-5
"Empty can" position for testing supraspinatus strength.

and muscle activity increases, from position 1 to position 3. Position 1 is a position of rest, with the arms at the side in neutral position. Position 2 has the hands on the hips, thumbs facing posteriorly, with the shoulders in 10° extension in the coronal plane. This position requires some muscle activity of the serratus and upper trapezius. Position 3 is one of 90° glenohumeral abduction and maximal glenohumeral internal rotation. Muscle contraction is necessary in the upper and lower trapezius, serratus, and rhomboids. Side-to-side differences greater than 1.2 cm have been statistically correlated with presence of shoulder pathology.[6,7]

A number of tests may be used in provocative testing of the glenohumeral joint. All rely on creating a situation in which the instant center of rotation of the glenohumeral joint is not constrained within normal confines. Pain, a feeling of movement or weakness, a feeling of apprehension, a feeling of reproduction of clinical symptoms, or a palpable or audible "clunk" or "pop" are the usual positive responses. The experience and personal preference of the individual examiner guides which of the tests to use. But enough tests should be used to check impingement, superior labral pathology, inferior capsular and labral pathology, and posterior pathology.

Impingement testing can be done in several ways, all of which are designed to compress the rotator cuff under the coracoacromial arch. Two more common testing procedures involve abduction above 90°, internal rotation, and forward movement or abduction to 90°, horizontal adduction, and internal rotation. Further testing can involve injection of xylocaine into the subacromial space. It has been

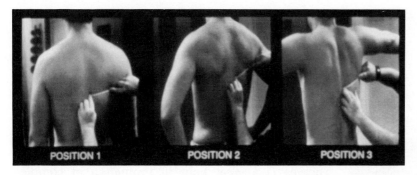

FIGURE 3-7
Scapular stability testing. Each position progressively loads the scapular stabilizing musculature. (*Used by permission from Contemporary Orthopedics, May 1991.*)

presumed that if all the symptoms are relieved by this maneuver, all the pathology can be attributed to the impingement. However, in younger athletes, most impingement is considered secondary to other shoulder pathology, usually some mild anterior or superior instability.[8,9] It therefore should be considered another clinical sign, rather than a complete diagnosis, and other causes should be sought.

Anterior and anterior-inferior instability can be checked by the apprehension test, the anterior drawer (Fig. 3-8), or the relocation test. The apprehension test is performed by raising the shoulder to 90° of abduction and then externally rotating the arm, palpating the anterior glenoid rim. Pain, apprehension, or a pop is a positive response. In the anterior drawer or relocation tests, anteriorly directed forces are used to test the restraints. In the anterior drawer, one hand holds the humeral head and the other hand is on the scapular neck and coracoid. The humeral head is directed anteriorly, and motion can be felt between the two bones. As Warren[10] has pointed out, different ligamentous structures are the major stabilizers at different positions of abduction and rotation, so the shoulder should be stressed at 0°, 45°, and 90° abduction, and neutral and 90° external rotation. Differential movement and symptoms can be found at each position. Posterior and posterior-inferior instability can be checked at the same time by directing a posterior force in each of the positions. Posterior instability can be further checked by a direct posteriorly directed force, with the athlete's arm and the examiner's hands in the same position as for anterior testing. Posterior-inferior testing, to check the integrity of the posterior portion of the inferior glenohumeral ligament, is best done with the shoulder internally rotated at a position of 40° of horizontal adduction (Fig. 3-9). A palpable protrusion or posterior pain is a positive test.

The sulcus sign probably checks superior constraints to inferior translation. This test is often positive in atraumatic multidirectional instability. It is performed by placing longitudinal traction on the arm in neutral position at the side. A positive test is signified by the appearance of a space between the acromion and humeral head.

Superior labral injuries are becoming more recognized as entities, either as separate pathologic problems or in combination with other shoulder problems. Testing for superior labral tears can be accomplished by either the "clunk" test of Andrews,[11] or the "anterior slide" test.[6] In the clunk test, the arm is abducted to 180° and an anterior force is placed on the humeral head while the arm is rotated. If a detached labral piece is caught, a clunk is felt. In the anterior slide test (Fig. 3-10), an anterior-superiorly directed force is applied to the elbow with the hands on the hips. In the presence of a superior labral tear the humeral head will not be constrained and will move over the labrum, causing anterior-superior pain and/or a pop.

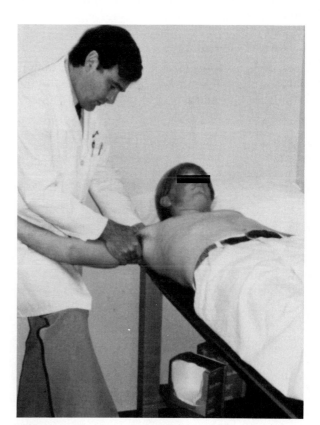

FIGURE 3-8
Anterior drawer test. Anterior force is applied to the shoulder in different positions of abduction and external rotation.

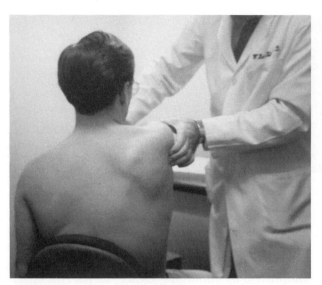

FIGURE 3-9
Posterior inferior ligament testing. Pain or soreness can be felt at the examiner's fingertips.

The AC joint may be tested by manipulation of the clavicle in an anterior-posterior or superior-inferior direction, to check the integrity of the coracoclavicular and acromioclavicular ligaments.

The biceps tendon can be palpated and stressed by placing the arm at 90° abduction and 15° internal rotation. Pain or a palpable click indicates tendon pathology or subluxability.

Neurovascular Testing

The complete clinical exam of the shoulder includes evaluation of the neurologic and vascular structures of the shoulder and arm. Many neurologic and vas-cular problems may mimic symptoms and signs of shoulder pathology. Screening tests may be used to see if more advanced diagnostic procedures should be done.

Local and distant neurologic problems should be checked. Local sensation can be examined for nerve injuries, primarily axillary nerve problems. Diffuse, nonanatomic sensory problems may suggest reflex sympathetic dystrophy. A familiarity with the anatomy of the brachial plexus and peripheral nerves is a great help in evaluation of complex problems around the shoulder. Specific well-documented motor nerve injuries, such as the long thoracic nerve (serratus anterior), axillary nerve (deltoid), or suprascapular nerve (infraspinatus and/or supraspinatus) should be kept in mind. More generalized neuropathies, such as traction plexopathies seen in traumatic shoulder dislocations, or peripheral neuropathy seen in diabetes, also may give rise to pain, weakness, or performance decrements. Distant problems, such as nerve root compression or avulsion, and compression neuropathies, such as tardy ulnar palsy or carpal tunnel syndrome, may refer pain to the shoulder.

Intermittent, partial, or complete vascular lesions can refer symptoms to the area of the shoulder. Local skin color changes may suggest sympathetic dystrophy or venous obstruction, while distal color changes or diminution of pulses may suggest arterial lesions. Effort claudication or positional claudication may suggest intermittent vascular embarrassment. Bruits or thrills may suggest partial injuries or fistulas. The Adson's maneuver (Fig. 3-11) should be

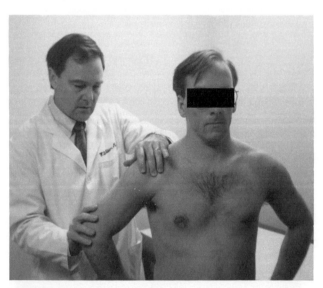

FIGURE 3-10
Anterior slide testing. Position of examiner's and patient's arms.

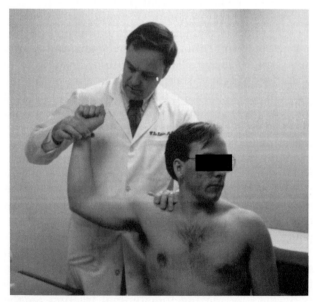

FIGURE 3-11
Adson's maneuver. Pulse is checked with arm in abduction and external rotation, with different positions of the neck and head.

done in heavily muscled athletes, because muscle hypertrophy is a common lesion producing intermittent partial vascular lesions.

Imaging

Imaging is not a part of the clinical exam. The type and extent of the imaging process for shoulder pathology is still the subject of debate. However, it is clear that whatever imaging is employed should be determined after, and as the result of, the clinical exam.

Working Diagnosis

The working diagnosis should reflect the spectrum of anatomic and functional alterations that exist in the kinetic chain for shoulder function. Most alterations will be in the vicinity of the shoulder joint, but other distant anatomic areas should be included. The working diagnosis should provide guidelines for initiation of treatment, should guide the development of the exercise prescription for rehabilitation, and, by highlighting all the components of the alterations, should set up criteria for return to athletic activity.[2,3] The anatomic alterations would include rotator cuff tears, Bankhart lesions, AC joint bone spurs, or axillary nerve lesions. The functional alterations would include force couple imbalance, internal rotation inflexibility, or throwing sidearm rather than overhand.[2,3]

CONCLUSIONS

The shoulder represents a complex balance of constraints working to allow mobility with stability. Because of its role as a funnel toward the end of a kinetic chain, high forces can be concentrated on the component parts of the shoulder, and alterations anywhere in the chain can cause problems at the shoulder. The clinician needs a systematic approach to this complex entity to be able to assemble the information necessary to arrive at a complete and accurate diagnosis of the shoulder problem. All the questions and tests discussed in this chapter would not be performed on every athlete on every clinical exam. However, the clinician should ask enough questions in the history to be comfortable with the context of the injury, and enough tests should be performed on the basis of the history to give the physical exam a high degree of sensitivity and specificity for a complete and accurate diagnosis.

REFERENCES

1. Leadbetter W: An introduction to sports induced soft tissue inflammation, in Leadbetter W, Buckwalter J, Gordon SL (eds): *Sports Induced Inflammation*. Park Ridge, IL, American Academy of Orthopaedic Surgeons, 1991, chap 1, pp 3–25.
2. Kibler WB, Chandler TJ, Pace BK: Principles of rehabilitation after chronic tendon injuries. *Clin Sports Med* 11:661, 1992.
3. Kibler WB: Concepts in exercise rehabilitation, in Leadbetter W, Buckwalter J, Gordon SL (eds): *Sports Induced Inflammation*. Park Ridge, IL, American Academy of Orthopaedic Surgeons, 1991, chap 52, pp 759–771.
4. Kibler WB, Chandler TJ: Racquet sports, in Fu F, Stone D (eds): *Sports Injuries: Mechanisms, Prevention, and Treatment*. Baltimore, Williams & Wilkins, in press.
5. Andrews J: Forces on the shoulder in the throwing motion. ACSM Meeting, Dallas, 1992.
6. Kibler WB: The role of the scapula in the throwing motion. *Contemp Orthop* 22:525, 1991.
7. Michell L: Moire Analysis of Scapulothoracic Dyskinesis in Shoulder Pain. ACSM Meeting, Salt Lake City, May 1990.
8. Jobe FW, Kuitine RS: Shoulder pain in the overhead throwing athlete. *Orthop Rev* 18:963, 1989.
9. Nirschl RP: Shoulder impingement syndromes. *Instr Course Lect*, Chicago, 1989.
10. Warren RF: Ligamentous constraints about the shoulder. ACSM Meeting, Dallas, 1992.
11. Andrews JR: Physical exam of the shoulder, in Andrews JR, Zarins BA (eds): *Injuries to the Throwing Arm*, Philadelphia, Saunders, chap 3, pp 51–65.

CHAPTER 4

Imaging of the Athlete's Shoulder: Evaluation with X-Ray, Ultrasound, Arthrography, CT, and MRI

Martha C. Nelson

The shoulder is a complex structure, and acute or chronic injury may involve a variety of abnormalities. These include fractures, dislocations, loose bodies, and injuries to the rotator cuff, capsular complex, and articular cartilage as well as surrounding soft tissues. Clinical examination of the patient may fail to reveal the precise extent of injury to the shoulder and may result in misdiagnosis.[70] Plain radiographic examination is usually necessary but can also be nonspecific.

PLAIN FILMS

Plain radiographs obtained close to the time of injury may reveal fractures, dislocations, and radiographic loose bodies.[24,50,66,81,93]

Fractures are usually visible in at least a single projection. Accompanying nonspecific soft tissue swelling and mild subluxation of the humerus may also be identified. However, if a fracture is suspected but not identified on the radiographs, the patient should be treated as if a fracture were present. Follow-up films in several weeks may reveal the fracture more clearly and show callus formation.[24,66]

Calcific and ossific densities are clearly seen on plain radiographs. Hydroxyapatite deposition (calcific tendinitis) is commonly encountered in the shoulder, particularly in the rotator cuff tendons near their site of attachment on the humeral head. Calcium pyrophosphate can be seen in chondroid structures such as articular cartilage and the joint capsule. Fracture fragments and intraarticular loose bodies may be localized and their exact number determined.[24,66,81]

One of the basic premises of orthopedists and radiologists alike is that plain film radiographic evaluation of the musculoskeletal system requires at least two x-rays of the area to be examined, perpendicular to each other. However, when evaluating the shoulder, this principle is often ignored. Frequently, the routine shoulder trauma series consists of two anteroposterior (AP) views with the humerus in ex-ternal and internal rotation. This series is limited and will not provide a total examination of the anatomically complex shoulder.[24,66,70]

The AP view of the shoulder is appropriate for diagnosing calcific deposits, loose bodies, and most dislocations with associated fractures and soft tissue swelling. In this procedure, the x-ray beam is directed in the plane of the thorax and the glenohumeral joint is oriented obliquely. The medial portion of the humeral head is superimposed over the glenoid, obscuring the joint space. For this reason the AP view is inadequate to visualize injuries and other disorders of the glenohumeral joint and scapula such as posterior dislocations and glenoid fractures. To compensate, it is often suggested that a trauma series of the shoulder include a true AP view (Grashey projection) of the shoulder and an axillary lateral view (Fig. 4-1).[66,81]

The true AP, or Grashey, view is obtained by medial to lateral angulation of the x-ray beam 35 to 45° or by rotation of the patient to the vertical x-ray beam. The x-ray beam is projected directly into the glenohumeral joint in the plane of the scapula. An advantage of this view is that the patient can be supine or erect with the arm at the side or in a sling. This view shows overlapping of the coracoid process and glenohumeral joint. Also, the glenoid is seen in profile with separation of the humeral head and the glenoid. Any overlapping of these two structures is compatible with a dislocation.[18,66]

The axillary view requires some degree of abduction of the arm, preferably 70 to 90°, and can be taken in a supine or erect position. The x-ray beam is directed superiorly through the axilla to the x-ray cassette. This view is particularly useful in evaluation of the glenohumeral joint, shows the relationship of the humeral head to the glenoid, and allows accurate visualization of the anterior and posterior margins of the glenoid. Additional fractures of the acromion and coracoid can be demonstrated and integrity of the acromioclavicular (AC) joint evaluated. If this view cannot be obtained because of pain or spasm, one of the modified axillary projections (a true scapulolateral view or transthoracic view) is

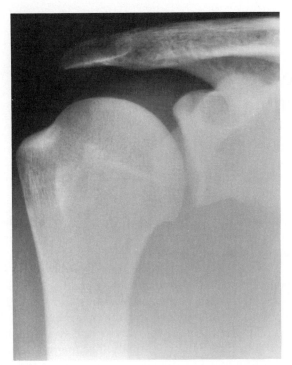

FIGURE 4-1
The normal Grashey view, or true AP view, separates the humeral head from the glenoid, allowing visualization of the glenohumeral joint. Any overlapping of these structures is abnormal and consistent with a dislocation.

necessary for complete evaluation of the posttraumatic shoulder.[66]

Cleaves modified the axillary view so less abduction of the arm is needed. A curved cassette is placed in the axilla and the x-ray beam is taken from superior to inferior through the axilla.[12,82] Most radiology departments do not have rolled cassettes available, thus limiting the use of this projection.

The scapular Y view (scapulolateral or Y lateral view) helps define the spatial relationship of the glenoid and humeral head. In this view, the x-ray beam passes parallel to the scapular spine from the posterior chest to a laterally placed cassette. The lateral view of the scapula should be seen as the letter Y. The limbs of the Y are formed superiorly and anteriorly by the coracoid process, superiorly and posteriorly by the acromion. The vertical lower limb is formed by the body of the scapula. At the intersection of these limbs lies the glenoid fossa (Fig. 4-2). A normal shoulder would reveal the humeral head superimposed over the glenoid fossa.[85,93]

An anterior dislocation is easily diagnosed on an AP x-ray so the scapular Y view is not needed to diagnose the dislocation but may enable better visualization of fractures of the greater tuberosity. The scapular Y view is quite useful in evaluating posterior dislocations. However, many radiologists prefer the axillary view as it will better define fractures of the glenoid, not seen on the scapular Y view. The transthoracic view may be used as a substitute for the scapular Y or axillary radiograph.[66]

Additional radiographic views to evaluate the injured shoulder include other modified axillary views: (1) The Velpeau axillary lateral view is taken with the patient erect, but the arm may be in a sling. The advantage is that no abduction is required as in the previously described axillary views.[1] (2) The trauma axillary lateral can be taken with the patient supine. Often this view is a great advantage in patients with multiple trauma.[66] (3) The West Point axillary lateral view allows evaluation of the anterioinferior glenoid rim, usually the portion of glenoid fractured with anterior dislocations and not always seen on true axillary views; yet it is obtained in a prone position. (4) The apical oblique view (in which the patient is posteriorly rotated 45° with 45° caudad beam angulation) demonstrates anteroinferior fractures as well as anteroinferior calcification. In addition to diagnosing dislocations, compression fractures of the posterolateral humeral head are well defined in this view.[26,43,84]

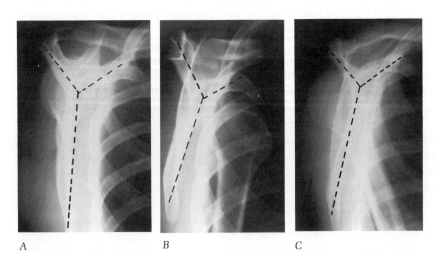

A   B   C

FIGURE 4-2
The scapular Y view may be substituted for the axillary view and is especially helpful in detecting dislocations. *A.* A normal shoulder shows the humeral head overlying the glenoid fossa. The Y is formed by the three extensions of the scapula as shown by the drawn lines. *B.* An anterior dislocation and (C) a posterior dislocation are easily distinguished by this view. Fractures of the greater tuberosity can be seen, but the glenoid cannot be totally visualized for integrity.

Additional special radiographic views to diagnose specific lesions are discussed under specific topic sections.

CONVENTIONAL TOMOGRAPHY

The role of conventional tomography in evaluation of the musculoskeletal system has decreased since the advent of newer, more sophisticated techniques such as CT and MRI. Yet plain film tomography serves an important role in certain clinical situations and is a helpful adjunct to plain film radiography. For instance, in evaluation of skeletal trauma, sets of tomograms obtained in planes perpendicular to each other (i.e., coronal and parasagittal) can detect and delineate subtle fractures, osteochondral defects, and evaluate healing of fractures. Loose bodies within a joint or periarticular osseous bodies can be visualized. In evaluation of septic arthritis vs. severe osteoporosis, tomography allows distinction between the two entities by allowing scrutiny of the subchondral bone to detect bony destruction. In chronic osteomyelitis, tomography can detect sequestra (often obscured by additional osseous abnormalities) that indicate active infection and thus alter patient treatment. The applications of tomography in tumor evaluation are well known: i.e., identification of tumor matrix or calcification, cortical destruction by tumor and soft tissue extension, and scrutiny of bone to identify the lone (or multiple) nidus of an osteoid osteoma especially when hidden by sclerosis.[73,81]

The role of conventional tomography in detection of soft tissue masses is limited; however, its application can be utilized to evaluate the area between a soft tissue lesion and the surface of underlying bone. Underlying subtle bony changes visible on tomograms would suggest a more aggressive lesion than probably suspected on plain radiographs.

Disadvantages of conventional tomography include lengthy examination times, large radiation dose to patient, and streak artifacts created if linear tomography is used instead of pluridirectional tomography. In this era of cost-effectiveness, many radiology centers have removed their infrequently utilized tomography machines to make room for those modalities that are more profitable and high in demand such as CT scanners or MR units.

FLUOROSCOPY

The importance of fluoroscopy and its many applications are usually not well appreciated. It is a fundamental diagnostic tool for many radiologic and orthopedic procedures, especially for evaluation of musculoskeletal problems.

When radiographic evaluation of the shoulder for trauma-related injuries is equivocal, maneuvering the patient under fluoroscopy into multiple positions while obtaining spot films will often prove very satisfactory. This approach is convenient, easy to perform, and inexpensive. Fluoroscopy will negate the lengthy process of obtaining multiple additional plain radiographs that often prove frustrating and unsatisfactory.[73]

The detection of a fracture, its extent, and its relationship to surrounding structures can be evaluated, as can the integrity of the articular surface. Follow-up of fracture healing and nonunion can easily be documented by fluoroscopy. Movement along fracture lines can be detected, especially if stress is applied.

Fluoroscopy is often combined with other diagnostic modalities. One example is videotaping a procedure while employing fluoroscopy to evaluate joint motion of the shoulder. Lack of smooth motion with abrupt changes can signify instability, as can a vacuum phenomenon or osteophytes that hinder normal motion.[65,69] The stability of the acromioclavicular joint can be evaluated by a carefully monitored fluoroscopic study. Applying stress may yield important information regarding the acromioclavicular and coracoclavicular ligaments in cases of posttraumatic instability.

Shoulder impingement syndrome is a common cause of shoulder pain. In addition to plain film evaluation of the shoulder, fluoroscopy may allow better visualization of subacromial spurs, osteophytes of the inferior AC joint, joint motion, and contact between the inferior surface of the acromion (or a spur) and the humeral head in abduction.[65,69,74] I find that a well-positioned AP film of the shoulder with the humerus externally rotated and abducted will usually give satisfactory results and allow the diagnosis of bony impingement.

Fluoroscopy is used for guidance in many radiologic procedures such as arthrography, biopsies, tenography, bursography, and aspirations.[27,28] Monitoring by fluoroscopy documents needle location, assures the arthrographer that injected contrast is indeed within the joint, and can localize a rotator cuff tear during an arthrogram injection of contrast and/or air. Fluoroscopic guidance is a requisite for a variety of neurosurgical and orthopedic procedures, and its utility is well recognized, i.e., insertion of screws and prosthetic devices and localization of desired operative level prior to surgery.

As an additional application in cases where plain films are equivocal, fluoroscopy can be employed to further evaluate the shoulder when a dislocation is suspected. A Hill-Sachs lesion may be better viewed tangentially under fluoroscopy than on an internally rotated AP view if the proper degree of rotation is not used. Loose bodies within the joint can be documented by their change in location upon altering patient position.[73]

ARTHROGRAPHY

Shoulder arthrography is helpful in evaluation of partial or complete rotator cuff tears, labral pathology, loose bodies, adhesive capsulities (or frozen shoulder), bicipital abnormalities, synovial pathology, and abnormalities of the joint capsule.[5,7,19,27,28,60,67,80] However, an arthrogram is an invasive procedure and not without risk. Complications, though rare nowadays, include infection, allergic reaction, and synovial effusions. Its utility is limited by many factors—positioning, technical skill of the radiologist and technologist, as well as number and quality of films obtained. An arthrogram, while technically simple, if performed properly allows direct visualization of the contrast-covered supraspinatus tendon, biceps tendon, articular cartilage, and labrum. A double-contrast arthrogram—an injection of several milliliters of soluble contrast medium followed by approximately 10 mL of air—is the preferred type of arthrogram to evaluate the shoulder and provides information not obtained from a positive (or single) contrast study. Contrast and air will be detected in a torn or deformed surface.[80]

Complete Rotator Cuff Tears

A complete rotator cuff tear allows communication of contrast and/or air between the glenohumeral joint and the subacromial-subdeltoid bursa through the torn area of the tendon. Performing fluoroscopy during the injection or videotaping of the procedure can identify the exact location of one or multiple tears within the tendon substance. AP views in internal and external rotation will document a complete rotator cuff tear. I generally repeat the AP x-rays after exercise, especially if the initial radiographs are negative. This helps avoid a false-negative diagnosis, especially if a tear is quite small (Fig. 4-3). Axillary and bicipital groove views provide additional information about the labrum and status of the biceps tendon.[27,28,60,80,99]

Partial Rotator Cuff Tears

Partial rotator cuff tears do not extend through the entire tendon thickness; thus no communication

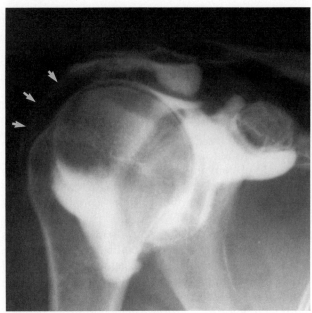

FIGURE 4-3
The most common site of a complete rotator cuff tear is of the supraspinatus tendon within 1 cm of its attachment on the greater tuberosity. As demonstrated here, extension of contrast material into the subdeltoid and subacromial bursae is the arthrographic criterion of a complete tear (arrows). The exact size of tear is not seen.

between the injected, contrast-filled glenohumeral joint and subacromial-subdeltoid bursa will be seen. Also only partial tears that extend to the glenohumeral joint (or involve the undersurface of the supraspinatus tendon) will be detected. A partial tear located in the superior supraspinatus surface adjacent to the subacromial bursa cannot be demonstrated by a shoulder arthrogram. Identification of linear or irregular collections of contrast within the tendon is compatible with a partial rotator cuff tear[27,28] (Fig. 4-4). Repetitive films taken after several bouts of exercise increase the sensitivity and specificity of this diagnosis and also of a complete rotator cuff tear if only a partial tear was identified on the initial films.

The arthrogram remains the best radiologic procedure to employ if adhesive capsulitis is suspected (Fig. 4-5). To date no published information is available without utilizing magnetic resonance imaging (MRI) for this diagnosis. Plain radiographs may only reveal focal demineralization of the humeral head and limited mobility of the arm in the AP abducted view. Upon injection of contrast media, the patient usually complains of immediate pain. The findings of adhesive capsulitis are a small joint space with an irregular "choppy" capsule and synovium. The axillary recess and subacromial bursa will contain little contrast within them. Adhesions may be contrast-covered and visible. In addition, contrast material frequently leaks from the joint or biceps tendon—not usually seen in a normal shoulder (unless there

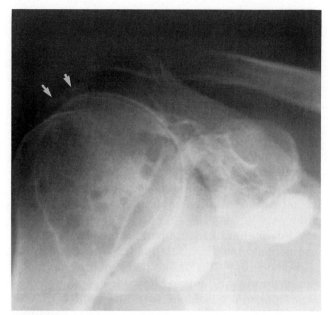

FIGURE 4-4
Partial rotator cuff tears (arrow) appear as abnormal collections of air or contrast that extend above the articular cartilage of the humeral head and appear as interruptions of the inferior tendon surface (which communicates with the contrast-filled joint). No contrast is seen in the subacromial-subdeltoid bursae. Note the multiple bubbles produced by injection of air, a pitfall of the double-contrast technique, that should not be mistaken for loose bodies.

is overinjection and overdistention of the normal joint)—into surrounding soft tissues. Sometimes the injection of contrast followed by air may actually alleviate the condition with immediate marked reduction of symptoms and improvement of mobility.[28,80]

Articular Cartilage Abnormalities

Abnormalities of the articular cartilage may be associated with rotator cuff pathology and are best seen on double-contrast arthrography. Cartilage defects not seen on plain x-rays will be clearly outlined by air or contrast and easily detected. Bankart deformities or Hill-Sachs defects that do not involve underlying bone

are easily appreciated. Cartilage degeneration and erosions will be seen. In addition, capsular deformities can be demonstrated, especially those following a shoulder dislocation.[5,7,13,16,19,28,38,40,52,80]

Loose osteocartilaginous bodies or fragments secondary to fractures, degenerative arthritis, or avascular necrosis can be localized within the joint space or biceps tendon sheath. They will be contrast-covered and visible.[27,28,80]

Biceps Tendon Abnormalities

Suspected abnormalities of the biceps tendon that are an indication for a double-contrast arthrogram include partial and complete tears of the long head of the biceps, tenosynovitis, or dislocation of the tendon. Contrast normally fills the intraarticular portion of the long head of the biceps tendon sheath, and the biceps tendon is visible within the distended capsule and its sheath. A complete tear is diagnosed when one cannot visualize the tendon within the capsule or sheath. A partial tear or tenosynovitis will result in increased diameter of the tendon and an indistinctness of the usually sharply defined tendon margin secondary to edema and inflammation.[66,77,80]

An abnormal location of the biceps tendon may be an anatomic variation or be a posttraumatic finding. An axillary or bicipital groove radiograph obtained after administration of contrast and air should reveal a normal biceps tendon in its intertubercular groove. A subluxed or dislocated tendon will not change its expected position with AP internal and external rotation. The diagnosis of abnormal position is best made on an axillary or bicipital groove view where the tendon will usually be seen medial to the humeral tuberosities.[77]

Pitfalls of Arthrography

What are the potential pitfalls of shoulder arthrography? A joint effusion prevents adequate contrast coating of surfaces, often leading to underdetection of abnormalities. The addition of epinephrine to the

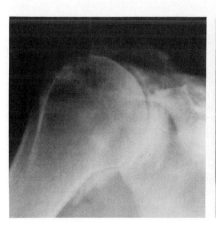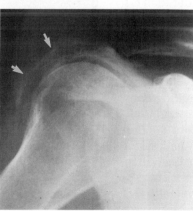

FIGURE 4-5
Two fluoroscopic views several minutes apart revealed (left) capsular contraction, reduced volume of the subscapularis bursa, and axillary recess consistent with adhesive capsulitis. Injection of air, even though resistance was felt (right), led to joint distention and detection of a complete rotator cuff tear (arrows).

47

contrast media delays resorption of contrast, which is necessary, especially if computed tomography follows the arthrogram and there is a time delay between the two parts of the study. Poor technique can lead to inadvertent injection of the subacromial-subdeltoid bursa, suggesting a complete rotator cuff tear, but no contrast will be seen in the normally filled glenohumeral joint. Air bubbles can mimic loose osteocartilaginous bodies within the joint. Overinjection of air may cause rupture of the joint capsule with leakage of contrast and air into surrounding soft tissue structures, distorting normal structures and preventing adequate visualization. The contrast-filled biceps tendon sheath may mimic fluid in the subacromial-subdeltoid bursa if the study limits the number of x-rays obtained to only AP views.

In summary, arthrography is dependent on good radiologic and technologic technique for the physician to make an adequate study of high diagnostic accuracy. Postarthrographic CT imaging (CTA) in the axial plane provides additional information and increases the accuracy of diagnosis.[20,27,28,39]

COMPUTED TOMOGRAPHY (CT)

CT can accurately depict fractures, dislocations, intraarticular loose bodies, radiopaque foreign bodies, intraarticular disorders, and to a limited extent can evaluate the surrounding soft tissue structures (Fig. 4-6).

Intraarticular abnormalities are best appreciated with postarthrographic CT imaging (CTA). Air, water-soluble iodinated contrast, or double contrast (a combination of air and contrast) can be injected into the glenohumeral joint, followed by thin-slice CT imaging with both soft tissue and bone algorithms employed.[38,39,40,50,52,71,75,78,79,92,99] In recent years, magnetic resonance (MR) imaging has become more widely accepted for imaging of the shoulder than CT or CTA.[38] MR doesn't require intraarticular contrast, soft tissue resolution is excellent, and there is no radiation exposure.

Computed tomography has excellent contrast resolution and is an excellent modality to assess musculoskeletal trauma when plain radiography fails to adequately assess a bone or periarticular abnormality. In the past 20 years since its introduction to clinical practice, modifications have made CT a frequently utilized diagnostic tool rather than alternative lengthy and invasive procedures.[76–78] This application is particularly beneficial in evaluation of complex anatomic structures, especially the shoulder. The ability to obtain thin-slice images, measure tissue attenuation coefficients, rapid scan time, reduced radiation exposure, markedly improved contrast resolution, and three-dimensional imaging capability make CT a highly useful tool for evaluating the musculoskeletal system. Computer manipulation of images at the video console allows variable reconstruction algorithms to be used that permit optimal visualization of high-contrast structures, such as bone.

Evaluation of the patient with shoulder trauma can be completed with the patient in a comfortable supine position. It is best to image both shoulders so the asymptomatic normal shoulder can be used as a comparison.[13,76] Rapid scanning combined with thin-section contiguous images provides maximum information and allows multiplanar reformatting of data to provide images in other planes of interest. Not every radiology center has three-dimensional reconstruction capabilities (Fig. 4-7). It is important to ask.

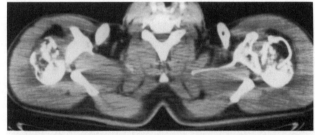
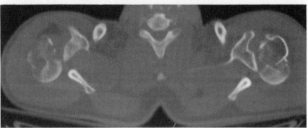

FIGURE 4-6
This 16-year-old soccer player was hit by lightning during a game. At time of hospital admission his chest x-ray was interpreted as normal and a right humeral fracture was seen. The left shoulder was not included on the x-ray. An AP x-ray of the right shoulder reveals a comminuted fracture of the surgical neck of the humerus. The axillary view demonstrates a posterior dislocation missed on the AP view. CT examination was performed to evaluate fracture fragment location, displacement, and integrity of the joint. Both soft tissue (top) and bone (bottom) algorithms were used. Note there are bilateral posterior dislocations. The fracture fragments can be identified for number, size, and location.

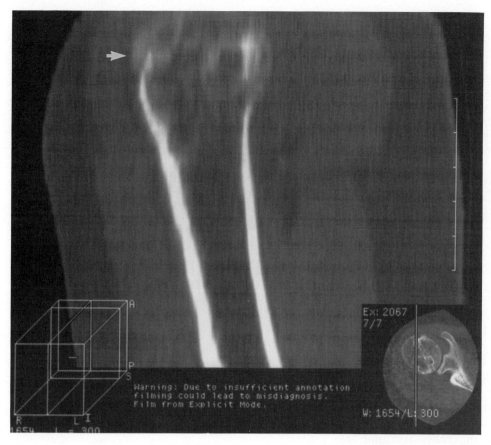

Warning: Due to insufficient annotation
filming could lead to misdiagnosis.
Film from Explicit Mode.

Ex: 2067
7/7

W: 1654/L: 300

FIGURE 4-7
This swimmer was felt to suffer from an overuse syndrome. Plain x-ray reveals epiphyseal lysis that crosses the closed growth into the metaphysis. Axial CT images (bone left, soft tissue right) show bony destruction and cortical breakthrough (arrow). A three-dimensional reconstructed image in the sagittal plane yields additional information about tumor location. This assists the orthopedist who wishes to biopsy the abnormal area. The line on the image in the lower right corner depicts the actual location of the sagittal slice. Diagnosis: chondroblastoma.

Fracture-dislocations, whether subtle or complex, can be adequately demonstrated and their extension into the articular surface well seen. The spatial relationships of fracture fragments can be evaluated to allow the orthopedist to plan treatment. CT can also assess postoperative changes and assess reduction of a dislocation. In cases of instability, maximum visualization of associated fractures, i.e., Bankart or Hill-Sachs lesions, can be delineated and measured[16] (Fig. 4-8). Associated soft tissue injuries can be seen as CT allows differentiation between soft tissues with slightly different contrast characteristics. Muscle, fat, blood, and fluid can be differentiated as can subtle calcifications.[77–79]

In cases of myositis ossificans, the early "eggshell" peripheral calcification can be identified. As this may not be seen on plain x-rays, the use of CT should prevent an otherwise extensive workup for a possible soft tissue tumor[34] (Fig. 4-9).

Intravenous contrast administration is advantageous to enhance vascular structures and delineate their anatomy. Traumatic transection of a vessel or a pseudoaneurysm can be seen. The muscular anatomy is highlighted and the relationship of any soft tissue mass to the adjacent or nearby vessel can be assessed.[76]

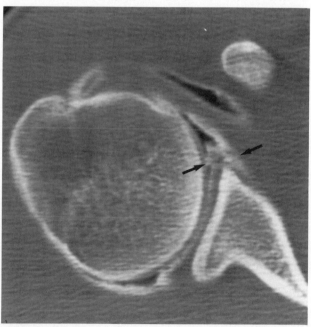

FIGURE 4-8
This example of anterior instability accurately depicts the avulsed anterior capsulolabral complex (arrows). The underlying bony anterior glenoid is normal. The articular cartilage and posterior labrum have smooth contrast-covered margins and are normal.

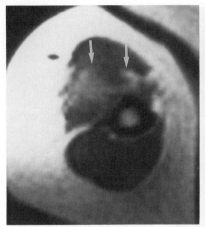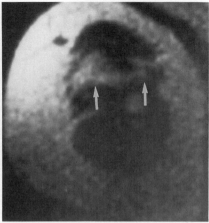

BONE SCAN

The bone scan does serve a limited role in traumatic and sports injuries of the shoulder, especially when initial routine radiographs fail to diagnose the abnormality. Additionally, some injuries that cannot be diagnosed by normally used x-ray methods will be easily detected by bone scan. These include: (1) Stress fracture or periosteal injury. (However, this application is most utilized in evaluation of weight-bearing bones where stress fractures are commonly encountered, i.e., the tibia.) (2) Occult fractures. A fracture may not be radiographically apparent until 7 to 10 days after an injury, whereas a bone scan will be positive within 72 h of injury. This modality is useful in youngsters and elderly osteoporotic patients where subtle fractures may not be apparent on plain radiographs.[73] (3) Joint abnormalities. Diagnostic radionuclide arthroscopy involves the injection of a minimal amount of intraarticular isotope, and the risk of synovitis or allergy is absent. However, contrast radiography or arthrography are more effective radiologic procedures. (4) Acute muscle injury. Bone-scanning agents will localize in areas of acutely necrotic muscle, i.e., electrical burn, excessive exercise, rhadomyolisis, etc. Most abnormalities demonstrate intense uptake on bone scan within 24 to 48 h of injury and generally resolve within a week. The intensity of bone scan abnormalities generally correlates with the amount of serum creatinine elevation. Abnormal serum level of the enzymes may suggest the diagnosis of myocardial infarction. Thus the same injection of isotope can be used to detect skeletal muscle necrosis and any myocardial injury if present. The findings of each of these categories of disorders usually allow differentiation between them. In addition, a bone scan may be helpful in evaluation of union of fractures, but it is used predominantly for lower-extremity fractures. Bone scanning is an important diagnostic tool in evaluation of intramedullary bone lesions and for a screening tool in evaluation of avascular necrosis and metastases in the appropriate clinical setting.[94,99]

ULTRASONOGRAPHY

The primary reason to use shoulder ultrasonography is to diagnose rotator cuff tears and associated abnormalities of the biceps tendon. Sonographic evaluation is less expensive than a shoulder arthrogram, is usually accessible, and allows evaluation of both shoulders for comparison (Fig. 4-10). The ultrasound examination can be completed within 15 to 20 min.

In the mid 1980s, there were many published studies describing the normal and abnormal sonographic appearances of the rotator cuff.[3,4,14,15,23] More recent publications have described in detail the

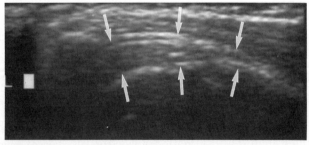

FIGURE 4-10

Ultrasound is a readily accessible tool to quickly evaluate the shoulder for the rotator cuff tear or biceps tendon abnormalities. The normal sonogram of a shoulder identified the rotator cuff tendon of uniform thickness and echogenicity (area between arrows). Inferior to the tendon is the humeral head which has a smooth cortical surface.

sonographic criteria for rotator cuff tears.[45,55] The technique for ultrasound examination has been refined and more recently described in the radiologic and orthopedic literature.[32] It is the modality of choice for the fastest noninvasive screening means of allowing appropriate diagnosis of rotator cuff tears and assessing the status of the biceps tendon.[3,5]

Sonography has comparable accuracy in diagnosing rotator cuff tears to arthrography. Its advantages are that an ultrasound examination is noninvasive, painless, and more pleasing to patients. Also, sonography permits a more complete examination of the shoulder, yielding more anatomic detail of a rotator cuff tear than a standard arthrogram.[18,23]

Limitations

There are limitations of sonography. Equipment, technique, and a thorough knowledge of the normal appearance of the shoulder can limit or enhance the examination. As Mack reported, there is a "substantial learning curve that exists with cuff sonography."[47,48] Many radiologists confirm the fact that shoulder sonography is one of the most difficult procedures to perform and master, and thus they hesitate to use it for shoulder examination.

Over the past 5 years, improvement of equipment has led to greater diagnostic accuracy of rotator cuff tears.[91,94,95] High-resolution linear array transducers are available, i.e., 7.5 MHz, and provide excellent images of the rotator cuff. For extremely well developed or large patients, lower-frequency transducers can be used. Linear array transducers are preferred over wedge-shaped images produced by mechanical scanners for better resolution and minimization of artifacts.[59]

Technique

Mack, Middleton, and Crass have published detailed studies that describe their techniques of sonographic examination of the shoulder. Generally, the patient is examined in a seated position. Each shoulder is examined as per protocol and compared for asymmetry. A detailed examination entails evaluation of the biceps tendon followed by ultrasound of the rotator cuff. Examination of the biceps tendon is crucial because abnormalities of both the biceps tendon and rotator cuff may coexist. Also, abnormalities of the biceps tendon may mimic rotator cuff lesions.[14,15,47,48,53–59]

Biceps Tendon Evaluation

An effusion of the biceps tendon is an important abnormality to identify. Middleton reported a 55 per-

cent correlation of biceps tendon sheath effusions and an associated rotator cuff tear.[56–58] Therefore, if an effusion is identified, a complete examination of the rotator cuff is required. An effusion may be seen with other abnormalities such as shoulder impingement, adhesive capsulitis, osteocartilaginous loose bodies, instability, and biceps tenosynovitis; so, if a cuff tear is not identified, arthrography or magnetic resonance imaging may be needed for further evaluation and diagnosis of these abnormalities that may not be identified by ultrasound.

Other biceps tendon abnormalities that can be detected by sonographic examination include biceps tendinitis (decreased tendon echogenicity and tendon enlargement), subluxation or dislocation of the tendon, and tendon rupture—usually seen with an associated rotator cuff tear.

Rotator Cuff Evaluation

A full-thickness rotator cuff tear is defined sonographically as "absence of the normal tendons on static and dynamic images."[45,55–59] Associated findings may include a glenohumeral joint effusion, fluid in the subacromial-subdeltoid bursa, an elevated location of the humeral head and decreased acromiohumeral space, humeral head irregularity, and alterations of the superior aspect of the supraspinatus tendon. Obviously the accuracy of ultrasound evaluation of the rotator cuff increases with large, complete tears and diminishes with small or fine tears.

Limitations of Sonography

What are the disadvantages of sonographic evaluation of the shoulder? Utilization of poor equipment can produce artifacts. Poor positioning is a common problem, and inexperienced sonographers can confuse normal structures for pathology. This examination is operator-dependent, and lengthy training is necessary to become a proficient shoulder sonographer. A thorough knowledge of shoulder anatomy is essential. Finally, discrepancies in criteria for ultrasound diagnosis of rotator cuff tears exist and can be confusing. Improvements in technique and equipment are occurring that will enhance diagnostic accuracy and allow sonography to become a good diagnostic choice for initial evaluation of suspected rotator cuff tears.[53,54,91]

ARTERIOGRAPHY

Angiography is useful for cases of suspected vascular injury that may result with shoulder dislocation or secondary to comminuted or open fractures. Indications for arteriography include an abnormal vascular examination (cold or pulseless extremity), bleeding, or ischemia. Arteriographic abnormalities include extravasation of contrast, vessel occlusion, intraluminal defects, focal vascular thickening, arteriovenous fistula, or lumen narrowing.

Arteriography is often used in the initial workup of tumors. Knowing the vascularity and origin of feeding vessels to a lesion greatly aids presurgical planning. Autologous donation of blood or presurgical embolization may follow if a very vascular lesion is detected and a high risk of surgical bleeding is expected to occur.

Recent MR advances allow angiographic sequences to be performed with or without intravenous administration of gadolinium. Computerized flow sequences that delineate vascular structures and allow interpretation of abnormalities are gaining recognition as a viable alternative to arteriography. While many trauma centers perform MR angiography (MRA) of large vessels close to the axial skeleton, arteriography remains the gold standard of suspected vascular injury until proved otherwise.[99] Future advances of MRA should prove helpful in the periphery and in small-vessel evaluation.

MAGNETIC RESONANCE IMAGING (MRI)

MR imaging has proved to be of great diagnostic value in the evaluation of acute or chronic shoulder injuries. Initial limitations of MR shoulder imaging have been improved upon, including the development of specialized surface coils that are specifically designed for different anatomic regions of the body. And software advances provide the ability to employ off-center fields of view (FOV) so that the body part to be imaged does not need to be placed in the center of the MR cylinder. In addition, the development of larger-size matrices and thus smaller pixel size have markedly improved the spatial resolution of MR images, allowing accurate detection of subtle abnormalities and close evaluation of small body parts.

MR allows multiplanar imaging with small fields of view (FOV), is noninvasive, and enables accurate evaluation of bone and soft tissue structures. Thus distinction between cortical and intramedullary bone, tendons, cartilaginous structures, muscle, fat, and fluid is accomplished owing to the superior MR contrast resolution of these structures compared with other imaging modalities.[5,11,17,33,35,37,44,87,88,90]

That is not to say MR imaging is not without technical difficulties or limitations. The limited magnet cylinder diameter precludes imaging of large or very muscular patients. The patient may become claustrophobic during a shoulder MR exam as the upper torso and head will be contained within the magnet for the duration of the examination, which may be as long as 1 h. The noise generated during the multiple sequences is fairly loud and compounds any tendency toward claustrophobia. Also, technical problems can arise, prolonging imaging time or requiring termination and rescheduling the patient.

Other limiting factors to be considered include the magnet strength and design. Is the person interpreting the images knowledgeable of the anatomy and familiar with MR criteria for pathology of the shoulder?

The technique for MR evaluation of the shoulder varies from institution to institution and can be modified depending on the patient's history.[2,17,22,37,86,88] Yet it is generally agreed that use of a specialized shoulder coil, a small field of view, larger matrix size, and a combination of imaging in at least two planes yields a study with enough information to carefully scrutinize the images and permit a highly accurate diagnosis.

The technique employed at our institution has been modified over the past 4 years as new software, coils, and magnet upgrades have allowed. The patient is placed in a supine position with a specialized shoulder coil (Helmholtz, Siemens, Iselin, NJ) centered over the shoulder to be examined. Axial localizing images are performed, and utilizing off-center field of view techniques, the images of the shoulder are centered on the console and filmed. From these images, the desired area to be examined and plane of imaging can be selected.

MR can provide information about the acutely injured shoulder that complements plain film radiography. Complex fractures may be visualized in a multiplanar fashion and surrounding soft tissue structures scrutinized for entrapment, disruption, hemorrhage, and edema. Intramedullary abnormalities such as bone edema (bruising) or bleeding can be evaluated and followed. Intrasubstance injuries of the rotator cuff can be easily visualized—i.e., tendon disruption or avulsions that are distinct from the more commonly seen supraspinatus tears in the "critical zone" of the tendon near its attachment to the greater tuberosity of the humerus. Falls and direct blows to the shoulder may avulse or tear the superior portion of the supraspinatus or subscapularis tendons and result in accompanying hematomas.[9,10,21,30,68]

Biceps tendon ruptures are easily detected by MR evaluation. Images will show lack of visualization of the tendon within its sheath, and usually a joint effusion can be identified as well.[9,10,21,30]

To date, the glenohumeral ligaments and capsular mechanism of the shoulder remain somewhat difficult to visualize and adequately evaluate by MR. Some studies claim to be able to accurately assess the joint capsule but with varying degrees of confidence. Future refinements of shoulder imaging may alter this.

Impingement

Impingement results in rotator cuff–related pain associated with abduction of the arm above shoulder level. Changes occur within the rotator cuff tendons, primarily the supraspinatus tendon. Neer proposed that supraspinatus tendon lesions resulting from chronic impingement are the result of impingement of the tendon by the inferior surface of the acromion, acromioclavicular (AC) joint, coracoid process, or coracoclavicular ligament.[65] Variations in anatomy as well as degenerative changes, i.e., osteophytes or spurs, result in repetitive trauma to the supraspinatus tendon and often the biceps tendon as well. Most researchers, including Neer, have divided impingement syndrome into three distinct stages that correlate with pathologic changes found within the rotator cuff tendons.[65,67,89,100]

In stage I impingement, reversible hemorrhage and edema may be found within the supraspinatus tendon. Usually patients are less than 25 years of age. Commonly associated sports activities leading to this finding are tennis, baseball, and swimming. Stage II impingement is usually found in a slightly older age group, and symptoms are usually more

chronic in duration than in stage I. Histologically, the tendon demonstrates fibrosis or more diffuse inflammatory changes. Stage III impingement is often seen in patients over 40 years of age. In stage III impingement, the previous changes of stages I and II have led to tendon degeneration and complete tendon rupture, usually within the "critical zone" of the supraspinatus tendon. The critical zone is considered to be the 1-cm avascular area of the supraspinatus tendon adjacent to its insertion onto the greater tuberosity of the humerus.[34,35,100]

Plain film radiography, fluoroscopy, and CT arthrography (CTA) are diagnostic of late-stage rotator cuff arthropathy, that is, a complete rotator cuff tear. Stage I and II impingement cannot be diagnosed by these radiographic studies and MR is an excellent modality to assess intrasubstance changes of the rotator cuff and to aid the clinician in determining the type of treatment to employ.

Magnetic resonance imaging is very useful in diagnosing shoulder impingement in all three stages and can distinguish between stages. However, adequate visualization of the rotator cuff tendons is dependent on magnet strength (higher field strength systems yield better images), choice of surface coil, arm position, FOV, and plane of imaging. The previously discussed axial localizing images determine location of off-center FOV. Serial coronal oblique images best identify tendons of the rotator cuff muscles; that is, the plane of imaging parallels the supraspinatus muscle and tendon so these structures are seen in continuity. T1-weighted (T1W) images best demonstrate normal anatomy. Proton density weighted (PDW) and T2-weighted (T2W) images better define pathology (Fig. 4-11).

In patients with stage I or II impingement ("tendinosis"), the tendons that comprise the rotator cuff are intact.[69] On T1W and PDW images, high signal within the tendon will be best appreciated owing to

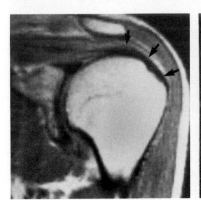 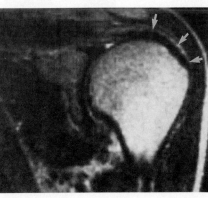

FIGURE 4-11
A normal T1W coronal oblique image (left) depicts a normal supraspinatus tendon as a continuous signal void (arrows). The bones are bright-signal on T1W owing to the high content of intramedullary fat. Fat is bright on T1W, i.e., subcutaneous fat. Cortical bone containing calcium is seen as a signal void or black. The T2W image (right) demonstrates decreased signal of fat-containing structures. There is no change in the signal void or low signal of normal tendons and cortical bone. Any fluid on T2W would become bright in signal.

better signal-to-noise ratio (S/N) and thus better resolution on these sequences rather than T2W images. Since the tendons are intact, no appreciable amount of fluid should be seen in the subacromial-subdeltoid bursa. Also, the subdeltoid fat stripe should be preserved and well defined. Some of these patients may have bony spurs that result in direct bony impingement of the supraspinatus tendon, the musculotendinosis junction, or muscle itself. These findings allow clinicians to plan effective therapy (Fig. 4-12).[89,100]

MR findings of a complete rotator cuff tear (stage III impingement) can be suggested by plain films. The elevated humeral head, lack of ability to actively abduct the arm for appropriate films, spur formation, and osteoarthritis (OA) of the AC joint with large inferior osteophytes are indications of a complete rotator cuff tear. Full-thickness tears may be seen by ultrasonography, arthrography, CTA, or MR.

MR findings of a complete tear include loss of homogeneity of signal of the usually black (signal void) or low-signal intact tendon. The subdeltoid fat line will be discontinuous or obscured. T2W images may reveal fluid in the glenohumeral joint as well as the subacromial-subdeltoid bursa, secondary to extravasation of fluid through the torn tendon (Fig. 4-13). In chronic tears, muscle atrophy, fatty replace-

ment of musculature, and tendon retraction may be identified. MR can accurately demonstrate the location, extent, and size of full-thickness rotator cuff tears. Secondary bony changes of impingement may be seen in almost 50 percent of these patients as well. Changes of advanced rotator cuff arthropathy, including humeral head collapse, cartilage degeneration, and erosion of the AC joint and acromion may accompany the above and be evaluated by MR.[5,22,35,41,42,44,54,64,67,76,100]

Partial Rotator Cuff Tears

Criteria to describe MR findings of partial tears are preliminary at this time. An area of increased signal on the inferior surface of the supraspinatus tendon may correlate with a partial tear. However, multiple studies have described the frustration in trying to distinguish between a small full-thickness tear, tendinitis, and a partial tear.[5,67,76,97] Further work in this area may solve this problem. Nirschl coined the term "tendinosis," a catchall term to encompass all three of the above conditions, and this term is frequently employed to describe the MR findings that cannot distinguish the above three abnormalities.[69]

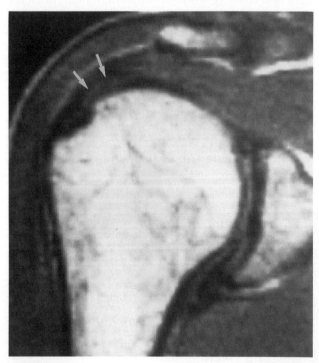

FIGURE 4-12
Examples of stage I impingement.

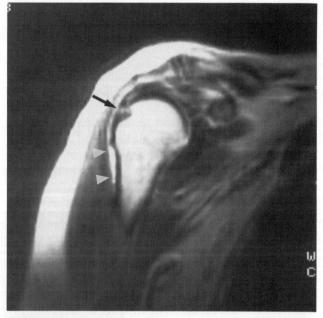

FIGURE 4-13
Stage III impingement or complete rotator cuff tear. Site of the tear is marked by arrows. The area of bright signal may be linear or irregular but traverses the entire tendon width. The subdeltoid fat line is distorted or obscured by fluid in the subacromial-subdeltoid bursae (arrowheads). Note the altered signal of the supraspinatus muscle secondary to AC joint impingement.

Instability

The anterior capsular mechanism of the shoulder is important for stability.[75,76,83,88,94,96,98] It consists of the glenoid labrum, glenohumeral ligaments, synovial membrane, joint capsule, subscapularis muscle and tendon, as well as the subscapularis bursa. Abnormalities of these structures are commonly seen with repetitive trauma—especially subluxations and dislocations. There is a range of abnormalities that can occur and lead to development of shoulder instability. Abnormalities include Hill-Sachs lesions, detachment, partial or complete tears of the labrum and capsule, laxity of the subscapularis muscle and tendon, and development of a large anterior pouch. The labrum is not the only stabilizing factor of the shoulder, but there is a frequent association of labral lesions and instability, thus making the detection of labrum abnormalities a reliable sign of instability.[2,6,8,13,29,38,44,46,49,50,51,72,79,99,100]

Abnormalities of the labrum and detection of instability have been well defined and are easily demonstrated by CTA and arthrotomography. While CTA is still considered to be the procedure of choice by many to examine patients with a history of subluxations and dislocations, the recent advances in MR imaging will probably let MR replace this modality in studying patients with a subluxation or dislocation history. This is because MR is noninvasive and allows multiplanar imaging of associated structural changes that accompany a subluxation or dislocation.[1,5,38,67,76,99]

Contiguous axial images demonstrate the humeral head–glenoid relationship, comparable with the axial images of computed tomography and CTA. The glenoid labrum and articular cartilage can be assessed. The normal anterior labrum is of low to moderate signal intensity and often triangularly shaped (though normal variations exist).[72,76,90,101] The posterior labrum is usually more rounded in shape. Articular hyaline cartilage is normally uniform in thickness and smooth at the articular surface. The subscapularis muscle and its tendon insertion onto the lesser tuberosity of the humerus are best seen on axial images. The long head of the biceps tendon can be evaluated for position, size, and any abnormalities. The biceps tendon itself is a normal signal void surrounded by a thin moderate signal sheath and located within the bicipital grove. Fluid collections in the subscapularis bursa are easily identified on T2W axial views, as fluid is bright in signal.

The normal anterior capsule and glenohumeral ligaments are low-signal structures adjacent to the subscapularis tendon. It is often not possible to differentiate these structures unless a joint effusion is present, and even then normal folds of tissue may be mistakenly identified as pathology. In addition, it is generally acknowledged that three types of anterior capsule insertions exist and that the type III capsular insertion, located more medially along the scapula, has a higher association with recurrent dislocations (cause or effect is disputed).[100,101]

Hill-Sachs lesions, also best evaluated on axial images, are wedge-shaped defects on the posterolateral surface of the humeral head. With MR, these lesions can be diagnosed and measured.

Legan et al. have reported a 95 percent sensitivity in detection of anterior labrum tears and deem MR imaging of the shoulder to be "a highly accurate" technique for evaluation of shoulder instability.[46] He and others have found MRI to be less effective in detection of labral tears in other locations.[5,46,67,88] Tears of the labrum by MR criteria include high-signal transecting the substance of this structure, truncation, absence of a normal labrum, detachment, or the "glenoid labrum oval mass" sign (GLOM)—detection of a soft tissue mass that gives an expanded appearance to the anterior labrum (Figs. 4-14 and 4-15).[46]

As the association of rotator cuff pathology and labrum abnormalities becomes better understood,

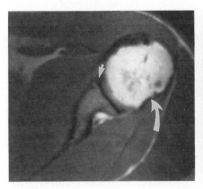 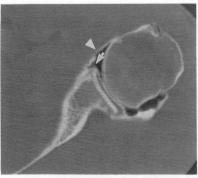

FIGURE 4-14

An axial T1W MR image is compared with an axial CTA image demonstrating anterior instability. In both images, the anterior labrum is amputated, suggesting instability. However, the CTA image best delineates the irregular anterior capsule (arrowhead), well seen because the joint is distended by air. The anterior capsule cannot be seen on the MR image. Note the posterolateral portion of the humeral head is flattened, representing a Hill-Sachs defect (curved arrow).

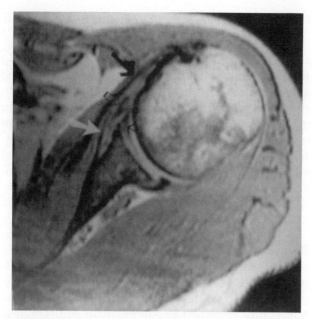

FIGURE 4-15
Three-dimensional gradient echo imaging is faster than the usually employed spin echo techniques, but many MR units are either not capable of obtaining good resolution images or can't utilize this technique when off-center FOV is needed, as in shoulder examinations.

MR imaging should become the study of choice to image the injured shoulder. Its multiplanar capabilities make MR ideal to image the rotator cuff and detect any other abnormalities to suggest associated instability.

Posterior instability of the shoulder is less commonly encountered than anterior instability and is also not as well understood. Acute posterior dislocations are infrequent and associated with seizures and high-voltage electrical burns. Recurrent posterior dislocations are common, especially when there are associated significant bony defects of the humerus and glenoid.

In athletes with overuse syndromes, recurrent posterior subluxations occur with or without a history of trauma. The posterior capsular mechanism consists of the posterior capsule, labrum, synovial membrane, superior and posterior rotator muscles,

and their tendons. As with anterior instability, associated findings of posterior instability include defects of the labrum (posteriorly) capsular abnormalities, and bony defects (generally an impaction defect of the anteromedial surface of the humeral head or "trough" lesion). The bony defect becomes larger with repeated dislocations, as does the Hill-Sachs lesion associated with anterior dislocations. While MR can detect the abnormalities of posterior instability, as stated previously, experience in this area is not as well developed as in evaluation of anterior instability.[46,88,94]

Patients with combined instability, i.e., anterior and posterior or multiplanar, are said to have multidirectional instability. This disorder is thought to be an abnormality of the soft tissues of the shoulder leading to ligamentous laxity that render the joint extremely mobile. Certain athletes are prone to this disorder, especially with repetitive episodes of trauma, i.e., football, wrestling, and gymnastics.[6,8,13,30,35,44,46,51,87,88,100]

MR findings may include single or multiple labrum abnormalities, capsule redundancy, and/or distention (Fig. 4-16). CTA is often a reliable diagnostic tool for evaluation of a lax or redundant capsule and ligamentous structure as the capsule is imaged after distention with air and contrast material and thus is easily seen.[38,72,78,79,92]

Contrast Agents

MR arthrography with contrast agents has been used in cadaver specimens to further evaluate and understand the shoulder. The procedure involves intraarticular injection of gadolinium-DTPA or saline into the glenohumeral joint. Gadolinium has T2 shortening effects and may obviate the need for T2W sequences to be obtained—therefore, imaging time is greatly reduced and image degradation from motion is reduced. There may be improved detection of complete rotator cuff tears and partial tears of the undersurface of the supraspinatus tendon utilizing contrast. Zlatkin has showed the beneficial effects of intraarticular injection of gadolinium to evaluate the

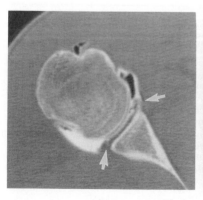 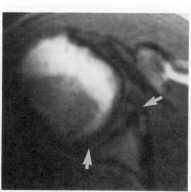

FIGURE 4-16
This case of multidirectional instability is a recurrent subluxer. Anterior and posterior defects (arrows) are detected, better seen on the CTA image (left) than the MR T1W image (right).

labrum and capsular structures due to the capsular distention obtained prior to imaging (similar to CTA).[101]

A disadvantage of this technique in live patients is coordination of the time of injection and delay until the MR exam, as well as the invasive nature of the technique. And in most radiology departments, the injection takes place in the fluoroscopy section, often a distance away from the MR center. Future developments in this area, particularly studies on actual patients, are needed to establish the role of this technique, but the initial results of cadaver studies are encouraging. MR arthrography may become the study of choice in those patients with rotator cuff abnormalities and clinically significant shoulder instability.

Biceps Tendon Abnormalities

Lesions of the long head of the biceps tendon include biceps tendinitis and instability (Fig. 4-17). Tendinitis may be divided into categories by pathoanatomy, but by MR evaluation, the findings within the tendon itself are identical. Most often, biceps tendinitis is secondary to impingement syndrome and tears of the rotator cuff. It is rare for biceps tendinitis to be an isolated entity.[58,59] The long head of the biceps tendon has an intimate relationship with the rotator cuff, and as both structures pass under the coracoacromial arch, both are involved in the impingement syndrome. MR findings include synovial edema and swelling as the tendon is involved with the same inflammatory process as the remainder of the synovium in cases of impingement. Biceps tendinitis is usually initiated by compression in young athletes, especially in activities that involve overhead motion. Plain films and arthrography are usually normal in this condition. Fluid may be seen on T2W images within the tendon sheath, but this is nonspecific. Fluid may be also secondary to tenosynovitis or from a joint effusion as the glenohumeral joint and biceps tendon sheath communicate.[6,21,45,76]

Discrete increased signal within the tendon substance may be observed on T1W and PDW images. Over time, the tendon may become thickened and frayed. One of the complications of biceps tendinitis is tendon rupture, usually seen at its weakest portion, just distal to its exit from the joint cavity. Ultrasound evaluation of the biceps tendon is an easily performed exam to detect a rupture. Its presence within the intertubercular groove cannot be seen. While biceps tendon ruptures are generally easy to recognize clinically, tears may occur in association with anterior rotator cuff tears.[6,21,45] A complete MR shoulder examination should well define both structures and include coronal oblique as well as axial images.

Biceps tendon subluxations and dislocations (instability) are rarely seen as an isolated entity but are more commonly encountered with fractures of the proximal humerus and external rotation injuries involving the lesser tuberosity and subscapularis tendon. (This dislocation is easily detected on axial MR images, and the dislocation is always medial.[9,21,30]) In addition, dislocations of the long head of the biceps tendon are frequently seen with large complete rotator cuff tears. The low-signal biceps tendon surrounded by its medium-signal tendon sheath will be displaced medial to the intertubercular groove with or without an intact subscapularis tendon.

Osteonecrosis

Osteonecrosis may be the etiology of shoulder pain in patients with a previous fracture, especially of the surgical neck of the humerus. Patients with predisposing factors of bone infarction, i.e., primary anemia or hemoglobinopathy, occlusive vascular disease, exogenous steroid usage, alcoholism, collagen vascular disease, etc., are prone to developing osteonecrosis as well. Numerous studies have reported the high sensitivity and specificity of magnetic res-

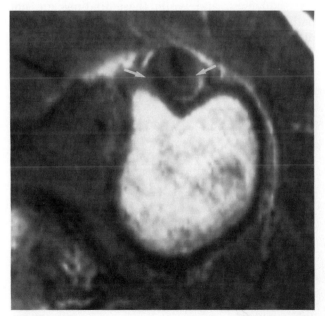

FIGURE 4-17
Biceps tendinitis examples. Axial T1W images show marked thickening of the low-signal long head of the biceps tendon (arrows) within its sheath.

onance imaging in detecting the early changes of osteonecrosis, facilitating treatment at an early stage (Fig. 4-18).[100]

MR is more sensitive to detection of early osteonecrosis than plain films or radionuclide imaging. Decreased signal intensity of subarticular bone on T1W1, PDW, and T2W images correlates with avascular bone, or one may see areas of dark signal band surrounding normal marrow (high signal on T1W images due to fat content). The "double-line" sign, which consists of bright granulation tissue within low-signal sclerotic bone, may also be identified. Articular collapse and fragmentation are easily detected as well as overlying deformities or irregularity of articular cartilage. A joint effusion (high or bright T2W signal) is seen in approximately half of all cases.

Synovial Disorders

Arthritis and related synovial disorders cause shoulder pain, and their inflammatory changes can be identified at an early stage by MR. Periarticular edema, synovial proliferation, and edema will be seen. Inflammatory changes may affect the surrounding soft tissues as well as tendons, muscles, and bursae. Fluid collections, atrophy, and cysts may be assessed. Progression of disease may lead to articular cartilage degeneration and destruction, bony erosions, and disruption of tendons, ligaments, and the joint capsule.[100,101]

An inflammatory arthritis may cause bone erosions and ultimately lead to rotator cuff tears. Some MR centers employ intravenous administration of gadolinium to separate a joint effusion from an acutely inflamed synovium—which will demonstrate increased signal intensity or enhancement if inflamed.[101] The effusion will lack enhancement.

Osteoarthritis of the shoulder (glenohumeral joint and AC joint) may be a complication of trauma. Subchondral cysts, loose bodies, cartilage damage, and bony proliferation can be seen by MR exam, but plain films often diagnose this condition. Utilization of gradient echo imaging parameters (i.e., GRASS, FISP, and FLASH), rather than the more commonly used spin echo technique, is helpful for evaluation of cartilaginous structures and detection of osteocartilaginous bodies. MR will detect the subtle or early changes of degenerative joint disease well before plain radiographs reveal any abnormalities. Though infrequent, ganglion cysts may accompany degeneration of the joint. Their detection is simply accomplished by MR. Their location, size, and origin can be assessed as well as secondary compressive changes or muscle atrophy. A common location of a shoulder ganglion is a branch of the suprascapular nerve.[25]

Synovial osteochondromatosis will demonstrate synovial metaplasia and intraarticular nodules that may or may not be calcified, bony erosion, and degenerative joint alterations. MR is helpful in assessing these patients after surgery for recurrence.[100]

Pigmented villonodular synovitis (PVNS) also causes synovial proliferation, bone cysts, and erosions. The soft tissue hemosiderin-laden nodules of synovium appear low to moderate signal on all image sequences, and while these findings are not pathognomonic of this disorder, the findings are highly suggestive. Synovitis or an effusion of the

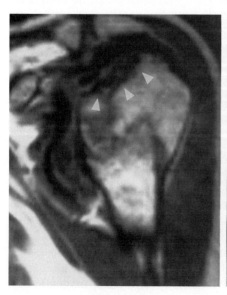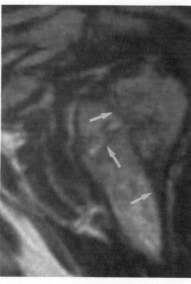

FIGURE 4-18
Follow-up of fractures by MR examination can detect multiple abnormalities as shown in this case. Coronal oblique T1 (left) and T2 (right) images define the sites of healed fracture lines, low signal due to calcification (arrows). There are low-signal areas of the articular portion of the humeral head (arrowheads) representing avascular necrosis and subchondral collapse.

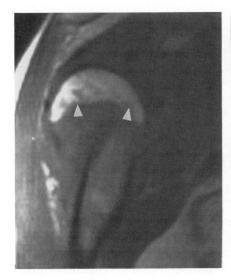 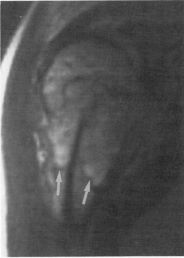

FIGURE 4-19
This semiprofessional tennis player fell and complained of shoulder pain. The plain film was fairly unremarkable. Because of continued symptoms, MR was performed. T1W (left) and T2W (right) coronal oblique images revealed low-signal T1 and bright-signal T2 marrow replacement of the proximal metadiaphyseal region of the right humerus. This process terminated at the growth plate (arrowheads). Breakthrough of cortex medially and laterally with tumor extension into soft tissue is seen (curved arrows). Arrows mark the poorly defined inferior border. Biopsy revealed non-Hodgkin's lymphoma. The patient received radiation therapy to this area.

joint becomes brighter in signal with increased T2W.[101]

Tumors

Tumors about the shoulder are not uncommon. Typically the patient presents with pain, swelling, and decreased range of motion as in the many other shoulder disorders. Often, diagnostic studies obtained at the time of an athlete's injury will demonstrate an otherwise undetected neoplasm of bone or soft tissue. MR is a valuable tool for evaluation of shoulder neoplasms because of the high resolution between normal and abnormal tissues. In some cases, plain films may allow a diagnosis of certain lesions and preclude additional expensive and lengthy workup.[25] Plain films are also an important addition to evaluation of any neoplasm evaluated by MR or CT (Figs. 4-19 and 4-20).

Short T_R/T_E sequences, T1W, best demonstrate the anatomy as well as definition between normal marrow fat and the lesion, whereas long T_R/T_E images, T2W, reveal maximum muscle-lesion contrast. MR is diagnostic of soft tissue lipomas that have bright, homogeneous T1 signal (as does subcutaneous fat) and decreases in brightness with T2 weighting. MR is limited in tissue diagnosis of most tumors. The utility of MR in lesions about the shoulder is to locate the tumor, determine size, and evaluate the neurovascular bundle and involvement of adjacent structures (Fig. 4-21). It also permits evaluation of spread of tumor to different soft tissue compartments. Preoperative evaluation and postsurgical therapeutic imaging is ideal to assess tumor response or recurrence.

Use of intravenous gadolinium (Gd-DTPA) has been tried to distinguish tumor from areas of reactive edema but has its pitfalls. Viable tumor will gener-

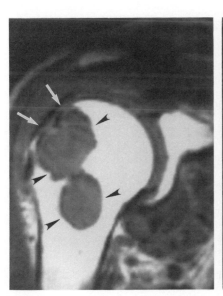 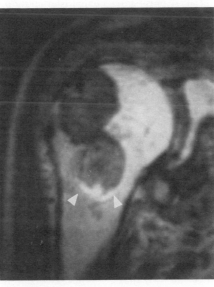

FIGURE 4-20
Because of unabated shoulder pain MR was decided upon for this patient. Coronal MR images (left is T1W and right is T2W) revealed low-signal areas of marrow replacement within the epiphysis and metaphysis of the proximal humerus (arrows). High-signal fluid can be identified at the rim of the lower nodular area (arrowheads). Biopsy revealed amyloidosis. Amyloid is low-signal on T1W and T2W.

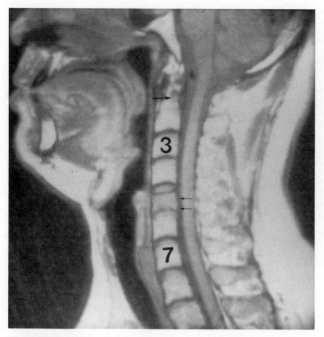

FIGURE 4-21
After a normal shoulder MR, examination of the brachial plexus was indicated. The T1W sagittal localizing view depicts low signal in the dens and the body of C_5, as compared with the bright T1 signal expected in normal vertebrae.

ally enhance with gadolinium injection, whereas edema will not. However, nonviable areas of tumor do not enhance either. MR is limited in detection of calcification and periosteal reaction, better detected by CT.[101] At times these two studies may complement each other in tumor workups. Future developments of dynamic gradient echo imaging, fat saturation techniques, and MR angiography should further aid in MR tumor evaluation.[2,51,53,61,94,99]

IN CONCLUSION

Multiple radiographic techniques are available to use individually or in combination to evaluate the acute or chronically injured athlete's shoulder. Employing the most efficient and least expensive diagnostic tools make sense in this era of rising medical costs. As described, each modality has its limitations as well as particular applications for the type of pathology suspected. But from experience, communication between the clinician and radiologist remains the most effective form of managing and working up a shoulder injury or other lesion in the best fashion possible.

REFERENCES

1. Bloom M, Obata W: Diagnosis of posterior dislocation of the shoulder with use of Velpeau axillary and angle up roentgenographic view. *J Bone Joint Surg (Am)* 49A:943–949, 1967.
2. Boorstein JM, Kneeland JB, Dalinka MK, et al. Magnetic resonance imaging of the shoulder. *Curr Probl Diagn Radiol* 21(1):3–27, 1992.
3. Brandt TD, Cardone BW, Grant TH, et al: Rotator cuff sonography: A reassessment. *Radiology* 173:323–327, 1989.
4. Bretzke CA, Crass JR, Craig EV, et al: Ultrasonography of the rotator cuff: Normal and pathologic anatomy. *Invest Radiol* 20:311–315, 1985.
5. Burk DL Jr, Karasick D, Kurtz AB, et al: Rotator cuff tears: Prospective comparison of MR imaging with arthrography, sonography, and surgery. *AJR* 153:87–92, 1989.
6. Burk DL Jr, Torres JL, Marone PJ, et al: MR imaging of shoulder injuries in professional baseball players. *Magn Reson Imaging J* 1(3):385–389, 1991.
7. Callaghan JJ, McNiesh LM, Dehaven JP, et al: A prospective comparison study of double contrast computed tomography arthrography and arthroscopy of the shoulder. *Am J Sports Med* 16:13–20, 1988.
8. Cartland JP, Crues JV 3d, Stauffer A, et al: MR imaging in the evaluation of SLAP injuries of the shoulder. Findings in 10 patients. *AJR* 159(4):787–792, 1992.
9. Cervilla V, Schweitzer ME, Ho C, et al: Medial dislocation of the biceps brachii tendon: Appearance at MR imaging. *Radiology* 180(2):523–526, 1991.
10. Chan TW, Dalinka MK, Kneeland JB, Chervrot A: Biceps tendon dislocation: Evaluation with MR imaging. *Radiology* 179(3):649–652, 1991.
11. Chandnani V, Ho C, Gerharter J, et al: MR findings in asymptomatic shoulders: A blind analysis using symptomatic shoulders as controls. *Clin Imaging* 16(1):25–30, 1992.
12. Cleaves E: A new film holder for roentgen examination of the shoulder. *AJR* 45:288–290, 1941.
13. Coumas JM, Waite RJ, Goss TP, et al: CT and MR evaluation of the labral capsular ligamentous complex of the shoulder. *AJR* 158(3):591–597, 1992.
14. Crass JR, Craig EV, Bretzke C, et al: Ultrasonography of the rotator cuff. *Radiographics* 5:941–953, 1985.
15. Crass JR, Craig EV, Feinberg SB: The hyperextended internal rotation view in rotator cuff ultrasonography of rotator cuff tears: A review of 500 diagnostic studies. *J Clin Ultrasound* 16:313–327, 1989.
16. Danzig L, Resnick D, Greenway G: Evaluation of unstable shoulders by computed tomography. A preliminary study. *Am J Sports Med* 10:138–141, 1982.

17. Davis SJ, Teresi LM, Bradley WG, et al: Effect of arm rotation on MR imaging of the rotator cuff. *Radiology* 181(1):265–268, 1991.

18. DeSmet A: Anterior oblique projection in radiography of the traumatized shoulder. *AJR* 134:515–518, 1980.

19. Deutsch AL, Resnick D, Mink JH, et al: Computed and conventional arthrotomography of the glenohumeral joint. Normal anatomy and clinical experience. *Radiology* 153:603–609, 1984.

20. El-Khoury GY, Albright JP, Yousef MMA, et al: Arthrotomography of the glenoid labrum. *Radiology* 131:333–337, 1979.

21. Erickson SJ, Fitzgerald SW, Quinn SF, et al: Long bicipital tendon of the shoulder. Normal anatomy and pathologic findings on MR imaging. *AJR* 158(5):1091–1096, 1992.

22. Evancho AM, Stiles RG, Fajman WA, et al: MR imaging diagnosis of rotator cuff tears. *AJR* 151:751–754, 1988.

23. Farin PU, Jaroma H, Harju A, et al: Shoulder impingement syndrome: Sonographic evaluation. *Radiology* 176:845–849, 1990.

24. Flinn RM, MacMillan CL Jr, Campbell DR, Fraser DB: Optimal radiography of the acutely injured shoulder. *J Can Assoc Radiol* 34:128–132, 1983.

25. Fritz RC, Helms CA, Steinbach LS, Genant HK: Suprascapular nerve entrapment: Evaluation with MR imaging. *Radiology* 182(2):437–444, 1992.

26. Garth WP Jr, Slappey CE, Ochs CW: Roentgenographic demonstration of instability of the shoulder: The apical oblique projection. *J Bone Joint Surg (Am)* 66-A:1450–1453, 1984.

27. Goldman AB, Dines DM, Warren RF: *Shoulder Arthrography: Technique, Diagnosis, and Clinical Correlation.* Boston, Little, Brown, 1982, pp 1–3.

28. Goldman AB, Gehlman B: The double-contrast shoulder arthrogram. *Radiology* 127:655–663, 1978.

29. Gross M, Seegler L, Smith J, et al: Magnetic resonance imaging of the glenoid labrum. *Am J Sports Med* 18(3):229–234, 1990.

30. Holder J, Kursunoglu BS, Flannigan B, et al: Injuries of the superior portion of the glenoid labrum involving the insertion of the biceps tendon: MR imaging findings in nine cases. *AJR* 159(3):565–568, 1992.

31. Holder J, Terrier B, Von-Schulthess GK, Fuchs WA: MRI and sonography of the shoulder. *Clin Radiol* 43(5):323–327, 1988.

32. Holder J, Fretz CJ, Terrier F, et al: Rotator cuff tears: Correlation of sonographic and surgical findings. *Radiology* 169:791–794, 1988.

33. Huber DJ, Sauter R, Mueller E, et al: MR imaging of the normal shoulder. *Radiology* 158:405–408, 1986.

34. Hudson T: *Radiologic-Pathologic Correlation of Musculoskeletal Lesions.* Baltimore, Williams & Wilkins, 1987, pp 582–583.

35. Iannotti JP, Zlatkin MB, Esterhai JL, et al: Magnetic resonance imaging of the shoulder. Sensitivity, specificity, and predictive value. *J Bone Joint Surg (Am)* 73(1):17–29, 1991.

36. Imhoff A, Hodler J: Arthroscopy and MR of the shoulder—A comparative retrospective analysis. *Z Orthop* 130(3):188–196, 1992.

37. Keift GJ, Bloem JL, Obermann WR, et al: Normal shoulder: MR imaging. *Radiology* 159:741–745, 1986.

38. Kieft GJ, Bloem JL, Rozing PM, Obermann WR: MR imaging of recurrent anterior dislocation of the shoulder: Comparison with CT arthrography. *AJR* 150:1083–1087, 1988.

39. Kinnard P, Tricoire JL, Levesque P, Bergeron D: Assessment of the unstable shoulder by computer arthrography. A preliminary report. *Am J Sports Med* 11:157–159, 1983.

40. Kleinman PK, Kanzaria PK, Goss TP, Pappas AM: Axillary arthrotomography of the glenoid labrum. *AJR* 142:993–999, 1984.

41. Kneeland JB, Middleton WD, Carrera GF, et al: Rotator cuff tears. Preliminary application of high resolution MR imaging with counter rotation current loop-gap resonators. *Radiology* 160:695–699, 1986.

42. Kneeland JB, Middleton WD, Carrera GF, et al: MR imaging of the shoulder: Diagnosis of rotator cuff tears. *Am J Roentgenol* 149:333–337, 1987.

43. Kornguth PJ, Salazar AM: The apical oblique view of the shoulder: Its usefulness in acute trauma. *AJR* 149:113–116, 1987.

44. Kursunglu-Bralime S, Resnick D: Magnetic resonance imaging of the shoulder. Imaging of joints. *Radiol Clin North Am* 28(5):941–954, 1990.

45. Lawson TL, Middleton AWD: MRI and ultrasound evaluation of the shoulder. *Acta Orthop Belg* 57(Suppl 1):62–69, 1991.

46. Legan JM, Burkhard TK, Goff WB 2d, et al: Tears of the glenoid labrum: MR imaging of 88 arthroscopically confirmed cases. *Radiology* 179(1):241–246, 1991.

47. Mack LA, Matsen FA III, Kolcoyne RF, et al: Evaluation of the rotator cuff. *Radiology* 157:205–209, 1985.

48. Mack L, Nyberg D, Matsen F: Sonographic evaluation of the rotator cuff in ultrasonography of the musculoskeletal systems. *Radiol Clin North Am* 26(1):161–177, 1988.

49. Masciocchi C, De BS, Barile A, et al: Acute instability of the shoulder in athletes. The role of magnetic resonance in therapy planning. *Radiol Med (Torino)* 82(6):751–756, 1991.

50. Masten FA, Thomas S, Rockwood C: Glenohumeral instability, in Rockwood CA, Matsen FA (eds): *The Shoulder.* Philadelphia, Saunders, 1990, chap 14, pp 526–622.

51. McCauley TR, Pope CF, Jokl P: Normal and abnormal glenoid labrum: Assessment with multiplanar gradient-echo MR imaging. *Radiology* 183(1): pp 35–37, 1992.

52. McGlynn FJ, El-Khoury G, Albright JP: Arthrotomography of the glenoid labrum in shoulder instability. *J Bone Joint Surg (Am)* 64:506–518, 1982.

53. Middleton WD: Ultrasonography of the shoulder. Ultrasonography of small parts. *Radiol Clin North Am* 30(5):927–940, 1992.

54. Middleton WD, Reinus WR, Nelson GL, et al: Pitfalls of rotator cuff sonography. *AJR* 146:555–560, 1986.

55. Middleton WD: Status of rotator cuff sonography. *Radiology* 173:307–309, 1989.

56. Middleton WD, Reinus WR, Tooty WG, et al: Ultrasonography of the biceps tendon apparatus. *Radiology* 157:211–215, 1985.

57. Middleton WD, Reinus WR, Totty WG, et al: Ultrasonographic evaluation of the rotator cuff and biceps tendon. *J Bone Joint Surg (Am)* 68(A):440–450, 1986.

58. Middleton WD, Edelstein G, Reinus WR, et al: Sonographic detection of rotator cuff tears. *AJR* 144:349–353, 1985.

59. Middleton WD, Kneeland JB, Carrera GF, et al: High-resolution MR imaging of the normal rotator cuff. *AJR* 148:559–564, 1987.

60. Mink JH, Harris E, Rappaport M: Rotator cuff tears: Evaluation using double-contrast shoulder arthrography. *Radiology* 157:621–623, 1985.

61. Mirowitz S: Normal rotator cuff: MR imaging with conventional fat-suppression techniques. *Radiology* 180:735–740, 1991.

62. Mirowitz S: Normal rotator cuff: MR imaging with conventional and fat-suppression techniques. *Radiology* 180:735–740, 1991.

63. Morrison D, Ofstein R: The use of magnetic resonance imaging in the diagnosis of rotator cuff tears. *Orthopedics.* 13(6):633–637.

64. Morrison D, Ofstein R: The use of magnetic resonance imaging in the diagnosis of rotator cuff tears. *Orthopedics* 13(6):633–637.

65. Neer CS II: Impingement lesions, in Nirschl RP: Shoulder Tendinitis. *American Academy of Orthopaedic Surgeons Symposium on Upper Extremity Injuries in Athletes. Clin Orthop* 173:70–77, 1983.

66. Neer CS II, Rockwood CA Jr: Fractures and dislocations of the shoulder, in Rockwood CA, Green DP (eds): *Fractures,* 2d ed. Philadelphia, Lippincott, 1984.

67. Nelson MC, Leather GP, Nirschl RP, et al: Evaluation of the painful shoulder. A prospective comparison of magnetic resonance imaging, computerized tomographic arthrography, ultrasonography, and operative findings. *J Bone Joint Surg (Am)* 73(5):707–716, 1991.

68. Neumann CH, Holt RG, Steinbach LS, et al: MR imaging of the shoulder appearance of the supraspinatus tendon in asymptomatic volunteers. *AJR* 158(6):1281–1287, 1992.

69. Nirschl RP: Pettrone FA (ed): Rotator cuff tendinitis: Basic concepts of pathoetiology. *Instruct Course Lect* 38:439–445, 1987.

70. Nirschl RP, Pettrone FA: Clinical examination of the shoulder. Read at the annual meeting of the American College of Sports Medicine, Salt Lake City, Utah, June 1990.

71. O'Brien SJ, Warren RF, Schwartz E: Anterior shoulder instability. *Orthop Clin North Am* 18:395–408, 1987.

72. Pappas AM, Goss TP, Kleinman PK: Symptomatic shoulder instability due to lesions of the glenoid labrum. *Am J Sports Med* 11:279–288, 1983.

73. Pavlov H, Freiberger RH: Fractures and dislocations about the shoulder. Seminars. *Roentgenology* 13:85–96, 1978.

74. Petersson CJ, Redlund J: The subacromial space in normal shoulder radiographs. *Acta Orthop Scand* 55:57–58, 1984.

75. Protzman RR: Anterior instability of the shoulder. *J Bone Joint Surg (Am)* 62-A:909–918, 1980.

76. Rafii M: Shoulder, in *MRI and CT of the Musculoskeletal System.* St Louis, Mosby-Year Book, 1992, pp 465–549.

77. Rafii M, Firooznia H, Bonamo JJ, et al: Athlete shoulder injuries: CT arthrographic findings. *Radiology* 162:559–564, 1987.

78. Rafii M, Firooznia H, Golimbu C, et al: CT arthrography of capsular structures of the shoulder. *AJR* 146:361–367, 1986.

79. Rafii M, Minkoff J, Bonamo J, et al: Computed tomography (CT) arthrography of shoulder instabilities in athletes. *Am J Sports Med* 16:352–361, 1988.

80. Resnick D: Shoulder arthrography. *Radiol Clin North Am* 19:243–252, 1981.

81. Richardson JB, Ramsay A, Davidson JK, Kelly IG: Radiographs in shoulder trauma. *J Bone Joint Surg (Br)* 70-B:457–460, 1988.

82. Rokous JR, Abbott HG: Modified axillary roentgenogram. A useful adjunct in the diagnosis of recurrent instability of the shoulder. *Clin Orthop* 82–84, 1992.

83. Rowe CR, Zarins B: Recurrent transient subluxation of the shoulder. *J Bone Joint Surg (Am)* 63-A:863–872, 1981.

84. Rozing PM, De Bakker HM, Obermann WR: Radiographic views in recurrent anterior shoulder dislocation. Comparison of six methods for identification of typical lesions. *Acta Orthop Scand* 57:328–330, 1986.

85. Rubin SA, Gray RL, Green WR: The scapular "Y": A diagnostic aid in shoulder trauma. *Radiology* 110:725–726, 1974.

86. Seeger LL: Magnetic resonance imaging of the shoulder. *Clin Orthop* 244:48–59, 1989.

87. Seeger LL: MRI of the musculoskeletal system. *Orthopedics* 159(4):437–442, 1992.

88. Seeger L, Gold R, Bassett L: Shoulder instability: Evaluation with MR imaging. *Radiology* 168:695–697.

89. Seeger LL, Gold RH, Bassett LW, Ellman H: Shoulder impingement syndrome: MR findings in 53 shoulders. *AJR* 150:343–347, 1988.

90. Seeger LL, Ruszkowski JT, Bassett LW, et al: MR imaging of the normal shoulder: Anatomic correlation. *AJR* 148:83–91, 1987.

91. Sell S, Konig H: Nuclear magnetic resonance tomography and ultrasound imaging of anatomic structures of the shoulder joint. *Sportverletz-Sportschaden.* 5(2):96–98, 1991.

92. Shuman WP, Kilcoyne RF, Matsen FA, et al: Double-contrast computed tomography of the glenoid labrum. *AJR* 141:581–584, 1983.

93. Silfverskiold J, Straehley D, Jones W: Roentgenographic evaluation of suspected shoulder dislocation: A prospective study comparing the axillary view and the scapular "Y" view. *Orthopedics* 13(1):63–69, 1990.

94. Silliman JF, Hawkins RJ: Current concepts and recent advances in the athlete's shoulder. *Clin Sports Med* 10(4):693–705, 1991.

95. Soble MG, Kaye AD, Guay RC: Rotator cuff tear: Clinical experience with sonographic detection. *Radiology* 173:319–321, 1989.

96. Townley C: The capsular mechanism in recurrent dislocation of the shoulder. *J Bone Joint Surg (Am)* 32A(2):370–380, 1950.

97. Traughber PD, Goodwin TE: Shoulder MRI: Arthroscopic correlation with emphasis on partial tears. *J Comput Assist Tomogr* 16(1):129–133, 1992.

98. Turkel SJ, Panio MW, Marshall JL, Girgis FG: Stabilizing mechanisms preventing anterior dislocation of the glenohumeral joint. *J Bone Joint Surg (Am)* 63-A:1208–1217, 1981.

99. Vellet AD, Munk PL, Marks P: Imaging techniques of the shoulder: Present perspectives. *Clin Sports Med* 10(4):721–756, 1991.

100. Zlatkin MB, Dalinka MK, Kressel HY: MRI of the shoulder. *Magn Reson Q* 5:3–22, 1989.

101. Zlatkin MB: *MRI of the Shoulder.* New York, Raven Press, 1991.

CHAPTER 5

Arthroscopy—Setup, Operative Indications

Frank A. Pettrone

INTRODUCTION

Shoulder arthroscopy has evolved from a purely investigational tool to a relatively common procedure with numerous surgical treatment options, all in the past decade. Its development has been similar to that of knee arthroscopy. In its initial stage the most common uses were to confirm a diagnosis, define pathology, or plan open treatment. Today, owing to the contributions of innovative surgeons and improved technology, arthroscopic surgery is utilized as the treatment modality of choice in many conditions. New arthroscopic surgery concepts are appearing regularly.

The advantages of shoulder arthroscopy over traditional open surgery are less morbidity due to less invasive surgery, better visualization of certain intra- and extraarticular pathologic conditions, adaptability to outpatient setting, and earlier and easier rehabilitation.[38,39]

Arthroscopists familiar with the knee have relatively easily added shoulder arthroscopy to their armamentarium. As with any new procedure, however, there is a distinct learning curve for the surgeon. The desire of surgeons to perform shoulder arthroscopy will increase in direct proportion to its applicability to a greater number of pathologic conditions.

HISTORY

The first arthroscopes were derived from cystoscopes. Takagi in Japan initiated the concept of arthroscopy by inspecting a cadaveric knee.[45] In 1931, Burman first examined the shoulder arthroscopically.[9] Watanabe is credited with initiating the modern era of arthroscopy in 1950 by his introduction of the number 21 arthroscope.[54] This innovative instrument consisted of a fragile, easily breakable frame with a tungsten bulb providing questionable lighting. The 1970s saw the introduction of a more rigid arthroscope with fiber-optic lighting. The 1980s saw even better picture control developed with smaller, lighter-color cameras that were sterilizable (soakable). Other advances were hand-held suction punches, power shaver burr equipment, and arthro-

scopic pumps (to provide more controlled flow and pressure). All of these have combined to make arthroscopy a much safer and dependable procedure, and all orthopedic surgeons are capable of performing it.

Numerous authors have made contributions in expanding the role of shoulder arthroscopy. Wiley in 1980 evaluated "frozen shoulders," distended the capsule, and manipulated the joint with good results.[59,60] Heiri and Maitland,[21] as well as Conti,[11] also used arthroscopy for manipulation of frozen shoulders.[11] Watanabe presented its use for identifying osteochondral fractures and loose bodies and evaluating rheumatoid arthritis.[56] Bateman commented on its uses in rotator cuff tears, snapping shoulders, humeral subluxations, and recurrent dislocations. Johnson described its usefulness in the removal of loose bodies, resection of remnants of the biceps tendon, removal of portions of a torn rotator cuff, synovectomy and rheumatoid disease, and staple fixation for subluxating shoulders.[23] Caspari has added improvements in equipment and in technique for the treatment of recurrent dislocation.[10] Andrews and Carson have commented on labral tears and partial rotator cuff tears treated arthroscopically in the throwing athlete.[2–4]

Arthroscopy of the shoulder is more technically demanding than knee arthroscopy. Its indications, though initially limited, are clearly expanding from the advances delineated above. However, a thorough knowledge of shoulder anatomy (gross as well as arthroscopic) is essential for the arthroscopist. This topic is covered in this text and will not be repeated here.

INDICATIONS

There are no clearly defined indications for shoulder arthroscopy. Most shoulder arthroscopies were initially performed as purely diagnostic before a more definitive open procedure was performed. Many new procedures have been described, but with questionable patient selection indications and limited follow-up, these all require further study as to their efficaciousness. I discuss current indications for shoulder arthroscopy in reference to specific pathologic conditions: (1) impingement and rotator cuff tears, (2) instability, (3) glenohumeral arthritis, (4) adhesive capsulitis and calcific tendinitis, and (5) loose bodies.

Impingement

Dr. Charles Neer coined the term "impingement syndrome."[36] This frequent cause of anterior shoulder pain is due to repetitive microtrauma to the rotator cuff (primarily supraspinatus) as it glides under the arch composed of the acromion and coracoacromial ligament.[46] There, a progressively thickened subacromial bursa forms and progressive degeneration of the rotator cuff and biceps tendon occurs. Treatment is dependent upon the stage of inflammation. Stage 1 consists of bursitis and inflammation of the rotator cuff. This stage is reversible and will respond to an appropriate exercise program. Stage 2 consists of bursitis and tendinitis with partial thickness tears. Again, appropriate nonsteroidal medication, supervised exercise to rehabilitate the rotator cuff, and avoidance of further overload strain (throwing or lifting overhead) is usually successful. Stage 3 changes entail a rotator cuff tear along with the reactive inflammatory bursal changes. The arthroscope can play a helpful role in diagnosis and guide to treatment. Since one can visualize both the intraarticular and subacromial spaces and hence these sides of the rotator cuff, the presence and extent of rotator cuff tear can then be seen. The extent of subacromial bursitis and the condition of the coracoacromial arch and the acromial clavicular joint can also be documented (Plates 2 and 3).

Neer originally described an open anterior acromionectomy for impingement syndrome (for stage 2 disease, unresponsive to 6 months of conservative treatment).[36] The arthroscope can now be used to avoid this open procedure, which entails taking down the anterior deltoid muscle.[34] This arthroscopic procedure was first described by Ellman in 1985.[16–18] Gartsman et al. reported that as effective an acromioplasty can be performed arthroscopically as openly (that is, the amount of acromion removed).[19] Early results of these series are encouraging, with the advantages being that they are performed as an outpatient procedure with earlier and easier rehabilitation.[17]

Andrews has described the use of arthroscopy in throwing athletes with partial rotator cuff tears.[2–4] Favorable results were reported with limited debridement of partial rotator cuff tears. The appropriate indications in these patients should be failure to respond to a well-supervised rotator cuff rehabilitation program and both examination under anesthesia

and arthroscopic confirmation of the absence of instability. If present and functionally disabling, instability should be corrected first. In those patients who have failed conservative therapy and do not demonstrate instability, arthroscopic rotator cuff debridement and concomitant subacromial arch decompression is appropriate.

The role of arthroscopic debridement and arch decompression in patients with full-thickness rotator cuff tears is more controversial. The results of this procedure have been inconsistent. It is my feeling that if pain is a primary indication in the elderly patient, then debridement and decompression is helpful. However, if weakness is the primary complaint in a younger, more active individual, then open rotator cuff repair is preferable.

Acromioclavicular arthritis can produce an impingement syndrome as well as pain in the cross-chest abduction or overhead position. An arthroscopic Mumford procedure can be performed for this indication. This is an expansion of the basic subacromial technique with the addition of a portal directly through the acromioclavicular joint through which a shaver or burr may be introduced.

Instability

The term *instability* and its definition with respect to the shoulder has become critical in the throwing athlete. Today it is recognized that glenohumeral stability is defined by the status of the capsule, glenohumeral ligaments, labrum, rotator cuff, humeral head, and glenoid.[6,7,35,37] The arthroscope is uniquely suited to diagnosing and defining these lesions. Recent advances are expanding its role into the treatment of instability.[47–49,58] First and foremost in the evaluation of instability is a thorough examination under anesthesia. This is a frequently overlooked benefit of arthroscopy.

It is to be emphasized that arthroscopy is not mandatory in the majority of patients with instability. Adequate information can be derived from the history and examination under anesthesia. Careful notation of the degree of abduction and internal and external rotation at which excessive anterior, inferior, or posterior humeral head translation occurs is essential in understanding the extent and directions of instability. A thorough arthroscopic exam then defines the competence of the capsule and glenohumeral ligaments as well as other bony or intraarticular pathology. With these two essential components of examination the surgeon can decide upon an arthroscopic vs. an open repair for instability. There is a complex relationship between the rotator cuff and biceps tendon and the capsule-labral-ligamentous complex in the control of humeral head translation. In the throwing athlete presenting with pain it is often difficult to distinguish the contributions of instability or impingement, if not both. With repetitive force loads the failure of one structure leads to changes in the other structures of the shoulder. In evaluating a throwing athlete under 35 years of age with impingement syndrome, instability should be considered as being present until proved otherwise. Arthroscopy may prove a valuable diagnostic aid in these patients to direct treatment to either an arthroscopic or open solution to the instability problem.

Detrisac and Johnson, Fu, Snyder, Warren, and others have all contributed to our understanding of the significance of the labrum and glenohumeral ligaments.[1,5,15,20,29–31] They have also been instrumental in surgical advances in the treatment of instability. Many procedures have evolved, all of which initially scarify the anterior glenoid neck, then affix the glenohumeral ligaments and labral complex to the edge of the glenoid. Johnson initially utilized a technique of arthroscopic staple capsulorrhaphy for this step.[22] Metal types of fixation intraarticularly, however, are discouraged today.[61] A newer dissolvable type of fixation (Suretak) may prove to be a helpful solution to this problem.[1] Caspari developed a suture punch to grasp the ligament and then pass these sutures through the scapular neck to be tied posteriorly.[10] A variety of other suture paths and tying techniques are available.[20,33,57] Newer techniques have employed various types of metal or plastic "tacks" for fixation. The published results of all these techniques are encouraging but have small numbers and short follow-ups. In general, also, they have a slightly increased incidence of recurrence vs. traditional open repairs. The ideal candidate for an arthroscopic stabilization would seem to be an active athlete's dominant arm with a traumatic Bankart lesion, competent ligaments and capsule, engaged in a noncontact sport. A second ideal candidate would be a nonathletically active individual with recurrent subluxation history. The "gold standard" should still be an open surgical repair that historically has resulted in only a 3 percent recurrence rate. There are also well-recognized problems with the use of metal devices in the shoulder.[22,61] Arthroscopic stabilization procedures are technically demanding (Plates 4 and 5).[24]

The structure and function of the labrum has been of great interest recently. Initially labral tears were described as producing only mechanical symptoms without instability. More recently labral findings in association with instability have been described.[25–27] Andrews described superior labral lesions causing pain or clicking in the throwing athlete.[3]

These in general responded well to arthroscopic debridement alone. A number of variations of normal in the anterior superior labrum, particularly about the biceps tendon insertion, have also been described. Snyder has called attention to superior labral tears and instability.[52] He has classified these disruptions with the more severe grade involving the biceps tendon also. The most critical area of labral pathology involves the anterior inferior glenoid (below the 3 o'clock position). Here labral tears are clearly related to functional instability. In this situation capsuloligamentous repair should be performed, not merely labral debridement alone.

Glenohumeral Arthritis

In early osteoarthritis, arthroscopic debridement of loose bodies, spurs, synovium, and chondral lesions can be useful. In early rheumatoid arthritis, arthroscopic synovectomy has proved encouraging. In the more severe osteoarthritis, particularly with restriction of motion, arthroscopic debridement has not provided consistent good results.

Adhesive Capsulitis and Calcific Tendinitis

Arthroscopy is also useful when combined with manipulation under anesthesia in patients with adhesive capsulitis.[1,21,32,40–42] Adjunctive bony pathology is rarely found, but the ability to debride synovium provides symptomatic relief and aids the aggressive physical therapy that is essential after manipulation. Heiri and Maitland found a decreased joint volume in adhesive capsulitis that can be improved with debridement and manipulation.[21]

Calcific deposits are amenable to arthroscopic needling and debridement. Localization subacromially with a needle is indicated by a cloudlike debris. Curetting or debriding with a shaver is then useful. Results have been gratifying.

Loose Bodies

Loose bodies, particularly if they are associated with catching of the shoulder, are amenable to arthroscopic retrieval. These can be seen in osteoarthritis, chondromatosis, osteochondral fracture fragments, or instability. Particularly with instability, treatment should be directed at stabilization rather than merely loose body removal.

TECHNIQUE

Anesthesia and Setup

General anesthesia is the most frequent type of anesthesia employed. Another option preferred by some is regional anesthesia (scalene block). General anesthesia has the advantage of allowing a thorough exam under anesthesia before surgery that is essential in the evaluation of instability. Regional anesthesia requires a skilled anesthesiologist but is ideal for outpatient surgery, particularly in the beach chair position. Both setups are described below.

LATERAL DECUBITUS

Patients are intubated and turned onto their side and held with a vacuum pack or bean bag. The operative shoulder and arm are held in longitudinal traction in a position of 15° forward flexion and approximately 60° of abduction with the trunk tilted somewhat posteriorly. Approximately 15 lb of traction is applied with Buck's traction. This position is for glenohumeral arthroscopy.[45] For subacromial arthroscopy, the arm is positioned somewhat lower at about 20° abduction. An additional modification we have employed that is particularly useful for arthroscopic stabilization procedures is the use of "double traction." A second traction is applied via a sling looped under the axilla and directed vertically. The sum of vector forces of this traction and the previously applied longitudinal force is approximately 45° abduction, which provides superb glenohumeral distraction. This increased space for viewing and operating is particularly useful with the cannula size and instrumentation necessary for arthroscopic stabilization procedures (Fig. 5-1).[45]

The primary advantages of the lateral decubitus position are: most surgeons are more familiar with the arthroscopic anatomy in this position vs. thinking at 90° turned as in a beach chair position; it provides excellent distraction capabilities for instrument clearance to operate in the glenohumeral joint; and the position of anatomic structures is constant,

not as changeable as with the beach chair position.[1,23,32,45]

The primary disadvantage of the lateral decubitus position is clearly the difficulty entailed in changing from an arthroscopic to an open procedure. The repositioning and redraping necessary require extra effort and time from both staff and surgeon. There have also been reports of transient neuropraxia from prolonged maintenance of this abducted position.[1,51]

BEACH CHAIR

The upright, seated, or beach chair position has been popularized by Warren.[50] This technique provides a choice of scalene block or general anesthesia. With a regional anesthesia the patient may be positioned upright facing a monitor for viewing. Similarly, after an exam under general anesthesia the patient is positioned with the trunk elevated 70° in the seated position with the knees flexed. The head is firmly secured to a headrest. The patient is placed with the affected shoulder freely accessible over the edge of the table. The arm, while draped freely, may be either held by an assistant or rested on an arm board (Fig. 5-2).

The primary advantage of the beach chair position for those comfortable with its use is the neutral or untensioned position of all the ligaments. In addition, ligament tautness can be readily evaluated by arm motion facilitated in this position. There is also an easy changeover for conversion to open surgery. The main disadvantages are the difficulty positioning patients securely in the upright position so that they do not slide down and lose their position during surgery, and the additional adjustment to the anatomic disorientation for those not accustomed to this less common position.[1,50]

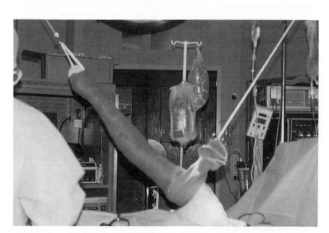

FIGURE 5-1
"Double" traction.

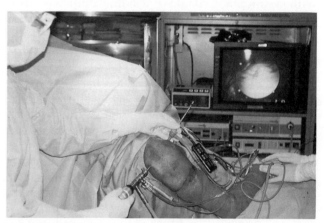

FIGURE 5-2
Beach chair position.

Portal Placement and Diagnostic Arthroscopy

The proper placement of portals for diagnostic and then operative shoulder arthroscopy is facilitated by outlining with a marking pen topographical anatomy (clavicle, acromioclavicular joint, acromion, and coracoid). The glenohumeral joint is palpated by grasping the humeral head between the thumb and index and middle finger and translating it anterior and posterior. The initial portal is made in this plane from posterior beginning two finger breadths down and two finger breadths posterior to the posterior inferior corner of the acromion. With experience one appreciates a soft spot at this posterior site. This spot corresponds to the interval between the infraspinatus and teres minor. The axillary nerve is the closest structure for potential complication but lies well inferior at the lower edge of the teres minor (Fig. 5-3).[8]

It is helpful to inject this portal site with 5 mL of 0.25% marcaine with epinephrine 1:200,000, make a stab wound, and then install 30 mL of the solution subacromially initially. Then place the spinal needle in the plane of the glenohumeral joint and push forward toward the coracoid, keeping a finger anteriorly on it for spatial orientation. A pop is felt as one enters the joint. Inject 30 mL of solution intraarticularly. Ease the arthroscopic sleeve and blunt trochar in the same path again, and similarly a pop is noted as the joint is entered. Free, easy mobility of the sheath superior and inferior indicates that correct placement has occurred, as does backflow of fluid. Next the light source is substituted for the trocar, after establishing fluid inflow through a side arm; then visualization of the joint commences.

Before making additional portals it is helpful to orient oneself anatomically and clear the joint. Using the inflow and draining sequentially, clarity of vision is established. One should then orient the joint beginning superiorly at the biceps insertion, our "north star." We follow this out the biceps group, then back down the anterior glenoid rim, identifying the subscapularis tendon. At this point we establish a second portal, for both diagnostic and operative arthroscopy. The second portal is placed anteriorly in a triangular space bounded superiorly by the biceps tendon, inferiorly by the subscapularis tendon, and medially by the glenoid rim. One can palpate lateral to the coracoid and use a spinal needle, then trocar to enter the joint in this triangular space (Plate 6). One must remain lateral and superior to the coracoid to avoid potential neurovascular complications. Matthews et al.[28] have demonstrated that the brachial plexus and axillary artery lie medial to the coracoid and the musculocutaneous nerve lies lateral and inferior to the coracoid. An alternative method is to push the arthroscope from posterior directly anteriorly into this triangular space, tenting the capsule. Then substitute a blunt rod (Wissinger) for the light source and force this forward through the capsule to the skin tenting it. A stab wound is then made and a disposable cannula with side arm for flow is introduced over the rod. Diagnostic arthroscopy can now be performed, viewing from posterior and introducing instruments from anterior.

Additional Portals

SUPERIOR

This portal was introduced as an adjunctive inflow or viewing portal. With adequate inflow through the side arm either with or without a pump, we rarely employ this portal now. The placement site is in the notch of the supraspinatus fossa between the clavi-

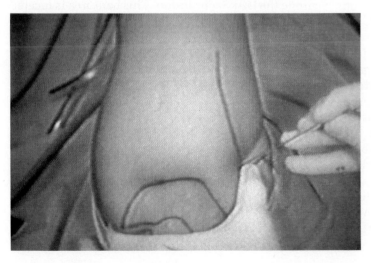

FIGURE 5-3
Posterior portal placement.

cle anteriorly, the spine of the scapula posteriorly, and the medial border of the acromion laterally. Again the spinal needle is helpful for orientation. It is directed approximately 30° lateral and slightly anterior. This enters the joint at the posterior superior corner through the supraspinatus muscle belly (a minor disadvantage).

LATERAL (SUBACROMIAL) PORTAL

This accessory portal is essential for viewing or instrumenting the subacromial space. The site is located approximately 3 cm inferior to the lateral edge of the acromion in line with the posterior border of the clavicle. As mentioned above, we have previously instilled the subacromial space with 30 mL of 0.25% marcaine with epinephrine 1:200,000 to facilitate hemostasis. When viewing from posterior this portal can be used with a probe for palpation, a shaver for debridement, instruments for resecting the coracoacromial ligament, and burrs for resecting the acromion and AC joint. The portal passes through the deltoid muscle but lies well above the axillary nerve, which passes anteriorly 5 cm below the lateral acromial border.

SUPERIOR (CLAVICULAR) PORTAL

An additional useful superior portal is located at the AC joint. With viewing established from posterior and after debriding the subacromial bursa, a spinal needle is introduced directly inferior through the AC joint. As the needle is visualized from inside, the portal is then enlarged with a stab wound, then trocar. Instruments can then be introduced, particularly for distal clavicular resections.

Equipment

A television monitor and all video equipment are best placed across the patient so that the surgeon may view it looking comfortably straight ahead. All video and pump controls are in direct vision of the surgeon. Normal saline is used for all arthroscopies even if electrocautery is to be used. Two 3-L bags of fluid each with 1 mL of epinephrine 1:1,000 added are hung to allow longer uninterrupted inflow. As a routine, additional equipment needed is a sterilizable (soakable) video camera, video control, 30° 4.5-mm arthroscope, a power suction shaver system, probe, or basic hand instruments (scissors, punches, graspers, etc.).

Optional additional equipment is a shoulder-holding traction device, a pump to deliver inflow at a pressure-controlled flow rate, video equipment for recording on either tape or still photography, spe-

cialized instruments (e.g., Caspari suture punch for arthroscopic stabilization) or equipment (e.g., Suretak), electrocautery, or more recently a laser.

Procedure

We perform diagnostic arthroscopy in a specific sequential fashion for completeness.[45] We begin superiorly at the biceps tendon at its superior glenoid insertion. This serves as our "north star," 12 o'clock, or primary orientation point. The tendon is visualized and probed, establishing its integrity at insertion as well as any flattening or fraying as we proceed laterally along the tendon. The labrum is next probed from superior both anterior and posterior to the biceps, then progressing anteriorly down the glenoid rim to the bottom or 6 o'clock position. A probe is essential here to evaluate the labrum for flaps, fraying, or frank detachment. Detrisac has documented in approximately 20 percent of individuals the presence of a labral sulcus as a normal variant.[15] This is usually in the 2 or 3 o'clock position. It is of smooth, uniform character to differentiate it from a detachment. In addition, there is a great variation in the thickness of the labrum. It is thin superiorly, becoming thicker inferiorly. In its thicker inferior portion it is triangular or wedge-shaped, appearing much like a knee meniscus. The articular cartilage of the glenoid is likewise examined. The humeral head is evaluated next with internal rotation and probing to study the anterior portion, external rotation to follow it more posteriorly, and abduction to evaluate it superiorly.

Special attention is given to the posterior superior portion of the humeral head, looking for a chondral or osteochondral defect of a Hill-Sachs compression fracture. Its presence is indicative of instability. There is also a variable "bare" area here that may mimic the Hill-Sachs lesion. This bare area is located lateral to the Hill-Sachs lesion. It is readily distinguished by its punctate-like appearance. It is said by DePalma not to be present in the young but progressively increased in size after the age of 30 (Plates 7 and 8).[12–14]

The rotator cuff is next viewed, with abduction beginning at the anterior margin of the supraspinatus, the biceps tendon, and progressively first superior then posterior along the cuff. Palpation is helpful as well as shaving away any debris. A thin layer of synovium is present here investing the supraspinatus, and fraying of this synovium should not be misdiagnosed as a frank rotator cuff tear.

The capsuloligamentous structures anteriorly are of critical importance and are viewed next. The superior glenohumeral ligament is variably seen, frequently being obscured by the biceps tendon. The subscapularis tendon, however, is invariably clearly seen and is most useful for orientation. It is a large distinct band entering the joint from lateral and is superior to the middle and inferior glenohumeral ligaments. It can be seen to clearly tighten with abduction and external rotation of the shoulder. The middle glenohumeral ligament crosses over the subscapularis tendon and is attached variably to the anterior glenoid labrum from superior to anterior on the scapular neck. It is probed and tested in external rotation (becoming tighter). The inferior glenohumeral ligament is next located. It is the most distinct and substantial of the glenohumeral ligaments and the prime stabilizer of the joint. Warren et al. have defined two discrete portions of this ligament, the thickened anterior or superior band of the inferior glenohumeral ligament (IGHL), a thickened inferior capsular pouch, and a posterior band of the IGHL.[1,5,43,53]

The posterior labrum and glenoid are lastly evaluated with a probe. If this proves difficult from posterior, a switch is made and we view from anterior and probe from posterior. This view is also helpful to view the posterior-inferior capsular area. We also employ this anterior viewing portal to clearly evaluate the anterior rim of the scapular neck and labrum when debriding this region for stabilization procedures.

Lastly, each shoulder arthroscopy is completed by viewing the subacromial space. As mentioned previously, the subacromial arthroscopy is aided by instilling 30 mL of 0.25% marcaine with epinephrine 1:200,000 to control bleeding. The arthroscope and sheath in the posterior portal are redirected more superiorly underneath the acromion. The lateral portal has been established previously and a shaver is inserted. The anterior portal is also repositioned either bluntly from anterior or from posterior inside out and recannulating over a rod. It should come to lie just under the coracoacromial ligament. Frequently a shaver must be employed to clear the subacromial bursa that obscures the field initially. This being done and the probe inserted laterally, we evaluate the rotator cuff for bursal site tears or calcific deposits. The coracoacromial ligament is then probed, looking for thickening or proliferation about it. Next the acromion is viewed and studied to ascertain if there is spurring or a hooklike (Bigliani type 3) process implicated in impingement syndromes. Lastly, the AC joint, particularly the inferior tip of the distal clavicle, is viewed again, inspecting for spurs or osteophytes that contribute to impingement syndromes.

CONCLUSION

Shoulder arthroscopy has made significant strides in the last 10 years. Its usefulness to orthopedic surgeons has dramatically increased. In spite of previous familiarity from knee arthroscopy, however, a definite learning curve is involved with shoulder arthroscopy. Utilizing appropriate indications for surgery with an awareness of arthroscopic anatomy, shoulder arthroscopy will become an integral part of the orthopedic surgeon's armamentarium.

REFERENCES

1. Altchek D, Warren R, Skyhar M: Shoulder arthroscopy, in Rockwood CA Jr, Matsen FA (eds): *The Shoulder*. Philadelphia, Saunders, 1990.
2. Andrews JR, Carson WG: The arthroscopic treatment of glenoid labrum tears in the throwing athlete. *Orthop Trans* 8(1):44, 1984.
3. Andrews JR, Carson WG, McLeod WD: Glenoid labrum tears related to the long head of the biceps. *Am J Sports Med* 13(5):337–341, 1984.
4. Andrews JR, Carson WG, Ortega U: Arthroscopy of the shoulder: Technique and normal anatomy. *Sports Med* 12(1):1–7, 1984.
5. Bach BR, Warren RF, Fronek J: Disruption of the lateral capsule of the shoulder. A cause of recurrent dislocation. *J Bone Joint Surg (Am)* 70B(2):274–276, 1988.
6. Bankart ASB: The pathology and treatment of recurrent dislocation of the shoulder. *Br J Surg* 26:23–29, 1938.
7. Blazina E, Saltzman JS: Recurrent anterior subluxation of the shoulder in athletes: A distinct entity. *J Bone Joint Surg (Am)* 51A:1037–1038, 1969.
8. Bryan WJ, Schauder K, Tullos H: The axillary nerve and its relationship to common sports medicine shoulder procedures. *Am J Sports Med* 14:113, 1986.
9. Burman MS: Arthroscopy on the direct visualization of joints: An experimental cadaver study. *J Bone Joint Surg (Am)* 8:669, 1931.

10. Caspari RB: Arthroscopic evaluation and reconstruction for shoulder instability. Unpublished data presented to Arthroscopy Association of North America, February 7, 1988, Atlanta, GA.

11. Conti V: Arthroscopy in rehabilitation. *Orthop Clin North Am* 10(3):709, 1979.

12. DePalma AF: Degenerative lesions of the shoulder joint at various age groups which are compatible with good function. *Instr Course Lect* 7:168–180, 1950.

13. DePalma AF: *Surgery of the Shoulder.* Philadelphia, Lippincott, 1973.

14. DePalma AF, Callery G, Bennett GA: Variational anatomy and degenerative lesions of the shoulder joint. *Instr Course Lect* 6:255–280, 1949.

15. Detrisac DA, Johnson LL: *Arthroscopic Shoulder Anatomy. Pathologic and Surgical Implication.* Thorofare, NJ, Slack, 1986.

16. Ellman H: Arthroscopic subacromial decompression: Analysis of one to three year results. *Arthroscopy* 3:173, 1987.

17. Ellman H: Arthroscopic subacromial decompression: 1–3 year follow-up study. *Instr Course Lect*, February 1988.

18. Ellman H: Shoulder arthroscopy: Current indications and techniques. *Orthopaedics* 11:45, 1988.

19. Gartsman GM, Blair ME, Noble MS, et al: Arthroscopic subacromial decompression. An anatomical study. *Am J Sports Med* 16(1):48–50, 1988.

20. Goldberg B, Nirschl R, Pettrone FA: Arthroscopic Transglenoid Suture Capsulolabral Repairs. AOSSM Meeting, Orlando, FL, July 1991.

21. Heiri GB, Maitland A: Arthroscopic findings in the frozen shoulder. *J Rheumatol* 8:149–152, 1981.

22. Johnson LL: Arthroscopic staple capsulorrhaphy. A preliminary report. Unpublished data presented at the American Shoulder and Elbow Surgeons Meeting, Atlanta, GA, February 7, 1988.

23. Johnson LL: The shoulder joint: An arthroscopist's perspective of anatomy and pathology. *Clin Orthop* 223:113–125, 1987.

24. Klein AH, France JC, Mutschler TA, Fu FH: Measurement of brachial plexus strain in arthroscopy of the shoulder. *Arthroscopy* 3(1):45–52, 1987.

25. Kohn D: The clinical relevance of glenoid labrum lesions. *Arthroscopy* 3(4):223–230, 1987.

26. Kummel BM: Arthrography in anterior capsular derangements of the shoulder. *Clin Orthop* 83:170–176, 1982.

27. Kummel BM: Spectrum of lesions of the anterior capsular mechanism of the shoulder. *Am J Sports Med* 7:111, 1979.

28. Matthews LS, Zarins B, Michael RH, Helfet DL: Anterior portal selection for shoulder arthroscopy. *Arthroscopy* 1(1):33–39, 1985.

29. McGlynn FJ, Caspari RB: Arthroscopic findings in the subluxating shoulder. *Clin Orthop* 183:173–178, 1984.

30. McGlynn FJ, El-Khoury G, Albright JP: Arthrotomography of the glenoid labrum in shoulder instability. *J Bone Joint Surg (Am)* 64A:506, 1982.

31. Mendoza FX, Nicholas JA, Reilly J: Anatomic patterns of anterior glenoid labrum tears. *Orthop Trans* 11:246, 1987.

32. Mendoza FX, Noskwa CA: Shoulder arthroscopy in the upper extremity. *Am J Sports Med* 18:159–168, 1990.

33. Morgan CD, Bodenstab AB: Arthroscopic Bankart suture repair: Technique and early results. *Arthroscopy* 3(2):111–122, 1987.

34. Morrison DS: Correlation of acromial morphology and the results of arthroscopic subacromial decompression. *Orthop Trans* 12:731, 1988.

35. Moseley HF, Overgaard B: The anterior capsular mechanism in recurrent anterior dislocation of the shoulder. *J Bone Joint Surg (Am)* 44B(4):913–927, 1962.

36. Neer CS: Anterior acromioplasty for chronic impingement syndrome in the shoulder. *J Bone Joint Surg (Am)* 54A(1):41–50, 1972.

37. Neer CS, Foster CR: Inferior capsular shift for involuntary inferior and multidirectional instability of the shoulder. *J Bone Joint Surg (Am)* 62A(6):897–908, 1980.

38. Nelson M, Leather G, Nirschl R, Pettrone FA: Evaluation of the painful shoulder. *J Bone Joint Surg (Am)* 73A(5):707, June 1991.

39. Neviaser TJ: Arthroscopy of the shoulder. *Orthop Clin North Am* 18(5):361–386, 1987.

40. Neviaser JS: Adhesive capsulitis of the shoulder: Study of pathological findings in periarthritis of the shoulder. *J Bone Joint Surg (Am)* 17A:219, 1945.

41. Neviaser RJ, Neviaser TH: The frozen shoulder: Diagnosis and management. *Clin Orthop* 223:59–64, 1987.

42. Olgilvie-Harris DJ, Wiley AM: Arthroscopic surgery of the shoulder: A general appraisal. *J Bone Joint Surg (Am)* 68B(2):201–207, 1986.

43. Pappas AM, Goss TP, Kleinman PK: Symptomatic shoulder instability due to lesions of the glenoid labrum. *Am J Sports Med* 11(5):279–288, 1983.

44. Paulos L: Arthroscopic subacromial decompression: Technique and preliminary results. Unpublished data presented to Arthroscopy Association of North America, April 1985.

45. Pettrone FA: *Shoulder Arthroscopy, AAOS Symposium—Upper Extremity Injuries in Athletes.* St Louis, Mosby, 1986, p 300.

46. Rathbun JB, Macnab I: The microvascular pattern of the rotator cuff. *J Bone Joint Surg (Am)* 52B(3):540–553, 1970.

47. Rowe CR, Patel D, Southmayd WM: The Bankart procedure. *J Bone Joint Surg (Am)* 60A(1):1–16, 1978.

48. Rowe CR, Zarins B: Recurrent transient subluxation of the shoulder. *J Bone Joint Surg (Am)* 63A(6):863–872, 1981.

49. Schwartz R, O'Brien SJ, Warren RF: Posterior stability of the shoulder. Presented to the American Shoulder and Elbow Surgeons Meeting, Atlanta, GA, February 7, 1988.

50. Skyhar MJ, Altcheck DW, Warren RF: Shoulder arthroscopy in the seated position. *Orthop Rev* 10:1033, 1988.

51. Small NC: Complications in arthroscopy: The knee and other joints. *Arthroscopy* 2:253, 1986.

52. Snyder S, Karzel R, DelPizzo W, et al: *Slap Lesions of the Shoulder, Arthroscopy.* New York, Raven Press, 1990, vol 1, p 274.

53. Turkel SJ, Panio MN, Marshall JL, Girgis FG: Stabilizing mechanisms preventing anterior dislocation of the glenohumeral joint. *J Bone Joint Surg (Am)* 63A(8):12108–12117, 1986.

54. Uthoff HU: Anterior capsular redundancy of the shoulder: Congenital or traumatic. *J Bone Joint Surg (Am)* 67B:363–366, 1985.

55. Watanabe M, Takeda S, Ikeuchi H: *Atlas of Arthroscopy,* 3d ed. New York, Igaku-Shoin, 1978.

56. Watanabe M: Arthroscopy: The present state. *Orthop Clin North Am* 10:505–522, 1979.

57. Watanabe M: The development and present status of the arthroscope. *J Jpn Med Inst* 25:11, 1954.

58. Warren RF: Subluxation of the shoulder in athletes. *Clin Sports Med* 2(2):339–354, 1983.

59. Wiley AM: Arthroscopy for shoulder instability and a technique for arthroscopic repair. *Arthroscopy* 4(1):25–30, 1988.

60. Wiley AM, Older MB: Shoulder arthroscopy: Investigation with a fiberoptic instrument. *Am J Sports Med* 8:18–31, 1980.

61. Zuckerman JD, Matsen FA III: Complications about the glenohumeral joint related to the use of screws and staples. *J Bone Joint Surg (Am)* 66A(2):175–180, 1984.

CHAPTER 6

Shoulder Instability—Overview with Surgical Indications and Treatment Options

Michael J. Pagnani
David W. Altchek

INTRODUCTION

The remarkable range of motion of the shoulder is permitted by a relative lack of bony constraint. The surrounding glenohumeral soft tissues are, as a result, the primary determinants of shoulder stability. In the athletic population, the shoulder is subjected to enormous loads that, not uncommonly, result in soft tissue injury and instability. Recent advancements in our understanding of the pathoanatomy of the unstable shoulder are helpful in the development of a scientific approach to the restoration of function in the athlete with shoulder instability.

ANATOMY AND BIOMECHANICS OF SHOULDER INSTABILITY

Only a small portion of the relatively large humeral head contacts the glenoid fossa in any shoulder position[12,49] and the bony architecture of the shoulder contributes little to stability. The surrounding soft tissue envelope is therefore the primary contributor to the stability of the normal glenohumeral joint. Normally, translation of the head on the glenoid is confined to only a few millimeters.[14,28,32,51,52,73]

The soft tissues surrounding the shoulder interact in a complex system that stabilizes the joint. Pathology that interferes with this intricate system leads to instability. The capsule contains discrete thickenings or capsular ligaments that are important in understanding the pathomechanics of shoulder instability. The ligaments come under tension when the joint is placed at the extremes of motion, and they protect against instability when all other mechanisms have been overwhelmed.[40] Three anterior glenohumeral ligaments have been described: the superior glenohumeral ligament (SGHL), the middle glenohumeral ligament (MGHL), and the inferior glenohumeral ligament complex (IGHLC)[62] (Fig. 6-1). The SGHL originates from the anterosuperior labrum

anteriorly to the biceps tendon and inserts superior to the lesser tuberosity near the bicipital groove. The MGHL arises adjacent to the SGHL and extends medially to attach on the lesser tuberosity in intimate association with the subscapularis tendon. The IGHLC extends from the anteroinferior labrum to insert just inferior to the MGHL. The IGHLC is actually composed of three functionally disparate parts: an anterior band, a posterior band, and an interposed axillary pouch.[48] DePalma[21] noted several variations in the composition of the glenohumeral ligaments. The MGHL is the most variable structure; it may be robust in some cases and completely absent in others.

The role of the anterior glenohumeral ligaments in preventing instability is complex and varies with shoulder position and with the direction of the translating force. Ligament cutting studies at our institution have helped to elucidate the complex function of the capsular ligaments.[20,73] It appears that the IGHLC is the primary static restraint against anterior, posterior, and inferior translation when the arm is abducted between 45 and 90° (Fig. 6-2). In the midrange of abduction, the MGHL and subscapularis assist the IGHLC in resisting anterior translation while the teres minor and infraspinatus help prevent posterior translation. With the arm adducted, the SGHL and the MGHL stabilize against anterior movement, the posterior capsule and the SGHL resist posterior motion, and the SGHL and IGHLC are the primary restraints against inferior translation.

Injury to the capsular ligaments can occur in one of three forms: ligament detachment, ligament stretch, or ligament stretch with concomitant detachment. Detachment lesions are generally observed after a discrete traumatic event. In contrast repetitive microtrauma rarely results in capsular detachment. Bigliani et al.[10] recently investigated the response of the IGHLC to tensile loading using bone-ligament-bone cadaveric specimens. They found that the IGHLC demonstrated considerable plastic deformation prior to failure. These data support the concept

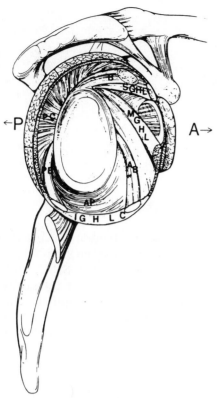

FIGURE 6-1
Capsuloligamentous anatomy of the glenohumeral joint. B = biceps tendon, SGHL = superior glenohumeral ligament, MGHL = middle glenohumeral ligament, AB = anterior band of inferior glenohumeral ligament complex, AP = axillary pouch of inferior glenohumeral ligament complex, PB = posterior band of inferior glenohumeral ligament complex, IGHLC = inferior glenohumeral ligament complex, PC = posterior capsule, A = anterior, P = posterior. (From O'Brien et al: The anatomy and histology of the inferior glenohumeral ligament complex of the shoulder. Am J Sports Med 18:449, 1990.)

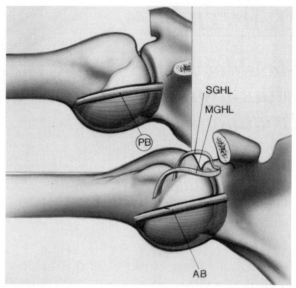

FIGURE 6-2
Illustration of the capsular ligaments with the humerus in 90° of abduction and neutral rotation. The bottom illustration depicts the glenohumeral joint from the anterior aspect. The top illustration is a mirrored view showing the posterior aspect of the joint. In this position, the inferior glenohumeral ligament complex is the primary static restraint against anterior, posterior, and inferior translation. Note that the anterior and posterior bands are taut in this position. PB = posterior band of inferior glenohumeral ligament complex, AB = anterior band of glenohumeral ligament complex, SGHL = superior glenohumeral ligament, MGHL = middle glenohumeral ligament. [From Bowen MK, Warren RF: Ligamentous control of shoulder stability based on selective cutting and static translation experiments. Clin Sports Med 10(4):757, 1991.]

that gradual stretching of the capsule can occur with repetitive microtrauma, which is a common etiologic factor in anterior subluxation.

While failure occurred most commonly at the glenoid insertion it was not uncommonly observed at the humeral insertion or in the midsubstance of the ligament. The authors pointed out that, even in cases where there was failure at the glenoid insertion, such failure occurred only after significant elongation of the IGHLC.

The importance of the anterior capsular stripping in relation to the labrum and the bony glenoid was stressed in the English literature by Bankart, beginning in 1923.[7-9] The term "Bankart lesion" has evolved to refer to capsular-periosteal separation at the glenoid neck.

It has been found that simulation of the Bankart lesion by detachment of the anterior half of the IGHLC from the glenoid results in only minimal increases in anterior translation.[66] It was therefore postulated that additional plastic deformation of the

IGHLC (and/or other portions of the capsule) is usually necessary to permit anterior dislocation.

Warren has formulated the "circle concept" of shoulder instability which states that abnormal glenohumeral translation in one direction requires capsular damage on both the same side and on the opposite side of the joint.[74] Both Blasier et al.[11] and Terry et al.,[69] in strain gauge analyses, have supported the circle concept in that both anterior and posterior capsular strain were noted to occur with anterior translation of the humeral head upon the glenoid.

The labrum is a fibrous structure that is attached to the glenoid rim.[19,45] Mobility of the labrum above the transverse equator of the glenoid is normal and not pathologic; in contrast, inferior mobility is abnormal. The long head of the biceps tendon inserts in association with the superior labrum, and the inferior glenohumeral ligament is adherent to the inferior labrum. It has[45,60] been shown that labral detachment by itself is insufficient to cause anterior dislocation unless accompanied by disruption of the anterior capsule. However, the labrum does have some role in anterior glenohumeral stability; the average anteroposterior depth of the glenoid fossa is doubled, from 2.5 to 5 mm, by the presence of the labrum,[33] and the labrum may serve as a "chock block" in controlling glenohumeral translation. Vanderhooft et al.[71] recently found that resection of the labrum reduced resistance to anterior translation by 20 percent. The presence of the labrum increases the articular surface area of the glenoid.[64] In addition, anteroinferior labral detachment is usually associated with some degree of capsular disruption from the glenoid neck. This capsular-periosteal separation creates laxity in an important stabilizer, the inferior glenohumeral ligament, which is intimately connected to the labrum.[43]

The term "rotator interval" has been used to describe the space between the superior border of the subscapularis and the anterior margin of the supraspinatus tendons over the anterior capsule.[48] The SGHL and the coracohumeral ligament are located in this region of the capsule. An enlarged rotator interval may be associated with increases in anterior, posterior, or inferior translation.[48,59] The size of the rotator interval should be assessed during operative repair; usually the interval is closed during the repair.

Some authors have implicated abnormalities in glenoid version or humeral torsion in the etiology of shoulder instability. However, Galinat et al.[25] found no association between glenoid version and anterior or posterior instability. Theories that attribute instability to abnormal humeral torsion also remain questionable.[39]

Bony defects of the humeral head or glenoid may be associated with glenohumeral instability (Fig. 6-3). The lesions represent impaction fractures that occur as the head moves over the glenoid rim. They are the effect, rather than the cause, of instability. Townley, in cadaveric experiments, showed that the Hill-Sachs lesion did not result in anterior dislocation unless it was accompanied by capsular disruption.[70] While these bony deficiencies alter the normal mechanics of the joint, we have found that stability can usually be achieved by the correction of associated soft tissue pathology without additional measures designed to compensate for the bone loss.

The rotator cuff tendons and the tendon of the long head of the biceps probably have an important role in controlling glenohumeral translation. Passive musculotendinous tension within the rotator cuff appears to have some static role in preventing translation.[34,68] As Rowe has pointed out, however, significant lesions of the subscapularis are uncommon surgical findings.[58] Instead, the primary mechanism by which these muscles affect glenohumeral stability appears to be a dynamic one, and is associated with a coordinated system of selective muscular contraction.

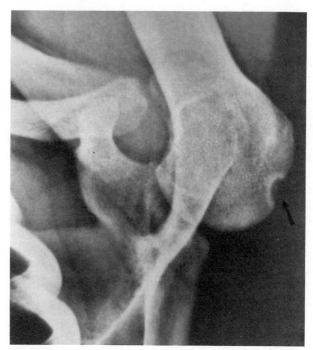

FIGURE 6-3
Stryker notch view demonstrating a Hill-Sachs lesion (arrow) in a patient with anterior instability.

The muscles of the rotator cuff adjust tension in the capsuloligamentous system by a selective process of contraction. Importantly, contraction of the rotator cuff and biceps muscles compresses the humeral head into the glenoid and increases the load needed to translate the head.[16] It has been estimated that the joint compressive load required to balance the abducted unloaded arm would be approximately 90 percent of body weight, or 680 N in a 70-kg person.[13] Bowen et al. have noted that joint compression in excess of 22 N significantly limits inferior translation of the humeral head.[13] Joint compression continued to stabilize the joint after venting of the capsule and sectioning of three-fourths of the joint capsule.

Blasier et al.,[11] in a biomechanical study in which rotator cuff tension was simulated, concluded that cuff contraction had an important stabilizing effect on the joint, but that the contributions of the individual components of the cuff did not differ from one another. If tension on any one of the components of the cuff were omitted, there was a substantial reduction in anterior joint stability compared with the case when tension was applied to all components. The degree of instability was independent of which portion of the cuff was not tensioned.

McKernan et al.[42] and Cain,[16] in cadaveric experiments, showed that simulated maximal contraction of the posterior rotator cuff muscles reduced anterior ligamentous strain. The rotator cuff may function as a secondary stabilizer in cases of capsuloligamentous deficiency. In a related study, McKernan et al.[41] have proposed that the ability of the cuff muscles to act as secondary stabilizers may be unable to completely counteract the degree of capsuloligamentous damage that is seen with the classic Bankart lesion. The stabilizing effect of a particular muscle is dependent on the position of the shoulder; a change in position may render a secondary stabilizer nonfunctional.

The role of the rotator cuff appears to be of increased importance in patients with atraumatic or microtraumatic subluxation.[15,24] In these patients, an intensive rehabilitation program designed to strengthen the rotator cuff may be effective in permitting an effective return to activities.

CLASSIFICATION OF SHOULDER INSTABILITY

Shoulder instability may be classified on the basis of frequency, chronology, direction, degree, etiology, and the presence or absence of voluntary control. The condition may be described as acute, recurrent, or chronic (i.e., fixed or locked). The instability may occur anteriorly, posteriorly, or inferiorly, or it may be multidirectional. The articular surfaces may become completely separated (dislocation), or symptoms may occur owing to abnormal translation without complete separation (subluxation).

An inciting traumatic event is less common in patients with posterior or multidirectional instability when compared with anterior dislocation. On the other hand, a microtraumatic etiology associated with repetitive use is common in anterior subluxation as well as in the posterior and multidirectional groups, especially in throwers and swimmers. Some patients are unable to relate the onset of their symptoms to either trauma or repetitive use; this atraumatic subgroup is more commonly of the multidirectional type.

Finally, the ability of the patient to voluntarily display instability should be determined. A certain number of these patients are psychologically disturbed. While classic teaching has been to avoid operation in all patients with voluntary instability,[57] there is recent evidence that there is a subgroup of patients who can voluntarily demonstrate their instability but who do not have underlying psychiatric disease. Generally, these patients have more of a positional type of posterior instability.[24]

PATIENT HISTORY

A careful history and physical examination remain the cornerstone of diagnosis in shoulder instability.

Acute and Recurrent Anterior Dislocation

Anterior instability of the glenohumeral joint is the most common type of shoulder instability. The diagnosis of acute or recurrent anterior dislocation is usually straightforward. Indirect forces that place the shoulder in a position of extreme external rotation are the most common cause of anterior dislocation.

Recurrent Anterior Subluxation

The diagnosis of recurrent anterior subluxation is often more difficult than that of recurrent anterior dislocation. The patient with recurrent subluxation is often unaware that the shoulder has "popped out." The chief complaint may be subtle, such as a sense of movement, pain, or clicking with certain activities. The pain is often poorly localized. Pain in the posterior aspect of the shoulder may occur because of traction on the posterior capsule and tendons in resisting anterior translation. In other patients, the pain may be anterior. Rowe et al.[59] have described the "dead-arm syndrome" in patients with anterior subluxation. In this situation, the patient experiences sharp pain when the arm is used in a position of abduction and external rotation. The patient may then lose control of the extremity and may drop any object that is held in the hand. After the acute episode, the severe pain usually subsides quickly, but the shoulder may remain sore and weak. In throwers, pain is often associated with the cocking or acceleration phases, but it may occasionally occur during follow-through. Swimmers commonly experience pain with the backstroke or during turns. Overhead serves and volleys are particularly likely to incite symptoms during racket sports. Volleyball and water polo are also commonly associated with recurrent anterior subluxation.

PHYSICAL EXAMINATION OF THE UNSTABLE SHOULDER

Examination of the glenohumeral joint is generally performed in two parts. The patient is initially in a standing position and later is examined in a supine position.

Cervical radiculopathy may cause shoulder pain and the cervical spine examination and neurovascular assessment should always be part of the routine. The shoulder region is inspected for deformity, asymmetry, and atrophy. Passive and active ranges of motion are measured, and the shoulder is checked for impingement. Ligamentous laxity is commonly associated with shoulder instability. Laxity may be assessed in a variety of ways. Index metacarpophalangeal extension in excess of 90°, elbow hyperextension, and knee hyperextension are indicators of generalized laxity. The degree of thumb hyperabduction with the wrist volar flexed can be noted by the distance between the thumb and volar forearm. If the thumb reaches the forearm, the test is considered positive.

The anterior apprehension test is performed by passively abducting the arm to 90° and then progressively increasing the degree of external rotation. Pain or discomfort is consistent with anterior instability.

Grading of the sulcus sign (Fig. 6-4) is based on the distance between the inferior margin of the lateral acromion and the humeral head when a downward traction force is applied to the adducted arm. Less than 1 cm of distance represents a 1+ sulcus, 1 to 2 cm indicates a 2+ sulcus, and more than 2 cm is a 3+.[2] An abnormal sulcus sign primarily reflects laxity of the superior capsular ligaments and is indicative of inferior instability. An extremely large

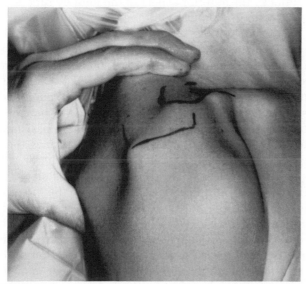

FIGURE 6-4
The sulcus sign. An extremely large sulcus is indicative of multidirectional instability. [*From Altchek et al: T-plasty modification of the Bankart procedure for multidirectional instability of anterior and inferior types. J Bone Joint Surg (Am) 73A:105, 1991.*]

sulcus is pathognomonic of multidirectional instability. Assessment of inferior translation with the arm abducted more than 45° may, however, more accurately reflect tension on the inferior capsule.[13,73]

The patient is then placed supine. The patient's shoulder is moved to the edge of the examination table. The humerus is elevated into the plane of the scapula. One of the examiner's hands is used to load to the humeral shaft while the opposite hand is placed on the elbow and used to compress the joint and to maintain neutral rotation. The examiner senses the degree of translation, the presence of crepitation, and whether or not distinct subluxation can be produced. The extremity is tested in both glenohumeral abduction and adduction in an attempt to selectively stress specific portions of the capsule. Translation is graded as 1+ if there is increased translation compared with the opposite shoulder. If the head can be subluxated over the glenoid rim but then spontaneously reduces, translation is graded as 2+. Complete dislocation without spontaneous reduction constitutes 3+ translation.[2] The opposite shoulder should be tested for comparison.

The posterior stress test is performed with the arm internally rotated and forward flexed to 90°. Pain or a "click" may be noted as the humerus is loaded in an anteroposterior direction and progressively adducted across the chest. If the arm is brought out of adduction, reduction of a subluxated shoulder may be distinctly palpated.

The relocation test[35] is helpful in evaluating anterior instability. The examiner's hand is placed over the anterior shoulder of the supine patient. A posteriorly directed force is applied with the hand in order to prevent anterior translation of the head. The shoulder is then abducted and externally rotated in a manner similar to the anterior apprehension test. A positive relocation test is obtained when this anterior pressure allows increased external rotation and diminishes associated pain and apprehension. The relocation test may not be specific for anterior instability.[65]

The findings on physical examination of a shoulder with recurrent anterior subluxation are often quite subtle. Tenderness may be noted over the posterior shoulder. The anterior apprehension test usually causes pain to a greater degree than it causes apprehension. This pain is usually relieved upon performance of the relocation test. Rotator cuff impingement symptoms frequently accompany anterior subluxation, particularly in throwers and overhead athletes.[36] In these patients, the examiner must try to use the physical examination to reproduce the patient's symptoms. If symptoms are more pronounced with maneuvers that stress the rotator cuff, diagnosis is weighted toward cuff pathology. If, on the other hand, translation manuevers more closely reproduce symptomatology, the diagnosis leans toward instability.

RADIOGRAPHY

Routine radiographic examination of the acutely injured shoulder includes anteroposterior (AP), transscapular (Y) lateral, and axillary views. Additional projections may reveal subtle signs of bony injury associated with instability. The West Point view[54] often reveals the presence of a fracture or ectopic bone production at the anterior glenoid rim that may not be visualized in other projections. The Stryker notch view[27] is especially helpful in demonstrating the Hill-Sachs lesion (Fig. 6-5).

The "apical oblique projection" described by Garth et al.[26] may be helpful in detecting Hill-Sachs and glenoid fractures, especially if the shoulder is acutely injured, since positioning for the West Point or Stryker notch views may be painful in these patients. This is essentially a true AP view (in the plane of the joint) modified by aiming the roentgenographic beam from above downward.

An arthrogram may be considered after dislocation in patients older than 45, especially if the patient seems to be slow to recover after dislocation. Computer tomography (with or without arthrogra-

phy) is also helpful in selected cases. Finally, magnetic resonance imaging (MRI) is emerging as a potentially helpful tool in the evaluation of labral and capsular lesions. We have found that MRI is particularly valuable in those patients with both rotator cuff signs and instability. MRI has proved to be highly accurate in staging the cuff pathology and is improving with regard to lesions of the glenoid labrum.

ACUTE ANTERIOR DISLOCATION

Anterior dislocation of the glenohumeral joint is the most common type of shoulder instability. After the diagnosis has been made, the shoulder should be reduced as quickly and as gently as possible. If such an injury is witnessed in a young athlete on the playing field, an immediate reduction maneuver may be performed with the arm in slight abduction, forward flexion, and gentle internal rotation.

If this maneuver is unsuccessful, the patient should be taken to the locker room and the reduction method described by Stimson[67] attempted. The patient is placed prone with the arm hanging free, and 5 lb (or more) of weight are attached to the upper extremity. With muscular relaxation the humeral head may spontaneously reduce. If the head fails to reduce spontaneously, a scapular rotation maneuver[5,47] is attempted. The scapula is manipulated to "unlock" the anterior aspect of the joint by functionally increasing the amount of glenoid anteversion.

If the shoulder remains unreduced after an attempt at scapular rotation, the patient is generally transported and radiographs are obtained. If there are no associated fractures, a modified Kocher maneuver may be employed.[38] The patient is positioned supine, and one sheet is tied around the patient's chest and axilla. This sheet is held by an assistant to provide countertraction. A second sheet is then wrapped around the caretaker's waist as he or she stands in the axillary region. The patient's elbow is flexed to 90°, and the sheet is applied to the forearm just distal to the antecubital fossa. Traction is then applied by the backward lean of the physician with the arm held in slight abduction. The arm is then gently moved in external and internal rotation until the shoulder reduces. The modified Kocher maneuver carries a risk of iatrogenic damage to bony and neurovascular structures.

In older or debilitated patients, radiographs should be obtained prior to attempts at relocation in order to rule out concomitant fracture. Radiographs of the injured shoulder should always be obtained

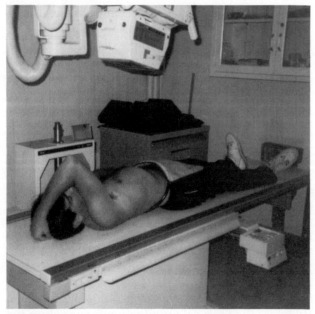

FIGURE 6-5
Patient positioning for the Stryker notch view.

after reduction. Greater tuberosity fractures occur in approximately 15 percent of anterior shoulder dislocations.[55]

A neurovascular examination should be performed before and after reduction. The axillary nerve is the most frequently damaged neurologic structure after an anterior dislocation.

Several factors may influence the rate of recurrence after an anterior dislocation. The age of the patient at the time of initial dislocation has been shown to have a major effect on the incidence of recurrence. Rowe and Sakellarides[56] noted a 94 percent recurrence rate in those patients under 20 years of age at primary dislocation but found that only 14 percent of those patients over 40 years of age had a recurrence. In addition, Rowe[55] noted increased recurrence in those patients who sustained an atraumatic dislocation when compared with traumatic dislocators. Simonet and Cofield noted that athletes tended to recur more commonly than nonathletes.[63] Concomitant greater tuberosity fractures greatly reduce the risk of recurrence.[31,55]

The effect of immobilization and rehabilitation on recurrence rates is also somewhat controversial. Rowe[55] noted a trend toward decreased recurrence in patients immobilized for 3 weeks, but no further decrease in patients immobilized for 6 weeks. Simonet and Cofield[63] reported that immobilization had no effect on recurrence, but they found that restricting sports or full activity for 6 weeks did reduce recurrence. Wheeler et al.[75] felt that rehabilitation had no effect on recurrence in army cadets after a primary dislocation.

We generally immobilize young patients who suffer a traumatic anterior dislocation for 4 to 6 weeks. The available basic science data[17] suggest that, for optimal capsular healing to occur, immobilization of this duration is required. This period is followed by a rehabilitative regimen that employs rotator cuff and scapular rotator strengthening. External rotator strengthening receives particular emphasis. Positions of extreme abduction and external rotation are avoided for 3 months after removal of the sling. A full range of motion, complete return of strength, and the absence of pain are prerequisites to the return to sports and overhead activities. When the patient returns to athletic activities, a harness that limits abduction may provide additional security against recurrent damage.

In older patients, especially those over than 40 years of age, immobilization is continued only until pain subsides. Seven to 10 days in a sling are usually required. Because of the diminished risk of recurrence and the difficulty in regaining motion in this age group, the rehabilitation program is started earlier.

If progress with therapy seems slow, an arthrogram (or MRI) should be obtained to rule out a rotator cuff pathology, particularly in the older age group. Evidence of deltoid weakness suggests the need for electromyographic studies to evaluate the axillary nerve.

Open reduction of acute anterior shoulder dislocations is necessary in those rare cases that are irreducible by closed methods and in dislocations that are more than 3 weeks old at the time of presentation. Displaced fractures of the greater tuberosity and large fractures of the glenoid rim may also require surgical treatment in the acute setting.

The role of operative stabilization of acute dislocations in young scholastic athletes is controversial. These patients appear to be at extremely high risk for recurrence. The acute dislocation often curtails sports activity for the current year, and the development of recurrent instability results in an extended period away from athletics and other activities. For some patients, this long absence from their sport may be extremely undesirable. Wheeler et al.[75] reported a dramatic decrease in the recurrence rate in army cadets after arthroscopic staple capsulorrhaphy or after simple arthroscopic debridement of the labrum and capsular insertion site. The treatment of these patients should be individualized on a case-by-case basis. The risk of recurrence should be explained as well as the potential risks of a surgical procedure. In some young athletes engaged in throwing or contact sports, early restoration of the disrupted anatomy would appear to provide the best opportunity to continue in their sport without losing a significant period of the following season.

RECURRENT ANTERIOR INSTABILITY

Patients who develop recurrence should have a complete radiographic evaluation for evidence of bony pathology.

The treatment of recurrent anterior instability begins with a period of rest. After an acute event, an arm sling is worn for a few days for comfort. Nonsteroidal anti-inflammatory medication is administered during this time. Prolonged immobilization after the second dislocation is of no apparent value. A rehabilitation program that emphasizes rotator cuff and periscapular muscle strengthening is then employed.

The indications for surgical treatment of recurrent anterior shoulder instability are highly subjective and include recurrence, pain, or activity limitation. Patients with atraumatic or microtraumatic forms of instability, particularly those with subluxation, may respond to a rotator cuff and periscapular strengthening program. Such a program should continue for 3 to 6 months prior to consideration for operation. Those patients with traumatic instability have a poorer prognosis with rehabilitation. In this population, operative treatment may be considered if symptoms interfere with activity. Patients with voluntary anterior instability are often poor operative candidates and require psychologic testing and a rigorous attempt at rehabilitation.[57]

The goals of operative treatment for shoulder instability are to stabilize the shoulder and to restore pain-free motion. In general, the surgeon should have a clinical sense of the direction and degree of instability from the office evaluation, and this impression should be confirmed by the examination under anesthesia (EUA). The surgeon should expect to note increased translation when the EUA is compared with the office examination. A finding of posterior subluxation that accompanies anterior instability is not unusual and does not alter the surgical approach. On occasion, the findings may be equivocal, and the arthroscope may add objective data to the evaluation.

Throwers with concomitant instability and rotator cuff symptoms are particularly good candidates for arthroscopy. The arthroscopic examination may help in identifying intraarticular pathology and in the detailed planning of an open or an arthroscopic stabilization procedure. However, the tendency to overemphasize minor changes that are noted arthroscopically should be avoided. Degenerative lesions of the labrum are common in patients older than 40.[6,21]

Our approach is to perform an arthroscopic examination in all traumatic types of anterior instability, since the likelihood of capsular-periosteal disruption of the anterior glenoid, which can be repaired arthroscopically, is high in these patients. In patients with an atraumatic etiology, an open technique is generally used. If the EUA reveals multidirectional instability as evidenced by a 3+ sulcus sign, we proceed directly to an open stabilization procedure.

Since 1986, we have performed arthroscopy in the modified "beach chair" position.[1] We feel that there are several advantages to the beach chair position. It allows the surgeon to examine the shoulder in various positions of abduction and rotation since there is no traction upon the arm. There is also a lower risk of neuropraxia[37] from traction, and the an-

terior structures are not placed in traction. In addition, an arthroscopic procedure can be simply converted to an open procedure without the need for extensive repositioning and redraping. The beanbag is simply deflated, and the head of the operating table is lowered to the appropriate level. Translatory forces may be delivered in both anterior and posterior directions to assess the relationship between the head and the glenoid.

Pathologic findings during the arthroscopic examination include detachment of the anteroinferior capsulolabral structures, stretching of the IGHLC, and fraying or tearing of the anteroinferior labrum. Laxity of the axillary pouch is present when the arthroscope is easily passed into the anteroinferior joint cavity without the normal restraint of the capsular tissues. This phenomenon is referred to as the "drive-through" sign.

Anteroinferior labral flaps are often associated with instability. Large labral flaps that appear nonfunctional can be debrided, but the surgeon must not destabilize the IGHLC. Altchek et al.[3] recently reported poor long-term results in patients who underwent arthroscopic debridement of labral flaps at all sites. This treatment provided temporary pain relief, but symptoms generally recurred upon resumption of normal activities and sports. Patients with evidence of labral detachment and instability did especially poorly. We do not recommend debridement of anteroinferior labral insufficiency as an isolated treatment.

Many operative procedures have been described for the treatment of anterior shoulder instability. From the discussion earlier, it is clear that limiting external rotation does not address the true pathology of the anteriorly unstable shoulder. Such functional restraint severely limits the patient in an unnecessary manner. The Putti-Platt procedure, in particular, may cause degenerative arthritis when the subscapularis is shortened excessively.[29,60]

Bone-block procedures, when done in isolation, also fail to address anteroinferior capsulolabral insufficiency. The concept of an anterior bony buttress (upon which these procedures are based) may be invalid, particularly in patients with subluxation.[61] These types of operations also tend to limit motion. When metal hardware is used to fix the bone block, there is a high risk of complications from penetration of the joint or loosening.[79] A revision stabilization procedure is especially difficult after a Bristow procedure owing to extensive scarring of the anterior capsule and subscapularis tendon.[78]

Regan et al.[53] noted limitation and weakness of external rotation in all patients after Bristow, Magnuson-Stack, and Putti-Platt procedures. Of these three procedures, the Putti-Platt affected external rotation to the greatest degree. Surprisingly, external rotation was better in patients who had undergone a Magnuson-Stack than in patients who had been treated with a Bristow. Excess capsular laxity is not addressed by these procedures.

The concept of repairing the capsular-periosteal separation at the anterior glenoid neck was first proposed by Perthes[50] and later expounded upon by Bankart.[7-9] This technique attacks the pathology at its most common site and is directed at reconstitution of the primary static stabilizer of the shoulder, the IGHLC. If abnormal capsular laxity is encountered, the procedure is easily modified to account for this pathologic factor as well. In a long-term review of 50 patients treated by Bankart and his colleagues between 1925 and 1954, recurrence occurred in only two patients.[23] Rowe et al.[58] noted a 3.5 percent recurrence rate in 145 patients after a Bankart procedure. When properly performed, the procedure results in a superior functional outcome compared with the previously discussed operations. In the series of Rowe et al., 69 percent of the patients regained full range of motion.[58]

Our basic procedure for the open surgical treatment of recurrent anterior glenohumeral instability is a modification of the Bankart procedure. The subscapularis tendon may be detached medial to its insertion at the greater tuberosity (Fig. 6-6), or it may be split longitudinally and stripped from the anterior capsule. A selective capsular repair is then employed. The presence or absence of a Bankart lesion is determined by previous arthroscopic examination or through a small transverse capsular incision. In patients with a demonstrated Bankart lesion or a traumatic etiology, the capsule is opened by a vertical incision medially at the glenoid margin[47] (Fig. 6-6). A medial capsular incision allows for repair of the detached capsule in combination with shifting of lax tissue. If no Bankart lesion is present or if the patient has an atraumatic etiology, a lateral capsular incision is generally utilized. The lateral incision facilitates the capsular shift when medial capsular detachment is absent. Bone blocks are considered only in those rare cases in which there is a severe deficiency (greater than 40 percent) of the anterior glenoid, and even then, the bone block is used in conjunction with a repair of the capsulolabral system. Procedures that are designed to limit external rotation are not a part of our armamentarium in the initial surgical treatment of anterior instability.

Arthroscopic stabilization techniques offer the advantage of less perioperative pain and morbidity, and they can be performed in an outpatient setting. At present, however, the risk of recurrence after arthroscopic stabilization is higher than that after an open procedure. Early reports revealed recurrence rates of between 15 and 20 percent after arthroscopic stabilization procedures.[30,76,77] Recently, Morgan[44] has reported a recurrence rate of only 5 percent after 1- to 7-year follow-up of 175 patients who had undergone an anterior stabilization using a transglenoid suture technique.

Techniques of arthroscopic stabilization are still in their infancy. At present, these procedures should be performed only by experienced arthroscopists in selected patients. A well-performed open stabilization is certainly preferable to a failed arthroscopic procedure. Patients treated arthroscopically may require a longer period of postoperative immobilization than patients treated by open techniques.[30]

In the authors' view, the ideal candidate for an arthroscopic stabilization is a patient with a recurrent anterior subluxation or dislocation who has a demonstrated detachment of a stout, well-defined IGHLC-labral complex on arthroscopic examination. Patients who appear to have an attenuated, patulous anterior capsule are better treated by an open stabilization.[4,22,72] There is a great hope that arthroscopic techniques will improve the results of the operative treatment of instability in throwers. In the series of Rowe et al.,[58] 69 percent of those patients treated by an open Bankart procedure regained full motion. Morgan[44] reported recovery of full range of motion in 87 percent of the first 55 patients that he treated arthroscopically. Less than one-third of the throwing athletes treated by Rowe et al. with an open Bankart repair were able to return to their premorbid level of pitching.[58] Coughlin et al.[20] have noted disappointing results (less than 50 percent success rate) in returning overhead athletes to their premorbid level of function after metal staple capsulorrhaphy. Warner et al.[72] reported that 9 of 12 overhead athletes who were stabilized arthroscopically with a biodegradable tack were able to return to their preinjury level of function.

Multidirectional instability and voluntary instability are absolute contraindications to an arthroscopic stabilization procedure. The finding of a poorly formed IGHLC or the lack of a Bankart lesion on arthroscopic examination is a relative contraindication. Some surgeons feel that an arthroscopic method should not be used in the presence of a large Hill-Sachs lesion.

We have experience with two forms of arthroscopic stabilization procedures. The first type of sta-

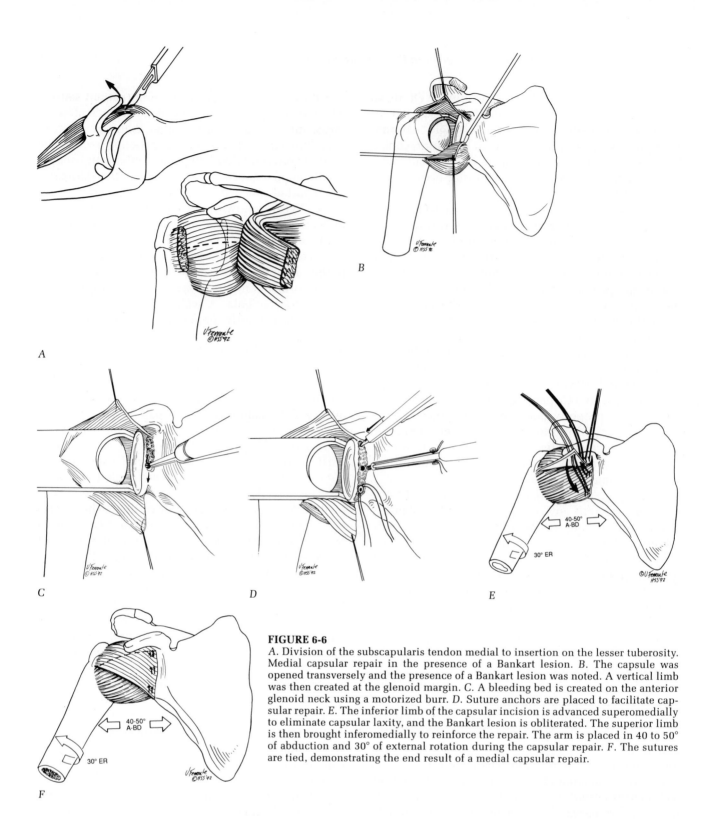

FIGURE 6-6
A. Division of the subscapularis tendon medial to insertion on the lesser tuberosity. Medial capsular repair in the presence of a Bankart lesion. B. The capsule was opened transversely and the presence of a Bankart lesion was noted. A vertical limb was then created at the glenoid margin. C. A bleeding bed is created on the anterior glenoid neck using a motorized burr. D. Suture anchors are placed to facilitate capsular repair. E. The inferior limb of the capsular incision is advanced superomedially to eliminate capsular laxity, and the Bankart lesion is obliterated. The superior limb is then brought inferomedially to reinforce the repair. The arm is placed in 40 to 50° of abduction and 30° of external rotation during the capsular repair. F. The sutures are tied, demonstrating the end result of a medial capsular repair.

bilization employs sutures that are passed through drill holes in the glenoid neck and are tied posteriorly (Fig. 6-7). The second technique involves the use of an absorbable tack (Fig. 6-8).[72] We have recently begun to experiment with the arthroscopic use of suture anchors. In some patients, a combination of the two techniques may be needed for optimal tensioning of the tissue. In this situation, sutures are used superiorly to tension the tissues, and then a tack is placed at the 4 o'clock position to close the

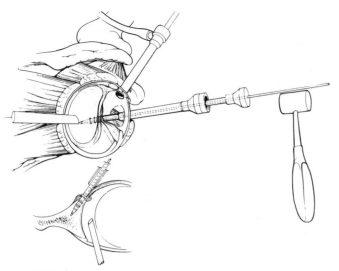

FIGURE 6-7
Arthroscopic stabilization using transglenoid suture technique. Sutures are passed through the labrum and anteroinferior capsule. A Beath pin is then drilled from the anterior glenoid neck and through the bony glenoid. The pin and one end of the sutures are recovered as they exit the skin posteriorly. The anterior halves of the sutures are paired together and tied. Tension is then placed on the posterior halves of the sutures to pull the capsulolabral structures to the glenoid neck. The posterior halves of the sutures are then tied over a fascial bridge.

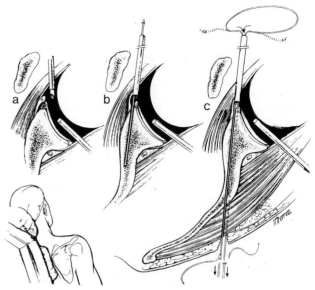

FIGURE 6-8
Arthroscopic stabilization using biodegradable tacks (Acufex Microsurgical). A cannulated drill bit and guide wire are used to advance the capsular tissues to the glenoid neck. After a hole is drilled into the anterior glenoid, the drill bit is removed and the guide wire is left in place. *A.* A biodegradable tack is then placed over the guide wire and impacted into place with a cannulated pusher. *B.* Illustration of the shoulder after placement of a single tack. Generally, two tacks are used to stabilize the shoulder.

defect. We do not recommend the routine use of metal hardware around the shoulder. The use of metal staples has consistently been associated with a high incidence of postoperative instability as well as frequent problems related to staple loosening.[18,20,22,76,77]

Patients with concomitant instability and impingement who fail conservative treatment should have surgical intervention to provide stability. Subacromial decompression is not recommended as a primary procedure in these patients. Occasionally, anterior acromioplasty may be required as a secondary part of treatment.

CONCLUSION

Glenohumeral stability is dependent upon the soft tissues surrounding the joint. If a primary stabilizer is attenuated or damaged, there appear to be secondary restraints to abnormal translation. The high loads incurred at the shoulder during athletic activity can overwhelm both primary and secondary mechanisms of stability. Our understanding of these intricate relationships has increased dramatically in recent years.

Many patients, particularly those with an atraumatic etiology, respond to nonoperative rehabilitation that emphasizes rotator cuff and periscapular strengthening. The operative treatment of instability should attend to damage to the capsulolabral system and to excess capsular laxity. A scientific approach that is directed at the restoration of normal capsular anatomy should be employed to prevent instability while retaining maximal function.

REFERENCES

1. Altchek D, Skyhar M, Warren R: Shoulder arthroscopy for shoulder instability, in Barr J (ed): *Instr Course Lect* vol 38, 1989.
2. Altchek D, Warren R, Skyhar M, Ortiz G: T-plasty modification of the Bankart procedure for multidirectional instability of anterior and inferior types. *J Bone Joint Surg (Am)* 73A:105–112, 1991.
3. Altchek D, Warren R, Wickiewicz T, Ortiz G: Arthroscopic labral debridement: A three-year follow-up study. *Am J Sports Med* 20:702–706, 1992.
4. Altchek D: Arthroscopic Anterior Stabilization in Patients without Labral Detachment. Presented at Annual Meeting of Arthroscopy Association of North America, Boston, 1992.

5. Anderson D, Zuirbulis R, Ciullo J: Scapular manipulation for reduction of anterior shoulder dislocation. *Clin Orthop* 164:181–183, 1982.

6. Andrews J, Carson W, McLeod W: Glenoid labrum tears related to the long head of the biceps. *Am J Sports Med* 13:337–341, 1985.

7. Bankart A: The pathology and treatment of recurrent dislocation of the shoulder joint. *Br Med J* 2:1132–1133, 1923.

8. Bankart A: The pathology and surgical treatment of recurrent dislocation of the shoulder. *Br J Surg* 26:23–29, 1938.

9. Bankart A: Discussion on recurrent dislocation of the shoulder. *J Bone Joint Surg (Br)* 30B:46–47, 1948.

10. Bigliani L, Pollock R, Soslowsky L, et al: Tensile properties of the inferior glenohumeral ligament. *J Orthop Res* 10:187–197, 1992.

11. Blasier R, Guldberg R, Rothman E: Anterior shoulder stability: Contributions of rotator cuff forces and the capsular ligaments in a cadaver model. *J Shoulder Elbow Surg* 1:140–150, 1992.

12. Bost F, Inman V: The pathological changes in recurrent dislocation of the shoulder: A report of Bankart's operative procedure. *J Bone Joint Surg (Am)* 24:595–613, 1942.

13. Bowen M, Deng X, Warner J, et al: The Effect of Joint Compression on Inferior Stability of the Glenohumeral Joint. Unpublished data.

14. Bowen M, Warren R: Ligamentous control of shoulder stability based on selective cutting and static translation experiments. *Clin Sports Med* 10(4):757–782, 1991.

15. Burkhead W, Rockwood C: Treatment of instability of the shoulder with an exercise program. *J Bone Joint Surg (Am)* 74A:890–896, 1992.

16. Cain P, Mutschler T, Fu F: Anterior stability of the glenohumeral joint: A dynamic model. *Am J Sports Med* 15:144–148, 1987.

17. Clayton M, Weir G: Experimental investigations of ligamentous healing. *Am J Surg* 98:373–378, 1959.

18. Cook M, Richardson A: Arthroscopic staple capsulorrhaphy for treatment of anterior shoulder instability. *Orthop Trans* 15:1, 1991.

19. Cooper D, Arnoczky S, O'Brien S, et al: Anatomy, histology, and vascularity of the glenoid labrum: An anatomical study. *J Bone Joint Surg (Am)* 74A:46–52, 1992.

20. Coughlin L, Rubinovich M, Johansson J, et al: Arthroscopic staple capsulorraphy for anterior shoulder instability. *Am J Sports Med* 20:253–256, 1992.

21. DePalma A, Callery G, Bennett G: Variational anatomy and degenerative lesions of the shoulder joint, in Blount W, Banks S, *Instr Course Lect* vol VI, 1949.

22. Detrisac D: Arthroscopic shoulder staple capsulorraphy for traumatic anterior instability, in McGinty J (ed): *Operative Arthroscopy*. New York, Raven Press, 1991.

23. Dickson J, Duvas M: Bankart's operation for recurrent dislocation of the shoulder. *J Bone Joint Surg (Br)* 39B:114–119, 1957.

24. Fronek J, Warren R, Bowen M: Posterior subluxation of the glenohumeral joint. *J Bone Joint Surg (Am)* 71A:205–216, 1989.

25. Galinat B, Howell S, Kraft T: The glenoid-posterior acromion angle: An accurate method of evaluating glenoid version. *Orthop Trans* 12:727, 1988.

26. Garth W, Slappey C, Ochs C: Roentgenographic demonstration of the shoulder: The apical oblique projection. A technical note. *J Bone Joint Surg (Am)* 66A:1450–1453, 1984.

27. Hall R, Isaac F, Booth C: Dislocations of the shoulder with special reference to accompanying small fractures. *J Bone Joint Surg (Am)* 41A:489–494, 1959.

28. Harryman D, Sidles J, Clark J, et al: Translation of the humeral head on the glenoid with passive glenohumeral motion. *J Bone Joint Surg (Am)* 72A:1334–1343, 1990.

29. Hawkins R, Hawkins R: Failed anterior reconstruction for shoulder instability. *J Bone Joint Surg (Br)* 67B:709–714, 1985.

30. Hawkins R: Arthroscopic stapling repair for shoulder instability: A retrospective study of 50 cases. *Arthroscopy* 5:122–128, 1989.

31. Hovelius L, Erikkson K, Fredin H, et al: Recurrences after initial dislocation of the shoulder: Results of a prospective study of treatment. *J Bone Joint Surg (Am)* 65A:343–349, 1983.

32. Howell S, Galinat B, Renzi A, Marone P: Normal and abnormal mechanics of the glenohumeral joint in the horizontal plane. *J Bone Joint Surg (Am)* 70A:227, 1988.

33. Howell S, Galinat B: The glenoid-labral socket: A constrained articular surface. *Clin Orthop* 243:122–125, 1989.

34. Jens J: The role of the subscapularis muscle in recurrent dislocation of the shoulder. *J Bone Joint Surg (Br)* 46B:780–781, 1964.

35. Jobe F, Bradley J: Rotator cuff injuries in baseball: Prevention and rehabilitation. *Sports Med* 6:377–386, 1984.

36. Jobe F, Kvitne R: Shoulder pain in the overhead athlete: The relationship of anterior instability and rotator cuff impingement. *Orthop Rev* 18:963–975, 1989.

37. Klein A, France J: Measurement of brachial plexus strain in arthroscopy of the shoulder. *Arthroscopy* 3:45–52, 1987.

38. Kocher E: Eine neue Reductionmethode für Schulterverrenkung. *Berl Klin Wochenschr* 7:101–105, 1870.

39. Kronberg M, Brostrom L-A: Humeral head retroversion in patients with unstable humero-scapular joints. *Clin Orthop* 260:207–211, 1990.

40. Matsen F, Thomas S, Rockwood C: Anterior glenohumeral instability, in Rockwood C, Matsen F (eds): *The Shoulder.* Philadelphia, Saunders, 1990.

41. McKernan D, Mutschler T, Rudert M, et al: Significance of a partial and full Bankart lesion: A biomechanical study. Presented at Annual Meeting of the Orthopaedic Research Society, Las Vegas, 1989.

42. McKernan D, Mutschler T, Rudert M, et al: The characterization of rotator cuff muscle forces and their effect on glenohumeral joint stability: A biomechanical study. *Orthop Trans* 14:237–238, 1990.

43. Morgan C, Bodenstab A: Arthroscopic Bankart suture repair: Technique and early results. *Arthroscopy* 3:111–122, 1987.

44. Morgan C: Arthroscopic transglenoid Bankart suture repair. *Operative Tech Orthop* 1:171–179, 1991.

45. Moseley H, Overgaard B: The anterior capsular mechanism in recurrent dislocation of the shoulder: Morphological and clinical studies with special reference to the glenoid labrum and glenohumeral ligaments. *J Bone Joint Surg (Br)* 44B:913–927, 1962.

46. Nobuhara K, Ikeda H: Rotator cuff interval lesion. *Clin Orthop* 223:44–50, 1987.

47. O'Brien S, Warren R, Schwart E: Anterior shoulder instability. *Orthop Clin North Am* 18:395–408, 1987.

48. O'Brien S, Neves M, Arnoczky S, et al: The anatomy and histology of the inferior gleno-humeral ligament complex of the shoulder. *Am J Sports Med* 18:449–456, 1990.

49. Perry J: Anatomy and biomechanics of the shoulder in throwing, swimming, gymnastics, and tennis. *Clin Sports Med* 2:247–270, 1983.

50. Perthes G: Ueber operationen der habituellen Schulterluxation. *Deut Z Chir* 85:199, 1906.

51. Poppen N, Walker P: Normal and abnormal motion of the shoulder. *J Bone Joint Surg (Am)* 58A:195–201, 1976.

52. Poppen N, Walker P: Forces at the glenohumeral joint in abduction. *Clin Orthop* 135:165–170, 1978.

53. Regan W, Webster-Bogaert S, Hawkins R, Fowler P: Comparative functional analysis of the Bristow, Magnuson-Stack, and Putti-Platt procedures for recurrent dislocation of the shoulder. *Am J Sports Med* 17:42–48, 1989.

54. Rokous J, Feagin J, Abbott H: Modified axillary roentgenogram: A useful adjunct in the diagnosis of recurrent instability of the shoulder. *Clin Orthop* 82:84–86, 1972.

55. Rowe C: Prognosis in dislocations of the shoulder. *J Bone Joint Surg (Am)* 38A:957–977, 1956.

56. Rowe C, Sakellarides H: Factors related to recurrences of anterior dislocations of the shoulder. *Clin Orthop* 20:40–48, 1961.

57. Rowe C, Pierce D, Clark J: Voluntary dislocation of the shoulder: A preliminary report on a clinical, electromyographic, and psychiatric study of twenty-six patients. *J Bone Joint Surg (Am)* 55A:445–460, 1973.

58. Rowe C, Patel D, Southmayd W: The Bankart procedure: A long-term end-result study. *J Bone Joint Surg (Am)* 60A:1–16, 1978.

59. Rowe C, Zarins B: Recurrent transient subluxation of the shoulder. *J Bone Joint Surg (Am)* 63A:863–872, 1981.

60. Samilson R, Prietom V: Dislocation arthropathy of the shoulder. *J Bone Joint Surg (Am)* 65A:456–460, 1983.

61. Schauder K, Tullos H: Role of the coracoid bone block in the Bristow procedure. *Am J Sports Med* 20:31–37, 1992.

62. Schlemm F: Ueber die Verstarkungsbander am Schultergelenk. *Arch Anat* 45:1853, 1853.

63. Simonet W, Cofield R: Prognosis in anterior shoulder dislocation. *Am J Sports Med* 12:19–24, 1984.

64. Soslowsky L, Flatow E, Bigliani L, Mow V: Articular geometry of the glenohumeral joint. *Clin Orthop* 285:181–190, 1992.

65. Speer K, Deng X, Borrero S, et al: A biomechanical evaluation of the Bankart lesion. Presented at Annual Meeting of American Shoulder and Elbow Surgeons, San Francisco, 1993.

66. Speer K: An evaluation of the relocation test. Presented at Annual Meeting of the American Shoulder and Elbow Society, San Francisco, 1993.

67. Stimson L: An easy method of reducing dislocations of the shoulder and hip. *NY Med Rec* 57:356–357, 1900.

68. Symeonides P: The significance of the subscapularis muscle in the pathogenesis of recurrent dislocation of the shoulder. *J Bone Joint Surg (Br)* 54B:476–483, 1972.

69. Terry G, Hammon D, France P, Norwood L: The stabilizing function of passive shoulder restraints. *Am J Sports Med* 19:26–34, 1991.

70. Townley C: The capsular mechanism in recurrent dislocation of the shoulder. *J Bone Joint Surg (Am)* 32A:370–380, 1950.

71. Vanderhooft E, Lippitt S, Harris S: Glenohumeral stability from concavity-compression: A quantitative analysis. Presented at Annual Meeting of American Shoulder and Elbow Surgeons, Washington, DC, 1992.

72. Warner J, Pagnani M, Warren R, et al: Arthroscopic Bankart repair with an absorbable, cannulated fixation device. *Orthop Trans* 15:761–762, 1991.

73. Warner J, Deng X, Warren R, Torzilli P: Static capsuloligamentous constraints to superior-inferior translation of the glenohumeral joint. *Am J Sports Med* 20:675–685, 1992.

74. Warren R, Kornblatt I, Marchand R: Static factors affecting posterior shoulder stability. *Orthop Trans* 8:89, 1984.

75. Wheeler J, Ryan J, Arciero R, Molinari R: Arthroscopic versus nonoperative treatment of acute shoulder dislocations in young athletes. *Am J Sports Med* 5:213–217, 1989.

76. Wiley A: Arthroscopy for shoulder instability and a technique for arthroscopic repair. *Arthroscopy* 4:25–30, 1988.

77. Yahiro M, Matthews L: Arthroscopic stabilization procedures for recurrent anterior shoulder instability. *Orthop Rev* 11:1161–1168, 1989.

78. Young D, Rockwood C: Complications of a failed Bristow procedure and their management. *J Bone Joint Surg (Am)* 73A:969–981, 1991.

79. Zuckerman J, Matsen F: Complications about the glenohumeral joint related to the use of screws and staples. *J Bone Joint Surg (Am)* 66A:175–180, 1984.

Anterior-Inferior Instability— Arthroscopic Stabilization

Bruce J. Goldberg
Robert P. Nirschl
Frank A. Pettrone

INTRODUCTION

Arthroscopy has had a profound impact on orthopedic surgery. It has contributed to a deeper understanding of normal and pathologic anatomy, improved our diagnostic ability, and added new dimensions to treatment options. The arthroscope has evolved from a simple diagnostic tool to a therapeutic tool with excisional and reconstructive options. In the shoulder, this evolution has progressed to the treatment of anterior glenohumeral instability.

Various surgical techniques for glenohumeral stabilization have developed as a result of equipment innovations and surgeon creativity. The success of early techniques[4,10,14–18,20–22,31,32,35,36,38–40] was not encouraging, but technical and equipment modifications along with surgeon experience have greatly improved on those early results.[5,8,12,13,19,24,25,33,37,40] At the present, however, all these encouraging modifications lack long-term follow-up and critical analysis of both the failures and successes.

Why consider an arthroscopic technique when open techniques are essentially a known commodity? Arthroscopic evaluation of the shoulder more precisely delineates the pathology, allows surgeons to specifically address the pathologic lesion, and minimizes the surgical trauma to otherwise normal tissue, thereby decreasing postoperative morbidity, decreasing periarticular fibrosis, minimizing loss of range of motion, and facilitating return to activity.

This chapter discusses the various anatomic and technical factors in the decision-making process, reviews the different arthroscopic techniques for glenohumeral stabilization, and reviews the available results.

INDICATIONS

The indication of surgical intervention is the presence of symptomatic anterior instability uncorrected by rehabilitation or instability that precludes effective participation in a rehabilitative effort. The de-
cision whether to use an arthroscopic technique of any variety depends on the specific pathoanatomy and the quality of tissue available for reconstruction. All the commonly used variations depend ultimately on the presence of a well-formed inferior glenohumeral ligament (IGHL). None of the arthroscopic techniques are recommended for individuals with multidirectional instability.

PATHOANATOMY

Arthroscopic evaluation allows for the recognition of the specific anatomic lesion, and the arthroscopic stabilization techniques provide the means to restore the normal anatomic relationships.

The pathoanatomy encountered is a combination of congenital and acquired factors. Congenital factors are the presence of generalized ligamentous laxity, multidirectional shoulder laxity, and normal variations in capsulolabral anatomy. Acquired factors are the type and anatomic location of the tissue injury, as well as the quality of capsulolabral tissue. There are multiple patterns of capsulolabral injury, and recognizing the patterns is critical to the decision making and success of the arthroscopic techniques.

CONGENITAL

Generalized ligamentous laxity has been characterized by the combination of greater than 10° of elbow hyperextension, greater than 10° of knee hyperextension, greater than 90° of extension of the metacarpal-phalangeal joint, and radial abduction of the thumb to the forearm.[16] The inherent tissue elasticity of an individual is not an all-or-none phenomenon. Somewhere along this continuum is the patient with multidirectional shoulder laxity who may not exhibit all the characteristics of generalized ligamentous laxity. It is not clear whether one must demonstrate all or a combination of the four to be considered a difficult candidate for shoulder reconstruction. From our experience, the presence of three out of four of these factors would identify a potential problem with any method of reconstruction, especially arthroscopic, where the periarticular scarring is minimized and does not contribute to the postoperative stability.

The distinction between the physical finding of laxity and the functional disruption of instability is important. The finding of multidirectional laxity is often but not always found in association with generalized ligamentous laxity. This patient population will have suffered a traumatic injury and demonstrate unidirectional instability and apprehension with functional disruption. Their contralateral shoulder will demonstrate an asymptomatic multidirectional laxity without apprehension or functional impairment. From our experience, these patients can be treated successfully with arthroscopic techniques if their acquired pathology shows evidence of acute capsuloligamentous failure without chronic attenuation.

Lastly, normal nonpathologic variations in the capsulolabral structures may contribute to glenohumeral stability. Many authors[9,27,28] have described variations in the presence and size of the middle glenohumeral ligament (MGHL). Rames[28] and DePalma[9] describe variants in which the anterior capsule is confluent without discernible ligaments. The absence of a well-formed IGHL may contribute to constitutional shoulder laxity. Morgan[27] described a higher incidence of a type III capsular anatomy (i.e., a cordlike MGHL) in clinically stable shoulders.

These congenital factors are difficult to quantify and do not fit nicely into a simple clear-cut decision-making process. They are concerns for both the open and arthroscopic methods of treating glenohumeral instability. As the arthroscopic techniques try to address the specific pathologic lesion and thereby restore the preinjury pattern rather than rely on additional periarticular scarring for stability, the arthroscopic procedure may be less successful in these individuals where their preexisting capsular anatomy or inherent tissue elasticity are contributing factors to the functional disruption after injury.

ACQUIRED

Acquired factors depend on the type of injury (acute or chronic, disruption or attenuation), anatomic location (glenoid or labral, labral or capsular, anteroinferior or anterosuperior or both) and the quality of the injured structure (degenerative or healthy, poorly formed or robust).

At any point along the glenoid-labral-capsular complex, the tissue may be disrupted at a single location and be of good quality, making anatomic restoration relatively simple, or may be complex with varying tissue quality and disruption at multiple levels, making anatomic restoration nearly impossible.[1–3,11,13]

Simple patterns involve disruption at the glenolabral interval ("true Bankart") or at the capsulolabral level. The most straightforward is the "true Bankart," with disruption at the glenolabral interval without IGHL compromise. Simple capsular disruption may involve only the IGHL or both the MGHL and IGHL. The IGHL may be detached with or without the MGHL. The quality of the remaining tissue is critical. A disrupted, robust, well-formed IGHL is very different from an attenuated or poorly formed, disrupted IGHL.

Complex lesions include simple disruption but at two anatomic levels (glenolabral and capsulolabral) or labral detachment with capsular attenuation or congenital laxity. Disruption at both the glenolabral and capsulolabral intervals requires both labral reapproximation and IGHL tensioning to restore capsulolabral anatomy. Another type of complex pattern is a degenerative labrum, detached or intact, and capsular disruption. The critical factor in this situation is reestablishment of both position and tension of the IGHL. The incompetent, degenerative labrum may be debrided away to advance and secure the IGHL to the decorticated anterior glenoid neck. An intraoperative assessment of the tissue quality and degree of needed superomedial shift will determine whether to proceed with an arthroscopic technique. In our experience, as long as the IGHL is well formed and competent, it can be mobilized and advanced adequately to provide a functional IGHL.

Capsular attenuation (i.e., redundancy and thinning) without labral injury is another pattern. However, its etiology is less clear-cut but nevertheless essential to the decision-making process for surgical reconstruction. Observed etiologies include (1) an old simple disruption that has healed in an elongated position with good tissue quality distal to an intervening segment of attenuated tissue (i.e., an attempted healing response); (2) congenital laxity without observable evidence of injury or healing; or (3) microscopic interstitial failure without observable disruption representing a chronic adaptation to repetitive overload physiologic stress. The distinction between an elongated ligament that has been subjected to chronic repetitive stress causing microrupture and a ligament that was frankly disrupted and healed with a thinned intervening segment is important. The previously disrupted ligament should have the thinned intervening segment resected and the competent segment of the IGHL advanced and secured to the anterior glenoid neck. When the ligaments demonstrated thinning and laxity without this intervening segment, a great deal of superomedial shift may be needed to reestablish appropriate tensioning of the IGHL. In this situation, the amount of superomedial shift and the inherent tissue qualities may exceed the capacities of the arthroscopic techniques. We have used the arthroscopic multiple suture technique successfully in this situation if the patient doesn't demonstrate any other findings of congenital joint laxity. If the patient demonstrates any other findings of joint laxity, we recommend proceeding with an open procedure. However, additional clinical investigations are needed to define the indications in this difficult subgroup.

TECHNIQUES

The arthroscopic stabilization techniques for anterior glenohumeral instability are evolving. The ongoing process of equipment development and technique modifications has created a number of different techniques. The goal of surgical reconstruction in anterior glenohumeral instability is the restoration of the anatomic and functional integrity to the gleno-labral-capsular complex.

General Principles

In spite of technical and equipment variations, all the arthroscopic techniques have basic similarities.

SURGICAL TECHNIQUE

The potential healing tissue surfaces must be debrided of scar and hypertrophied synovium, an attempted healing response, to provide freshened surfaces. The capsulolabral tissue must be mobilized off the glenoid to the 6 o'clock position to allow the necessary superomedial shift.

The anterior glenoid rim and neck must be debrided and decorticated, providing a bleeding cancellous bone surface for healing. Attention to detail is important, often requiring the use of a 70° scope or visualization from an anterior portal to ensure adequate decortication (Plate 9).

The point of fixation on the anterior glenoid should be as close to the articular rim as possible without violating the articular surface or compromising fixation strength, usually 3 to 5 mm medial to the articular edge. Overmedialization should be

avoided. The prepared and mobilized capsulolabral complex must be firmly secured to the anterior glenoid neck.

POSITIONING

The lateral decubitus or modified beach chair positions can be used with any of these techniques. Each has its various advantages, disadvantages, and advocates. In either case, the patient must be positioned and draped to provide access to the entire posterior shoulder including the medial border of the scapula. When using the lateral decubitus position, allowing the patient to "roll-back" 20 to 30° will increase the accessibility of the anterior shoulder.

PORTAL PLACEMENT

The placement of the anteroinferior portal is important to the access needed to mobilize the capsulolabral tissues down to the 6 o'clock position and inferior suture placement needed to advance the IGHL superomedially. The anteroinferior portal should be created caudal in the biceps-subscapularis safe triangle, hugging the edge of the subscapularis tendon (Plate 10). A second anterior portal may be established cephalad in the safe triangle.

Equipment

Innovative equipment has been integral to the development and expansion of these arthroscopic techniques.

SUTURE PLACEMENT

The suture punch (Linvatec, Largo, FL) has an arthroscopic type handle with a movable upper jaw and an immobile lower jaw (Fig. 7-1A). The mobile upper jaw is fenestrated. The lower jaw has a cannulated tine. The cannula extends through the instrument shaft to the handle. With the aid of a feeder wheel, the suture is placed in the hole at the back of the handle, advanced through the shaft and out the tine of the lower jaw. The fenestra in the upper jaw accepts the tine of the lower jaw when the jaws are closed. The punch grabs the tissue; the tine pierces the tissue and into the hole of the upper jaw. The suture is then fed through the tine and thus through the tissue. The jaws are opened, the tine disengaged, and the suture punch withdrawn, delivering both sutures ends out the cannula.

The shoulder stitcher (Acufex, Mansfield, MA) (Fig. 7-1B), the suture hook (Linvatec, Largo, FL) (Fig. 7-1C), and the suture passer (Mitek, Norwood, MA) (Fig. 7-1D) are cannulated devices with a

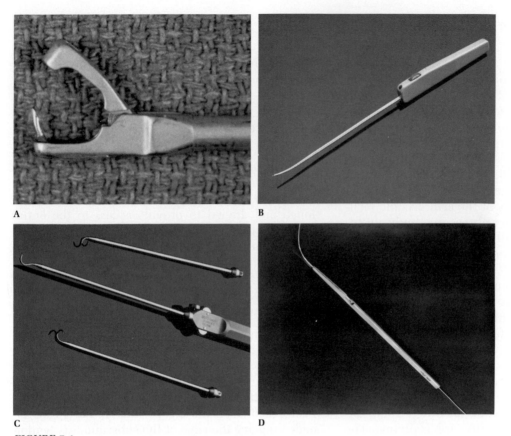

A   B

C   D

FIGURE 7-1
Equipment—suture placement. *A.* Suture punch (Linvatec, Largo, FL) allows for suture placement and retrieval in one step. Other cannulated devices allow arthroscopic suture placement with varying angles of approach to the tissues. With these devices, the free suture end must be retrieved in a second step. *B.* Shoulder stitcher (Acufex, Mansfield, MA). *C.* Suture hook (Linvatec, Largo, FL). *D.* Suture passer (Mitek, Norwood, MA).

needlelike tip for tissue puncture. The tip pierces the tissue and the suture is inserted into the cannula at the back of the instrument handle and fed through the cannula into the joint by means of a roller system, feeder wheel, or by hand. Then the free end of the suture is retrieved with a grasper or suture retrieval loop and brought back out the arthroscopic cannula.

SUTURE TYING

The knot pusher and knot cutter (Arthrex, Naples, FL) are used for intraarticular suturing. A multiple-hitch slip knot is made extraarticular. The suture ends are passed individually through the two fenestrae at the tip of the knot pusher. With tension applied to the suture ends, the knot is pushed down the arthroscopic cannula into the joint. Additional throws are created by repeating this sequence. The knot cutter has the same fenestrae and a sliding outer sleeve that is advanced to cut the suture ends intraarticularly.

FIXATION DEVICES

Mitek GII (Mitek, Norwood, MA) (Fig. 7-2A) is a suture anchor consisting of a titanium body, a nitenol memory arc, and an eyelet for the suture. The memory arc can be elastically deformed. After creating a drill hole, the Mitek II is placed, causing the memory arms to deform and spring back into the cancellous bone, providing firm fixation in the bone and preventing the Mitek II from pulling out.

Suretac (Acufex, Mansfield, MA) (Fig. 7-2B) is cannulated biodegradable implant, made of polyglyconate. It consists of a shaft and a flat head. The shaft has ridges to increase its fixation strength and the flat head captures the soft tissues.

CANNULAS

The suture punch cannula (Linvatec, Largo, FL) is a large oblong cannula that allows access for all the reconstructive equipment. It has a cannulated obturator for insertion over a Wissinger rod and a rubber

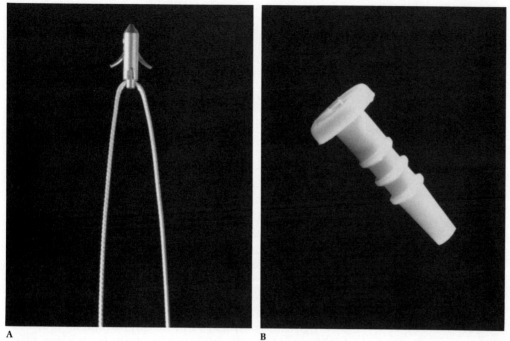

A   B

FIGURE 7-2
Fixation devices. *A.* Mitek GII (Mitek, Norwood, MA). *B.* Suretac (Acufex, Mansfield, MA).

diaphragm to prevent fluid escape, maintaining intraarticular distention pressure.

DRILLING

The suture punch drill bit (Linvatec, Largo, FL) is a 3.3-mm-diameter stepped drill bit with a 2.0 shaft and proximal eyelet for sutures. It creates a drill hole slightly larger than the size of the eyelet and sutures, allowing for easier transglenoid passage of the multiple sutures.

Suture pins (Bowen, Rockville, MD) are 2.2-mm-diameter pins with a sharp pointed tip and multiple eyelets on the opposite end for sutures. The sharp tip allows for tissue spearing and prevents the pin from "walking" on the anterior glenoid neck when drilling. The diameter of the tip is larger than the shaft to allow easier transglenoid passage. The multiple eyelets deliver the sutures transglenoid and allow for easy separation into multiple bundles.

The suture punch drill guide (Linvatec, Largo, FL) (Fig. 7-3A) is a double-barreled instrument with a gunlike handle. The distal ends of the barrels are beveled inward to allow proper orientation on the glenoid rim. It places the drill hole about 3 to 5 mm medial to the glenoid margin and orients the transglenoid drilling to exit in the infraspinatus fossa.

The shoulder guide (Acufex, Mansfield, MA) (Fig. 7-3B) is a rectangular outrigger-type guide. The suture pin cannula has a flange which is placed on the anterior glenoid surface and prevents inadvertent medial migration. The outrigger is used to direct and control the posterior exit of the transglenoid drilling.

COMBINATION

The grasping stitcher (Arthrex, Naples, FL) (Fig. 7-4) combines suture placement, tissue tensioning, and transglenoid drilling. The instrument is inserted through the anterior portal. The tissue is grasped, tensioned, and pierced with a 1.7-mm suture pin. The outrigger drill guide is positioned to ensure appropriate direction and exit site for the transglenoid drilling.

Specific Techniques

The various techniques can be grouped according to the need for transglenoid drilling. The anterior only (nontransglenoid) techniques avoid the potential risks of suprascapular nerve injury and infraspinatus tissue entrapment. Proponents of the transglenoid techniques have found the occurrence of this potential risk to be small and have noted the improved ability to tension and advance the IGHL more completely.

Current anterior only techniques use the biodegradable fixation device[34] and the suture anchor.[38] The current transglenoid techniques are the multiple suture technique[8] and the horizontal mattress technique with intraarticular knots.[20,26]

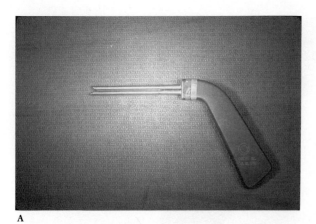

A

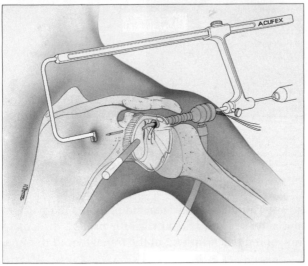

B

FIGURE 7-3
Drill guides. *A.* Suture punch drill guide (Linvatec). *B.* Shoulder guide (Acufex).

TRANSGLENOID TECHNIQUES

General

The major disadvantage of the transglenoid techniques is the potential for supraspinatus nerve injury. The direction of the drilling is critical. Exiting in the middle portion of the infraspinatus fossa 5 to 10 cm caudal to the midpoint of the scapular spine will minimize this potential. Entrapment of the infraspinatus fascia is a potential problem. If absorbable suture is used, at approximately 3 months the patients will often feel the sutures pop in this area.

Multiple Suture Technique[8]

The indications are traumatic anterior or anteroinferior instability in which a well-formed IGHL is present. In the face of increased IGHL laxity, a portion can be resected, approximately 5 to 10 mm, so that the superomedial advancement will restore adequate tension. A degenerative labrum may be resected to better advance the IGHL and restore its anatomic position and functional integrity. Contrain-

dications include multidirectional instability, generalized ligamentous laxity, poorly formed IGHL, or thin and atrophic anterior capsule.

Multiple suture technique is performed in the lateral decubitus position with 20 to 30° of roll-back in a single traction setup. Standard posterior and anterior arthroscopic portals are established. The tissue surfaces are prepared in the usual manner. The suture punch cannula is placed in the anterior portal over an arthroscopic exchange rod. Using the suture punch through the anterior portal, multiple 0 or 2-0 PDS or Maxon sutures are placed in the capsulolabral structures (Fig. 7-5A). An average of three to seven sutures are used. Each suture is brought out the anterior cannula. Then a suture punch drill or suture pin is drilled transglenoid starting at the 2 o'clock position, just below the glenoid rim and exiting posteriorly in the infraspinatus fossa. The drilling may be done freehand or with the suture punch drill guide. In either case, the direction and posterior exit site is critical to avoid supraspinatus nerve injury. The drill must exit in the infraspinatus fossa 5 cm caudal to the midpoint of the scapular spine. The drill is advanced to tent the skin posteriorly, and a small incision is made. A plane is established between the subcutaneous fat and the infraspinatus fascia on either side of the incision for about 2 cm. The sutures are then threaded through the eyelets on the proximal end of the drill and delivered posteriorly by advancing the drill transglenoid by hand (Fig. 7-5B). The suture ends are separated and isolated, tensioning them both collectively and separately while releasing the shoulder traction and observing capsulolabral reapproximation to the anterior glenoid neck. The suture ends are separated into two bundles and each bundle is passed back un-

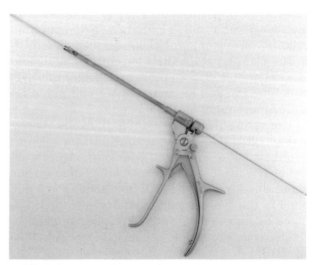

FIGURE 7-4
Grasping stitcher (Arthrex).

94

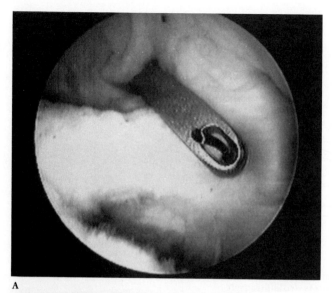

A

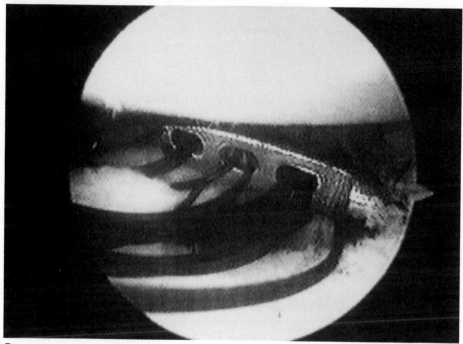

B

FIGURE 7-5
Multiple suture technique. *A.* The sutures are placed with the suture punch. *B.* The suture punch drill bit is drilled transglenoid. The sutures are delivered transglenoid through the eyelets.

derneath the infraspinatus fascia with a free needle, resulting in a 2- to 3-cm fascia bridge over which the sutures are then tied. The IGHL is advanced by virtue of the suture placement and by the tensioning of the sutures.

Horizontal Mattress Technique[20,25,26]
The horizontal mattress technique is an arthroscopic modification of the open technique described by Reider and Inglis.[29] This technique is recommended only for shoulders with a Bankart lesion and an intact, nonattenuated IGHL. One modification[26] uses a stitcher-grasper that allows for increased shifting of the capsule while placing the suture pin. However,

no results have been reported for its use in situations with capsular disruption, capsular attenuation, or with a degenerative labrum that is excised and the IGHL advanced.

The patient is placed in the lateral decubitus and standard arthroscopic portals are used. A single large horizontal mattress suture (1-PDS) is placed. Two modified Beath suture pins are used to place the sutures. The inferior pin is used to "spear" the capsulolabral tissue obliquely and then is reoriented to advance the anteroinferior labral tissue up to its anatomic position (Fig. 7-6*A*). Then this pin is drilled transglenoid and is angled 30 to 40° inferior and medial to exit 7 to 10 cm inferior to the midpoint of the

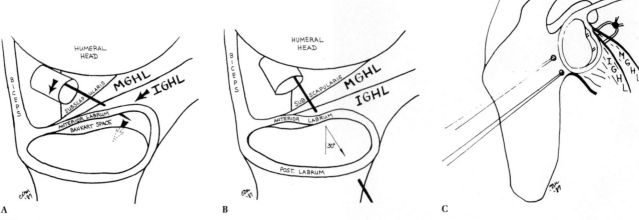

A   B   C

FIGURE 7-6
Horizontal mattress technique. *A.* The suture pins spear the capsulolabral tissue. The tissue is advanced superomedially, by reorienting the pin. *B.* The pin is drilled transglenoid. *C.* The anterior knot is delivered through the anterior cannula. The sutures are tensioned and tied posteriorly over the infraspinatus fascia, thereby reapproximating and securing the capsulolabral tissue against the decorticated glenoid rim. (*Reprinted with permission.*[26])

scapular spine in the infraspinatus fossa (Fig 7-6B). The upper pin is placed about 1.5 cm cephalad to the first pin in the area of the MGHL through the labrum and drilled transglenoid in a similar manner. Both pins are placed approximately 3 mm off the glenoid rim to better recreate the labral buttress and deepening of the glenoid. Both pins are advanced, each delivering two 1-PDS sutures through small posterior incisions. An anterior knot is created and drawn in through the anterior cannula, securing the capsulolabral structures against the anterior glenoid neck by tensioning the sutures from posterior (Fig. 7-6C). One set of sutures is brought subcutaneously to the other incision and the sutures are tied over an infraspinatus fascial bridge.

A modification of this technique has been developed by both Morgan[24] and Maki,[19] utilizing intraarticular knots to avoid entrapment of the infraspinatus fascia. After delivering four ends of the 1-PDS posteriorly, two with each pin, 5-mm "Mulberry-type" knots are tied posteriorly and then advanced retrograde, back into the joint to the posterior glenoid neck by applying tension through the anterior portal (Fig. 7-7A). Then the anterior capsulolabral structures are secured to the anterior glenoid neck by tying one strand of the upper pair to a strand of the lower pair with the arthroscopic knot pusher (Fig. 7-7B). The tying process is repeated for the other strands, producing a double-layered horizontal mattress.

As an alternative method of suture placement, a grasping stitcher allows for the grasping, tensioning, and shifting of the capsular tissue while placing the suture pin. It also provides an aim guide to assist in directing and exiting the pin in the infraspinatus fossa, away from the suprascapular nerve (Fig. 7-7C).

ANTERIOR ONLY (NONTRANSGLENOID) TECHNIQUES

General
Anterior only techniques avoid potential suprascapular nerve injury, as well as posterior tissue damage and entrapment. Current techniques use the Suretac, a cannulated biodegradable fixation device,[34] and the Mitek GII suture anchor.[38]

Suture Anchor Technique[38]
The suture anchor technique provides secure anterior fixation without transglenoid drilling. It is recommended for patients with Bankart lesions without capsular compromise.

The patient is positioned in the lateral decubitus with a bean bag and placed in a double-traction setup. The arm is also internally rotated to relax the anterior capsular structures. Four portals are established: anterior superior (ASP), anterior inferior (AIP), posterior superior (PSP), and posterior inferior (PIP). The PSP is placed at the posterolateral corner of the acromion, just at the bony margin, at the level of the glenohumeral joint. This is slightly more cephalad than the standard posterior arthroscopic portal. AIP is created in an inside-out manner at the inferior border of the safe biceps-subscapularis triangle, along the superior edge of the subscapularis tendon. The PIP, used primarily for the arthroscopic pump cannula, is made 3 cm caudal to the PSP portal. The ASP is created in an outside-in manner in

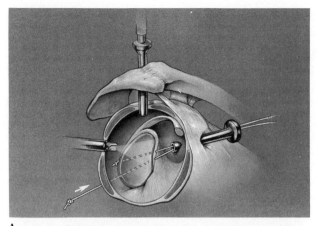

A

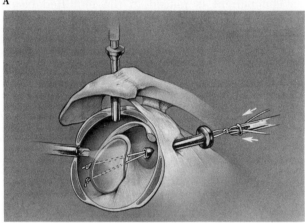

B

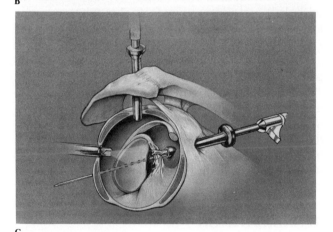

C

FIGURE 7-7
Modified horizontal mattress technique. *A.* After two sutures are placed transglenoid, "Mulberry knots" are tied in each suture posteriorly. *B.* Using the intraarticular knot pusher, the capsulolabral tissue is reapproximated to the glenoid rim. *C.* The grasping stitcher may be used to assist in tissue advancement and in directing the transglenoid drilling. (*Reprinted with permission.*[20])

the rotator cuff interval. Once the four portals are established, the capsulolabral lesion and anterior glenoid neck are prepared in the usual manner. The soft tissue is debrided, capsulolabral complex mobilized, and anterior glenoid neck decorticated with motor-

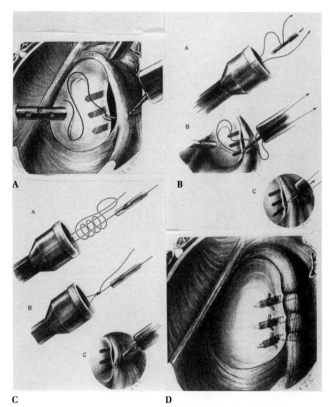

A   **B**

C   **D**

FIGURE 7-8
Suture anchor technique. *A.* Sutures are placed with the suture hook. Holes in the anterior glenoid are drilled with the Mitek drill. *B.* The Mitek GII is advanced along the "inside" end of the suture and into the drill hole. *C.* Using the intraarticular knot pusher, a multiple-hitch slip knot is slid down, reapproximating the capsulolabral tissue to the glenoid rim. *D.* Three anchors are recommended. (*Reprinted with permission.*[38])

ized burr. Then three Mitek drill holes are placed, paying careful attention to the direction, which should be angled 15 to 30° medially to avoid articular surface penetration. Then 0-PDS suture is placed through the capsulolabral tissue with a suture hook or punch (Fig. 7-8A). Both suture ends are brought out the anterior cannula. Both the ASP and AIP can be used for suture placement, with the ASP providing more inferior access. As an alternative the ASP can be used to steady and tension the capsulolabral tissue for suture placement through the AIP. Both the ASP and PSP may be used for the arthroscope, providing good visualization for both drill and suture placement. A 70° angle arthroscope is useful in the PSP. The "inside" end of the suture is threaded through the Mitek device. The Mitek is then slid down the suture into the previously made drill hole (Fig. 7-8B). Then an intraarticular arthroscopic knot pusher is used to secure the capsulolabral tissue to the anterior glenoid neck (Fig. 7-8C). This process is repeated for all three sutures (Fig. 7-8D). Capsulolabral advancement or plication can be accomplished

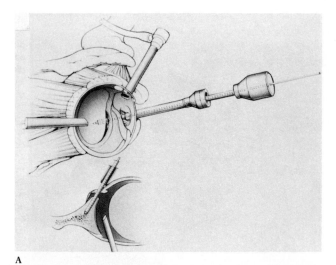

A

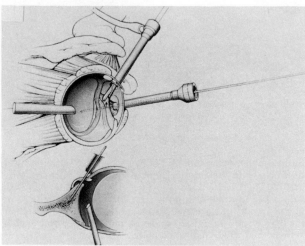

B

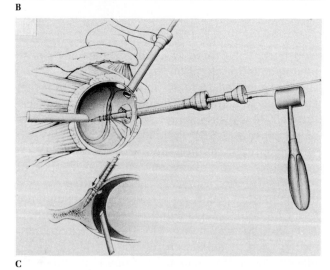

C

FIGURE 7-9
Suretac technique. *A.* The capsulolabral tissue is advanced superomedially and speared with the Suretac wire and cannulated drill. They are both advanced into the anterior glenoid for about 1 cm. *B.* The cannulated drill is disengaged, leaving the wire in the glenoid rim. *C.* The cannulated Suretac is advanced over the wire, reapproximating the capsulolabral tissue to the decorticated anterior glenoid rim. (*Reprinted with permission.[34]*)

by placing the sutures into the IGHL distal to the labrum and then again through the labrum.

Suretac Technique[34]

The anterior only technique popularized by Russell Warren utilizes the Suretac, a cannulated biodegradable fixation device. This technique avoids the potential hazard of transglenoid drilling and infraspinatus tissue entrapment and the potential complications of metal implants. The "ideal" patient is one with a labral detachment and a "robust" IGHL. It is not recommended in patients with thin or poorly formed IGHL, which Warren states are best managed with an open technique.

The patient is placed in the modified beach chair position. Three arthroscopic portals are established. A standard posterior portal is made inferior to the posterolateral corner of the acromion. An anterior superior portal is positioned lateral and superior to the coracoid process. An anterior inferior portal is created at the superior edge of the subscapularis tendon in the biceps-subscapularis safe triangle. The capsulolabral lesion and scapular neck are prepared in the usual manner with debridement, mobilization, and decortication. The Suretac cannulated drill with a wire extending a few millimeters beyond the tip of the drill are assembled. The capsulolabral tissue is speared with the wire and advanced superomedially either by reorienting the wire-drill assembly or by tensioning the tissue with a grasper from the anterosuperior portal prior to the spearing process. The wire tip is positioned on the anterior glenoid neck and the drill is advanced manually or by power to a depth of 10 mm (Fig. 7-9*A*). The drill and wire assembly are disengaged, drill removed, leaving the wire in the bone (Fig. 7-9*B*). The Suretac is advanced over the wire and impacted into the drill hole, capturing and securing the capsulolabral tissue against the glenoid neck (Fig. 7-9*C*). Suretacs are used at the 2 and 4 o'clock positions.

REHABILITATION[5,7,8,13,20,25,34,38]

The arthroscopic techniques are less traumatic to the surrounding soft tissues than the open techniques, and postoperative pain subsides more quickly. Nevertheless, the basic principles of tissue healing must be taken into consideration.

An initial period of immobilization and protection for 3 to 4 weeks is recommended. During this time, some protocols allow removal for hygiene, isometrics, or pendulum exercises to 90°. The second phase of the rehabilitative program starts at 3 to 4 weeks and addresses ROM and strength development. ROM exercises consist of pendulum, active-assist, UBE (upper body exerciser, Cybex) and active ROM. Some authors recommend restricting the extremes of abduction and external rotation for up to 3 months. Full or near-full ROM is achieved between 6 and 12 weeks. Progressive resistance exercises involve isometrics, isotonics, Theraband, and submaximal endurance work. Phase three of the rehabilitative process initiated at about 8 to 10 weeks intensifies strength development with increased isotonic, Isoflex tension cord, heavier Theraband, and submaximal isokinetics. Phase four starts at about 4 months with maximal isokinetics, controlled plyometric, and light sport activities. Initiation of this phase depends on the achievement of ROM and basic strength development. Full sport participation with contact and vigorous throwing are allowed at 6 months, provided the other rehabilitation goals have been achieved.

REVIEW OF RESULTS

The results of the currently used modifications of the arthroscopic techniques are encouraging. This improvement is the result of improved equipment, improved technical expertise, and better understanding of the capsulolabral pathology. Restoration of functional stability, range of motion, return to activity, and complications are important considerations in the review of these procedures.

The horizontal mattress technique has been reported by Morgan,[23-26] Maki,[20] and Rose.[30] Morgan[26] reported on 55 recurrent traumatic dislocators with 4 to 7 years of follow-up. Two patients (4 percent) experienced a return of their instability, but only after a second traumatic injury. Full range of motion was obtained in 87 percent with near full ($< 10°$ loss of external rotation) in the remaining 13 percent. In this group, 53 patients (96 percent) experienced complete resolution of their preoperative apprehension, full or near full ROM, and return to their preinjury level of activity without symptoms of instability. In a second series of 120 recurrent traumatic dislocators or subluxors with a follow-up of 1 to 3 years, there were 9 failures (6 percent). Seven of these 9 failures were collision athletes. Further subgrouping revealed a failure rate of 16 percent in the collision athletes and 1.5 percent in the throwers or noncollision athletes. Maki[20] reported only 1 failure (7 percent) in 15 noncollision athletes, with all patients resuming their previous level of activity. Rose[30] reported on 50 patients with 2 failures (4 per-

cent), with an average loss of external rotation of 4° at 0° of abduction and 8° at 90° of abduction.

The multiple suture technique has been reported by Caspari[6-8] and Goldberg.[12,13] Caspari[8] reported a 4 percent redislocation and a 4 percent "one-time" resubluxation rate, on 49 shoulders with 2- to 4-year follow-up. All shoulders regained 90 percent of their external rotation, measured at 90° of abduction. The average postoperative Bankart score[31] was 90. Goldberg, Nirschl, McConnell, and Pettrone[12] reported an 11 percent recurrence of functional instability, no redislocations, and a 5 percent "one-time" resubluxation rate on 49 shoulders with 2- to 4-year follow-up. Ninety-two percent of the shoulders obtained full or near-full ROM; 75 percent of the competitive and 70 percent of the recreational athletes returned to their same type and same level of activity. Only the 4 failures (i.e., postoperative functional instability) cited their shoulder as the reason for not returning to their previous activity level. Fifteen of 17 high-demand athletes returned to the same type and same level of activity, including 5 of 6 collision, 4 of 4 throwing, and 6 of 7 "other" (kayaking, rock climbing, military obstacle course, weight lifting). The average postoperative Bankart score[31] was 91.

The suture anchor technique has been reported by Wolf.[38] He reported no failures on 20 patients with a 12-month follow-up.

Using the Suretac technique, Warren and Warner[33,34] reported an 8 percent recurrence rate in 26 patients with 2- to 4-year follow-up. An average of 7° external rotation at 90° of abduction was lost. Five of 8 throwers and all 4 swimmers returned to their premorbid level of activity.

For the transglenoid techniques (n = 328), 6 complications were reported: 3 transient neuropraxias,[12,26] 1 superficial wound infection,[12] 1 partial infraspinatus atrophy,[12] and 1 synovial fistula from a nonabsorbable suture tied over a button.[8] All reported these early in their "learning curve" without recent problems. Neither of the anterior techniques has reported any complications.[34,38]

DISCUSSION

The arthroscopic treatment of anterior and anteroinferior glenohumeral instability is evolving. Initial techniques involved the placement of a metallic fixation device to reapproximate a Bankart lesion or shift the inferior capsule. A high rate of recurrence and complications from the implanted hardware prompted the development of the techniques discussed above.

The restoration of functional stability using these current arthroscopic techniques is between 90 and 100 percent, depending on the report.[8,12,13,20,26,30,34,38] A higher rate of success is reported by those who restrict their indications to traumatic instability with a Bankart lesion without IGHL involvement (94 to 100 percent), while those who have expanded their indications to include IGHL lesions report a slightly lower rate of success (89 to 94 percent). These results compare favorably with the results of open techniques.

The arthroscopic techniques offer profound advantages with regard to the range of motion and return to activity. This is illustrated in the higher Bankart scores, with authors reporting an average over 90,[6,13,26] all authors reporting at least 90 percent of the patients obtaining full or near-full ROM, with the biggest difference in the external rotation at 90° of abduction.[8,12,13,20,26,34,38] The ability of the arthroscopic technique to address the specific pathology without causing additional trauma to the anterior structures, thereby preventing anterior periarticular scarring, can explain this improvement in postoperative range of motion. In addition, this allows the throwers and overhead athletes to return to their activity in a higher percentage of cases.[13,34]

Patient selection is the key factor in the success of the arthroscopic stabilization procedures. Recognition of acquired and congenital factors correlated with clinical history is an essential element in the decision-making process. All the arthroscopic techniques work well with the traumatic, unidirectional dislocator who has a Bankart lesion and a well-formed, uncompromised IGHL. None of the techniques are recommended for the patient with multidirectional instability, generalized ligamentous laxity, and a poor IGHL. Where between these two extremes the arthroscopic techniques will find their niche in shoulder reconstruction is yet unclear. The presence and quality of the IGHL is a central factor to this analysis. The horizontal mattress and multiple suture techniques work well with a capsular disruption needing simple reattachment back to its anatomic location. The anterior only technique, using the suture anchor and the Suretac, have the potential ability to reapproximate the IGHL to the glenoid neck, but the clinical experience in these situations is limited. When confronted with a redundant IGHL, requiring a capsular shift, most authors have recommended an open technique. A history of chronic instability, instability resulting from relatively minor trauma, or constitutional laxity should alert the surgeon to the possibility of tissue inadequacies that exceed the capacity of the arthroscopic techniques. The patient with multidirectional laxity and traumatic anteroinferior instability can be treated arthroscopically if a true Bankart without capsular compromise or a simple IGHL avulsion is identified. However, the arthroscopic techniques have the advantage and disadvantage of addressing the specific pathologic lesion and restoring the preexisting anatomy without the adjunctive side effect of periarticular scarring. In this subgroup, restoring a stable but constitutional lax shoulder may carry with it the same disadvantages of the "original shoulder" and may be inappropriate. From our experience, the multiple suture technique is capable of shifting the capsule substantially to tighten the anterior capsule but may result in posterior instability due to the new imbalance created and the inability of the posterior structure to adequately compensate. The delicate balance, both passive and dynamic, as well as the inherent tissue quality is a clear limit to the successful application of the arthroscopic techniques in these patients.

With further clinical investigation, the effect of the normal nonpathologic capsulolabral variants on the success of the arthroscopic reconstruction of shoulder instability will be delineated. At this time, a well-formed IGHL is critical. A confluent but discernible MGHL-IGHL combination must be positioned more superiorly on the glenoid "clock," keeping in mind that the superior edge represents the MGHL component. A confluent anterior capsule without discernible ligaments is not amenable to arthroscopic reconstruction.

Collision athletes have a high rate of recurrence with both arthroscopic and open techniques. Certain activities place the shoulder at greater risk. The large impact forces of collision sports and the moderate forces applied in extreme positions of wrestling place both the uninjured as well as the reconstructed shoulder at high risk. A number of authors[20,26,34] have reported higher recurrence rates in their collision athletes and wrestlers using the arthroscopic techniques. Goldberg, Nirschl, McConnell, and Pettrone didn't find the return to collision athletics a factor in the analysis of their failures. None of the reviews analyzes the reason for the higher failure rate in these high-risk athletes. Did these athletes return to the same high-risk activity to suffer a similar trauma that caused their original injury? Given the arthroscopic technique's ability to identify and address the specific pathologic lesion without causing periarticular scarring, did we simply reestablish the individual's anatomy that may have predisposed him to the original injury? Did the repair fail at the site of reattachment or at a new interval? Was it a failure of the fixation method or inadequate strength at the healing interface? The strength of the various arthroscopic repairs has not been tested and compared with uninjured capsulolabral strength. Was the original repair tensioned adequately to restore stability without the aid of periarticular scarring? Nevertheless, the patients involved in high-risk activities may require the additional strength and the motion restrictions of the periarticular scarring of the open techniques.

As a corollary to this line of thought, the activities requiring full range of motion such as the throwing sports, tennis, and volleyball are clearly more amenable to the arthroscopic techniques. The ability to restore stability without interfering with ROM is critical to full return to activity in these sports.

CONCLUSION

The preliminary experience of all the arthroscopic techniques is promising. Using these techniques, the relief of apprehension, full range of motion, and return to athletic activity can be achieved safely and effectively in appropriately selected patients.

REFERENCES

1. Adolfsson L, Lysholm J: Arthroscopy and stability testing for anterior shoulder instability. *Arthroscopy* 5(4):315–320, 1989.
2. Baker CL: Arthroscopic evaluation of the unstable shoulder. *Operative Tech Orthop* 1(2):164–170, 1991.
3. Baker CL, Uribe JW, Whitman L: Arthroscopic evaluation of acute initial anterior shoulder dislocation. *Am J Sports Med* 181:25–28, 1990.
4. Burger RS, Stengel D, Bonatus T, Lewis J: Arthroscopic staple capsulorrhaphy for recurrent shoulder instability. *Orthop Trans* 14:596–597, 1990.
5. Cash JD: Recent advances and perspectives on arthroscopic stabilization of the shoulder. *Clin Sports Med* 10(4):871–886, 1991.
6. Caspari RB, Savoie FH, Meyers JP, et al: Arthroscopic management of the unstable shoulder. Presented at the American Academy of Orthopaedic Surgeons, Las Vegas, 1988.
7. Caspari RB, Savoie FH: Arthroscopic reconstruction of the shoulder: The Bankart repair, in McGinty JB (ed): *Operative Arthroscopy*. New York, Raven, 1991.
8. Caspari RB: Arthroscopic reconstruction for anterior shoulder instability, in Paulos LE, Tibone JE (ed): *Operative Techniques in Shoulder Surgery*, Gaithersburg, MD, Aspen, 1991.
9. DePalma AF: *Surgery of the Shoulder*. Philadelphia, Lippincott, 1983, pp 55–58.
10. Detrisac DA: Arthroscopic staple capsulorrhaphy for traumatic anterior shoulder instability, in McGinty JB (ed): *Operative Arthroscopy*. New York, Raven, 1991.
11. Detrisic DA, Johnson LL: *Arthroscopic Shoulder Anatomy*. Thorofare, NJ, Slack, 1968.
12. Goldberg BJ, Nirschl RP, McConnell JP, Pettrone FA: Arthroscopic transglenoid suture capsulolabral repair—Preliminary results. Presented at the 17th Annual Meeting of the American Orthopaedic Society for Sports Medicine, Orlando, 1991.
13. Goldberg BJ, Nirschl RP, McConnell JP, Pettrone FA: Arthroscopic transglenoid suture capsulolabral repair—Preliminary results. *Am J Sports Med* 21(5):656–665, 1993.
14. Gross RM: Arthroscopic shoulder capsulorrhaphy: Does it work? *Am J Sports Med* 17(4):495–500, 1989.
15. Hawkins RB: Arthroscopic stapling repair for shoulder instability: A retrospective study of 50 cases. *Arthroscopy* 5(2):122–128, 1989.
16. Hawkins RJ, Hobeika P: Physical examination of the shoulder. *Orthopaedics* 10:1270–1278, 1983.
17. Johnson LL: Shoulder arthroscopy, in Johnson LL (ed): *Arthroscopic Surgery: Principles and Practice*. St Louis, Mosby, 1986.
18. Kaveney MF, Wilson FD: Arthroscopic staple capsulorrhaphy for recurrent shoulder instability. *Orthop Trans* 12:728, 1988.
19. Maki NJ: Arthroscopic stabilization for recurrent shoulder instability. *Orthop Trans* 13:508, 1989.
20. Maki NJ: Arthroscopic stabilization—Suture technique. *Operative Tech Orthop* 1(2):180–183, 1991.
21. Matthews LS, Helfet DL, Spearman J, et al: Arthroscopic staple capsulorrhaphy for anterior instability of the shoulder. *Arthroscopy* 2:116, 1986.
22. Matthews LS, Vetter WL, Oweida SJ, et al: Arthroscopic staple capsulorrhaphy for recurrent anterior shoulder instability. *Arthroscopy* 4(2):106–111, 1988.
23. Morgan CD, Bodenstab AB: Arthroscopic Bankart suture repair: Technique and early results. *Arthroscopy* 3(2):111–122, 1987.

24. Morgan CD: Arthroscopic Bankart repair. Presented at the 9th Annual Meeting of the Arthroscopic Association of North America, Orlando, 1990.

25. Morgan CD: Arthroscopic transglenoid Bankart suture repair, in Paulos LE, Tibone JE (ed): *Operative Techniques in Shoulder Surgery.* Gaithersburg, MD, Aspen, 1991.

26. Morgan CD: Arthroscopic transglenoid Bankart suture repair. *Operative Tech Orthop* 1(2):171–179, 1991.

27. Morgan CD, Rames RD, Snyder SJ: Arthroscopic assessment of anatomic variations of the glenohumeral ligaments associated with recurrent anterior shoulder instability. Presented at the 59th Annual Meeting of the American Academy of Orthopaedic Surgeons, Washington, DC, 1992.

28. Rames RD, Morgan CD, Synder SJ: Anatomical variations of the glenohumeral ligaments. Presented at the 7th Open Meeting of the American Shoulder and Elbow Surgeons, Anaheim, CA, 1991.

29. Reider B, Inglis AE: The Bankart procedure modified by the use of Prolene pullout sutures. *J Bone Joint Surg (Am)* 64A:628–629, 1982.

30. Rose DJ, Moyer RA, et al: Arthroscopic suture capsulorrhaphy for anterior shoulder instability. Presented at the 57th Annual Meeting of the American Academy of Orthopaedic Surgeons, New Orleans, 1990.

31. Rowe CR, Patel D, Southmayd WW: The Bankart procedure. A long-term end-result study. *J Bone Joint Surg (Am)* 60A:1–16, 1978.

32. Sweeney HJ: Arthroscopic repair for recurrent dislocation of the shoulder. *Orthop Trans* 12:164, 1988.

33. Warner JD, et al: Arthroscopic Bankart repair utilizing an absorbable cannulated fixation device. Presented at the 58th Annual Meeting of the American Academy of Orthopaedic Surgeons, Anaheim, 1991.

34. Warner JP, Warren RF: Arthroscopic Bankart repair using a cannulated, absorbable fixation device. *Operative Tech Orthop* 1(2):192–198, 1991.

35. Weber SC: A prospective evaluation comparing arthroscopic and open treatment in the management of recurrent anterior glenohumeral dislocation. Presented at the 58th Annual Meeting of the American Academy of Orthopaedic Surgeons, Anaheim, 1991.

36. Wiley AM: Arthroscopy for shoulder instability and a technique for arthroscopic repair. *Arthroscopy* 4(1):25–30, 1988.

37. Wolf EM: Arthroscopic anterior shoulder capsulorrhaphy, in Paulos LE, Tibone JE (eds): *Operative Techniques in Shoulder Surgery.* Gaithersburg, Aspen, 1991.

38. Wolf EM, Wilk RM, Richmond JC: Arthroscopic Bankart repair using suture anchors. *Operative Tech Orthop* 1(2):184–191, 1991.

39. Wolin PM: Arthroscopic glenoid labrum suture repair. *Orthop Trans* 14:597, 1990.

40. Yahiro MA, Matthews LS: Arthroscopic stabilization procedures for recurrent anterior shoulder instability. *Orthop Rev* 18(11):1161–1168, 1989.

CHAPTER 8

Posterior Instability

Richard J. Hawkins
William D. Morin
Jeffrey S. Noble

INTRODUCTION

Posterior glenohumeral instability is a poorly understood pathologic entity infrequently seen in an athletic population. The true incidence of posterior shoulder instability is uncertain but has been reported to represent 2 to 4 percent of those patients who present with shoulder instability.[5,35] Because of its relatively uncommon occurrence, treatment of this variant of shoulder instability remains controversial. Diagnostic and therapeutic difficulty arises in part from the confusion in terminology. Confusion also exists between posterior subluxation and dislocation. True posterior dislocation is an acute entity that is rare and most commonly associated with a low incidence of recurrence. A more common presentation of this traumatic onset is with an impression defect as described by McLaughlin that requires careful treatment based on the size of the defect and duration of the dislocation.[21,25] Recurrent posterior subluxation is a common but distinct and separate entity, often not associated with trauma, and is troublesome related to therapeutic implications.

Historically, early reports in the literature failed to distinguish recurrent posterior dislocation from subluxation and involved small, poorly defined patient populations. Reported surgical options for recurrent posterior instability have included glenoid[5,9,13,19,24,31,40,45] and humeral osteotomies,[7,24] posterior bone blocks,[1,11,12,28] posterior Bankart repairs,[22] posterior-inferior capsular shifts,[4,15,18,20,26] staple capsulorrhaphy,[43,44] and posterior capsular plication with infraspinatus advancement[8,16,32,41] or biceps tendon transfers.[5] With the locked posterior dislocation, utilizing an anterior approach, procedures of subscapularis or tuberosity transfer as well as arthroplasty have been described.[21]

In 1967, Scott reported on three cases utilizing a posterior glenoid osteotomy to diminish glenoid retroversion in patients with recurrent posterior instability.[40] One of these actually was dislocated in the recovery room. Subsequent authors have reported variable results with this procedure.[3,11,28] Associated complications are worrisome and include joint contracture,[19] subcoracoid impingement,[13] intraarticular fracture,[23] and eventual development of glenohumeral arthritis,[23] particularly with violation of the joint surface.

In 1949, Fried reported satisfactory results in a small series of patients utilizing an extracapsular bone block for "habitual posterior dislocation of the shoulder joint."[11] More recently, Mowery and associates reported excellent results in four of five patients utilizing an intraarticular posterior bone block from the posterior iliac crest.[28]

Hindenach,[22] as well as Rowe,[35] authored case reports utilizing "Bankart's method of repair" for recurrent posterior dislocation of the shoulder. Both papers reported favorable outcome following posterior capsular reattachment through drill holes in the posterior glenoid rim.

The posterior-inferior modification of the inferior capsule shift as described by Neer and Foster[29] resulted in successful outcome in the series of Bigliani and associates,[4] and in the series of Goss and Costello.[15]

Tibone and associates reported less than satisfactory results with posterior staple capsulorrhaphy in 20 athletes.[44] Although their stability was reasonably well restored, only one patient returned to his preoperative throwing level.

Fronek and associates reported a success rate of 91 percent utilizing posterior capsulorrhaphy for posterior subluxation of the glenohumeral joint.[12] Despite the low recurrence rate, 70 percent of these athletes participated at a diminished level of competition or were forced to change to a less demanding situation.

PATHOANATOMY

Stability of the glenohumeral joint can be divided into static and dynamic components. Static stability is divided into that provided by the capsuloligamentous structures and the congruence of the articular surfaces. Dynamic stability of the glenohumeral joint is related to the complex interaction of the glenohumeral ligaments, rotator cuff musculature, and the large muscles of the shoulder, such as the deltoid.

The static stabilizers, which control posterior translation, have been studied by capsular cutting experiments on cadaveric specimens.[38,39,46,47] Using such experiments, Warren et al. evaluated the stability of the shoulder to posterior displacement in two positions: (1) the neutral position, and (2) the classic position for posterior dislocation—that of flexion, adduction, and internal rotation.[46] They noted that no posterior subluxation or dislocation occurred in the classic position after incising the infraspinatus, teres minor, and the entire posterior capsule from the 12 to 6 o'clock positions. In addition, no posterior dislocation occurred with simply incising the anterior inferior and middle capsule from the 6 to 3 o'clock position. It was only after incising the anterior superior capsule from the 3 to 12 o'clock position that posterior dislocation occurred. Schwartz et al. evaluated specimens positioned at 90° of abduction or adduction and neutral humeral rotation.[38] Variation of horizontal abduction was then used to simulate clinical examination. Through these studies, they concluded that the posterior inferior capsule provided the primary posterior restraint to posterior dislocation. In addition, the anterior superior capsule and superior glenohumeral ligaments provided secondary restraints to posterior dislocation. Recently, Harryman et al. evaluated the role of the rotator interval in instability of the shoulder, using selective cutting studies, and concluded that a major component in resisting posterior and inferior glenohumeral displacement was provided by an intact rotator interval capsule.[17] Their studies revealed that sectioning of the rotator interval capsule increased, and imbrication of these structures decreased, the translation seen on sulcus and posterior drawer tests. Furthermore, dislocation of the glenohumeral joint occurred both inferiorly and posteriorly when the interval capsule had been sectioned.

Clinically, Nobuhara and Ikeda, in characterizing lesions of the rotator cuff interval, noted in their experience that symptomatic posterior inferior instability of the glenohumeral joint substantially decreased after closing and reinforcement of the rotator cuff interval capsule.[30]

In addition to stability offered by capsuloligamentous and bony structures, Gibb et al. evaluated the concept of stability due to a limited joint volume.[14] Such a limited joint volume is able to resist translational forces when applied to the glenohumeral joint by creating a relative vacuum intraarticularly. Clinical testing, using anterior and posterior load-and-shift maneuvers and sulcus testing, were used both in the intact shoulder and after capsular venting. Simple capsular venting was shown to reduce the force necessary to translate the humeral head posteriorly by 10.8 N (43 percent).

The importance of dynamic stability has been theorized to aid in glenohumeral stability, either by pulling the head of the humerus posteriorly during external rotation or by compressing the humeral head congruently into the glenoid. Currently, a number of investigators are attempting to quantify and identify the crucial role dynamic stability plays in both posterior and overall glenohumeral stability.

It is apparent that many questions about posterior instability remain unsolved. Future emphasis will undoubtedly center around dynamic shoulder modeling to better delineate the restraints to posterior displacement.

CLASSIFICATION

The classification of posterior instability is presented in Table 8-1. Categories include traumatic vs. atraumatic and subluxation vs. dislocation. This is almost always a subluxation. The traumatic part of the classification is further subdivided into acute posterior dislocation (rarely without an impression defect) and a further subclassification of an acute posterior subluxation with an impression defect. When a traumatic posterior subluxation with an impression defect remains locked and undiagnosed, it becomes a "missed" chronic posterior dislocation.

Atraumatic recurrent posterior subluxation is subdivided into voluntary and involuntary, with four subtypes emerging: voluntary habitual (emotionally disturbed), voluntary—not willful (muscular control), involuntary positional (demonstrable by

TABLE 8-1
Classification of Posterior Instability

1. Acute posterior dislocation
   a. Without impression defect
   b. With impression defect
2. Chronic posterior dislocation locked (missed) with impression defect
3. Recurrent posterior subluxation
   a. Voluntary
      i. Habitual (willful)
      ii. Muscular control (not willful)
   b. Involuntary
      i. Positional (demonstrable)
      ii. Nonpositional (not demonstrable)

the patient with arm position), and involuntary (not demonstrable by the patient by arm position or muscular contraction). Direction of instability may be described as unidirectional (posterior), which is the subject of this chapter, but one must also be aware of the variants of multidirectional (posterior-inferior) or global instability that must be considered with unidirectional posterior instability.

The habitual subluxor was described by Rowe and associates in 1973.[36] The classic patient is an adolescent female with a psychiatric or personality disorder. Also described as "willful subluxors," these patients will not be helped by surgery and often require psychiatric evaluation. Although rare, it is important to distinguish this subset of patients in that they possess a subconscious desire to frustrate attempts at treatment and should not be considered surgical candidates.

Voluntary muscular and involuntary positional subluxors should not be confused with the previously described habitual subluxor. Although these patients can demonstrate their instability, they do not have a willful desire to do so, and exhibit no underlying psychiatric or personality disorder. Most often, these patients have a component of involuntary instability with certain movements or activities. The instability is termed voluntary muscular if demonstrable by muscular contractions and involuntary if posterior subluxation occurs with arm positioning. Some patients are both voluntary and involuntary.

The final subset of recurrent posterior subluxors is termed involuntary but is not demonstrable by the patient. Confirmation of this entity is difficult. As a diagnostic aid, "symptomatic translation" is useful in establishing the diagnosis clinically. During the load-and-shift maneuver, posterior translation of the proximal humerus on the glenoid rim may reproduce the patient's symptoms, strongly suggesting the diagnosis of posterior instability.

Acute Traumatic Posterior Dislocation

Acute posterior dislocation of the glenohumeral joint without an impression defect is extremely rare.[34,35] The subgroup of a locked posterior subluxation with an impression defect, sometimes termed a dislocation, is discussed in the next section.

HISTORY

The history of an acute posterior dislocation without an impression defect is that of either indirect violent trauma associated with seizures, electrical shock, motor vehicle accident, or more commonly, a blow pushing posteriorly on the forward outstretched extremity with the arm in a position of flexion, adduction, and internal rotation. This may occur in a football lineman with posteriorly directed force. Most commonly, the humeral head subluxes posteriorly and reduces spontaneously, although occasionally an actual dislocation may occur and remain temporarily locked out of the joint.

PHYSICAL EXAMINATION

In the majority of circumstances the acute posterior subluxation spontaneously reduces, as does the acute posterior dislocation, thus making it difficult to distinguish the two. With acute posterior dislocation presenting to the emergency department, the arm is in a fixed position, painful, with no motion and with the arm adducted and internally rotated. The patient is unable to externally rotate actively or passively.

RADIOGRAPHIC EXAMINATION

Appropriate radiographic examination is critical in diagnosing this entity. In all patients, a standard trauma series should be obtained, consisting of a true anteroposterior (AP) view of the shoulder at a right angle to the scapula, a transscapular lateral taken parallel to the scapula, and an axillary view. The axillary view provides the most accurate roentgenographic evidence of dislocation. It also identifies an impression defect should it be present,[20] which is a different subset, i.e., locked posterior subluxation. Axial plane computed tomography may be helpful in assessing glenoid version, glenoid rim changes, impression defects in the humeral head, and associated glenoid fractures.

TREATMENT

Closed treatment is usually effective in the acute setting. Following initial clinical and radiographic evaluation, reduction is facilitated by appropriate analgesia and muscular relaxants. The reduction is performed by flexion and adduction with longitudinal and lateral traction on the shoulder. Direct pressure may be applied to the humeral head from the posterior aspect of the shoulder to facilitate reduction. After successful reduction, stability of the shoulder should be assessed. If stable, the arm might be immobilized with the shoulder in mild extension and slight external rotation for 4 weeks. In fact, immobilization may be unnecessary. If unstable, the extremity should be immobilized in slight extension of the humerus and slight external rotation of the forearm for 6 weeks. Following immobilization, physiotherapy emphasizes rotational strengthening. Although accurate epidemiologic data are lacking, recurrent instability seems to be uncommon following an acute posterior dislocation if immediately diagnosed and appropriately managed. This fact is unknown in that acute posterior dislocations without impression defects diagnosed and reduced are rare.

Chronic Posterior Dislocation (Locked or Missed Posterior Dislocation)

A locked posterior dislocation of the shoulder results when an acute posterior dislocation exists in the presence of an impression defect and the humeral head remains in actual fact subluxed posteriorly. If diagnosed immediately, the term is a locked posterior subluxation. If the diagnosis becomes delayed, some refer to this as a missed posterior subluxation. The term dislocation has been applied, but, in fact, really this represents a subluxation with some of the humeral head outside the joint and some inside the joint. Unfortunately, if left untreated, progressive destruction of the humeral head may occur and glenoid changes may result, changing the prognosis and treatment.

HISTORY

The initial mechanism of injury may be related to multiple trauma, a seizure disorder, or an alcohol-related incident. When patients present acutely, they are very painful with limited motion, and appropriate roentgenographic investigation (particularly an axillary view) confirms the diagnosis. At late presentation, pain is diminished and patients complain of a functional deficit. The chief complaint is that of inability to externally rotate the arm, or in actual fact, an internal rotation deformity. These patients have difficulty combing their hair, washing their face, shaving, and even eating.[37] When physiotherapy does not improve their external rotation, these patients are often referred to the orthopedic surgeon with the diagnosis of "frozen shoulder."

PHYSICAL EXAMINATION

On clinical inspection, the humeral head appears prominent posteriorly, while the coracoid process is prominent anteriorly. The acromion process may appear squared off anteriorly and laterally. The key physical sign in establishing the diagnosis is the internal rotation deformity (Fig. 8-1).[20,21] The size of the impression defect correlates directly with the magnitude of the internal rotation deformity. This loss of external rotation significantly limits function of the extremity at the level of the head and neck. Rowe and Zarins also reported the inability of these patients to supinate the forearm when the arm is flexed forward.[37]

RADIOGRAPHIC EXAMINATION

Routine radiographs obtained initially in the absence of an axillary view may be interpreted as nor-

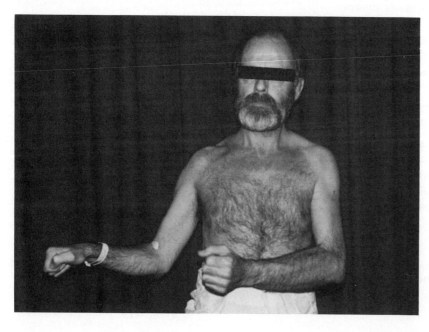

FIGURE 8-1
Clinical photograph of internal rotation deformity.

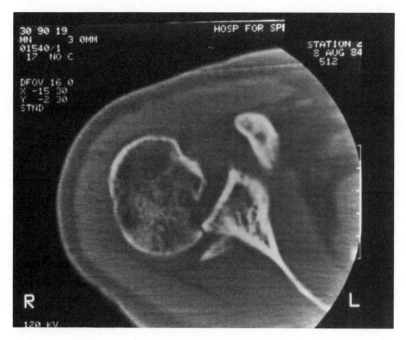

FIGURE 8-2
CT scan of chronic posterior dislocation with impression defect.

mal.[21] Frequently, radiographs are not obtained at the time of injury, especially if associated with seizure or alcoholism. The trauma series, as previously described, is essential in establishing the diagnosis of a locked posterior dislocation. The axillary view remains the key investigation to clearly demonstrate the posterior subluxation and delineate the size of the impression defect. The true AP and scapular lateral view are often difficult to interpret. The reason is that this is only a subluxation (some of the head in, some out). Several signs have been described on the AP view that suggest the diagnosis. These include internal rotation of the humerus, the vacant glenoid sign (reflecting a void in the anterior half of the glenoid fossa), and a "trough" line due to impaction of the humeral head. Nearly half of these patients will exhibit an undisplaced fracture of the greater tuberosity or proximal humerus.[20] These fractures may cause the reader not to focus on the glenohumeral joint. Computed tomography may be useful to elucidate the extent of the impression defect,

as well as to delineate associated glenoid changes (Fig. 8-2).

TREATMENT

Appropriate management of a locked posterior dislocation depends upon a variety of factors, including the duration of the dislocation, the size of the impression defect, the presence of changes in the glenoid, the functional disability of the patient, pain, and the general condition of the patient. Operative intervention is usually indicated in the active patient (Table 8-2).

When the duration of the dislocation is less than 6 weeks and the impression defect involves less than 20 percent of the articular surface, a gentle closed reduction as described in the previous section may be attempted. This reduction method may be successful in up to 50 percent of these delayed cases.[21] If stability is restored after reduction, the extremity might be immobilized in slight external rotation for

TABLE 8-2
Treatment Recommendations for Chronic Posterior Dislocation

Size of impression defect, %	Duration of dislocation	Treatment
20	<6 weeks	Closed reduction immobilization*
20–50	6 weeks to 6 months	Subscapularis transfer
>50	<6 months	Hemiarthroplasty† (20° retroversion)
>50	<6 months	Hemiarthroplasty† (0° retroversion)

*If unstable postreduction, proceed to subscapularis transfer.

†If significant concomitant glenoid erosion, may require total shoulder arthroplasty.

107

4 to 6 weeks. Perhaps immobilization is unnecessary. If instability with internal rotation persists after closed reduction, surgical reconstruction may be entertained.

When surgical reconstruction is necessary, the type of procedure depends upon the amount of intact articular cartilage remaining to be reduced into the glenoid fossa. If more than 50 percent of the articular cartilage is viable and can be reduced, a subscapularis transfer (described by McLaughlin and modified by Neer to include a portion of the tuberosity) is indicated.[26] Utilizing an anterior approach, the subscapularis insertion is identified and osteotomized from the lesser tuberosity. The humeral head is inspected and gently manipulated into the glenoid fossa. The subscapularis is then sutured into the defect via drill holes in bone. Postoperatively, immobilization in slight external rotation is maintained for 6 weeks.

With dislocation of greater than 6 months, progressive degeneration of the humeral head may ensue. When this occurs, or when the impression defect involves more than 50 percent of the articular surface, hemiarthroplasty may be indicated. When concomitant glenoid erosion with secondary degenerative changes is present, total shoulder arthroplasty may be warranted. To ensure stability when inserting the humeral component, retroversion should be decreased from the normal 35 to 40°. In general, if the posterior dislocation has been present less than 6 months, the component might be positioned in approximately 20° of retroversion. If the dislocation has been present for greater than 6 months, the humeral component might be placed in neutral version.[21] Using these guidelines, the final version can be adjusted with trial components in place. Plication of the posterior capsule may augment stability, preventing posterior subluxation or dislocation of the humeral component. If stability is achieved following arthroplasty, early motion may be initiated. If there is concern regarding stability of the implant, immobilization in external rotation is indicated.

Recurrent Posterior Subluxation

HISTORY

Recurrent posterior subluxation is the most common form of posterior instability and may be symptomatic, especially with athletic endeavors. Reports in the literature have referred to this entity as recurrent dislocation when, in fact, in most circumstances it represents only a subluxation. Unlike recurrent anterior instability, most patients with recurrent posterior instability do not present with an initial episode of significant trauma requiring reduction.[19,36] The most common scenario is that of an overuse endeavor with the shoulder, followed by an appreciation that it is slipping out of joint with arm positioning. With time, patients often learn to duplicate this maneuver and demonstrate the instability. Occasionally, it may progress so that the patient can sublux the shoulder with muscular contraction posteriorly. Most patients are only mildly symptomatic, and rehabilitation is the appropriate treatment regimen. Clinical laxity or excessive translation may be present in both shoulders, but it is usually the dominant shoulder that is symptomatic.[33] Patients often present to the doctor because of painful tendinitis of the shoulder associated with instability. This is especially so in overhead athletes such as throwers, swimmers, and volleyball players.[39] In the rare patient refractory to rehabilitation, surgery may be warranted.

PHYSICAL EXAMINATION

In contrast to anterior instability, most patients with recurrent posterior subluxation can demonstrate the instability. This is either by a muscular contraction, termed voluntary, or by arm positioning, termed involuntary. In the usual situation, as the patient elevates the arm, the shoulder subluxes posteriorly, and as it approaches the coronal plane of the body, in either elevation or horizontal abduction, the shoulder visibly reduces (Fig. 8-3). Scapular winging is very common with posterior instability, especially as the joint subluxes. Eliminating this winging may lessen or eliminate the posterior instability. Sometimes patients cannot demonstrate the instability and further testing is done to determine direction. Also, in contrast to anterior instability, patients with recurrent posterior subluxation do not usually exhibit an apprehension sign. Frequently, when stressed posteriorly, they are uncomfortable, but they are usually not apprehensive as applied to anterior instability. Patients who have involuntary posterior instability and cannot demonstrate it by any means usually have a reproduction of their symptom complex when the humeral head is translated posteriorly in the glenoid fossa. They often have a greater degree of posterior translation going at least to the rim when compared with the normal population, but not as excessive as one might expect. There is no muscle wasting, usually a full range of motion, minimal tenderness, and very occasional crepitus, particularly with translation maneuvers. Occasion-

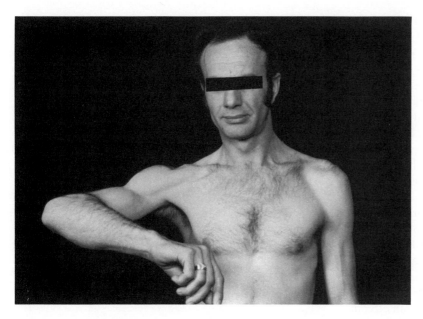

FIGURE 8-3
Clinical demonstration of posterior subluxation by arm positioning in the plane of adduction, internal rotation, and forward flexion.

ally, these patients have excessive flexibility in their joints, probably best assessed by abducting the thumb toward the forearm. Strength is often normal, but if there is a painful tendinitis, there may be pain-related weakness.

Assessment of posterior translation is carried out with the "load-and-shift" maneuver. With the patient sitting, the examiner grasps the humeral head between the thumb and index finger. While gently applying a compressive load to the glenoid with the humeral head, an attempt is made to translate the humeral head posterior and anteriorly. The extent of translation is then compared with the contralateral shoulder. Symptomatic posterior translation is helpful in confirming the diagnosis of posterior instability. When the humeral head is translated posteriorly, almost all patients with posterior instability appreciate that translation is their problem. Excessive translation in the absence of symptomatic reproduction must be interpreted cautiously. It is not uncommon for many normal patients to translate posteriorly almost to the glenoid rim.[27] The sulcus sign is determined by longitudinal traction on the upper arm, noting how far the humeral head moves away from the undersurface of the acromion. It is important to examine for this sign because it may be suggestive of an associated multidirectional instability pattern, rather than unidirectional posterior instability.

Other parameters for hyperflexibility in such patients besides thumb to forearm are extension of the middle finger parallel to upper arm, hyperextension of the elbows, patellar hypermobility, and an ability to touch the palms to the floor without bending the knees.

RADIOGRAPHIC EXAMINATION

There are seldom any plain film radiographic changes, although posterior rim erosive defects may rarely be observed. Stress radiographs are often useful in that an axillary view with the shoulder subluxed helps determine excessive translation. This can also be documented fluoroscopically. Computed axial tomography and MRI have not proved to date very helpful, although there are recent publications of MRI changes with posterior instability located in the posterior capsular area. In difficult cases, diagnostic arthroscopy, associated with an examination under anesthesia, may be helpful.

TREATMENT

Fortunately, most patients with recurrent posterior subluxation of the shoulder have minimal pain and functional disability. Physiotherapy continues to form the cornerstone of treatment, consisting of a rotational and scapular strengthening program. Rotational strengthening may be achieved utilizing a resistant rubber cord, emphasizing eccentric and concentric, external and internal rotation of the shoulder. Scapular strengthening may be achieved with seated rows for serratus and the rhomboids, and shrugs for the trapezius, in both a concentric and an eccentric mode. Rockwood, along with Fronek and Warren, have reported success of a structured rehabilitation program in the treatment of recurrent posterior instability.[10,12,33]

Operative treatment may be considered in patients who remain symptomatic and functionally disabled despite an adequate trial of physiotherapy and activity modification. This may be particularly

109

applicable in the athlete who has difficulty with overhead throwing, swimming, volleyball, and other sporting endeavors because of posterior instability. Pain may be an associated component, increasing the disability of the instability. These patients present to the orthopedic surgeon as either a painful shoulder with a disability or a functional disability related to the instability or a combination of the two. The usual indication for surgical treatment is pain. It is important for the surgeon to identify habitual or willful voluntary subluxors, since these patients will thwart any surgical intervention.

Arthroscopy may be useful diagnostically and sometimes therapeutically, especially in throwing athletes who have posterior instability.[39] Frequently other findings in the joint exist in the overhead athlete, and sometimes minor debridement or labral debridement may prove beneficial, at least temporarily, in terms of relieving pain. However, it seldom affects the instability pattern.

There are several described operative procedures in the literature, all with varying success.[2] One must be cautious to rule out multidirectional instability, or else a specific operative procedure, consisting of a shift, from either the back or the front, probably is indicated. For unidirectional posterior instability, however, there are several described procedures. In situations in which there is excessive glenoid version or glenoid deficiency, certain procedures may be entertained. Unlike anterior instability, where many surgeons correct the pathology frequently with unidirectional posterior instability, most surgeons perform one operative procedure, which is their favorite. However, in certain circumstances, for example, if one performs a capsular tenodesis posteriorly and there is an associated reverse Bankart lesion, it also requires correction.

Common operative procedures applied for posterior unidirectional instability are some form of capsulorrhaphy, a reverse Putti-Platt, or a posterior glenoid osteotomy. A posterior inferior capsular shift is reserved for patients who have multidirectional instability with an associated inferior component.

SURGICAL PROCEDURES

Posterior Capsular Infraspinatus Tenodesis

It is our preference in a patient who has recurrent unidirectional posterior subluxation to perform a soft tissue procedure employing the capsule and infraspinatus tendon (Figs. 8-4, 8-5, 8-6). At the joint level, with the arm in neutral position, the posterior capsule is often thin and translucent and the infra-

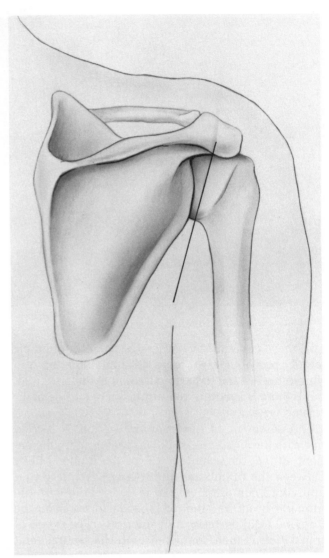

FIGURE 8-4
Posterior capsular infraspinatus tenodesis/posterior glenoid osteotomy. A longitudinal incision is made starting 2 cm medial to the posterolateral aspect of the acromion and extending along the posterior axillary line.

spinatus muscular. The secret to the procedure employed is to move more laterally toward the greater tuberosity where the capsule is thicker and the infraspinatus more tendinous.

Preoperatively, the patient may be placed into an outrigger shoulder spica cast with a long arm component and a detachable spica bar. Immediately postoperatively while in the operating suite, the spica bar can be incorporated with the arm positioned in 5° extension, 10 to 20° abduction, and 20° of external rotation. The difficulty in doing this is that the weight of the cast on the arm sometimes interferes with the surgery. It also poses some difficulties in draping, so frequently we put on only the waist band portion of the spica.

110

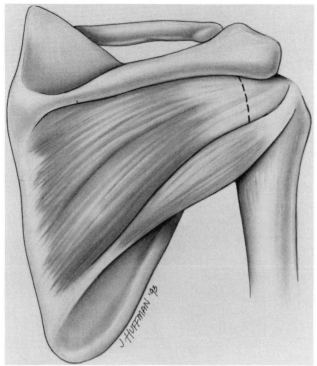

FIGURE 8-5
After the deltoid fibers are split bluntly, a vertical incision is made through both the infraspinatus tendon and capsule 1 cm lateral to the glenohumeral joint with the arm held in neutral rotation.

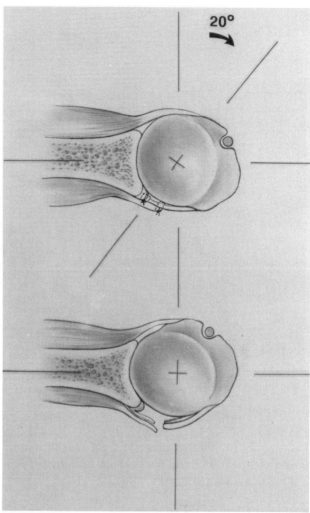

FIGURE 8-6
The capsulotomy is performed with the arm in neutral rotation. (Top) With the arm then positioned in 20° of external rotation, the lateral portion of the infraspinatus tendon and underlying capsule is sutured into the intact labrum. The medial infraspinatus tendon and capsule is then reflected laterally and sutured into place on the remaining capsule. (Bottom)

The surgery is performed in the lateral decubitus position with the operative shoulder draped free. A longitudinal incision commences just at the posterolateral corner of the acromion and extends distally to the posterior axillary crease (Fig. 8-4). The underlying deltoid is identified and split in line with its fibers, utilizing blunt digital dissection. Appropriate retractors are placed under the deltoid, under the acromion, to retract superiorly, and a large right-angle retractor to retract inferiorly. This reveals the underlying infraspinatus and teres minor fibers, which run at right angles to the deltoid. With the arm positioned in neutral rotation, a vertical incision approximately 3 to 4 mm parallel to the glenoid is made directly through the infraspinatus tendon and through the capsule to identify the joint surfaces (Fig. 8-5). It is critical that the incision not be made too far laterally or when repairing down to the posterior glenoid labrum, the shoulder will be too tight. Likewise, too far medially, the tissue is not of sufficient quality to allow an adequate repair.

The posterior glenoid labrum is identified. Rarely it may be detached and must be repaired to the glenoid through drill holes. Usually it is not detached, and the lateral flap of the infraspinatus and capsule is sutured down to the posterior glenoid labrum with approximately four strong sutures (Fig. 8-6). When this is completed and the arm is internally rotated, it usually comes to about 20° of internal rotation and stops at that point, secured there by the repair. In our experience, that seems to be appropriate.

Finally, the infraspinatus is overlapped, but it is mostly muscle fibers at this level and does not provide much of a substantial repair. The deltoid fibers fall together, subcutaneous tissue and skin are closed in the usual fashion, and the patient may be positioned in the splint in the above-described position. Occasionally, we simply bolster the arm with pillows, keeping the patient quiet for a day, until he or she can sit up and a spica can be applied (Fig. 8-7).

111

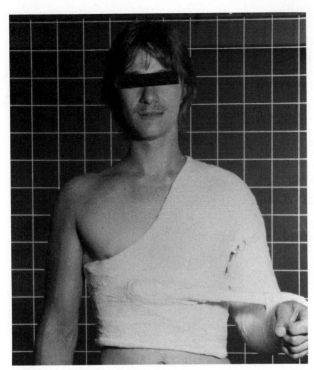

FIGURE 8-7
Postoperative spica cast immobilization.

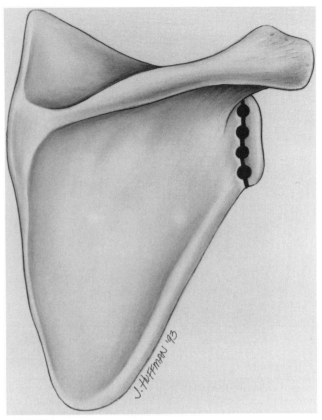

FIGURE 8-8
Bicortical drill holes placed through both the anterior and posterior cortex are made in a line 1 cm medial to the glenoid surface to mark the osteotomy site. An oscillating saw is used to connect the drill holes posteriorly, leaving an intact anterior cortex.

The time of immobilization is 4 weeks for traumatic posterior instability and 6 weeks for atraumatic posterior instability patients.

Posterior Glenoid Osteotomy

There are surgeons in North America and Europe who prefer a glenoid osteotomy for recurrent posterior instability (Figs. 8-4, 8-8, 8-9, 8-10). The concern with posterior glenoid osteotomy relates to the previously mentioned complications (especially an intraarticular fracture) that can occur. It may also be risky to change version in such patients for fear of creating another instability. If this procedure is to be employed, it should be combined with a capsule and infraspinatus reconstruction, appropriate postoperative immobilization, and very careful attention to detail regarding the osteotomy itself. The patient may be positioned in the spica preoperatively as described or may be left to the postoperative state, as described as an alternative option.

The incision is a straight-line incision, as previously described for the capsular infraspinatus repair (Fig. 8-8). The deltoid is similarly retracted. The infraspinatus is identified and reflected 1 cm medial to its tuberosity insertion. With the arm in neutral position, a vertical capsulotomy is made 1 cm lateral to the palpable glenoid rim. The medial capsule is reflected sharply from the glenoid neck. The poste-

rior labrum is left attached to the posterior glenoid rim.

A humeral head retractor facilitates visualization and allows determination of orientation of the joint surface. The line of the posterior osteotomy is selected at least 1 cm from and parallel to the glenoid articular surface and bicortical drill holes are created to delineate the osteotomy site. The drill holes in the glenoid neck are depth gauged and recorded. A small oscillating saw is used to connect the drill holes posteriorly, being mindful of the previously recorded depth measurements (Fig. 8-8). The anterior cortex should be maintained. Once the osteotomy is completed, a ½-in osteotome is gently placed and the osteotomy site is hinged upon the anterior cortex and periosteum (Fig. 8-9). A tricortical bone graft is harvested from the posterior acromion.

The osteotomy is hinged open with an osteotome, and a tricortical graft fashioned from the posterior acromion is inserted appropriately, usually allowing immediate stability (Fig. 8-10). Usually, no hardware is necessary.

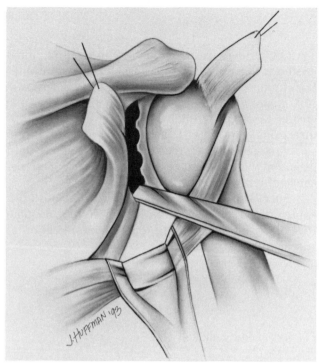

FIGURE 8-9
A ½-in osteotome is used to open up the osteotomy, hinging it upon the anterior cortex and periosteum.

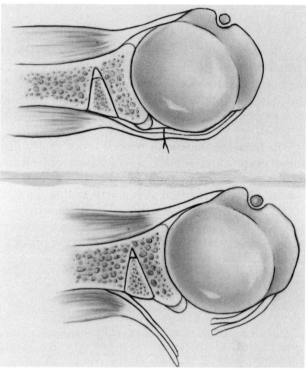

FIGURE 8-10
With the osteotomy opened, fashioned tricortical bone graft is positioned in the osteotomy, allowing early stability. (Top) The posterior soft tissue repair of capsule and infraspinatus is then completed. (Bottom)

With the arm positioned in neutral rotation, the capsule and infraspinatus are overlapped to the posterior labrum, the deltoid is allowed to close, and the remainder of the wound is closed in the usual fashion.

Posterior Inferior Capsular Shift

This procedure is reserved for multidirectional instability patients and is described appropriately in that section. It is, however, important to realize that some patients with posterior instability have an inferior component and therefore the shift should be performed. It is actually our preference, in the presence of inferior and posterior instability, to operate from the front because of the ability to close the superior interval and reconstruct the superior coracohumeral ligament more advantageously, restoring superior and anterior stability.

REHABILITATION

Following the initial period of spica cast immobilization, the rehabilitation proceeds in a similar fashion for all three surgical techniques. A three-phase program is initiated upon removal of the spica cast. Phase I consists of gentle passive motion emphasizing internal rotation, external rotation, and forward elevation and proceeds for approximately 4 weeks. Phase II follows and consists of active motion with terminal stretch, again emphasizing external rotation, internal rotation, and forward elevation. This phase continues for 2 to 4 weeks. Phase III consists of a strengthening program utilizing an elastic resistance cord, usually beginning 10 to 12 weeks postoperatively. This strengthening program includes external rotators, internal rotators, shoulder shrugs, and narrow grip seated rows and emphasizes the eccentric as well as the concentric contraction phase. Overhead athletic activity is allowed at 4 months postoperatively, with return to contact sports permitted at 6 months.

SUMMARY

An acute traumatic posterior dislocation without an impression defect requiring reduction is rare.

Locked posterior dislocation with an impression defect requires special clinical examination and an axillary view for diagnosis and its treatment depends upon the size of the impression defect and the duration of the dislocation. It is very rare in the athletic population, but if diagnosed, appropriate treatment will hopefully restore function.

113

Recurrent posterior subluxation is the most common form of posterior instability, perhaps not as uncommon as previously thought in the athlete. Fortunately, most patients with this pathology respond to a regimen of physiotherapy and activity modification.

In those patients who remain functionally disabled, despite an adequate trial of conservative treatment, operative intervention may prove helpful. Careful patient selection is essential in that the voluntary willful subluxor will not be helped by surgery. The best results are obtained in normal patients with normal tissues who have a traumatic onset to their instability pattern.

Our preference in patients with unidirectional posterior instability is to perform a capsular and infraspinatus tenodesis type of operation to the posterior glenoid labrum, utilizing the tissue near the greater tuberosity, which is of better quality. Multidirectional instability must be ruled out and, if present, an alternative procedure performed. Glenoid osteotomy is preferred by some but is of concern because of potential complications.

Successful management for recurrent posterior subluxation requires accurate diagnosis, an adequate trial of physiotherapy, and judicious application of surgical reconstruction.

REFERENCES

1. Ahlgren SA, Hedlund T, Nistor L: Idiopathic posterior instability of the shoulder joint: Results of operation with posterior bone graft. *Acta Orthop Scand* 49:600, 1978.
2. Bell RH, Noble JS: An appreciation of posterior instability of the shoulder. *Clin Sports Med* 10(4):887, 1991.
3. Bestasrd E: Glenoplasty: A simple reliable method of correcting recurrent posterior dislocation of the shoulder. *Orthop Rev* 5:29, 1976.
4. Bigliani LU, Endrizzi DP, McIlveen SJ: Operative management of posterior shoulder instability. *Orthop Trans* 13:232, 1989.
5. Boyd HB, Sisk TD: Recurrent posterior dislocation of the shoulder. *J Bone Joint Surg (Am)* 54A:779–786, 1972.
6. Brewer BJ, Wubbern RC, Carrera GF: Excessive retroversion of the glenoid cavity. *J Bone Joint Surg (Am)* 68A:724, 1986.
7. Chaudhuri GK, Sengupta A, Saha AK: Rotation osteotomy of the shaft of the humerus for recurrent dislocation of the shoulder. *Acta Orthop Scand* 45:193, 1974.
8. Dugas RW, Scerpella TA, Clancy WG: Surgical treatment of symptomatic posterior shoulder instability. *Orthop Trans* 14:245, 1990.
9. English E, Macnab I: Recurrent posterior dislocation of the shoulder. *Can J Surg* 17:147, 1974.
10. Farek J, Pavlov BH, Warren RF: Posterior subluxation of the glenohumeral joint: Nonsurgical and surgical treatment. *Orthop Trans* 10:220, 1986.
11. Fried A: Habitual posterior dislocation of the shoulder joint: A report on five operated cases. *Acta Orthop Scand* 18:329, 1949.
12. Fronek J, Warren RJ, Bower M: Posterior subluxation of the glenohumeral joint. *J Bone Joint Surg (Am)* 71A:205, 1989.
13. Gerber C, Ganz R, Vinh TS: Glenoplasty for recurrent posterior shoulder instability. *Clin Orthop* 216:70, 1987.
14. Gibb TD, Sidles JA, Harryman DT II, et al: The effect of capsular venting on glenohumeral laxity. *Clin Orthop* 268:120–127, 1991.
15. Goss TP, Costello G: Recurrent symptomatic posterior glenohumeral subluxation. *Orthop Rev* 17:1024, 1988.
16. Greenhill BJ: Persistent posterior shoulder dislocation: Its diagnosis and treatment by posterior Putti-Platt repair. *J Bone Joint Surg (Am)* 54B:763, 1972.
17. Harryman DT II, Sidles JA, Harris SL, et al: Role of the rotator interval capsule in passive motion and stability of the shoulder. *J Bone Joint Surg (Am)* 74A:53–66, 1992.
18. Hawkins RJ: Unrecognized dislocations of the shoulder, in Stauffer ES (ed): *Instructional Course Lectures*, The American Academy of Orthopaedic Surgeons. St Louis, Mosby, 1984, vol 34, p 258.
19. Hawkins RJ, Koppert G, Johnston G: Recurrent posterior instability of the shoulder. *J Bone Joint Surg (Am)* 66A:169, 1984.
20. Hawkins RJ, McCormack RG: Posterior shoulder instability. *Orthopaedics* 11:101, 1988.
21. Hawkins RJ, Neer CS, Planta RM, et al: Locked posterior dislocation of the shoulder. *J Bone Joint Surg (Am)* 69A:9, 1987.

THE COLOR PLATES

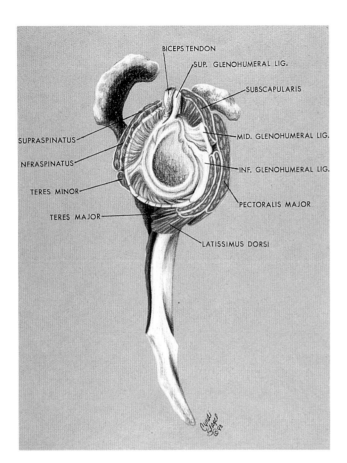

1 The anatomic relationships of the superior, middle, and inferior glenohumeral ligaments.

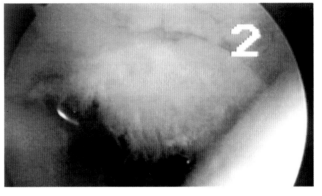

3 Rotator cuff tear.

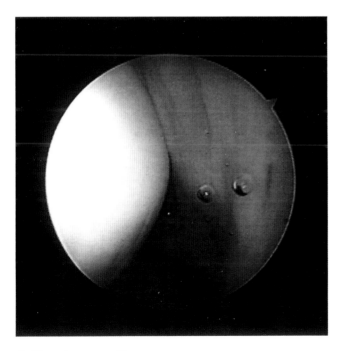

2 Normal rotator cuff.

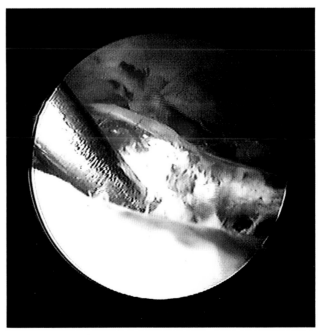

4 Bankart lesion prerepair.

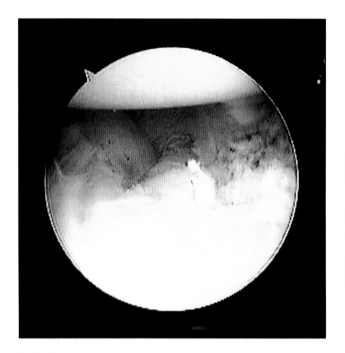

5 Bankart lesion postrepair.

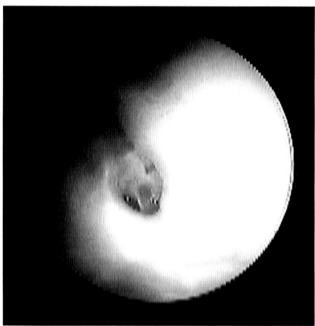

7 Punctate bare area.

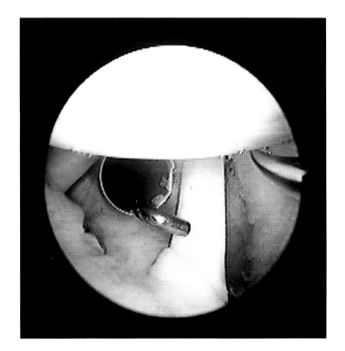

6 Triangular space.

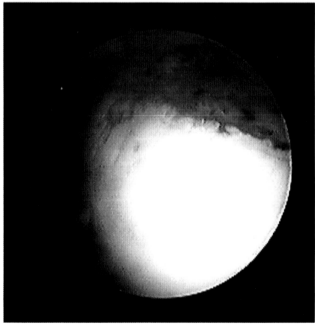

8 Hill-Sachs lesion.

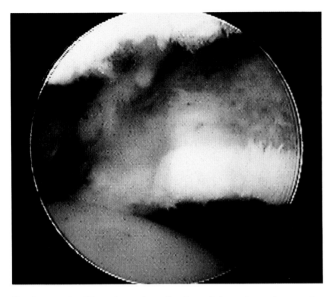

9 A motorized burr is used to abrade and decorticate the anterior glenoid neck and rim. This step requires attention to detail to ensure an adequate decorticated cancellous surface.

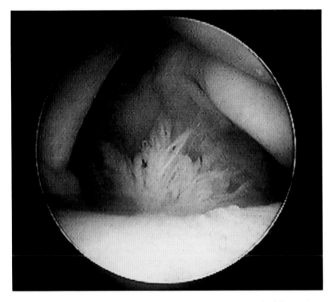

10 Portal placement. The "safe triangle" is formed by the biceps tendon (left), the subscapularis tendon (right), and the glenoid (bottom).

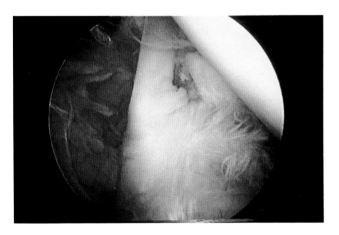

11 Intraoperative photograph of type I SLAP lesion.

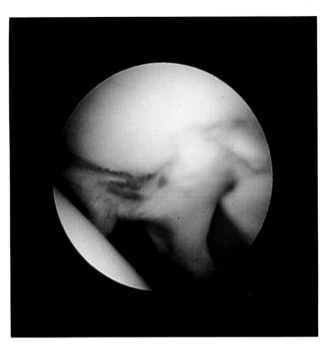

12 Intraoperative photograph of type II SLAP lesion.

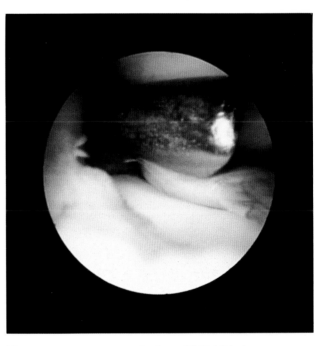

13 Intraoperative photograph of type III SLAP lesion.

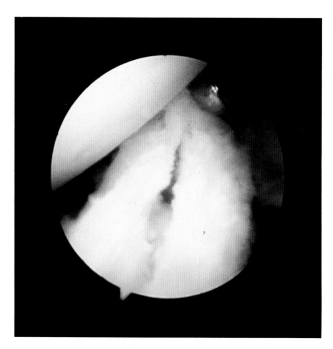

14 Intraoperative photograph of type IV SLAP lesion.

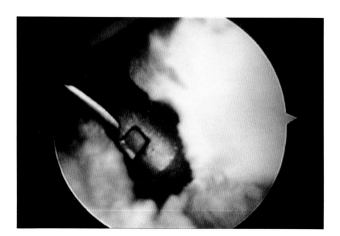

15 The suture Shuttle Relay is a device that will pass easily through a spinal needle or suture punch and that is used to pull non-absorbable suture through soft tissue.

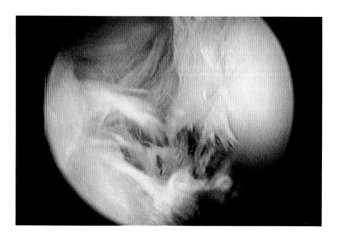

16 A large articular surface partial tear of the supraspinatus tendon is visualized arthroscopically.

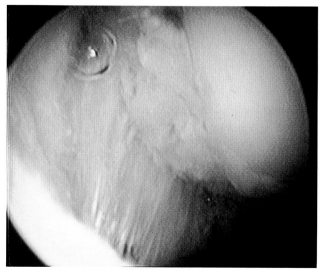

17 The same supraspinatus tendon as in Plate 16 following arthroscopic debridement of the tear. Note the remaining intact fibers.

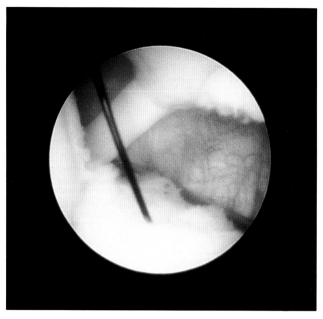

18 The suture marker is passed through the area of partial rotator cuff tearing to allow identification of the corresponding area of the rotator cuff when the bursal surface is examined.

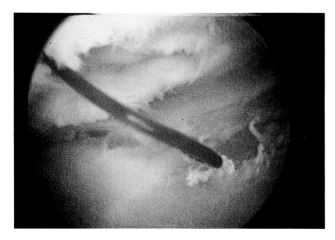

19 The suture marker passes through a partial tear on the bursal surface of this supraspinatus tendon.

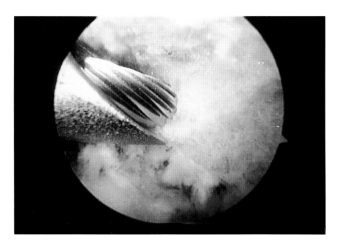

20 The width of the Acromionizer burr may be compared with the anterior acromial edge to determine the amount of bone resected.

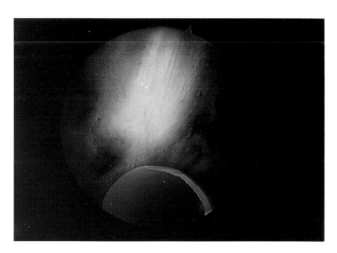

21 Arthroscopic view of normal coracoacromial ligament. Insertion of ligament at anteromedial corner of acromion. Cannula is at left of acromial anteromedial corner.

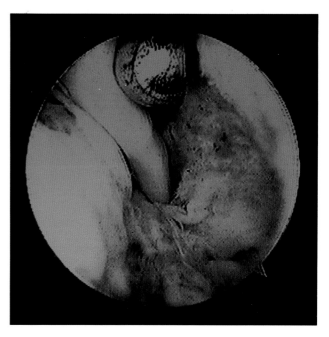

22 Arthroscopic view of angiofibroblastic rotator cuff tendinosis. Normal biceps tendon is seen passing past major changes in supraspinatus tendon.

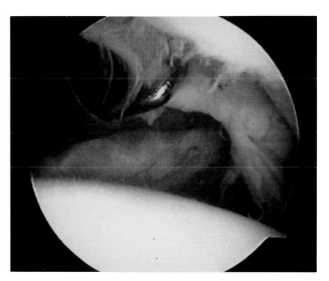

23 Arthroscopic view of partial detachment of degenerated labrum. Probe retracts labrum from glenoid rim.

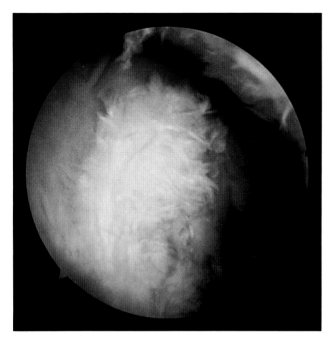

24 Arthroscopic demonstration of the classic area of abrasion of the undersurface of the acromion.

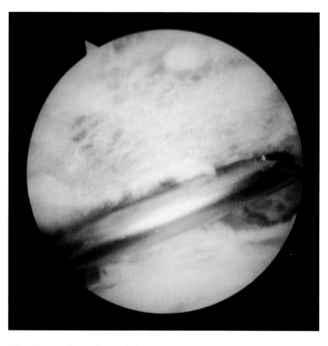

26 The undersurface of the acromion is flat and smooth and in the plane of the posterior acromion.

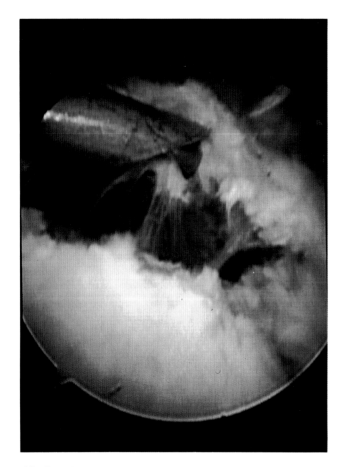

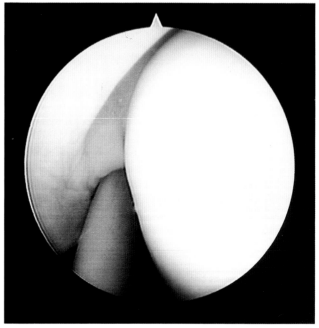

27 Arthroscopic view of a normal shoulder with biceps tendon, rotator cuff, and humeral head in view.

25 Completed coracoacromial ligament release.

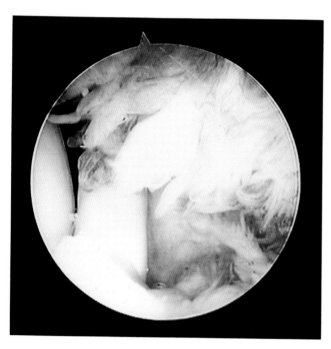

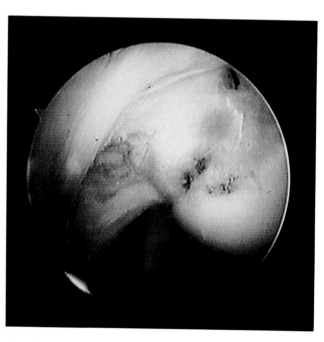

28 Arthroscopic view of an acute synovitis stage with patient involved with frozen shoulder. Portions of the biceps tendon is covered with proliferative synovial fringes.

30 After arthroscopic debridement of the tear shown in Plate 29.

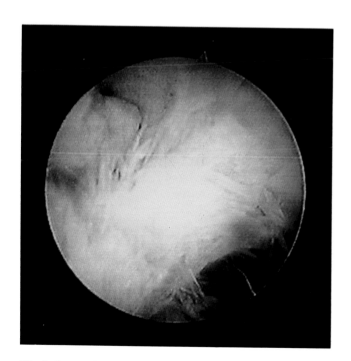

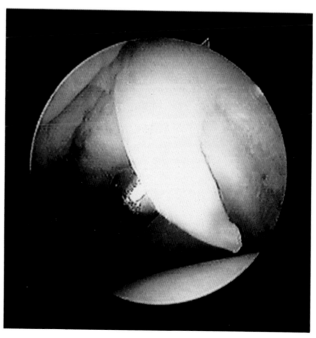

29 Arthroscopic view of a right shoulder from the posterior portal. An undersurface tear of the supraspinatus in a professional baseball player.

31 Arthroscopic view of a right shoulder from the anterior portal. An anterior labral flap tear in a professional pitcher.

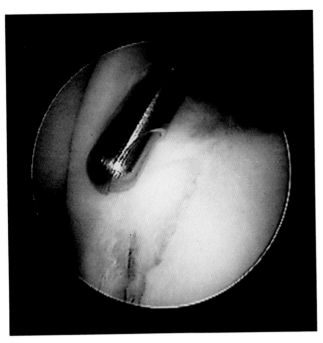

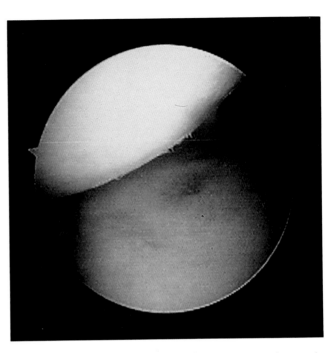

32 Arthroscopic view of a right shoulder from a posterior portal. Superior anterior labral tear at the biceps insertion after debridement in a professional pitcher.

34 Arthroscopic view of a right shoulder from the anterior portal. Defect in the glenoid is a normal finding, a "centering lesion," as seen in this professional pitcher.

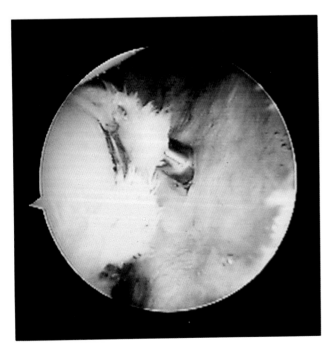

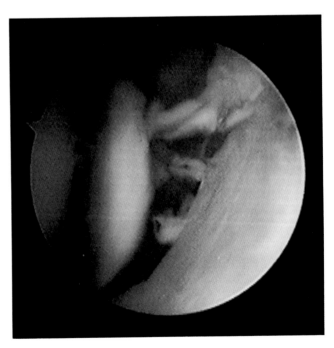

33 Arthroscopic view of a right shoulder from the anterior portal. Posterior labral tear in a professional pitcher.

35 Arthroscopic view of a right shoulder from the anterior portal. Osteochondrotic lesion displaced from the posterior glenoid is seen in a 22-year-old professional baseball player.

22. Hindenach JCR: Recurrent posterior dislocation of the shoulder. *J Bone Joint Surg (Am)* 29A:582–586, 1947.
23. Johnston GH, Hawkins RJ, Haddad R, et al: A complication of posterior glenoid osteotomy for recurrent posterior shoulder instability. *Clin Orthop* 187:147, 1984.
24. Kretzler HH Jr: Scapular osteotomy for posterior shoulder dislocation. Proceedings of the Western Orthopaedic Association. *J Bone Joint Surg (Am)* 56A:197, 1974.
25. McLaughlin HL: Locked posterior subluxation of the shoulder: Diagnosis and treatment. *Surg Clin North Am* 43:1621, 1963.
26. McLaughlin HL: Posterior dislocation of the shoulder. *J Bone Joint Surg (Am)* 34A:584, 1952.
27. Morton KS: The unstable shoulder: Recurring subluxation. *Injury* 10:304, 1978.
28. Mowery CA, Garfin SR, Booth RE, et al: Recurrent posterior dislocation of the shoulder: Treatment using a bone block. *J Bone Joint Surg (Am)* 67A:777, 1985.
29. Neer CS, Foster CR: Inferior capsular shift for involuntary inferior and multidirectional instability of the shoulder. *J Bone Joint Surg (Am)* 62A:897, 1980.
30. Nobuhara K, Ikeda H: Rotator interval lesion. *Clin Orthop* 223:44–50, 1987.
31. Norwood LA, Terry GL: Posterior shoulder subluxation. *Am J Sports Med* 12:25, 1984.
32. Roberts A, Wickstrom J: Prognosis of posterior dislocation of the shoulder. *Acta Orthop Scand* 42:328, 1971.
33. Rockwood CA Jr: Subluxation and dislocations about the shoulder, in Rockwood CA, Green DP (eds): *Fracture in Adults*. Philadelphia, Lippincott, 1984, pp 722–860.
34. Rockwood CA Jr: The diagnosis of acute posterior dislocation of the shoulder. *J Bone Joint Surg (Am)* 48A:1220, 1966.
35. Rowe CR: Prognosis in dislocations of the shoulder. *J Bone Joint Surg (Am)* 38A:957–977, 1956.
36. Rowe CR, Pierce DS, Clark JG, et al: Voluntary dislocation of the shoulder: A preliminary report on a clinical, electromyographic and psychiatric study of 26 patients. *J Bone Joint Surg (Am)* 55A:445, 1973.
37. Rowe CR, Zarins B: Chronic unreduced dislocations of the shoulder. *J Bone Joint Surg (Am)* 64A:494, 1982.
38. Schwartz E, O'Brien SJ, Warren FR, et al: Capsular restraints to anterior-posterior motion of the shoulder. *Orthop Trans* 12:727, 1988.
39. Schwartz E, Warren RF, O'Brien SJ, et al: Posterior shoulder instability. *Orthop Clin North Am* 18:L409–419, 1987.
40. Scott DJ Jr: Treatment of recurrent posterior dislocations of the shoulder by glenoplasty. *J Bone Joint Surg* 49A:471, 1967.
41. Severin E: Anterior and posterior recurrent dislocation of the shoulder: The Putti-Platt operation. *Acta Orthop Scand* 23:14, 1953.
42. Surin V, Blader S, Boras GM: Rotational osteotomy of the humerus for posterior instability of the shoulder. *J Bone Joint Surg (Am)* 72A:181, 1990.
43. Tibone JE, Prietto C, Jobe FW: Staple capsulorrhaphy for recurrent posterior shoulder dislocation. *Am J Sports Med* 9:135, 1981.
44. Tibone JE, Ting A: Capsulorrhaphy with a staple for recurrent posterior subluxation of the shoulder. *J Bone Joint Surg (Am)* 72A:999, 1990.
45. Vegter J, Marti RK: Treatment of posterior dislocation of the shoulder by osteotomy of the neck of the scapula. *J Bone Joint Surg (Am)* 63B:288, 1981.
46. Warren RF, Kornblatt IB, Marchand R: Static factors affecting posterior shoulder stability. *Orthop Trans* 8:89, 1984.
47. Weber SC, Caspari RB: A biomechanical evaluation of the restraints to posterior shoulder dislocation. *Arthroscopy* 5:115–121, 1989.

CHAPTER 9

Superior Labral Injuries

Ronald P. Karzel
Stephen J. Snyder

INTRODUCTION

Injuries to the superior glenoid labrum of the shoulder joint are frequently overlooked in the differential diagnosis of shoulder pain in the athlete. However, with the increased use of preoperative imaging studies such as magnetic resonance imaging, computed tomographic arthrography, and more recently, magnetic resonance arthrography, it is now possible to diagnose such problems preoperatively in many cases. Even more important, refinements in diagnostic shoulder arthroscopy have led to an improved understanding of the normal variations in labral anatomy, as well as improved visualization of labral pathology. It is now possible to treat most labral pathology with arthroscopic techniques.

Pathology involving the superior labrum of the shoulder is particularly common. Large tensile forces are exerted on the superior labrum by the attached biceps tendon, and in fact, the biceps tendon insertion blends into the superior labrum, which in turn is attached to the superior glenoid neck. Not only does the force of the biceps tendon contribute to the initial injury, but once an avulsion type of injury has occurred, continued pull of the biceps tendon on the detached labrum may prevent apposition of the labrum to the glenoid, and therefore interfere with the healing process. A second factor contributing to superior labral injury is the "meniscoid" configuration of the superior labrum that is often present. There is normally significant variation in labral size and appearance among individuals. Detrisac and Johnson have classified the pattern of labral attachment to the glenoid into two types.[1] In one type of labral attachment, the labrum is firmly anchored, both peripherally and centrally to the underlying glenoid, and there is no free labral edge. In these cases, the labrum has the appearance of a thin rim of fibrous tissue. In the other type, the labrum is attached peripherally to the glenoid but has a central free edge. The labrum is often quite substantial in size and has an appearance similar to that of the knee meniscus, resulting in the term "meniscoid" labrum (Fig. 9-1). This meniscoid labrum pattern is most likely to be seen in the superior glenoid, and when present, a large hypermobile labrum may be more likely to be injured.

A recent study[2] of labral vascularity has shown that the superior and anterior superior parts of the glenoid labrum have less vascularity than the other portions of the labrum. The vascularity that is present is limited to the peripheral labrum. This means that a meniscoid labrum is again similar to the knee meniscus, with limited potential for healing of tears occurring in the central avascular portion. Finally, there appears to be a relationship between the superior labral complex and anterior glenohumeral instability. Rodsky and coworkers studied strain on the inferior glenohumeral ligament and the torsional rigidity of shoulders before and after the creation of superior labral detachments.[3] In patients who had superior labral detachments, the strain on the inferior glenohumeral ligament was significantly greater than in normal shoulders. A 33 percent increase in glenohumeral ligament strain was found if no biceps force was applied; a 17 percent increase was noted with full biceps force. This study suggests that the long head of the biceps contributes to anterior stability by resisting external rotation forces in the abducted externally rotated position, and is consistent with electromyographic studies in throwing athletes showing that the biceps tendon is most active in the late cocking phase of pitching, and that increased biceps tendon activity is seen in pitchers who have anterior instability.[4] It appears from this study that the presence of superior labral pathology predisposes the athlete to increased strain on the inferior glenohumeral ligament and possibly leads to the development of anterior instability. It is also possible that in an athlete with an unstable shoulder, the increased biceps activity that is required to help maintain shoulder stability may also result in increased stresses on the superior labrum and be more likely to cause superior labral injury. Theoretically, a cycle of injury may ensue in which the athlete initially has mild anterior instability and compensates by increasing the force on the biceps tendon during the external rotation phase of throwing. This may, in turn, lead to increased stresses on the superior labrum, which may ultimately detach from the superior glenoid. Once this detachment occurs, increased stresses are placed on the anterior glenohumeral ligaments and may lead to propagation of the detach-

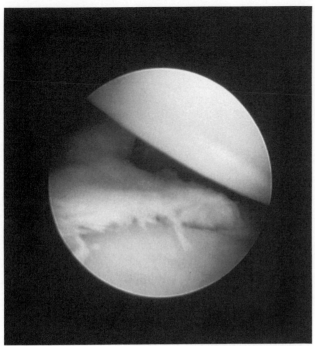

FIGURE 9-1
A "meniscoid" superior labrum has a prominent size and free central edge that gives an appearance similar to the knee meniscus.

ment down into the anterior labrum, resulting in the classic Bankart lesion. Likewise, if a Bankart lesion occurs first, it is possible that the labral detachment will propagate superiorly as well to involve the base of the biceps anchor. These theories may help to explain the association that is often noted between lesions of the superior labrum and glenohumeral instability.

TYPES OF SUPERIOR LABRAL PATHOLOGY

Andrews and Carson[5] first described a lesion of the anterior superior labrum associated with avulsion and fraying of these labral tissues in high-level throwing athletes. They studied 73 athletes with a superior labral lesion, which also involved partial tearing of the biceps tendon in some cases and in other cases a partial tearing of the rotator cuff tendon. They believed that the mechanism of injury was traction to the anterior superior labrum from the long head of the biceps tendon, which occurred in the deceleration phase of throwing. These lesions were treated arthroscopically with debridement of the loose fragments of the labrum, rotator cuff, and biceps tendon, followed by a vigorous rotator cuff and throwing rehabilitation program. Eighty-one percent of their patients were able to return to their previous level of throwing for at least one additional season.

More recently, a different pattern of injury to the superior glenoid labrum has been described.[6] This lesion involves the superior aspect of the glenoid labrum, beginning posterior to the biceps tendon and extending anterior to the biceps tendon, ending at or above the midglenoid notch. Such lesions are important because pathology in this area involves the insertion of the long head of the biceps tendon onto the superior glenoid. This injury has been labeled a "SLAP" lesion (superior labrum anterior and posterior).[6] SLAP lesions are not common but when present, they may be a source of significant disability to the patient, may be difficult to diagnose without the use of arthroscopy, and may often be successfully managed using arthroscopic techniques. SLAP lesions have been classified into four distinct types by Snyder and coworkers.[6] In type I lesions, the superior labrum is frayed and degenerated. Flaps and fragments of labral tissue may be present, but the peripheral labral edge remains firmly attached to the glenoid, and the biceps tendon anchor to the labrum is therefore secure (Fig. 9-2 and Plate 11). The type I lesion in an older individual may be considered a "normal" phase of the degenerative process, much like a degenerative meniscal tear.[7]

In type II lesions, fraying and degenerative changes may or may not be noted similar to those seen in type I lesions. The important difference in type II lesions, however, is that the superior labrum and the attached biceps tendon are also stripped off the superior glenoid neck, resulting in instability of the biceps labral anchor (Fig. 9-3 and Plate 12). The detachment of the superior labrum may be complete or partial, and it is important to distinguish this detachment from normal anatomic variations. Type II SLAP lesions are often overdiagnosed. As noted previously, a normal superior labrum may have a meniscoid-like appearance with a free inner edge, and this may give the appearance of the labrum's being pathologically loose. In acute superior labral avulsions, hemorrhage around the superior labral tissue and glenoid neck is easily recognized, appearing much like an acute Bankart lesion of anterior instability, and helps to make the diagnosis. However, in a chronic situation, the natural healing tendency of the avulsed tissues may cover the bony bed of the glenoid with smooth fibrous scar tissue, thereby concealing the underlying pathology. Also, with a normal meniscoid superior labrum, articular cartilage of the superior glenoid extends beneath the labrum to the level of the labral attachment, which may be quite peripheral on the glenoid neck. This normal variation must be distinguished from a true SLAP lesion, in which exposed cortical bone exists between the articular cartilage margin and the attachment of the superior labrum. In addition, with a type II SLAP

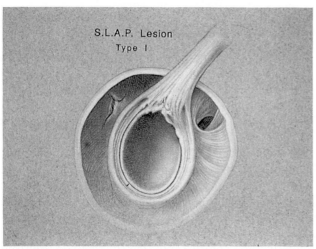

FIGURE 9-2
Schematic and intraoperative photograph (see Plate 11) of type I SLAP lesion. (*Schematic photograph reproduced with permission from Rames RD, Karzel RP: Injuries to the glenoid labrum, including SLAP lesions. Orthop Clin North Am 24:45–54, 1993.*[18])

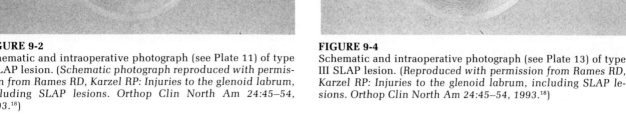

FIGURE 9-4
Schematic and intraoperative photograph (see Plate 13) of type III SLAP lesion. (*Reproduced with permission from Rames RD, Karzel RP: Injuries to the glenoid labrum, including SLAP lesions. Orthop Clin North Am 24:45–54, 1993.*[18])

lesion, the superior labrum should be seen to arch away by at least 3 to 4 mm from the superior glenoid owing to the continued pull of the biceps tendon on the detached superior labrum. A somewhat lax superior labral attachment in otherwise normal position is therefore *not* generally considered to be a SLAP lesion, but rather a normal variation.[7]

In type III SLAP lesions, the superior labrum has a vertical tear through its central portion analogous to a bucket handle tear in the meniscus (Fig. 9-4 and Plate 13). The torn fragment often displaces into the joint and may lead to mechanical symptoms. However, the remaining peripheral rim of labral tissue re-

mains well anchored to the glenoid, and the biceps tendon anchor is therefore intact. The type III or type IV tears obviously can occur only when a meniscoid labrum is present. Additionally, the bucket handle fragment may develop a central split resulting in two flaps—anterior and posterior.

In type IV SLAP lesions, the pathology also involves a vertical tear of the superior labrum, but in this case the superior labral tear extends up into the biceps tendon as well (Fig. 9-5 and Plate 14). The biceps tendon is partially torn, and the torn biceps tendon displaces into the shoulder joint with the labral flap. Usually the remaining biceps tendon is

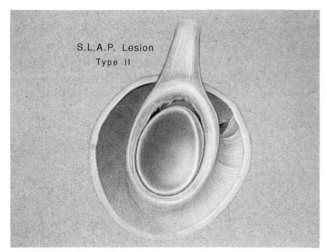

FIGURE 9-3
Schematic and intraoperative photograph (see Plate 12) of type II SLAP lesion. (*Reproduced with permission from Rames RD, Karzel RP: Injuries to the glenoid labrum, including SLAP lesions. Orthop Clin North Am 24:45–54, 1993.*[18])

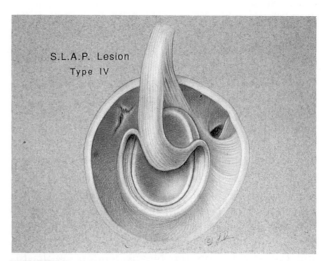

FIGURE 9-5
Schematic and intraoperative photograph (see Plate 14) of type IV SLAP lesion. (*Reproduced with permission from Rames RD, Karzel RP: Injuries to the glenoid labrum, including SLAP lesions. Orthop Clin North Am 24:45–54, 1993.*[18])

119

firmly anchored to the superior glenoid, but in some cases, the anchor itself may also be partially detached.

Other variations of SLAP lesions may occur. Burkhart and Fox[8] have described two cases in which SLAP lesions were associated with complete ruptures of the long head of the biceps tendon. Iannotti and Wang[9] have described a variation of the SLAP lesion in which a superior glenoid tubercle fracture is associated with a SLAP lesion. When present on x-ray, a superior glenoid tubercle fracture may suggest the diagnosis of SLAP lesion. Likewise various combinations of SLAP lesions type I through IV may also occur, not to mention the occurrence of these lesions associated with Bankart tears or instability, and variants such as sublabral holes and the Buford complex.

DIAGNOSIS OF SLAP LESIONS

The injured athlete with a SLAP lesion often presents a diagnostic challenge. In general, findings on history and physical examination are nonspecific, and even sophisticated imaging studies may fail to make the diagnosis. A high index of suspicion is required to allow the lesion to be diagnosed properly. SLAP lesions are frequently associated with other pathology, such as instability and rotator cuff tears, and these entities need to be ruled out. When taking a history on such patients, particular attention should be directed to the mechanism of injury. Two main mechanisms of injury are seen in patients with SLAP lesions. One particularly common cause of SLAP lesions is a history of a fall onto a slightly abducted and forward flexed arm. With axial loading of the arm in this position, forces appear to be transmitted through the humeral head into the superior glenoid, and as the humeral head slides superiorly on the loaded superior glenoid, the superior labral tissues may be avulsed off the glenoid. In these situations, a localized area of chondromalacia may be seen as well on the superior humeral head, corresponding to the area of loading at the time of impact. A second mechanism of injury involves traction from the biceps tendon. This may be seen in patients who report a sudden pulling or distraction force on the arm, particularly when the hand is in a supinated position with the elbow extended, thereby increasing the stresses on the biceps tendon. With this mechanism of injury, the biceps tendon appears to pull the superior labrum off the glenoid in a traction-type injury. Repeated traction of the biceps tendon on the labrum may also lead to SLAP lesions in the

throwing athlete or gymnast. Finally, patients with instability may develop SLAP lesions, or as noted previously, SLAP lesions may in fact lead to instability.

Patients with SLAP lesions complain primarily of pain and disability, often with difficulty performing their normal athletic activities. Symptoms are nonspecific, with many patients complaining of pain with overhead activities, suggestive of impingement syndrome. Other patients may complain of locking, snapping, or feelings of pseudo-subluxation suggestive of instability. In addition, many patients have pain over the anterior shoulder that may be confused with biceps tendinitis.

Findings on physical examination are also usually nonspecific. When the biceps anchor is involved with the SLAP lesion, resisted forward flexion of the arm in a supinated position (biceps tension test) may be painful. If a displaced labral fragment is present, the joint compression rotation test may be positive. This test is performed similar to MacMurray's test in the knee with the patient supine, and involves axially loading the humeral head into the glenoid and labrum while rotating the humeral head. If the labrum is subluxed into the joint, the labral tissue may become trapped between the humeral head, producing pain and/or clicking. It is also important to determine the presence of associated injuries to the rotator cuff tendons or associated glenohumeral instability during physical exam.

Diagnostic imaging studies are often nonspecific. Plain radiographic evaluation is usually negative, except as noted previously in the rare cases where fracture of the superior glenoid tubercle is seen with a SLAP lesion.[9] Improved experience with computed tomographic arthrography and magnetic resonance imaging has been helpful in many cases in diagnosing labral pathology, including SLAP lesions.[10–12] Unfortunately, however, other studies have shown that significant variation occurs in the radiographic appearance of the glenoid labrum in normal volunteers, and that many of these imaging techniques overdiagnose labral pathology.[13,14] In an attempt to improve on these results, a technique termed "magnetic resonance arthrography" has been employed recently.[15] In the magnetic resonance arthrography technique, an intraarticular injection of a magnetic contrast agent, gadolinium, is administered prior to performing magnetic resonance imaging. This technique was able to detect SLAP lesions in cases where conventional MRI scanning was not (Fig. 9-6). Although early results are encouraging, even with this technique, the tendency is to overdiagnose labral pathology in some cases, while in other

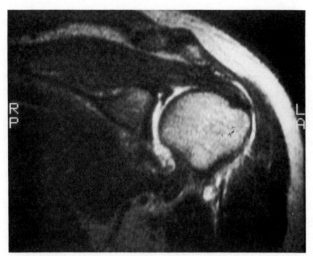

FIGURE 9-6
Intraarticular injection of gadolinium, a magnetic contrast agent, reveals the detachment of the superior labrum from the superior glenoid.

cases, a false-negative result is obtained. Because of these limitations in diagnosing SLAP lesions by history, physical examination, and diagnostic studies, a high degree of suspicion needs to be maintained, particularly in the patient whose symptoms and physical findings are not easily attributed to more common causes of shoulder pathology. Since many patients with persistent shoulder pain whose symptoms do not fit readily into one of the more commonly recognized causes of shoulder pain will in fact be found at the time of surgery to have labral pathology, the ultimate diagnosis of labral pathology therefore often requires performance of accurate diagnostic arthroscopy.

SURGICAL TREATMENT OF SLAP LESIONS

The method of surgical treatment of SLAP lesions varies depending on the type of SLAP lesion that is present. In type I lesions, arthroscopic debridement of the torn and frayed labral tissue back to intact labrum is performed. The attachment of the superior labrum and biceps tendon to the superior glenoid is carefully inspected, and if this attachment is intact, no additional treatment is required. In type III lesions, the bucket handle portion of the superior labral tear is excised in a manner similar to that used when excising a bucket handle tear of the knee meniscus.

Treatment of type IV SLAP lesions is somewhat more complicated and depends on the extent of biceps tendon pathology, the age of the patient, and the functional demands of that patient. In patients with a biceps tendon tear that involves less than half of the biceps tendon, particularly in patients who are

older and have less demand on the shoulder, treatment is similar to that for a type III lesion. In these cases, the superior labral fragment and the attached biceps tendon fragment are simply excised arthroscopically, often using an electrocautery electrode tip to cut the remaining attachments and allow removal of the fragment as a single piece. Further smoothing may then be performed with a shaver. If the biceps tendon tear is large, involving more than 50 percent of the tendon, and especially if the patient has symptoms of biceps pain, a biceps tenodesis may be performed at the same time. However, as noted previously, the biceps tendon has an important role in stabilizing the glenohumeral joint during the late cocking phases of throwing and other overhead activities. Performing a tenodesis in these cases may lead to increased glenohumeral instability and further damage to the shoulder. Likewise, if a small remaining portion of the biceps tendon is preserved, the increased stresses on this tendon may lead to further biceps tendinitis and possibly to eventual biceps tendon rupture. In younger, high-demand patients, we therefore prefer to repair the biceps tendon anchor surgically if possible, thereby preserving biceps tendon function. The remaining biceps tendon is first conservatively debrided with a shaver, removing only damaged fibers. The split in the biceps tendon and the superior labral tear can then be reapproximated using sutures placed arthroscopically in a mattress fashion through these tissues.

Treatment for type II SLAP lesions must be directed not only at the torn labral tissue but also at the reattachment of the biceps anchor to the superior glenoid neck. In our initial study,[6] the superior glenoid neck was simply debrided and abraded to achieve a bed of bleeding bone, and the arm was then placed in a sling for several weeks with the arm held in internal rotation and the elbow flexed in an attempt to promote healing of the superior labral tissue to the superior glenoid. Several of these patients underwent a second-look arthroscopy and at the time of arthroscopy were noted to have healed their lesions. However, in many cases, early motion is desirable, particularly when a SLAP lesion is present with additional pathology such as rotator cuff impingement or a partial rotator cuff tear. Also, continued pull of the biceps tendon may prevent healing if the labrum is not closely reapproximated to the glenoid. It appears, therefore, that some type of fixation of the superior labrum to the glenoid is desirable to promote an increased chance of healing and also to allow for earlier active motion.

Several different methods have been reported for reattachment of the superior labrum. Field and Savoie reported on 20 patients with type II and type IV SLAP lesions repaired using a transglenoid suture fixation technique and absorbable monofilament suture.[16] They had excellent or good results in all patients at an average of 21 months of follow-up. In another study, Yoneda and coworkers reported on 10 young athletes with type II SLAP lesions who were treated with abrasion of the superior glenoid neck and arthroscopic staple fixation of the superior labrum to the glenoid.[17] All these patients had a second arthroscopic evaluation at 3 to 6 months after surgery for staple removal. The authors report that in all 10 cases, the superior labrum had healed solidly to the glenoid. Excellent or good results were reported in 80 percent of their patients at 24 months of follow-up. Those patients with unsatisfactory results were felt to have problems with additional unrelated shoulder pathology.

At the Southern California Orthopedic Institute, we have utilized a repair technique that allows for fixation of the superior labrum to the glenoid with permanent mattress sutures, thereby avoiding the risk of placing metallic hardware near the glenohumeral joint. We have primarily used the Mitek GII suture anchor (Fig. 9-7A) for this purpose; more recently we have also used the Revo screw (Concept, Largo, Florida), which is a 4-mm headless cancellous threaded screw with a suture attached (Fig. 9-7B). One advantage of the Revo screw is the ability to remove it if the suture breaks or the knots do not seat well. In our technique, the torn and degenerated labral tissue is first debrided back to a stable rim. The next step is to debride the superior glenoid neck of soft tissue and abrade the cortical bone using a burr

to create a bleeding bone surface. Two anterior portals are used. The first portal is a standard anterior superior portal that is created near the intersection of the biceps tendon and the humeral head. The second anterior portal is created more inferiorly, just above the level of the leading edge of the subscapularis tendon. This portal can be appropriately created using a blunt-tipped obturator in an operating cannula passed from outside the shoulder into the glenohumeral joint while viewing from within the joint. The cannula remains well lateral to the coracoid process, and is in fact lateral to the articular cartilage of the glenoid. This portal is easily placed and avoids possible damage to the neurovascular structures passing beneath the coracoid.

After the abrasion is completed on the superior glenoid neck, the burr is used to create a pilot hole or target indentation in the superior glenoid neck just below the biceps anchor where the drill hole is to be made. By creating an indentation in this area, wandering of the drill due to the acute angle of drilling into the glenoid can be avoided. The appropriate drill is then passed through the operating cannula in the anterior superior portal, and a drill hole is made in the glenoid rim at the junction of the articular cartilage and the abraded glenoid neck, directing the drill at an angle approximately 45° posteriorly and 45° medially. After drilling to the appropriate depth, a suture anchor is loaded with no. 2 nonabsorbable suture and placed through the superior cannula into the drill hole. The Mitek anchor or Revo screw is gently seated into the hole using a mallet or screw-

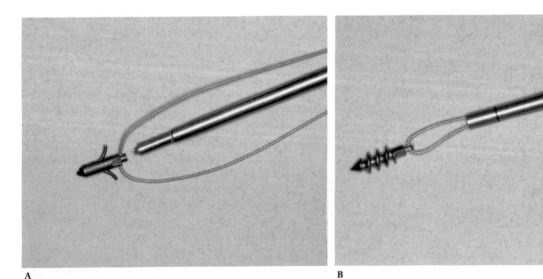

A   B

FIGURE 9-7
The Mitek GII suture anchor (*A*) and Revo screw (*B*) may be used to anchor suture in the superior glenoid.

driver to ensure firm fixation. The introducer is removed and tension is applied to the suture, testing to ensure that the anchor has been firmly seated.

A crochet hook is passed through the anterior inferior portal and is used to grab one limb of the suture passing through the anchor (Fig. 9-8). This suture is pulled out through the anterior inferior operating cannula. A 17-gauge, 6-in epidural needle is then placed through the anterior superior portal and passed through the biceps tendon and superior labral tissue, attempting to exit through the avulsed biceps anchor. Care is taken to ensure that a satisfactory amount of tissue for solid fixation has been obtained. Through the epidural needle, a suture Shuttle Relay (Concept, Largo, FL) is passed from outside the joint exiting on the inferior aspect of the superior labrum. The suture Shuttle Relay is a braided wire that has been fashioned so that there is a central open loop, and that has been coated with a smooth polypropylene surface except in the area of the central loop (Plate 15). The Shuttle Relay is grasped by a grasper inserted through the anterior inferior portal and pulled out of the shoulder joint adjacent to the previously passed suture. The suture is then placed into the eyelet of the shuttle, and the shuttle is then pulled back out the anterior superior portal (Fig. 9-9). This carries the nonabsorbable suture back through the labrum from inferior to superior, and out the anterior superior cannula. The second limb of the previously placed suture is passed through the labrum in a similar fashion, leaving a 6- to 8-mm space between the suture limbs, to provide an adequate soft tissue bridge.

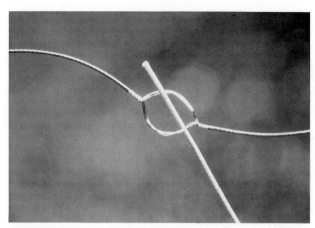

FIGURE 9-9
The suture Shuttle Relay is loaded with the suture and pulled back through the labrum and out the superior cannula. (*Reproduced with permission from Rames RD, Karzel RP: Injuries to the glenoid labrum, including SLAP lesions. Orthop Clin North Am 24:45–54, 1993.*[18])

Both limbs of the suture now pass from the Mitek anchor through the superior labral tissue and exit out the anterior superior portal. Multiple knots are tied using an arthroscopic suturing device (Concept, Largo, FL) (Fig. 9-10). The superior labrum must be maintained in a reduced position on the glenoid while the sutures are tied to ensure good approximation. For large SLAP tears, a second suture anchor may also be placed in a similar fashion, and multiple anterior suture anchors may also be placed in pa-

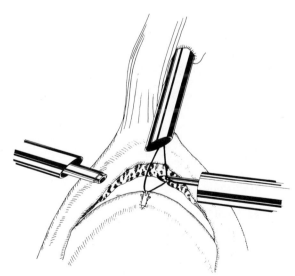

FIGURE 9-8
One limb of the suture is grasped and pulled out the anterior inferior cannula. (*Reproduced with permission from Rames RD, Karzel RP: Injuries to the glenoid labrum, including SLAP lesions. Orthop Clin North Am 24:45–54, 1993.*[18])

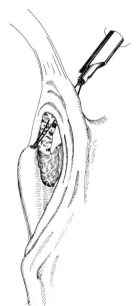

FIGURE 9-10
After the second suture is passed in a similar fashion to the first, a knot pusher is placed over the sutures. (*Reproduced with permission from Rames RD, Karzel RP: Injuries to the glenoid labrum, including SLAP lesions. Orthop Clin North Am 24:45–54, 1993.*[18])

tients who have a combined Bankart lesion. After the sutures have been tied, the labrum is carefully probed to ensure that it has been well attached to the glenoid. The ends of the suture are cut using a basket forceps inserted through the anterior superior cannula.

POSTOPERATIVE REHABILITATION

For tears in which debridement or excision of the labral tissue alone has been performed, the patient is allowed immediate motion as tolerated. When a type II lesion has been treated with abrasion of the glenoid neck alone, the patient is maintained in a sling with the elbow in a flexed position for the first 3 weeks. If a technique has been used to fix the superior labrum to the glenoid, the patient is placed in a sling for 1 week postoperatively but is allowed to remove the sling for full extension of the elbow as tolerated. After the first week, the patient is allowed to remove the sling to perform active range-of-motion exercises but is instructed to avoid external rotation of the shoulder beyond a neutral position and extension of the arm behind the body with the elbow extended for an additional 4 weeks to prevent stresses from the biceps tendon from disrupting the repair. Patients are generally restricted from activities placing a significant stress on the biceps tendon, such as most athletic activities, until 3 to 4 months after surgery.

Results of these techniques are still preliminary, as follow-up is short and the number of patients is still relatively small. In addition, many of these patients will have coexisting pathology such as impingement or instability that makes it difficult to determine precisely the role of the SLAP lesion in causing symptoms. In four of our cases, repeat arthroscopy of lesions fixed with these methods has been performed; in all cases healing of the superior labrum to the glenoid neck has occurred. Further follow-up and more patients with isolated SLAP lesions will be necessary before the efficacy of these procedures can be better defined.

SUMMARY

Although lesions of the superior labrum are often difficult to diagnose preoperatively, they may be a significant source of disability in the athlete. Recent advances in imaging techniques have improved our ability to diagnose these problems, but the definitive diagnostic tool remains diagnostic shoulder arthroscopy. When these lesions are detected by shoulder arthroscopy, arthroscopic treatment appears to be effective in allowing patients to resume their previous level of function with minimal morbidity. As long-term follow-up studies become available, and as new techniques for fixation of the superior labrum continue to be developed, our ability to correct these problems should increase even further in the future.

REFERENCES

1. Detrisac DA, Johnson LL: *Arthroscopic Shoulder Anatomy: Pathology and Surgical Implications.* Thorofare, NJ, Slack, 1986.
2. Cooper DE, Arnoczky SP, O'Brien SJ, et al: Anatomy, histology and vascularity of the glenoid labrum. An anatomical study. *J Bone Joint Surg (Am)* 74A:46–52, 1992.
3. Rodsky MW, Rudert MJ, Harner CD, et al: The role of the long head of the biceps and superior glenoid labrum in anterior instability of the shoulder. Presented at the American Academy of Orthopaedic Surgeons Annual Meeting, Anaheim, CA, 1991.
4. Glousman R, Jobe F, Tibone J, et al: Dynamic electromyographic analysis of the throwing shoulder with glenohumeral instability. *J Bone Joint Surg (Am)* 70A:220–226, 1988.
5. Andrews JR, Carson WG, McLeod WD: Glenoid labrum tears related to the long head of the biceps. *Am J Sports Med* 13:337–341, 1985.
6. Snyder SJ, Karzel RP, Del Pizzo W, et al: SLAP lesions of the shoulder. *Arthroscopy* 6:274–279, 1990.
7. DePalma AJ: *Surgery of the Shoulder*, 3d ed. Philadelphia, Lippincott, 1983, pp 212–245.
8. Burkhart SS, Fox DL: SLAP lesions in association with complete tears of the long head of the biceps tendon: A report of two cases. *Arthroscopy* 8:31–35, 1992.
9. Iannotti JP, Wang ED: Avulsion fracture of the supraglenoid tubercle: A variation of the SLAP lesion. *J Shoulder Elbow Surg* 1:26–30, 1992.
10. Nelson ML, Leather GP, Nirschl RP, et al: Evaluation of the painful shoulder. A prospective comparison of magnetic resonance imaging, computerized tomographic arthrography, ultrasonography and operative findings. *J Bone Joint Surg (Am)* 73A:707–716, 1991.
11. McCauley TR, Pope LF, Jokl P: Normal and abnormal glenoid labrum: Assessment with multiplanar gradient-echo MR imaging. *Radiology* 183:335–337, 1992.

12. Coumas JM, Waite RJ, Goss TP, et al: CT and MR evaluation of the labral capsular ligamentous complex of the shoulder. *AJR* 158:591–597, 1992.

13. Neumann CH, Petersen SA, Jahnke AH: MR imaging of the labral-capsular complex: Normal variations. *AJR* 157:1015–1021, 1991.

14. Chandnani V, Ho C, Gerharter J, et al: MR findings in asymptomatic shoulders: A blind analysis using symptomatic shoulders as controls. *Clin Imaging* 16:25–30, 1992.

15. Karzel RP, Snyder SJ: Magnetic resonance arthrography of the shoulder: A new technique of shoulder imaging. *Clin Sports Med* 1:123–136, 1993.

16. Field LD, Savoie FH: Arthroscopic suture repair of superior labral detachment lesions of the shoulder. Presented at American Orthopaedic Society for Sports Medicine Specialty Day, 59th Annual Meeting of the American Academy of Orthopaedic Surgeons, Washington DC, 1992.

17. Yoneda M, Hirouka A, Saito S, et al: Arthroscopic stapling for detached superior glenoid labrum. *J Bone Joint Surg (Am)* 73B:746–750, 1991.

18. Rames RD, Karzel RP: Injuries to the glenoid labrum, including SLAP lesions. *Orthop Clin North Am* 24:45–54, 1993.

Multidirectional Instability in the Athlete

Michael J. Pagnani
Russell F. Warren

INTRODUCTION

The shoulder is a common source of complaints in the athletic population. High loads are generated at the glenohumeral joint in throwing, swimming, and racket sports. Pathologic changes often occur in the athletes who repetitively perform these activities. The large forces directed upon the shoulder in contact sports are also a significant cause of injury. Multidirectional instability is increasingly recognized as an important subtype of shoulder disability in the athletic population. The signs and symptoms associated with multidirectional instability are often subtle, and the results of treatment have often been less than satisfactory.

Recent advances involving the recognition and pathoanatomy of the multidirectionally unstable shoulder have led to an improved outlook with regard to the treatment of this condition.

PATHOPHYSIOLOGY OF MULTIDIRECTIONAL SHOULDER INSTABILITY

The shoulder has the greatest range of motion of all the joints in the human body. Bony restraints to motion are minimal. It is the surrounding soft tissue envelope that primarily confers stability on the normal glenohumeral joint. This stability is due to both the static effect of ligaments and tendons and the dynamic mechanisms associated with muscular contraction.

It is generally believed that the basic lesion in multidirectional instability is excessive joint volume with laxity of the capsular ligaments. In the athlete, this laxity may be an inherent condition that becomes more pronounced with the superimposed trauma of sport. In addition, multidirectional instability may occur owing to extensive capsulolabral trauma in patients who do not appear to have laxity of other joints.

The pathology of the multidirectionally unstable shoulder of the *atraumatic* type usually consists of a large inferior capsular pouch that extends both posteriorly and anteriorly.[42] Anterior capsulolabral detachment is generally not associated with this capsular redundancy. In contrast, a *traumatic* type of multidirectional instability exists and will be seen to a varying degree depending on the physician's patient population. In loose-jointed athletes, particularly, a traumatic event may damage the shoulder tissue to the degree that the result is a shoulder with both multidirectional instability and a Bankart lesion of varying size.

While the shoulder capsule normally contains numerous synovial recesses, *abnormal* capsular redundancy is an important factor in the pathogenesis of multidirectional instability.[42] Gradual stretching of the capsule may occur with repetitive microtrauma, which is a common etiologic factor in multidirectional instability.[52] On the other hand, capsular laxity most commonly is due to inherent soft tissue laxity. These patients may have a mild form of a generalized connective tissue disorder. Belle and Hawkins[6] cultured fibroblasts from the skin of patients with multidirectional instability and discovered a significant increase in the relative amount of collagen produced in the multidirectional group.

The shoulder capsule is large, loose, and redundant to allow for the large range of shoulder motion. The capsule contains discrete ligaments that are important in understanding the pathomechanics of shoulder instability (Fig. 10-1). Three anterior glenohumeral ligaments have been described: the superior glenohumeral ligament (SGHL), the middle glenohumeral ligament (MGHL), and the inferior glenohumeral ligament complex (IGHLC).[17] The posterior capsule includes the area posterior to the biceps and superior to the posterior band of the IGHLC. This area is the thinnest part of the capsule; there is no direct posterior ligamentous reinforcement.

The role of the anterior glenohumeral ligaments in preventing instability is complex and varies with shoulder position and with the direction of the translating force. In most cases, it appears that the integrity of these ligaments is the key to stability of the joint. Conversely, laxity or injury to these structures seems to be the primary mechanism of instability.

Static ligamentous cutting studies have helped to elucidate the roles of the various anatomic structures in the production of glenohumeral instabil-

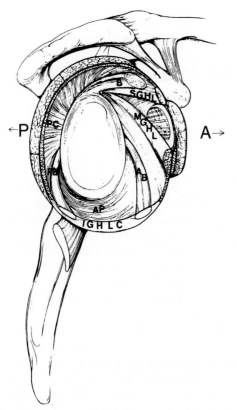

FIGURE 10-1
Capsuloligamentous complex of the shoulder. A = anterior, P = posterior, B = biceps tendon, SGHL = superior glenohumeral ligament, MGHL = middle glenohumeral ligament, AB = anterior band of inferior glenohumeral ligament complex (IGHLC), PB = posterior band of IGHLC, AP = axillary pouch, PC = posterior capsule. (*Used with permission from O'Brien SJ, Neves MC, Arnoczky SP, et al: The anatomy and histology of the inferior glenohumeral ligament complex of the shoulder. Am J Sports Med 18:449–456, 1990.*)

ity.[9,50] It appears that the IGHLC is the primary static restraint against anterior, posterior, and inferior translation when the arm is abducted between 45 and 90°.[9,46,47,57,60,64] In the midrange of abduction, the MGHL and subscapularis assist the IGHLC in resisting anterior translation while the teres minor and infraspinatus help prevent posterior translation.[50,60,66] With the arm adducted, the SGHL and the MGHL stabilize against anterior movement,[46–48] the posterior capsule and the SGHL resist posterior motion,[66] and the SGHL and IGHLC are the primary restraints against inferior translation.[9,26,64,65] These findings help to determine which specific area of the capsule requires additional tensioning when operative treatment is employed in the treatment of the multidirectionally unstable shoulder.

Uhthoff and Piscopo[61] have suggested that a congenitally abnormal insertion of the capsule into the glenoid neck may predispose to capsular redundancy. This theory is based on anatomic dissections of fetal and embryonic shoulders.

The space between the superior border of the subscapularis and the anterior margin of the supraspinatus has been termed the rotator interval[45] (see Fig. 10-2). The SGHL is located in this region of the capsule. A relatively large interval has been associated clinically with inferior instability[45] as well as anterior instability.[55] Harryman et al. recently found that this portion of the capsule plays a significant role in preventing inferior subluxation of the adducted shoulder and acts as a secondary restraint against posterior translation.[22] These findings correlate with the function of the SGHL. Enlargement of the rotator interval appears to result in abnormal inferior translation and may also be related to in-

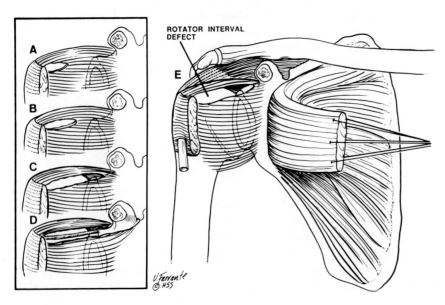

FIGURE 10-2
After division of the subscapularis tendon, a rotator interval defect may become visible. The interval may be variable in size (inset, *A–D*). In some cases, the superior glenohumeral ligament will be seen crossing through the defect (inset, *E*).

128

creases in anteroposterior motion. Assessment of the presence and size of the rotator interval is extremely important during operative repair for multidirectional instability. Closure of the interval will often significantly diminish excess capsular laxity.

The glenohumeral joint fluid aids in holding the articular surfaces together with viscous and intermolecular forces.[39] Additionally, the normal intraarticular pressure is negative, creating a relative vacuum that resists translation.[11,30,34] If these properties are disrupted by venting the capsule and introducing air or fluid, subluxation tends to occur.[34,65] Habermeyer et al.[20] found that traction on the arm caused an increase in negative pressure in normal shoulders but that no increase occurred in unstable shoulders; this suggests that the vacuum effect is somehow lost in the unstable shoulder. Excess capsular volume could, in theory, lead to a loss of these stabilizing properties.

The glenoid labrum is a fibrous structure that is intimately attached to the bony glenoid rim.[8,15,41] The superior attachment of the labrum is loose and "meniscal-like" while the inferior attachment is firm. The fibers of the biceps tendon intermingle with the superior labrum, and the inferior glenohumeral ligament blends into the inferior labrum.

The labrum increases the depth of the glenoid.[29] Vanderhooft et al.[62] recently reported that resection of the labrum reduced resistance to anterior translation by 20 percent in shoulders that were subjected to a compressive load. Separation of the labrum from the glenoid rim decreases the concavity of the socket. In addition, anteroinferior labral detachment is usually associated with laxity or disruption of an important stabilizer, the inferior glenohumeral ligament.[3–5,58]

The rotator cuff tendons and the tendon of the long head of the biceps may have important roles in controlling glenohumeral translation. The effect of passive musculotendinous tension within the rotator cuff appears to have some static role in preventing translation. However, the primary mechanism by which these muscles affect glenohumeral stability appears to be a dynamic one and is associated with a coordinated system of selective muscular contraction. It is likely that the muscles of the rotator cuff serve a complementary function in order to adjust tension in the capsuloligamentous system. Contraction of the rotator cuff and biceps muscles causes the humeral head to be compressed into the glenoid and increases the load needed to translate the head.[13,28,29] This function has been the basis for the conservative treatment of shoulder instability that incorporates strengthening of the rotators.

A second group of muscles affects glenohumeral stability. The scapular rotators (trapezius, rhomboids, latissimus dorsi, serratus anterior, and levator scapulae) position the scapula to provide a stable "platform" beneath the humeral head. This allows the glenoid to adjust to changes in arm position.

CLASSIFICATION

Three basic types of multidirectional instability can be differentiated on the basis of the direction and degree of abnormal translation. We have recently noted a fourth type. Type I is comprised of patients who have global instability and dislocate in all three directions. Type II patients demonstrate anterior and inferior dislocation as well as mild posteroinferior subluxation. Patients with posterior and inferior dislocation and mild anteroinferior laxity are classified as type III. In rare cases (type IV), patients appear to have abnormal anterior and posterior translation, both to the point of dislocation, without significant inferior translation. These cases, while uncommon, present a difficult management problem as the inferior component of instability is absent at both 0 and 45° of abduction.

The athlete who presents with instability in more than one direction should also be classified on the basis of etiology. Classically, the patient with multidirectional instability gives no history of significant traumatic injury. These individuals have generalized ligamentous laxity and usually are found to have capsular laxity without labral injury upon surgical exploration. There are patients (particularly athletes) with multidirectional instability who have had a significant traumatic injury to the shoulder. This injury is sometimes, but not always, superimposed on inherent soft tissue laxity. This group of patients may have a labral injury in addition to abnormal capsular redundancy. The labral injury may be a minor one, but in some cases, the entire inferior labrum may be disrupted. Finally, many of the athletes who present with multidirectional instability have a history of microtrauma associated with repetitive use of the arm and shoulder. This group includes many throwers, swimmers, and racket-sport athletes. Often these individuals present with signs and symptoms associated with subluxation rather than frank dislocation.

PATIENT HISTORY

Most athletes with multidirectional instability present with a sense of "looseness" and associated discomfort of the shoulder. Symptoms tend to occur with overhead and contact activities. Those patients with an atraumatic history or a loose capsule usually are able to reduce their shoulders spontaneously without assistance. Repetitive-use injury (often throwing) commonly results in symptoms consistent with subluxation. In the traumatic setting or with repeated injury, complete dislocation may occur.

Pain is an uncommon complaint except when associated with an acute event. However, the occasional patient will have pain while carrying a bag or with overhead activity. We have noted that patients with multidirectional instability often have a history of paresthesia in the involved upper extremity. Sensory symptoms tend to occur when the patient is carrying a bag or other load or is reaching overhead. Symptoms of thoracic outlet syndrome are frequently associated with multidirectional instability and may be due to traction on the brachial plexus associated with increased inferior translation of the shoulder.

These patients often present with bilateral complaints. Morrey and Janes[40] reported an increased failure rate after standard anterior stabilization in patients with bilateral instability and in those with a family history of instability. These groups of patients may have generalized ligamentous laxity and require a careful evaluation for evidence of multidirectional instability.

PHYSICAL EXAMINATION OF THE MULTIDIRECTIONALLY UNSTABLE SHOULDER

Examination of the athlete with suspected shoulder instability is generally performed in two parts. During the initial portion of the exam, the patient is asked to stand. In the second part, the patient lies supine with the shoulder placed on the edge of the examining table.

Several examination maneuvers have been developed to specifically address the issue of shoulder instability. Drawer tests are designed to assess translation of the humeral head on the glenoid. The degree of translation is noted in anterior, posterior, and inferior directions. Normally, translation is equal anteriorly and posteriorly and is greatest in neutral flexion-extension and neutral rotation. These tests are best performed with the patient in both the supine and standing positions. The arm is generally examined in 0 and 90° of abduction and in neutral rotation. Other positions of abduction and rotation may also be examined in an attempt to correlate pa-

thology with the existing basic science data presented earlier. Translation is graded as 1+ if there is increased translation compared with the opposite shoulder but if subluxation or dislocation does not occur. If the head can be subluxated over the glenoid rim but then spontaneously reduces, translation is graded as 2+. Frank dislocation without spontaneous reduction constitutes 3+ translation.[1] It is essential that the opposite shoulder be tested for comparison.

Grading of the sulcus sign is based on the distance between the inferior margin of the lateral acromion and the humeral head when a downward traction force is applied to the adducted arm. Less than 1 cm of distance represents a 1+ sulcus, 1 to 2 cm indicates a 2+ sulcus, and more than 2 cm is a 3+.[1] A 3+ sulcus sign reflects laxity of the SGHL and IGHLC and is indicative of inferior instability. It is pathognomonic of multidirectional instability. Assessment of inferior translation with the arm abducted more than 45° more accurately reflects tension on the inferior capsule.[9,64] Helmig et al., in a cadaveric study, noted that maximal inferior humeral migration occurred with the arm in 20° of abduction and neutral rotation.[26] We generally assess inferior stability at 0 and 90° of abduction with the arm in neutral rotation.

The patient with multidirectional instability usually exhibits symptomatic inferior instability in addition to anterior and/or posterior instability. The sulcus sign is therefore positive in these patients. The presence of inferior instability has been considered to be a requirement for the diagnosis of multidirectional instability.[44] However, we have noted a select group of patients who demonstrate marked anterior and posterior translation without significant inferior laxity.

Apprehension tests are designed to induce anxiety and protective muscular contraction as the shoulder is brought to a position associated with instability. The anterior apprehension test is performed with the arm abducted and externally rotated. The examiner progressively increases the degree of external rotation and notes the development of patient apprehension. We feel that the term "posterior apprehension test" is inappropriate since the patient with posterior instability usually exhibits discomfort rather than apprehension when the shoulder is stressed posteriorly. The posterior stress test is performed with the arm internally rotated and forward flexed to 90° (Fig. 10-3). Discomfort may be noted as the humerus is loaded in an anteroposterior direction and progressively adducted across the chest. Physical examination of the athlete with

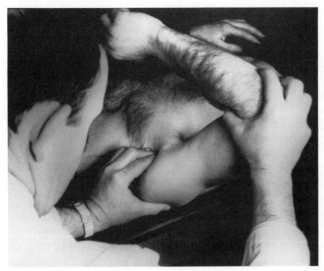

FIGURE 10-3
Posterior stress test. The arm is forward flexed and internally rotated. The humerus is loaded with a posteriorly directed force, and the arm is adducted across the chest.

atraumatic multidirectional instability usually reveals little or no pain or apprehension in any direction. Those with a *traumatic* etiology and anterior subluxation are more likely to have positive apprehension signs and associated pain.

Ligamentous laxity is commonly associated with shoulder instability and can be measured objectively on physical examination. The degree of thumb hyperabduction with the wrist volar flexed can be noted by the distance between the thumb and volar forearm. If the thumb reaches the forearm, the test is considered positive. An assessment is also made for index metacarpophalangeal extension in excess of 90°, elbow hyperextension, and knee hyperextension. Approximately 50 percent of patients with multidirectional instability have evidence of generalized ligamentous laxity.[1] Increased ligamentous laxity is not uncommon in recurrent posterior subluxation. Patients with recurrent posterior subluxation should be carefully evaluated for concomitant inferior instability to rule out multidirectional instability.

Concomitant findings of impingement occur in approximately 20 percent of patients with multidirectional instability.[1]

Examination under anesthesia (EUA) is a valuable tool since the awake patient often guards against vigorous attempts to evaluate translation. Under anesthesia, the shoulder is stressed inferiorly at 0 and 90° of elevation with the arm in neutral rotation. To assess anteroposterior laxity at 90° of elevation, one of the examiner's hands is used to deliver a translatory load to the humerus. The opposite hand is used to sense the degree of translation and/or the presence of crepitation. By placing the arm in neutral rotation,

translation is maximized. One must be careful in interpreting translation in the anesthetized patient; normal posterior translation may be as much as 50 percent of the glenoid diameter.[23] During the EUA, the head may be noted to displace to the posterior edge of the glenoid, and a "jump" may be noted. While a similar degree of *anterior* translation is normally present, the examiner usually perceives anterior translation to be less than posterior translation. The reason for this perception is unclear.

RADIOGRAPHY

In the general assessment of chronic shoulder instability, special views are helpful in the determination of bony anatomy and pathology. The "instability series" consists of anteroposterior (AP) views in internal and external rotation, a West Point axillary view, and a Stryker Notch view.[51] The West Point axillary view[54] often reveals the presence of a fracture or ectopic bone production at the anterior glenoid rim that may not be visualized in other projections. The Stryker Notch view[21] is especially helpful in demonstrating the Hill-Sachs lesion[27] when it is not visualized in the internal rotation AP view. In the athlete with atraumatic multidirectional instability, it is unusual to see a bony abnormality. If trauma is an etiologic factor, the development of radiographic abnormalities is more likely.

We have not found stress or traction films[43] to be necessary in delineating inferior instability. While weighted views may reveal inferior subluxation when the glenohumeral muscles are relaxed, clinical examination with simple inferior traction is sufficient to demonstrate a sulcus sign. Computed tomography (with or without arthrography) may be helpful in selected cases. Magnetic resonance imaging (MRI) is emerging as a potentially helpful tool in the evaluation of labral and capsular lesions, particularly when performed shortly after a dislocation when the attendant joint effusion permits better visualization of these structures.[63] In the absence of an effusion, intraarticular injection of gadolinium may improve the resolution of these tissues. MRI is also a valuable aid when significant cuff injury is associated with instability.

NONOPERATIVE TREATMENT OF MULTIDIRECTIONAL INSTABILITY

To paraphrase Neer,[44] "Not all loose shoulders are painful and not all require treatment." Symptomatic patients with multidirectional instability should be given a thorough trial of internal and external rotator strengthening. Patients with atraumatic multidirectional instability often respond to nonoperative therapy.

The treatment of multidirectional instability begins with a period of rest. After an acute event, an arm sling is worn for a few days for comfort. Nonsteroidal anti-inflammatory medication is administered during this time. Prolonged immobilization after a second traumatic dislocation is of no apparent value. In patients with atraumatic instability, immobilization may be of little value even after the initial dislocation.

A rehabilitation program that emphasizes rotator cuff and periscapular muscle strengthening is then employed. Kronberg et al., in an electromyographic study of patients with generalized ligamentous laxity, have noted decreased activity of the anterior and middle deltoid with abduction and flexion of the shoulder as well as increased activity of the subscapularis during internal rotation.[33] Isokinetic testing can help identify specific muscular weakness and can provide a baseline for comparison during the rehabilitative process.[31,59] Rotator cuff strengthening begins with rubber tubing exercises, progresses to spring exercises, and then advances to Nautilus or isokinetic exercises. We also emphasize elevation with weights in the scapular plane and seated push-ups in which the body is lifted from a chair by extension of the upper extremities with the hands placed upon the seat. Weights should be held so that they do not create an inferior traction force on the shoulder. If there is a positional component to the instability, that position should be avoided.

In the early phase of therapy, especially in patients with concomitant impingement, these activities should be performed with the arm adducted or in the lower ranges of abduction to protect the rotator cuff.[67] Later these exercises may be performed in 90° of elevation in the scapular plane as well. Muscular endurance should be emphasized in addition to strengthening. The scapular rotators are conditioned by a combination of shoulder shrugs, horizontal adduction exercises, pull-downs, chin-ups, and push-ups with the elbows kept at the sides.[31]

Throwing is not allowed until strength and motion are normal. Throwing is slowly progressed in distance, velocity, frequency, and duration. The patient's pitching mechanics should be adjusted to provide efficient energy transfer from the lower extremities and thorax to the shoulder. Specific activities that seemed to incite pain prior to the institution of therapy are withheld for longer periods of time.

A rehabilitative program often succeeds in patients with atraumatic instability. Traumatic dislo-

cators appear to respond less favorably. Recently, Burkhead and Rockwood[12] reported that an exercise program led to a good or excellent result in 80 percent of shoulders with atraumatic anterior subluxation, but in only 16 percent of shoulders with traumatic subluxation.

OPERATIVE TREATMENT OF MULTIDIRECTIONAL INSTABILITY

The indications for surgical treatment of multidirectional instability are highly subjective and include recurrence, pain, or activity limitation after a thorough trial of nonoperative management. Candidates for surgical stabilization of multidirectional instability should be well motivated since adherence to the postoperative rehabilitative program is extremely important to achieving a successful result. Voluntary dislocators often fare poorly after an operation. It should also be noted that atraumatic types of multidirectional instability appear to have higher postoperative recurrence rates than traumatic types. Thus, in the athlete, etiology should be considered when discussing the possibility of a return to sports.

The decision to operate on the athlete with multidirectional instability is based on careful consideration of the degree of instability, the etiology, and the symptoms experienced during athletic activity. If the patient has generalized laxity with no history of significant trauma, pain may be present, but often the chief complaint is a sense of looseness or movement with associated weakness during a specific activity. Lifting heavy objects may create a sensation of inferior looseness. In repetitive activities, rotator cuff fatigue or damage may be present and may mimic the impingement syndrome.

The degree of instability and the interference with sport will help to determine the level of treatment. While exercises are the basic initial treatment for all types of multidirectional instability and are successful in the majority (60 to 80 percent) of atraumatic cases, the overhead athlete who places high stresses upon the shoulder may fare less well with rehabilitation than with surgery.

In cases with a traumatic etiology, whether superimposed upon generalized laxity or not, our impression is that exercises are less helpful. These patients will note a specific event that produced their symptoms. As was mentioned earlier, traumatic conditions are more frequently associated with capsulolabral disruption (the Bankart lesion) that may be extensive enough to result in multidirectional instability. These patients frequently note a significant degree of pain and apprehension. Thus a thrower who is injured while sliding into a base may have pain and anterior apprehension in the cocking position while a patient with an atraumatic etiology usually does not have much pain or apprehension in this position. A football player injured while blocking may note posterior and inferior pain with stand-up blocking techniques.

Arthroscopy

Arthroscopy presently plays little role in the treatment of multidirectional instability, particularly of the atraumatic type. In general, if there is a significant component of inferior instability or subluxation, arthroscopy is avoided and an open procedure is performed. One exception to this rule would occur in a thrower who had generalized laxity with subluxation in an inferior direction as well as rotator cuff symptoms. In this setting, arthroscopic evaluation with debridement and rehabilitative exercise may provide the basis for initial treatment. If this treatment fails, as it well may, an open procedure addressing the instability is performed.

At present, in our opinion, there is no role for an arthroscopic stabilization procedure in the treatment of multidirectional instability. Current techniques of arthroscopic stabilization do not permit sufficient mobilization of capsular laxity, do not address the rotator interval, and thus are associated with a high failure rate in the treatment of multidirectional instability.[2,16,18]

Open Stabilization

The type of operative approach for multidirectional instability should be determined by the patient's history and physical findings. Generally, the approach should be made on the side associated with the greatest amount of clinical instability. In general, we prefer to approach the shoulder anteriorly since the soft tissues are of better quality, the capsular shift is more easily performed, and an enlarged rotator interval can be identified and addressed. However, if the clinical evaluation reveals that the principal direction of instability is posteroinferior with only mild anterior subluxation, a posterior approach is utilized.

Patients with inferior laxity may fail standard operative procedures designed for unidirectional instability. Excess capsular laxity is not addressed by procedures that limit external rotation (e.g., Putti-Platt,[49] Magnuson-Stack[38]). In some cases, these procedures may cause excessive tightness on one side of the hypermobile shoulder. Subluxation or disloca-

tion will then occur in the opposite direction, and glenohumeral arthritis may ensue. Bone-block procedures, such as the Bristow technique,[25] also fail to correct the capsular redundancy associated with multidirectional instability, allowing the humeral head to glide under the bone block.

ANTERIOR APPROACH

Our basic procedure for the surgical treatment of multidirectional glenohumeral instability in patients whose instability is primarily anterior is the T-plasty modification of the Bankart procedure.[1] The patient is positioned supine with the head of the bed raised 30° and the arm abducted 45° on an arm board. A folded towel is placed between the scapulae to rotate the scapula on the involved side laterally.

The skin incision is started just lateral to the coracoid and extended approximately 6 cm distally. (The axillary approach of Leslie[37] requires a considerable subcutaneous dissection and offers a limited view when dealing when multidirectional instability.) The deltopectoral interval is identified. The cephalic vein is retracted laterally, since there are fewer branches on the medial side. The surgeon must take care not to damage the vein as it crosses the superior aspect of the wound.

After dissection through the deltopectoral interval, the coracoid process and the clavipectoral fascia are identified. The fascia is incised lateral to the muscle belly of the short head of the biceps. To facilitate exposure in some cases, a partial, oblique incision is made in the conjoined tendon just distal to the coracoid. Avoid the musculocutaneous nerve, which may enter the tendon as close as 1 cm distal to the coracoid. We do not recommend coracoid osteotomy or complete detachment of the tendon.

The arm is then externally rotated, and the insertion of the subscapularis tendon is revealed. Three small branches of the anterior circumflex vessels ("the three sisters") lie near the inferior edge of the tendon and may require ligation. A small transverse incision (3 to 4 mm in length) is made at the inferior border of the tendon at the musculotendinous junction. The anterior capsule is visualized through this incision. A Kelly clamp or a periosteal elevator is then passed from inferomedial to superolateral in the interval between the anterior capsule and the tendon. The medial portion of the tendon is tagged with heavy, nonabsorbable sutures. The tendon is then incised obliquely over this clamp. The medial portion of the tendon is dissected from the capsule with a periosteal elevator.

Jobe et al.[32] have noted that the ability to throw commonly diminishes after operative treatment for shoulder instability. They have developed an approach in which the subscapularis tendon is split longitudinally rather than divided. We recommend this method in throwers and overhead athletes with unidirectional anterior subluxation or dislocation, but not for the treatment of true multidirectional instability. While a variation of this approach may be utilized in patients with greater degrees of instability, it is difficult to detect and correctly tension an enlarged rotator interval with this method.

Once the capsule is exposed, the exact type of repair is determined by the size of the rotator interval, the degree of capsular laxity, and the presence or absence of a Bankart lesion. After exposure of the anterior capsule by division of the subscapularis tendon, a search is made for the presence of a rotator interval (Fig. 10-2). The rotator interval is, in essence, a hiatus for passage of the subscapularis toward its insertion on the lesser tuberosity. Generally, the interval is small, but if it extends to the coracoid process, the superior capsule is left open. On occasion, we have noted the SGHL passing across the rotator interval (Fig. 10-2). An enlarged rotator interval will allow abnormal anteroinferior or posteroinferior translation of the humeral head. If present, an enlarged interval must be closed to create adequate tension in the capsular system. Otherwise a repair that advances tissue superiorly may stretch out. At times, closure of the interval alone may be sufficient to control excessive translation. In many cases, however, additional tensioning of the capsule is required. The interval may be closed prior to the creation of a formal capsulotomy, or the joint may be inspected through the interval if the interval is sufficiently large. When closure of the interval alone is insufficient to control translation and the joint has been inspected via the rotator interval, the interval can be incorporated into the capsulotomy by creating vertical capsular incisions on the medial and/or lateral sides of the interval and then advancing the capsule proximally (Figs. 10-4 and 10-5). In this method, the interval forms the transverse base for the capsular repair. Closure of the interval is accomplished with multiple nonabsorbable no. 1 sutures running from the base of the coracoid laterally to the humeral head.

Excess capsular laxity may be dealt with on the medial side of the joint, the lateral side of the joint, or both sides of the joint. If a Bankart lesion is present, we prefer a medial T-plasty capsulorrhaphy to allow correction of both the Bankart lesion and the capsular laxity. If only capsular laxity is found, it is technically easier to perform a lateral capsular shift as described by Neer.[14,35,42]

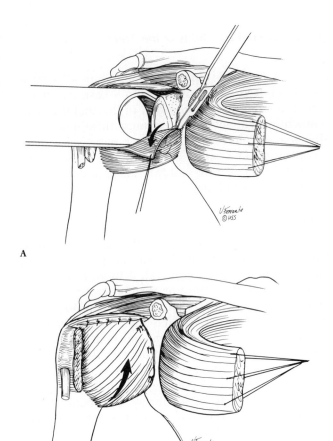

A

B

FIGURE 10-4

A. If a Bankart lesion is encountered in a patient with multidirectional instability, the rotator interval can be connected to a medial capsular incision in order to eliminate both the Bankart lesion and the abnormal capsular laxity. *B.* After creation of the medial limb of the capsular incision, the capsule is shifted superomedially and the rotator interval is closed with nonabsorbable sutures.

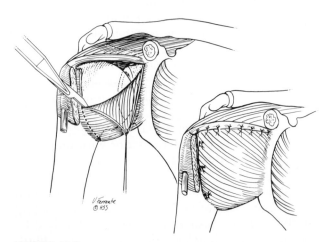

FIGURE 10-5

In cases with a large rotator interval in which no Bankart lesion is found, the interval may be incorporated into a lateral capsular shift. In this case, the capsule is shifted superolaterally.

If the rotator interval is not used to inspect the joint, the labrum is viewed via an oblique capsulotomy that is created proximal to the IGHLC (Fig. 10-6). This nearly transverse incision can then be extended either medially or laterally, depending on the presence or absence of a Bankart lesion. If a Bankart lesion is noted, the capsulotomy is converted to a T by creating a vertical limb at the glenoid margin that extends back to the posterior capsule (Fig. 10-6). The axillary nerve is vulnerable during this portion of the procedure and must be protected. The anterior glenoid margin is exposed and is roughened to a bleeding surface with a small osteotome or burr.[56] Drill holes are created at the glenoid margin for the passage of heavy nonabsorbable sutures. The inferior flap is then advanced superiorly to eliminate inferior laxity and medially while the arm is held in 30 to 45° of external rotation and 40 to 50° of abduction. In a thrower or swimmer, the maximum degree of external rotation that maintains stability of the

shoulder is preferable. The sutures are passed through the inferior limb and are tied. Next the superior flap is advanced distally, and the sutures are passed a second time. The goal is not to overtighten the capsule medially but to tension it superiorly.

Recently, we have used TAG suture anchors (Acufex Microsurgical, Inc., Mansfield, MA) to allow direct suture placement and to obviate the need for drill holes[53] (Fig. 10-6). If suture anchors are used, they must be prestressed by pulling on the sutures prior to passage through the capsule. The anchors should be placed at the glenoid margin and not medially along the glenoid neck.

If no Bankart lesion is found, the vertical limb of the T is placed laterally near the humeral neck (Fig. 10-7). The lateral limb allows easier and safer access to the posterior capsule and is preferable if there is no evidence of capsulolabral stripping from the anterior glenoid. The lateral incision is made directly on the bone if the humeral attachment of the

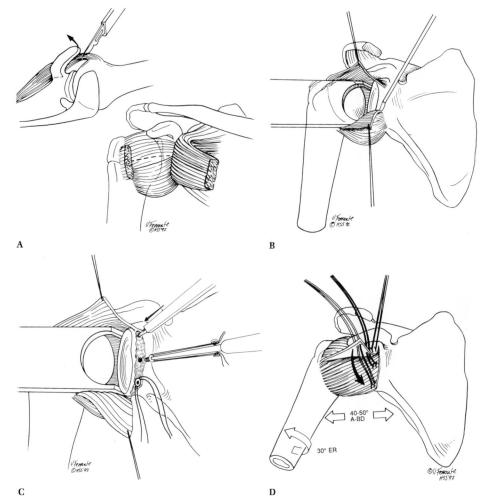

A

B

C

D

FIGURE 10-6
If a rotator interval lesion is not found, the joint is viewed through an oblique (almost transverse) capsular incision (*A*). If a Bankart lesion is encountered, the capsular incision is converted to a T by creating a vertical limb medially at the glenoid margin (*B*).

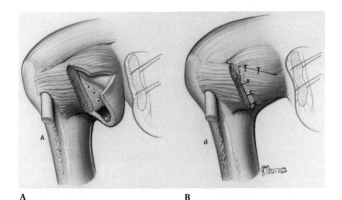

FIGURE 10-7
If no Bankart lesion is found, the capsule is shifted laterally. The vertical capsular incision is made laterally at the humeral neck. The superior flap of the capsule is shifted inferolaterally and the inferior flap is moved superolaterally.

capsule is attenuated or if there is stripping of the capsule from the humeral neck. In this situation, drill holes in the proximal humerus may be used for suture placement, but these are difficult to position, particularly inferiorly. Suture anchors are an excellent alternative, but the quality of the bone must be assessed following their placement, particularly in the superior portion of the humeral head.

In some cases with extreme inferior laxity, an anterior H-plasty may be necessary to allow sufficient mobilization of the capsule. This is accomplished by creating both medial and lateral vertical limbs in the capsulotomy and then advancing the inferior flap superiorly (Fig. 10-8).

It is important to note that an axillary contracture can occur after the performance of a capsular shift. These contractures tend to occur when the re-

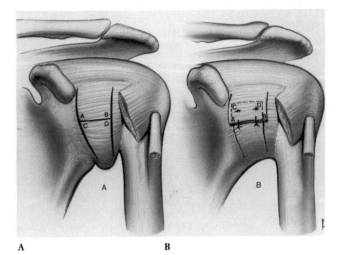

FIGURE 10-8
In cases with extreme capsular laxity, the anterior capsular incision may be converted into an H by creating both medial and lateral vertical incisions. The inferior capsular flap is then moved superiorly while the superior flap is brought inferiorly.

pair is performed in less than 45° of abduction. Once these contractures have occurred, restoration of elevation and rotation is extremely difficult.

In patients who have failed an attempt at anterior stabilization and are found to have evidence of multidirectional instability, extensive scarring may make it especially difficult to shift the capsule.[24]

After the capsule has been satisfactorily addressed, the subscapularis tendon is reapproximated but not tightened. If the conjoined tendon was partially released, it is repaired. A subcutaneous drain is placed, and the wound is closed.

After an anterior capsulorrhaphy for multidirectional instability, the patient is placed in a shoulder immobilizer, and the arm is kept in adduction and internal rotation for 6 weeks. We formerly placed these patients in an Orthoplast splint in slight abduction and internal rotation, but we have found that this is not necessary if the inferior instability has been eliminated when the repair is tested in the operating room. Pendulum exercises are initiated soon after surgery. Gentle passive flexion exercises to 90° are instituted after 3 weeks. At 6 weeks, active-assisted range of motion exercises are begun. When full range of motion is obtained, active resistance exercises are started in order to strengthen the internal and external rotators and the deltoid. Light throwing and sidearm racket sports are permitted after 6 months. At 6 to 9 months, patients with a traumatic etiology may return to contact sports, hard throwing, and overhead racket sports. Patients of the atraumatic type are protected from these activities for 9 to 12 months.

POSTERIOR APPROACH

Although some surgeons prefer an anterior approach for all types of multidirectional instability, we feel that a posterior approach should be used when the predominant clinical direction of instability is posterior.

The technique of posterior T-plasty capsular shift is as follows:[19] The patient is placed in either the lateral decubitus or, more recently, the modified beach chair position (Fig. 10-9). Initially, a horizontal skin incision was used. The horizontal incision is placed 1 cm inferior to the scapular spine, and allows the surgeon to obtain a bone graft from the scapular spine if indicated. We have gradually given up the use of a graft and have found that the transverse incision leaves a wide, uncosmetic scar.

A vertical incision is presently used in most patients. This incision is made midway between the lateral border of the acromion and the posterior axillary crease. The superficial deltoid fascia is identified, and the deltoid is split in the direction of its fibers to expose the infraspinatus and teres minor

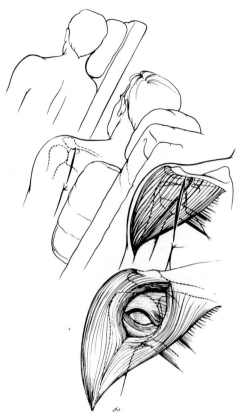

FIGURE 10-9
In cases with predominately posterior instability, the glenohumeral joint may be approached with the patient in the modified beach chair position. A longitudinal skin incision is used. The deltoid is split in the direction of its fibers. An interval is then created within the infraspinatus tendon to expose the joint. If the capsule is of poor quality, the infraspinatus may be tenotomized and used to reinforce the capsular repair.

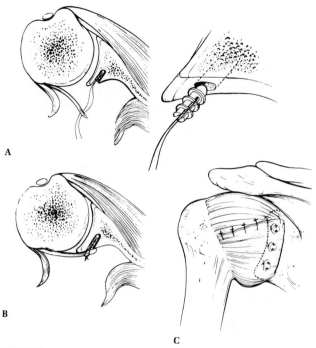

A

B

C

FIGURE 10-10
Posterior laxity may be eliminated by performing a T-plasty capsular incision and shifting the capsule. Suture anchors are used to fix the capsule.

tendons. Division of the deltoid begins at the scapular spine and proceeds inferiorly, staying proximal to the axillary nerve.

Next the infraspinatus tendon may be incised vertically with a large portion of the tendon remaining laterally. Alternatively, especially in throwers, the capsule may be exposed by developing an interval within the infraspinatus tendon without division of the tendon. The surgeon should be mindful of the axillary nerve and the posterior circumflex humeral vessels that exit the quadrilateral space immediately inferior to the teres minor.

A T-shaped capsular incision is then made (Fig. 10-10). If there is a doubt as to the presence of a Bankart lesion, an oblique capsular incision can be made to allow inspection of the joint. The incision may then be extended vertically on the medial or lateral margin of the joint in order to diminish the joint volume. If a posterior Bankart lesion is present, the vertical limb of the incision is placed medially, near the glenoid margin, to facilitate a concomitant Bankart repair. With the arm in neutral rotation and 30 to 40° of abduction, the capsule is reattached to the glenoid

through drill holes or using suture anchors. Prior to reattachment, the inferior limb of the capsule is advanced medially and superiorly to eliminate laxity in the posteroinferior capsule.

In cases without a Bankart lesion, the vertical portion of the T-plasty may be performed on the lateral side of the joint, and the capsule may be shifted at the humeral neck.

If marked capsular laxity is noted with the arm in a position of abduction despite the medial T-plication, a second vertical capsular incision is placed laterally to create an "H-plasty." In the patient with multidirectional instability, conversion of the capsulotomy to an H-plasty is often necessary in order to advance the inferior capsule further. It is important to dissect inferiorly to a degree that is sufficient to allow advancement of the posterior band of the IGHLC. The inferior capsule is then brought superiorly so that posterior laxity is eliminated with the arm in neutral rotation.

The capsular repair may be reinforced with the infraspinatus tendon if local tissue is felt to be insufficient. This tendon is of variable quality. Its proximal aspect tends to be its most prominent part. Often the healthy part of the tendon is quite short. When this is the case, attachment of the lateral portion of the tendon to the glenoid would unduly restrict internal rotation. Instead the tendon is simply sutured directly to the posterior capsule to reinforce the capsular repair.

137

The anterosuperior capsule has been shown to be an important stabilizer against posterior translation of the humeral head.[66] In our experience, it has not been necessary to specifically address the anterior structures at the time of reconstruction; however, the surgeon may have to consider the role of the anterosuperior capsule in posterior instability. Additional tensioning of this area may be especially applicable to cases with an atraumatic etiology. Inferior laxity with the arm in adduction may indicate that the superior structures need additional tensioning. Tensioning of the superior structures may be technically difficult from a posterior approach. This difficulty has led some surgeons to consider an anterior approach in selected cases.

The patient is maintained in an Orthoplast splint with the arm in extension and neutral rotation for the first 6 weeks after operation. In throwers, early passive motion may be instituted with rotation from neutral to full external rotation. Full internal rotation should be avoided. Flexion is best avoided for 6 weeks, but elevation in the plane of the scapula will allow healing to occur without undue stress to the repair.

COMBINED APPROACHES

Both anterior and posterior approaches may be required on rare occasions.[44] The combined approaches are indicated when significant anterior labral detachment is noted after a posterior approach, when there is doubt concerning the adequacy of stabilization after capsular repair of the first side, or when prior surgery has resulted in a contracture on the opposite side of the joint and release is required before a capsular shift can be performed.

Clinical Results

The results of the surgical treatment of shoulder instability in the face of capsular laxity have historically been less successful than those for unidirectional anterior instability. Results have improved with current techniques, however.

Neer and Foster, in their classic 1980 article[42] describing inferior capsular shift, reported a successful outcome in 36 of 37 shoulders with multidirectional instability. Neer has subsequently written that he has performed more than 100 additional inferior capsular shifts "with similar satisfactory results."

Bigliani et al.[7] presented the results of inferior capsular shift in 74 athletes with anterior and inferior instability. In this series, 89 percent of the athletes returned to their major sport and 73 percent were able to maintain their premorbid level of com-

petition. Seventy-one percent of overhead athletes returned to their premorbid level. Only 2 of 79 shoulders dislocated postoperatively. Average loss of external rotation was 7°.

Altchek et al.[1] noted four recurrences in 40 patients (42 shoulders) and a 95 percent patient satisfaction rate at 2-year minimum follow-up after T-plasty repair for anteroinferior multidirectional instability. One of the patients had a single postoperative episode of anterior subluxation, while three patients developed signs of posterior instability. In one of these three, a subsequent posterior stabilization was required. No patient lost more than 5° of abduction, forward flexion, or internal rotation. Approximately one-half of the patients regained external rotation to a degree that was equal to the opposite side. The vast majority of patients who lost motion were noted to have diminished motion preoperatively. No patient lost more than 20° of external rotation. Thirty-three of the patients reported full return to sports.

Brems and Bergfeld[10] reported on 20 patients (24 shoulders) treated with an inferior capsular shift and followed for 21 to 57 months. None of these patients has postoperative instability. Eighty-five percent were able to return to their premorbid level of function. Average motion loss was 17° of elevation, 15° of external rotation, and two spinal segments of internal rotation. Average rotator cuff strength was 73 percent of that on the opposite side.

Hawkins et al.[24] reported on 31 patients followed 2 to 5 years after an inferior capsular shift. Nineteen patients had a satisfactory result, only two of whom had significant posterior instability. Twelve patients had unsatisfactory outcomes. Of these 12, 7 had significant posterior instability, 10 had undergone a previous attempt at surgical stabilization, and 6 had osteoarthritic changes in the shoulder. The authors concluded that patients with primarily posterior instability fared more poorly, particularly if they had undergone previous surgery. It should be noted that, in contrast to the series of Altchek et al., most of the patients in Hawkins' series had the more classic findings of an atraumatic etiology and no Bankart lesion. This population tends to produce excessive collagen that may have poorer strength characteristics.

Lebar and Alexander[36] followed 10 active military personnel for an average of 28 months after inferior capsular shift. One patient required reoperation for recurrent instability. Losses of elevation and external rotation were minimal. There was an average loss of internal rotation of three spinal segments. The authors felt that prognosis was improved in patients who gave a history of a significant traumatic event and worsened if there was a history of a previous instability repair.

Complications

Recurrent instability is the most common complication after an attempt at operative stabilization for multidirectional instability. Neer has reported three cases of neuropraxia of the axillary nerve after inferior capsular shift.[43] We have had a brachial plexus palsy that involved multiple nerves, but fortunately the neuropraxia resolved over an 8-month period. As mentioned earlier, contractures can occur after capsular shifts and may result in pain, limited motion, and arthritis. One should not assume that all patients with multidirectional instability will automatically regain full motion regardless of the type of capsular tightening. While it is true that most of these patients tend to stretch out their repairs and gain motion (especially those with an atraumatic etiology), we have treated patients with marked contractures following capsular shifts that overtightened the axillary recess. Treatment of these patients is extremely difficult.

Reflex sympathetic dystrophy and thoracic outlet symptoms may occur after operative treatment of multidirectional instability. Often thoracic outlet symptoms are present preoperatively and may or may not resolve after surgery. It appears that excessive scar formation is a characteristic of some of the patients in the atraumatic group, and this scarring may result in pressure in the brachial plexus and outlet symptomatology.

CONCLUSIONS

Glenohumeral instability is a common cause of disability in the athletic population. The shoulder joint is extremely mobile, and bony stability has been sacrificed to allow for this motion. Glenohumeral stability is dependent upon the soft tissues surrounding the joint. These soft tissue stabilizers operate in a complex pattern that varies with shoulder position and activity. Multidirectional instability of the glenohumeral joint is increasingly recognized as an important cause of shoulder disability. Diagnostic signs may be subtle. Evidence of inferior laxity is the hallmark of diagnosis in most cases.

Nonoperative treatment and rehabilitation are based on the principle of secondary mechanisms of restraint. If operative intervention is employed, the surgeon should carefully define the problem and address the pathologic anatomy accordingly. Standard procedures for unidirectional anterior instability are likely to fail in the treatment of posterior or multidirectional instability and may, in fact, worsen the problem. A scientific approach that is directed at the restoration of normal capsular anatomy should be employed to prevent instability while retaining maximal function. This involves a careful assessment of the direction and degree of instability and a knowledge of the structures that primarily restrain these abnormal motions. Lax or damaged tissues can thus be repaired or tensioned to recreate a stable and functional joint.

REFERENCES

1. Altchek D, Warren R, Skyhar M, Ortiz G: T-plasty modification of the Bankart procedure for multidirectional instability of anterior and inferior types. *J Bone Joint Surg (Am)* 73A:105, 1991.
2. Altchek D, Warren R: Arthroscopic anterior stabilization in patients without labral detachment. Presented at Annual Meeting of Arthroscopy Association of North America, Boston, 1992.
3. Bankart A: The pathology and treatment of recurrent dislocation of the shoulder joint. *Br Med J* 2:1132, 1923.
4. Bankart A: The pathology and surgical treatment of recurrent dislocation of the shoulder. *Br J Surg* 26:23, 1938.
5. Bankart A: Discussion on recurrent dislocation of the shoulder. *J Bone Joint Surg (Br)* 30B:46, 1948.
6. Belle R, Hawkins R: Collagen typing and production in multidirectional instability of the shoulder. *Orthop Trans* 15:188, 1991.
7. Bigliani L, Kurzwell P, Schwartzbach C, et al: Inferior capsular shift procedure for anterior-inferior instability in athletes. *Orthop Trans* 13:560, 1989.
8. Bost F, Inman V: The pathologic changes in recurrent dislocation of the shoulder: A report of Bankart's operative procedure. *J Bone Joint Surg (Am)* 24:595, 1942.
9. Bowen M, Warren R: Ligamentous control of shoulder stability based on selective cutting and static translation. *Clin Sports Med* 10:757, 1991.
10. Brems J, Bergfeld J: Multidirectional shoulder instability. *Orthop Trans* 15:84, 1991.
11. Browne A, Hoffmeyer P, An K, Morrey B: The influence of atmospheric pressure on shoulder stability. *Orthop Trans* 14:259, 1990.

12. Burkhead W, Rockwood C: Treatment of instability of the shoulder with an exercise program. *J Bone Joint Surg (Am)* 74A:890, 1992.

13. Cain P, Mutschler T, Fu F: Anterior stability of the glenohumeral joint: A dynamic model. *Am J Sports Med* 15:144, 1987.

14. Cooper R, Brems J: Inferior capsular shift for multidirectional instability. Presented at Annual Meeting of the American Academy of Orthopaedic Surgeons, Washington, DC, 1992.

15. Cooper D, Arnoczky S, O'Brien S, et al: Anatomy, histology, and vascularity of the glenoid labrum. *J Bone Joint Surg (Am)* 73A:46, 1992.

16. Coughlin L, Rubinovich M, Johansson J, et al: Arthroscopic staple capsulorrhaphy for anterior shoulder instability. *Am J Sports Med* 20:253, 1992.

17. DePalma A, Callery G, Bennett G: Variational anatomy and degenerative lesions of the shoulder joint in Blount W, Banks S (eds): *The American Academy of Orthopaedic Surgeons Instructional Course Lectures*. Ann Arbor, JW Edwards, 1949, p 255.

18. Detrisac D: Arthroscopic shoulder staple capsulorrhaphy for traumatic anterior instability, in McGinty J (ed): *Operative Arthroscopy*. New York, Raven Press, 1991, p 517.

19. Fronek J, Warren R, Bowen M: Posterior subluxation of the glenohumeral joint. *J Bone Joint Surg (Am)* 71A:205, 1989.

20. Habermeyer P, Schuller U: Die Bedeutung des Labrum glenoidale für die Stabilitat des Glenhumeralgelenkes. *Unfallchirurg* 92:1989.

21. Hall R, Isaac F, Booth C: Dislocations of the shoulder with special reference to accompanying small fractures. *J Bone Joint Surg (Am)* 41A:489, 1959.

22. Harryman D, Sidles J, Harris S, Matsen F: Role of the rotator interval capsule in passive motion and stability of the shoulder. *J Bone Joint Surg (Am)* 72A:53, 1992.

23. Hawkins R, Koppert G, Johnston G: Recurrent posterior instability (subluxation) of the shoulder. *J Bone Joint Surg (Am)* 66A:169, 1984.

24. Hawkins R, Kunkel S, Nayak N: Inferior capsular shift for multidirectional instability of the shoulder: 2–5 year follow-up. *Orthop Trans* 15:765, 1991.

25. Helfet A: Coracoid transplantation for recurring dislocation of the shoulder. *J Bone Joint Surg (Br)* 40B:198, 1958.

26. Helmig P, Sojbjerg J, Kjaersgaard-Andersen P, et al: Distal humeral migration as a component of multidirectional shoulder instability: An anatomical study in autopsy specimens. *Clin Orthop* 252:1990, 1990.

27. Hill H, Sachs M: Grooved defect of the humeral head: A frequently unrecognized complication of dislocation of the shoulder joint. *Radiology* 35:690, 1940.

28. Howell S, Iombersteg A, Seger O, Marone P: Clarification of the role of the supraspinatus muscle in shoulder function. *J Bone Joint Surg (Am)* 68A:398, 1986.

29. Howell S, Galinat B: The glenoid-labral socket. A constrained articular surface. *Clin Orthop* 243:122, 1989.

30. Humphry G: *A Treatise on the Human Skeleton (Including the Joints)*. Cambridge, Macmillan, 1858.

31. Jobe F, Kvitne R: Shoulder pain in the overhead or throwing athlete: The relationship of anterior instability and rotator cuff impingement. *Orthop Rev* 18:963, 1989.

32. Jobe F, Giangarra C, Kvitne R, Glousman R: Anterior capsulolabral reconstruction of the shoulder in athletes in overhead sports. *Am J Sports Med* 19:428, 1991.

33. Kronberg M, Brostrom L-A, Nemeth G: Differences in shoulder muscle activity between patients with generalized joint laxity and normal controls. *Clin Orthop* 269:181, 1991.

34. Kumar V, Balasubramianum P: The role of atmospheric pressure in stabilizing the shoulder. An experimental study. *J Bone Joint Surg (Br)* 67B:719, 1985.

35. Lambrechts A, de Villiers C, de Beer J: Neer capsular shift for treatment of recurrent dislocation of the shoulder. *J Bone Joint Surg (Br)* 73B (suppl II):141, 1991.

36. Lebar R, Alexander A: Multidirectional shoulder instability: Clinical results of inferior capsular shift in an active-duty population. *Am J Sports Med* 20:193, 1992.

37. Leslie J, Ryan T: Anterior axillary approach to the shoulder joint. *J Bone Joint Surg (Am)* 44A:1193, 1962.

38. Magnuson P, Stack J: Recurrent dislocation of the shoulder. *JAMA* 123:889, 1943.

39. Matsen F, Thomas S, Rockwood C: Anterior glenohumeral instability, in Rockwood C, Matsen F (eds): *The Shoulder*. Philadelphia, Saunders, 1990, 526.

40. Morrey B, Janes J: Anterior dislocation of the shoulder: Long-term follow-up of the Putti-Platt and Bankart procedures. *J Bone Joint Surg (Am)* 58A:252, 1976.

41. Moseley H, Overgaard B: The anterior capsular mechanism in recurrent dislocation of the shoulder: Morphological and clinical studies with special reference to the glenoid labrum and glenohumeral ligaments. *J Bone Joint Surg (Am)* 44B:913, 1962.

42. Neer C, Foster C: Inferior capsular shift for involuntary inferior and multidirectional instability of the shoulder: A preliminary report. *J Bone Joint Surg (Am)* 62A:897, 1980.

43. Neer C: Involuntary inferior and multidirectional instability of the shoulder: Etiology, recognition, and treatment, in Stauffer E (ed): *American Academy of Orthopaedic Surgeons Instructional Course Lectures.* St Louis, Mosby, 1985, p 232.

44. Neer C: Dislocations, in *Shoulder Reconstruction.* Philadelphia, Saunders, 1990, p 273.

45. Nobuhara K, Ikeda H: Rotator cuff interval lesion. *Clin Orthop* 223:44, 1987.

46. O'Brien S, Schwartz R, Warren R, Torzilli P: Capsular restraints to anterior/posterior motion of the shoulder. *Orthop Trans* 12:143, 1988.

47. O'Brien S, Neves M, Arnoczky S, et al: The anatomy and histology of the inferior glenohumeral ligament complex of the shoulder. *Am J Sports Med* 18:449, 1990.

48. O'Connell P, Nuber G, Mileski R, Lautenslager E: The contribution of the glenohumeral to anterior stability of the shoulder joint. *Am J Sports Med* 18:579, 1990.

49. Osmond-Clarke H: Habitual dislocation of the shoulder: The Putti-Platt operation. *J Bone Joint Surg (Br)* 30B:19, 1948.

50. Oveson J, Nielson S: Posterior instability of the shoulder: A cadaver study. *Acta Ortho Scand* 57:436, 1986.

51. Pavlov H, Warren R, Weiss C, Dines D: The roentgenographic evaluation of anterior shoulder instability. *Clin Orthop* 194:153, 1985.

52. Pollock R, Bigliani L, Flatow E, et al: The mechanical properties of the inferior glenohumeral ligament. *Orthop Trans* 14:259, 1990.

53. Richmond J, Donaldson W, Fu F, Harner C: Modification of the Bankart reconstruction with a suture anchor. Report of a new technique. *Am J Sports Med* 19:343, 1991.

54. Roukos J, Feagin J, Abbott H: Modified axillary roentgenogram: A useful adjunct in the diagnosis of recurrent instability of the shoulder. *Clin Orthop* 82:84, 1972.

55. Rowe C, Zarins B: Recurrent transient subluxation of the shoulder. *J Bone Joint Surg (Am)* 63A:863, 1981.

56. Rowe C, Zarins B, Ciullo J: Recurrent anterior dislocation of the shoulder after surgical repair. *J Bone Joint Surg (Am)* 66A:159, 1984.

57. Terry G, Hammon D, France P, Norwood L: The stabilizing function of passive shoulder restraints. *Am J Sports Med* 19:26, 1991.

58. Townley C: The capsular mechanism in recurrent dislocation of the shoulder. *J Bone Joint Surg (Am)* 32A:370, 1950.

59. Townsend H, Jobe F, Pink M, Perry J: Electromyographic analysis of the glenohumeral muscles during a baseball rehabilitation program. *Am J Sports Med* 19:264, 1991.

60. Turkel S, Panio M, Marshall J, Girgis F: Stabilizing mechanisms preventing anterior dislocation of the glenohumeral joint. *J Bone Joint Surg (Am)* 63A:1208, 1981.

61. Uhthoff H, Piscopo M: Anterior capsular redundancy of the shoulder: Congenital or traumatic? An embryological study. *J Bone Joint Surg (Br)* 67B:363, 1985.

62. Vanderhooft E, Lippitt S, Harris S: Glenohumeral stability from concavity-compression: A quantitative analysis. Presented at Annual Meeting of American Shoulder and Elbow Surgeons, Washington, DC, 1992.

63. Vellett A, Munk P, Marks P: Imaging techniques of the shoulder: Present perspectives. *Clin Sports Med* 10:721, 1991.

64. Warner J, Deng X, Warren R, et al: Static capsuloligamentous restraints to superior-inferior translation of the glenohumeral joint. Presented at Annual Meeting of the Orthopaedic Research Society, Anaheim, 1991.

65. Warner J, Deng X, Warren R, et al: Superior-inferior translation in the intact and vented glenohumeral joint. Presented at Annual Meeting of American Shoulder and Elbow Surgeons, Anaheim, 1991.

66. Warren R, Kornblatt I, Marchand R: Static factors affecting posterior shoulder stability. *Orthop Trans* 8:89, 1984.

67. Zarins B, Rowe C, Stone J: Shoulder instability: Management of failed reconstructions, in Barr J (ed): *American Academy of Orthopaedic Surgeons Instructional Course Lectures.* Park Ridge, IL, American Academy of Orthopaedic Surgeons, 1989.

CHAPTER 11

Rotator Cuff Impingement in Athletes

Ronald P. Karzel
Wilson Del Pizzo

INTRODUCTION

In 1972, Neer first introduced the concept of rotator cuff impingement into the surgical literature.[1] Neer believed that the majority of rotator cuff lesions were the result of a mechanical impingement of the rotator cuff tendons beneath the anterior inferior portions of the acromion, particularly when the shoulder was placed in a position of forward elevation and internal rotation. Neer[1,2] described three stages in the impingement process. In stage I lesions, the rotator cuff is acutely inflamed, without mechanical disruption. He felt that these lesions occurred commonly in patients younger than 25 years old and that these lesions were generally reversible with rest and appropriate conservative management. If inflammation continued, stage II patients developed chronic scarring and fibrosis in the rotator cuff tendon, and many of these patients failed to improve with conservative measures. These patients, who were generally between the ages of 25 and 40 years old, often required surgery to decrease the stresses on the rotator cuff and allow the patients to return to activities. The operation proposed by Neer was an open anterior acromioplasty, in which the anterior inferior acromion and coracoacromial ligament were removed. Patients untreated at the early stages of impingement progressed into stage III impingement, which is characterized by mechanical disruption of the rotator cuff tendon, and changes in the coracoacromial arch such as osteophyte formation along the anterior acromion. These older patients generally required anterior acromioplasty and rotator cuff repair for appropriate treatment. In all these stages, the etiology of rotator cuff pathology was felt to be impingement of the rotator cuff tendons under a rigid coracoacromial arch. Tearing and degenerative changes within the rotator cuff were felt to be secondary to this primary impingement problem.

The influence of acromial morphology on the presence of rotator cuff lesions was studied further by Bigliani and Morrison,[3,4] who classified acromial shape into three types. A type I acromion is flat without significant narrowing of the subacromial space. A type II acromion has a smooth curve that parallels the humeral head. In a type III acromion, there is an anterior hook on the acromion that narrows the anterior subacromial space. They found a low incidence of complete rotator cuff tears in their cadaver study in patients with a type I arch, while most patients having complete rotator cuff tears had a type II or III arch configuration. These concepts of impingement syndrome as the primary cause of rotator cuff pathology have been widely accepted and have been useful for standardizing the approach to rotator cuff tears. In many cases, patients diagnosed as having impingement syndrome will do well after anterior acromioplasty and will be able to return to their previous activities. However, it has become increasingly clear that many patients previously diagnosed with impingement syndrome actually have other etiologies for their shoulder symptoms. This has resulted in additional theories regarding the causes of rotator cuff symptoms in athletes.

SECONDARY IMPINGEMENT

Many young athletes, particularly athletes involved in throwing and other overhead sports activities, develop symptoms that have been classically labeled as impingement syndrome. Despite symptoms of rotator cuff tendinitis and impingement findings on physical examination, many of these patients do not have findings consistent with impingement at the time of surgery, and subacromial decompression is often not helpful in relieving symptoms in these athletes and allowing them to return to full sports activities. Glousman[5] summarized the results of surgical treatment of rotator cuff dysfunction in athletes at the Kerlan-Jobe Orthopaedic Clinic. Elite athletes were studied, all of whom were felt to have primarily rotator cuff pathology and all of whom had failed a conservative rehabilitation program for at least 9 to 12 months or had a documented complete tear of the rotator cuff prior to proceeding with surgery. These patients were treated with an open anterior inferior acromioplasty, resection of the coracoacromial ligament, and rotator cuff repair if a tear was present. Only 50 percent of the athletes obtained a good result. When broken down into categories of participation, only 25 percent of swimmers obtained a good result, and only 34 percent of pitchers and throwers were able to return to their previous level of sports activities. When this group was separated further into skilled pitchers and throwers including collegiate and professional pitchers, only 27 percent obtained a good result. When results from the three different groups of impingement and complete rotator cuff tears were compared, the degree of rotator cuff pathology had no influence on the ultimate result. The second group of patients at their institution was reviewed following arthroscopic subacromial decompression, which also allowed for evaluation of the glenohumeral joint for associated pathology. None of these patients had a full-thickness rotator cuff tear. Although 77 percent of patients were able to return to sports, only 46 percent were able to return to the same level of overhead athletic activity following arthroscopic subacromial decompression. Only 25 percent of those who were found to have either capsular laxity or labral pathology were able to return to the same level of activity. In the arthroscopically treated group, none of the pitchers or swimmers were able to return to their same competitive status. The authors concluded that the ultimate results of arthroscopic subacromial decompression were comparable with those of open rotator cuff surgery. Such procedures resulted in excellent pain relief and reduced morbidity but did not allow predictable return to high-level competitive overhead sports.[6,7,8]

Several authors have noted the high incidence of anterior instability in the overhead athlete.[9–11] This has led to the concept of secondary impingement which is defined as rotator cuff impingement that occurs secondary to a functional decrease in the space in the supraspinatus outlet due to underlying instability of the glenohumeral joint. It appears that secondary impingement may be the most common cause of rotator cuff symptoms in younger patients, particularly throwing athletes. Overhead athletes frequently place large stresses on the dynamic and static stabilizers on the glenohumeral joint. These repetitive stresses may result in microtrauma to the glenohumeral ligaments. This eventually leads to attenuation of these structures, and the development of mild glenohumeral instability. Such instability places increased stress on the dynamic stabilizers of the glenohumeral joint, including the rotator cuff tendons. These increased demands on the rotator cuff may lead to rotator cuff pathology such as partial tearing or tendinitis, and as the rotator cuff muscle fatigues, the humeral head translates anteriorly and superiorly, impinging on the coracoacromial arch. This also leads to rotator cuff inflammation. In these patients, treatment should be directed at the underlying instability problem. This includes initial exercises for rotator cuff and parascapular strengthening in an effort to decrease fatigue and improve the dynamic stabilization of the shoulder. Also important is a program to maintain shoulder flexibility with stretching, particularly of a tight posterior capsule. Most athletes will respond well to such a program, and surgery will not be required. If rehabilitation is not successful, and the athlete desires to return to overhead athletics, surgical stabilization may be required. A recent study of anterior shoulder reconstructions in overhand athletes has shown that approximately 75 percent of overhand athletes treated with this approach have been able to return to their previous levels of sports activities.[12,13]

GLENOID IMPINGEMENT

The presence of partial-thickness rotator cuff tears in throwing athletes, particularly those involving the articular surface of the rotator cuff tendon, has been difficult to explain with previous concepts of impingement. In many of these athletes, articular surface tears are noted but are not accompanied by any tearing of the bursal surface or evidence of impingement when the subacromial bursa is examined. Such tears might occur in the presence of instability due to increased tensile stresses on the rotator cuff tendon either from abnormal motion of the glenohumeral joint or from the increased forces on the rotator cuff necessary to stabilize the shoulder. Recently, the concept of glenoid impingement has been advanced as a possible cause of such lesions. Walch and coworkers[14] studied 17 athletes with unexplained shoulder pain during throwing activities. The mean age of these athletes was 25 years, with a range from 15 to 30 years. None of these athletes had clinical, radiologic, or arthroscopic evidence of anterior instability, and all had positive impingement findings. When these patients were arthroscoped and the shoulder was placed in the abducted and externally rotated position, impingement was noted in all patients between the posterior superior edge of the glenoid and the insertion of the rotator cuff tendon with the arm in the throwing position. Contact occurred between 90 and 150° of abduction in the area between 9 and 11 o'clock on the posterior edge of the glenoid. In these patients, lesions were often noted in the area of impingement along the posterior aspect of the labrum. Many of these patients also had partial articular surface rotator cuff tears of the supraspinatus tendon. These investigators felt that this posterior contact was a normal finding and could be found in varying degrees in healthy subjects. It was felt that with repetitive hard throwing, however, such repeated contact could lead to pathologic changes on the posterior glenoid labrum as well as to tearing of the supraspinatus tendon.

Sidles and coworkers[15] attempted to visualize impingement of the supraspinatus tendon by obtaining MRI views of the shoulder with the arm in the overhead position. Six normal subjects were studied, and it was found that when the arm was maximally elevated, the acromion did not impinge on the supraspinatus tendon. Instead, the acromion impinged on the shaft of the humerus. However, in maximal elevation, the undersurface of the supraspinatus tendon did impinge on the superior glenoid rim. They suggested that undersurface impingement of the supraspinatus tendon against the superior glenoid occurs when the arm is maximally elevated, and that impingement of this type may potentially cause both the undersurface tearing of the supraspinatus tendon, as well as acromial roughening consequent to humeral impingement.[15] Taken together, these two preliminary studies suggest that our present concept of impingement may need to be refined and expanded further in the future. Many athletes previously considered to have classic subacromial impingement syndrome may in fact have other causes for their shoulder pain that need to be addressed.

Clearly, not all athletes with shoulder symptoms can be considered to have impingement problems. However, many athletes seen in clinical practice will in fact have impingement of the supraspinatus tendon. This is particularly likely to occur in recreational athletes, particularly those over the age of 30. In these athletes, repetitive overhead trauma such as when playing tennis or when weightlifting may lead to classic symptoms of rotator cuff tendinitis without the patient's having any findings of instability. As has been noted previously, it is important to always remember the differential diagnosis for patients with shoulder symptoms and exclude other causes of pain. The remainder of this chapter, however, is dedicated to the diagnosis, conservative treatment, and surgical treatment of those athletes who do in fact have a primary subacromial impingement as the source of their shoulder symptoms.

DIAGNOSIS OF IMPINGEMENT SYNDROME

History

A careful history regarding the onset of symptoms as well as an attempt to characterize the relationship of pain to specific phases of the athletic event performed is often helpful. A sudden onset of sharp pain in the shoulder with a tearing sensation is more suggestive of a rotator cuff tear, while the gradual onset of increasing pain in the shoulder, related to overhead activities, is more suggestive of an impingement problem. Activities placing the arm in an elevated and internally rotated position are most likely to cause pain with impingement, while activities placing the arm in an externally rotated and abducted position are most likely to cause a feeling of pain and instability in patients with anterior glenohumeral laxity. It should also be determined if there are any other symptoms suggestive of instability such as dead-arm symptoms, although such symptoms are only occasionally seen in patients with subluxation. With throwing activities, patients with anterior subluxation of the shoulder may complain of posterior capsular pain in the shoulder, which is sometimes confused with an infraspinatus tendinitis. It is also helpful to know if the patient has any stiffness, numbness, or parasthesias. The treatment that has already been provided and the response to that treatment should also be determined.

Physical Examination

Physical examination of the shoulder joint generally begins with inspection, which should be performed with the entire shoulder and scapula well visualized. Muscle mass should be compared bilaterally in order to aid in the detection of atrophy. Active range of motion should be assessed, and the scapula should be observed for the presence of scapular winging. Stiffness should be checked, particularly by determining the extent of external and internal rotation in the shoulder with the patient's shoulder abducted 90°. Average external rotation and internal rotation is approximately 90°. It is helpful to test external and internal rotation with the patient supine to prevent increased scapular motion that may mask a deficit in glenohumeral motion. Most high-level pitchers will be found to have increased external rotation in the dominant pitching side compared with the nondominant side, and many will also have a loss of internal rotation. In patients with adhesive capsulitis, it may be difficult to move the shoulder at all into an externally rotated position.

Palpation is performed along the joints, paying particular attention to the biceps tendon, the supraspinatus and subscapularis tendon, and the anterolateral corner of the acromion. The acromioclavicular joint should also be assessed for tenderness as well as the posterior capsule of the shoulder. The suprascapular nerve should be palpated in the area of the suprascapular notch, as tenderness in this area may indicate suprascapular nerve entrapment that may cause supraspinatus atrophy and masquerade as a rotator cuff tear. Strength should also be assessed manually. The supraspinatus tendon may be isolated by having the patient rotate the upper extremity so that the thumb is facing toward the floor, and then resistance is applied to the arms in a position of 30° of forward flexion and 90° of abduction. Both weakness and the production of pain should be assessed.

Special tests may also be performed to determine if impingement syndrome is present. Neer described the classic impingement sign, consisting of the occurrence of pain when the arm is placed in a forward flexed position, and then forced farther upward, impinging the supraspinatus tendon under the acromion.[2] Hawkins has described a similar test in which the shoulder is forward flexed to 90° in a neutral position and then internally rotated.[16] The production of pain is a positive impingement sign. Neer also described an impingement test,[2] in which 10 mL of local anesthetic is injected into the subacromial bursa. In patients with impingement, this procedure should result in an immediate, significant decrease in the patient's pain. However, even if these tests are positive, it only means that the patient has irritation of the rotator cuff tendon and subacromial bursa. The underlying cause of this irritation and whether this irritation is a primary or secondary problem cannot be determined.

As noted previously, tests should also be performed to rule out instability. Subtle instability may be appreciated by using the apprehension relocation test first described by Jobe.[12] To perform the apprehension relocation test, the patient's arm is placed in a 90° abducted position, with the patient supine on the table. The standard apprehension test is per-

formed, and many patients with subluxation will complain of pain, particularly in the posterior aspect of the shoulder. Pressure is then placed with the examining hand over the anterior aspect of the shoulder, pushing the humeral head back into the glenohumeral socket. If the pain disappears with this maneuver, this is suggestive of the presence of anterior glenohumeral instability. At the Southern California Orthopedic Institute, we have also used a related test that is called the "apprehension-suppression" test (Fig. 11-1). Anterior pressure is first placed over the shoulder joint, and then the arm is maximally externally rotated. Most patients will be comfortable in this position. When pressure is suddenly removed from the anterior aspect of the shoulder, patients with instability will often note sudden pain and a feeling of instability as the humeral head suddenly slides anteriorly. The patient again becomes more comfortable when anterior pressure is applied. However, although these tests are suggestive of instability, a recent study has concluded that patients with a positive apprehension relocation test have findings of actual instability at surgery only approximately 50 percent of the time.[17] Patients with rotator cuff irritation without instability may also have a positive test. Shoulder stability should be carefully assessed by manual palpation, which we prefer to do with the patient lying on a side and with the shoulder to be examined supported in a position of 90° of abduction to allow for a slight axial loading of the glenohumeral joint. This allows for stabilization of the scapula and a more precise determination of the presence of instability. It is important that a comparison be made between the two shoulders. It should be noted that many throwing athletes will have slightly increased laxity in the affected shoulder that may not be pathologic.

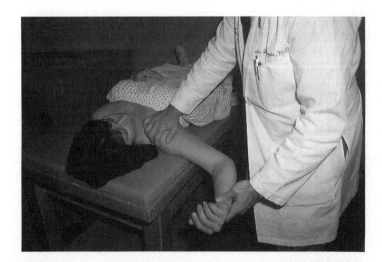

FIGURE 11-1
The "apprehension-suppression test" is performed by placing the arm into an apprehension position while maintaining pressure over the anterior humerus. The sudden release of pressure causes pain in a positive test.

Other tests are routinely performed including evaluation of the cervical spine, neurovascular examination to rule out problems such as thoracic outlet syndrome, and evaluation of the biceps tendon and the remainder of the upper extremity.

IMAGING TESTS

Particularly in the middle-aged athlete, routine radiographic studies of the shoulder may be helpful in diagnosis. We routinely use four views of the shoulder, consisting of an anterior-posterior view of the glenohumeral joint, an internal rotation view of the humerus with a 20° upward angulation to show the acromioclavicular joint, an axillary view, and a supraspinatus or arch view as described by Bigliani and Morrison.[3] These x-rays are used to rule out arthritis in the acromioclavicular joint or glenohumeral joint, and the axillary view is helpful for looking for subtle signs of instability such as glenoid avulsion fracture or Hill-Sachs defect. An os acromionale is also best visualized on the axillary view. The most important view in evaluating impingement is the arch view, which helps to determine the adequacy of the subacromial space. In a patient with a type III acromion who has a large anterior subacromial spur, there appears to be a much higher likelihood of primary impingement syndrome than is seen in those individuals with a type I acromion. In addition, we believe it is important to measure the width of the acromion on the arch view preoperatively prior to any type of subacromial decompression to ensure that the correct amount of bone is removed to allow for an adequate decompression, but

also to prevent an acromial fracture from excessive bone removal (Fig. 11-2).

When a patient fails to respond to appropriate conservative treatment for impingement syndrome, further diagnostic testing is indicated. Our test of choice at present is magnetic resonance imaging, which has essentially replaced arthrograms in our practice. MRI scans offer advantages over an arthrogram, in that they are noninvasive, do not require radiation, and can detect intrasubstance degeneration within the tendon or partial rotator cuff tears that are not readily detectable on conventional arthrography. In addition, MR scans do not result in postinjection pain and inflammation that may be caused by arthrogram contrast material. At present, we use an arthrogram only when the patient is claustrophobic, is physically too large to fit in the MRI scanner, or has a pacemaker or other contraindication to high-magnetic-field exposure. In our experience, MRI scanning is a useful and reliable test. However, good results with an MRI scan depend upon the quality of the imaging machine, with best results generally obtained using a 1.5-tesla magnet with dedicated shoulder coils and sophisticated software. Radiologists experienced in magnetic resonance imaging are also essential in evaluating the rotator cuff properly, but it is important that the shoulder surgeon review the films personally. In our experience, radiologists may misrepresent the actual condition of the rotator cuff, and reports from the radiologists may include the statement that the patient has impingement syndrome. Generally, this means that the patient had some evidence of impression of the acromioclavicular joint on the supraspinatus muscle belly and this may be a normal finding

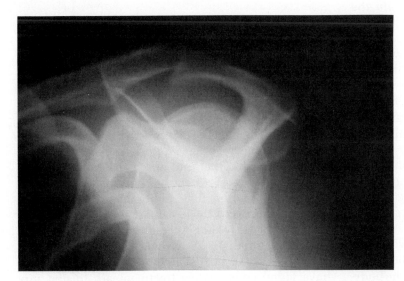

FIGURE 11-2
The "arch view" is obtained preoperatively to look for the presence of an anterior acromial spur and to determine the acromial thickness. This patient has a type III arch.

in many individuals. A diagnosis of impingement syndrome should be made on the basis of findings on history, physical examination, and imaging studies. Determining whether a patient has impingement syndrome from magnetic resonance imaging studies alone is not possible.

The best results appear to be obtained in magnetic resonance imaging by using three standard sequences including coronal, sagittal oblique, and axillary views. If the images are arranged so that the corresponding T1 and T2 images are placed side by side on the film, interpretation of the MRI scan is simplified, and it is less likely that subtle fluid collections that may indicate tears will be missed. The MRI scan in general is very sensitive in detecting rotator cuff pathology, even in the absence of mechanical disruption of the rotator cuff tendon. The biggest problem with MRI scans is often that the test is overly sensitive, and increased signal intensity due to tendinitis or partial tearing may be misinterpreted as a complete tear. In some cases, the use of an intraarticular contrast agent, gadolinium, in combination with MRI scans may improve the ability to detect partial rotator cuff tears.[19]

NONOPERATIVE TREATMENT OF IMPINGEMENT SYNDROME

As originally noted by Neer,[1] the majority of patients with impingement syndrome will recover with appropriate conservative measures without the need for surgery. Conservative treatment consists initially of rest from activities that cause pain, particularly repetitive overhead activities. Generally, antiinflammatory medications and ice will be used in an effort to decrease swelling and irritation. It is important to maintain conditioning activities while the athlete rests the shoulder to allow the quickest return to competition once the shoulder is healed. Many patients with rotator cuff tendinitis will also have mild degrees of stiffness in the shoulder, and initial stretching exercises for the shoulder to help regain full range of motion, particularly in forward flexion and internal rotation, are begun. Particular emphasis is placed on gentle, slow stretching maneuvers performed by the patient.

When irritation in the rotator cuff tendon has resolved and the patient has essentially normal motion, a program of rotator cuff muscle strengthening is begun. These exercises may be performed satisfactorily by the patient at home using an elastic tubing. Initially, internal and external rotation strengthening are performed against resistance from the rubber tubing with the elbow maintained at the side of the body

during these exercises to prevent impingement. As strength increases and pain diminishes, increased resistance is added, and strengthening exercises with the arm in a more abducted position may be allowed.

When the patient has regained full range of motion and strength in the shoulder, sports-specific exercises are begun and the patient is gradually allowed to return to sports activities. It is important to work at this point with the patient's coach or trainer to make sure that there is not a problem with technique that leads to impingement. With throwers, the patient with impingement syndrome frequently is overly abducting the shoulder from the ideal 90° abducted position during throwing. Correcting the throwing style may minimize the chances of recurrent impingement. Similarly, swimmers may need to increase their side-to-side roll when swimming freestyle to help minimize impingement. In addition, it is important to emphasize to the patient the necessity for maintaining a good rotator cuff strengthening and stretching program even after recovery from symptoms to prevent reinjury.

Generally, conservative measures are continued for at least 3 to 6 months or longer if the patient is improving. If the patient remains significantly disabled and has had no improvement after 3 months of conservative treatment, additional diagnostic testing such as an MRI is often indicated to rule out rotator cuff tearing. In those patients having a significant tear, surgery is recommended at this time. In the absence of a significant tear, further conservative treatment is continued. Corticosteroid injections into the subacromial bursa are used sparingly and are generally not repeated if no improvement is noted after an initial injection.

OPERATIVE TREATMENT OF CHRONIC IMPINGEMENT SYNDROME

As noted previously, most patients will respond well to a conservative treatment program. Indications for surgery are those patients who have failed at least 3 and preferably 6 months of appropriate conservative treatment, who have a full unrestricted passive range of motion, and who have a positive response to injection of lidocaine into the subacromial space. Surgery may be particularly likely to benefit those patients with a type III acromion having a large subacromial spur, and those patients in whom changes are noted in the rotator cuff tendon on MRI scanning.

At the Southern California Orthopedic Institute, patients with suspected rotator cuff problems who have failed conservative treatment are treated initially with examination under anesthesia and diagnostic arthroscopy. In general, an interscalene block anesthetic is placed by the anesthesiologist prior to the procedure, which is then performed in the lateral decubitus position with the patient under general anesthesia. The initial step is careful evaluation of the shoulder for range of motion and stability. In a patient with significant limitation of motion, manipulation of the shoulder is performed, and although diagnostic arthroscopy may also be performed, arthroscopic subacromial decompression is generally not performed on patients with significant preoperative stiffness because of the increased risk of postoperative adhesive capsulitis. It is also important to carefully document the presence of any instability. The shoulder is then arthroscoped and a systematic evaluation is performed within the glenohumeral joint. Particular attention is paid to the rotator cuff, especially the supraspinatus tendon near its insertion onto the greater tuberosity. The rotator cuff tendon is visualized both from the posterior portal and also from an anterior portal. The subscapularis tendon is also well visualized through the anterior portal. In addition, the shoulder is also inspected for other sources of pathology including labral tearing, or changes suggesting glenohumeral instability.

A partial tearing of the supraspinatus tendon along its articular surface is a common finding in symptomatic throwing athletes (Plate 16). Partial rotator cuff tears are carefully debrided using a 4.5-mm shaver to remove all fragmented and torn tissue but preserving all intact rotator cuff tendon (Plate 17). This allows a more accurate determination of the size and thickness of the rotator cuff tear and may help to reduce symptoms of catching and pain. If there is a question about rotator cuff integrity, the lateral arthroscopic portal is created, and a blunt obturator probe is used to palpate the entire surface of the rotator cuff while visualizing from within the glenohumeral joint. If the probe penetrates the rotator cuff, the diagnosis of a complete rotator cuff tear is confirmed. If the patient does not have a complete rotator cuff tear but does have a partial tear, the location of the partial tear is marked with a suture to allow for identification of the corresponding area of the rotator cuff on the bursal surface. A suture marker is placed by passing an 18-gauge spinal needle percutaneously through the lateral subacromial area, passing directly through the area of the rotator cuff tear into the glenohumeral joint. When the needle has been appropriately positioned, a no. 1 monofilament nonabsorbable suture is passed through the needle and into the glenohumeral joint. The needle is removed, taking care to maintain the suture within the joint (Plate 18). This leaves a readily visualized suture marker that crosses the subacromial space and enters the bursal surface of the rotator cuff tendon at the area of the damage that was noted on the articular surface.

BURSAL SIDE EVALUATION OF THE ROTATOR CUFF

Following the completion of glenohumeral arthroscopy, the arm is changed from a position of approximately 70° of abduction to 15° of abduction, and the traction weight may need to be increased slightly to approximately 12 lb. A cannula is inserted into the bursa, which is located below the anterior third of the acromion and anterior deltoid. A guide rod is used to place a second cannula in the anterior acromial portal. When both cannula are positioned correctly, the posterior cannula should be passing deep within the bursa, and the anterior cannula should be inserted only 2 to 3 cm. The bursa is also evaluated in a systematic fashion, and if the cannula has been properly positioned, it should be possible to evaluate the bursa prior to performing any shaving. This allows the surgeon to accurately assess the bursal surface for evidence of fraying as well as assessing the amount of clearance between the anterior inferior acromion and the supraspinatus tendon. Also noted are any signs of fraying or wear changes on the undersurface of the coracoacromial ligament. The marker suture may be visualized and shows whether any additional tearing is present on the bursal surface that might make the extent of tearing more significant than was appreciated from articulate side evaluation alone (Plate 19). If there is not evidence of bursal rotator cuff disruption, and the coracoacromial ligament is smooth with an apparently adequate space between the anterior acromion and rotator cuff, then the diagnosis of subacromial impingement is unlikely. In these cases, subacromial decompression is not performed. In a patient who has merely a small partial-thickness rotator cuff tear on the articular side, without evidence of impingement, only the glenohumeral debridement of this tear is performed. If, however, the patient has changes suggestive of impingement syndrome, an arthroscopic subacromial decompression is performed as well.

TECHNIQUE OF ARTHROSCOPIC SUBACROMIAL DECOMPRESSION

Many authors have described their techniques of subacromial decompression.[20–23] At the Southern

California Orthopedic Institute, we have modified several of these techniques to develop a system that allows for reproducible acromioplasty resulting in a measured amount of acromial resection. The technique begins with the arthroscope viewing posteriorly, and with instruments inserted through a lateral portal. This lateral portal is created on a line perpendicular to the lateral border of the acromion and intersecting the posterior aspect of the acromioclavicular joint in the supraspinatus fossa , (Fig. 11-3). This portal is created approximately 3 cm distal to the lateral acromial border. If following subacromial decompression open rotator cuff repair is necessary, this repair may be performed through a lateral deltoid splitting incision that also follows the same line and incorporates the lateral portal. An operating cannula is placed in this lateral border, and through this cannula a 5.5-mm full-radius resector is inserted and used to remove any bursal tissue. A nonconductive surgical irrigant is used, and an electrosurgical instrument is inserted through the lateral portal. The tip of this instrument is used to checkerboard the undersurface of the coracoacromial ligament and then to release the coracoacromial ligament from the anterior and lateral border of the acromion, taking care not to incise the overlying deltoid fascia. Soft tissues are cleared medially until the acromioclavicular joint is visualized. Further removal of soft tissue is performed using a full-radius resector. Electrocautery is used as required to maintain hemostasis. Visualization may be improved in many cases by using hypotensive anesthesia and by using an arthroscopy irrigation pump.

A high-speed Acromionizer burr (Dyonics Inc., Andover, MA) is then inserted through the operating cannula on the lateral portal. Generally, if the acromial width was 12 mm or thicker on a preoperative

arch view, a 5.5-mm Acromionizer is used. If the thickness is less than 12 mm, a smaller 4.0-mm Acromionizer burr is used instead. With posterior viewing the burr is inserted laterally and used to remove the anterolateral corner of the acromion for a distance of approximately 5 mm and then to smooth and bevel down the lateral margin of the acromion posteriorly back to the level of the previously created orientation line. An orientation trough is then created, beginning at the lateral border of the acromion just medial to the lateral subacromial portal, extending along the undersurface of the acromion to the posterior edge of the acromioclavicular joint (Fig. 11-4). The burr should be in line with the lateral orientation line on the skin as the trough is created. The proper depth of the orientation trough is determined from the preoperative arch x-ray view. In a thin acromion, a minimal trough is created, while for a thick acromion, a deep trough measuring up to 4 mm may be cut. While performing the bony resection, a large 5.5-mm cannula inserted through the anterior portal is used to section debris from the subacromial space. By not sucking debris through the Acromionizer, clogging of the Acromionizer burr and the need to interrupt the procedure for repeated cleaning of the burr is diminished.

Once the orientation trough has been completed, the arthroscope is transferred into the lateral portal and the operating cannula is moved to the posterior portal. The full-radius resector is used first to remove any bursal tissue that may be obstructing the view of the anterior acromion. The Acromionizer burr is then inserted and used to flatten the posterior edge of the orientation trough. The resection proceeds forward from the trough progressing from posteriorly to anteriorly, using the posterior aspect of the acromion as a "cutting block" to ensure a com-

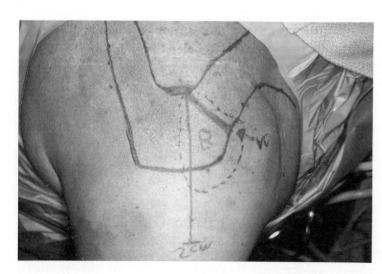

FIGURE 11-3
The lateral portal for subacromial decompression is created on a line drawn perpendicular to the lateral edge of the acromion, intersecting the posterior aspect of the acromioclavicular joint. The lateral portal is 2 to 3 cm distal to the lateral acromial edge.

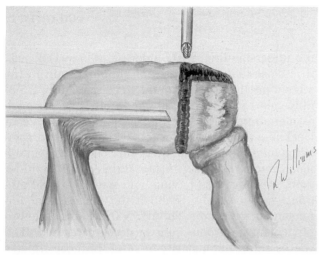

FIGURE 11-4
With viewing through the posterior portal, the lateral acromial edge is thinned, and an orientation trough is created from lateral to medial.

pletely smooth resection from posterior to anterior. The orientation trough ensures that a similar amount of bone is removed medially and laterally. Cuts are generally made by sweeping from medially to laterally as the burr is slowly advanced anteriorly. A thin bony edge of the anterior acromion is preserved initially, allowing the surgeon to estimate the amount of bone removed anteriorly by comparing the thickness of the lip with the thickness of the Acromionizer burr (Plate 20). The anterior spur is then removed beginning at the inferior edge. At the completion of the decompression, the patient has a completely flat acromion from medial to lateral and from posterior to anterior. Further smoothing may be performed with a full-radius resector.

The arthroscope is then shifted back to the posterior portal to make sure that the resection has been

adequately performed. Further smoothing may be performed as necessary. If the patient has a bony spur beneath the acromioclavicular joint as well, this may be easily removed following the subacromial decompression. With posterior viewing the electrocautery device is inserted through the lateral portal and used to incise the capsule below the acromioclavicular joint and expose the distal clavicle. Further soft tissues are removed with a shaver, and then the Acromionizer burr is used to resect the inferior distal clavicle until it is flush with the resected undersurface of the acromion. Resection is continued medially, approximately 1 cm, with beveling of the distal acromion medially and inferiorly.

Following completion of the subacromial decompression and resection of the inferior distal clavicle, if necessary, large partial tears of the rotator cuff tendon or complete rotator cuff tears may be repaired. Repairs may be performed using either an arthroscopic technique or an open technique through a lateral deltoid splitting. The details of this technique are beyond the scope of the present chapter. By initially performing the decompression arthroscopically, a small incision may be used, and a rapid rehabilitation program instituted.

Postoperatively, an arch view should be obtained, to document the adequacy of the subacromial decompression. The appearance on the postoperative arch view should be of a type I acromial arch without any residual spurring (Fig. 11-5).

POSTOPERATIVE REHABILITATION

Following subacromial decompression, the patient is placed in a sling but is encouraged to remove the sling when comfortable and begin active and passive range of motion exercises. When pain has decreased

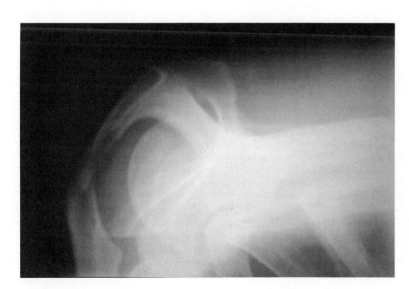

FIGURE 11-5
The patient should have a flat type I acromion on the postoperative arch view (same patient as in Fig. 11-2).

151

significantly and range of motion has returned toward normal, a program of strengthening similar to the previously mentioned conservative management for rotator cuff tears is instituted. Patients cannot begin sports-specific activities until they have full active range of motion in the operated shoulder and normal strength. For the middle-aged recreational athlete, it will generally be 3 to 4 months until the patient may return to previous sports activities.

As has been noted, subacromial decompression results are generally poor in young, high-performance overhand athletes. However, results are generally good for properly selected middle-aged patients with evidence of impingement on history and physical examination and at the time of arthroscopy. The general consensus in the literature is that arthroscopic subacromial decompression will result in a good return to the previous level of function in approximately 85 to 90 percent of patients.[20,21,24,25]

SUMMARY

The concept of impingement syndrome resulting in damage to the supraspinatus tendon from repetitive overhead activities has been an important advance in the understanding of shoulder pathology. However, it is clear that many cases of shoulder pain in the athlete previously considered to be secondary to impingement may in fact be due to other causes such as glenohumeral instability, rotator cuff fatigue or weakness, and mechanical abrasion of the supraspinatus tendon on the superior surface of the glenoid. It is therefore critical in the athlete with shoulder pain, even in those having pain with overhead motions, to accurately establish the diagnosis of impingement syndrome. Following the diagnosis of impingement syndrome, conservative treatment will be successful in the majority of cases. In those athletes having well-defined impingement syndrome, including findings consistent with impingement syndrome at arthroscopy, and who have also failed appropriate conservative management, arthroscopic subacromial decompression may result in a return to the previous level of function with minimal morbidity in a large number of cases. Arthroscopic subacromial decompression is a technically demanding procedure, with a significant learning curve, and a reproducible systematic technique such as that presented in this chapter should be helpful to ensure a high percentage of good results with a reproducible, accurate amount of subacromial bone resection.

REFERENCES

1. Neer CS: Anterior acromioplasty for the chronic impingement syndrome in the shoulder. *J Bone Joint Surg (Am)* 54A:41–50, 1977.
2. Neer CS: Impingement lesions. *Clin Orthop* 173:70–77, 1983.
3. Bigliani LU, Morrison DS, April EW: The morphology of the acromion and its relationship to rotator cuff tears. *Orthop Trans* 10:216, 1986.
4. Marian DS, Bigliani LU: The clinical significance of variations in acromial morphology. *Orthop Trans* 11:234, 1987.
5. Glousman RE: Instability versus impingement syndrome in the throwing athlete. *Orthop Clin North Am* 24:89–99, 1993.
6. Tibone JE, Elrod B, Jobe FW, et al: Surgical treatment of tears of the rotator cuff in athletes. *J Bone Joint Surg (Am)* 68A:887–891, 1986.
7. Tibone JE, Jobe FW, Kerlan RR, et al: Shoulder impingement syndrome in athletes treated by anterior acromioplasty. *Clin Orthop* 198:134–140, 1985.
8. Fly WR, Tibone JE, Glousman RE, et al: Arthroscopic subacromial decompression in athletes less than 40 years old. Abstract presented at the American Shoulder and Elbow Surgeons Sixth Open Meeting, New Orleans, LA, February 1990.
9. Garth WP, Allman FL, Armstrong WS: Occult anterior subluxations of the shoulder in non-contact sports. *Am J Sports Med* 15:579–585, 1987.
10. Warren RF: Subluxation of the shoulder in athletes. *Clin Sports Med* 2:339–354, 1983.
11. Jobe FW, Kvitne RS: Shoulder pain in the overhand or throwing athlete: The relationship of anterior instability and rotator cuff impingement. *Orthop Rev* 18:963, 1989.
12. Jobe FW, Giangarra CE, Kvitne RS, et al: Anterior capsulolabral reconstruction of the shoulder in athletes in overhand sports. *Am J Sports Med* 19:428–434, 1991.
13. Andrews JW, Broussard TS, Carson WG: Arthroscopy of the shoulder in the management of partial tears of the rotator cuff: A preliminary report. *Arthroscopy* 1:117–122, 1985.
14. Walch G, Boileau P, Noel E, Donell ST: Impingement of the deep surface of the supraspinatus tendon on the posterosuperior glenoid rim: An arthroscopic study. *J Shoulder Elbow Surg* 1:238–245, 1992.

15. Sidles JA, Harryman DT, Gillespy T, et al: Impingement of the supraspinatus tendon with the arm in maximal elevation. Presented at the American Shoulder and Elbow Surgeons Annual Meeting, Vail, CO, Sept 10–12, 1992.

16. Hawkins RJ, Abrams JS: Impingement syndrome in the absence of rotator cuff tears. *Orthop Clin North Am* 18:373–382, 1992.

17. Speer KP, Hannafin JA, Altchek DW, Warren RF: An evaluation of the shoulder relocation test. Presented at the 18th Annual Meeting of the American Orthopaedic Society for Sports Medicine, San Diego, CA, July 6–9, 1992.

18. Seeger LL, Gold RH, Bassett LW, Ellman H: Shoulder impingement syndrome: MR findings in 53 shoulders. *AJR* 150:343–347, 1988.

19. Karzel RP, Snyder SJ: Magnetic resonance arthrography of the shoulder. A new technique of shoulder imaging. *Clin Sports Med* 12(1):123–136, 1993.

20. Ellman H: Arthroscopic subacromial decompression: Analysis of one to three year results. *Arthroscopy* 3:173–183, 1987.

21. Esch JC, Ozerkis LR, Helgager JA, et al: Arthroscopic subacromial decompression—Results according to degree of rotator cuff tear. *Arthroscopy* 4:241–249, 1988.

22. Paulos LE, Harner CD, Parker RD: Arthroscopic subacromial decompression for impingement syndrome of the shoulder. *Tech Orthop* 3:33–39, 1988.

23. Sampson TG, Nisbet JK, Glick JM: Precision acromioplasty in arthroscopic subacromial decompression of the shoulder. *Arthroscopy* 7:301–307, 1991.

24. Gartsman GM: Arthroscopic acromioplasty for lesions of the rotator cuff. *J Bone Joint Surg (Am)* 72A:169–180, 1990.

25. Paulos LE, Franklin JL: Arthroscopic shoulder decompression development and application: A five-year experience. *Am J Sports Med* 18:235–244, 1990.

CHAPTER 12

Rotator Cuff Disease: Etiology, Pathology, Treatment

Robert P. Nirschl

The pathologic changes and etiologic factors that clinicians have associated with rotator cuff disease are being reassessed. Codman's[1] initial contributions have been augmented by the subsequent contributions of Moseley,[2] McLaughlin,[3] De Palma,[4] Rathbun and McNab,[5] Neer,[6] and Jobe and Jobe.[7] The influence of Neer and the concept of impingement on the current generation of orthopedic surgeons has been particularly pervasive.[6] The advent of arthroscopy and the increasing number of swimming, racket, and throwing-sport athletes who require diagnosis and treatment for rotator cuff disease has resulted in objective analysis that is at variance with the concepts associated with the impingement theory. In addition, surgical treatment protocols dedicated to the coracoacromial arch often fail to return the athletically active patient to a prior level of athletic activity. On the basis of these observations, it is clear that the theory of impingement alone is either too simplistic or often incorrect, thereby requiring the development of alternate or associate etiologic and treatment models.

FUNCTIONAL ANATOMY OF ROTATOR CUFF

The functional anatomy of the shoulder joint is quite complex and sophisticated. This sophistication includes but is not restricted to the rotator cuff. Inman and associates[8] demonstrated a complex interrelationship of shoulder movement. Saha[9] stated that locking of the greater tuberosity against the acromion never takes place "in any position of abduction" if healthy relationships exist. He further noted that a rolling-down movement of the humeral head in the glenoid cavity inevitably takes place with active humeral flexion or abduction. Saha's greatest contribution to shoulder mechanics, however, was in recognizing the "zero position" of approximately 150° of forward elevation and 45° of forward flexion where the shear and compression forces generated by the deltoid and rotator cuff are equally balanced.

Sarrafin[10] noted that compression at the level of the glenohumeral joint is essential for stability. At

less than 90° of shoulder abduction, the forces generated by the deltoid pass outside the joint, thereby causing upward humeral displacement unless counteracted by the counterforcing joint compression forces of the transversely positioned rotator cuff muscles. My arthroscopic observations of a small area of glenoid articular erosion suggest that normal glenohumeral compression occurs just caudal to an equatorial line drawn across the glenoid at midline in the AP plane. Sarrafin[10] confirmed Saha's report[9] that compression and shear forces are maximum at 90° and essentially nonexistent at 150° of abduction. Clinical experience in reference to the rotator cuff in throwing and swimming athletes confirms that the most punishing position is 90° of abduction in association with aggressive internal and external rotation. Conversely, sports techniques utilizing abduction above 135° (basketball, for example) are clinically less punishing to the rotator cuff. This observation correlates well with Saha's report of "zero balance" at higher humeral elevations.

Hollingshead[11] stated that the supraspinatus is a shoulder abductor. Jobe, Tibone, Perry, et al.[12] identified the role of the supraspinatus as a primary humeral head depressor, as well as a possible external rotator. Scarpinato, Bramwall, and Andrews[13] and Blatz[14] have suggested that the long head of the biceps may also act as a humeral head depressor. It is likely that scapular and upper thoracic muscle groups also act as a humeral head depressor. Kibler[15] has expressed the opinion as well that the scapular muscles stabilize the scapula to act as a firm platform for glenohumeral function and humeral head control. Scarpinato, Bramwall, and Andrews[13] have pointed out the vulnerability of the superior glenoid labrum in the acceleration phase of baseball throwing. Guidi and Nirschl[16] have also noted a clear relationship between partial thickness rotator cuff disease and anterior superior labrum pathologic changes including detachment. These observations strongly support the concept that anterior-superior glenohumeral instability plays a major role in rotator cuff disease.

Present evidence clearly indicates that the rotator cuff is important in the overall control of the glenohumeral joint. Instability of the joint (upward or anterior-superior humeral migration) is very likely to occur when the normal balance of strength, flexibility, and overall stability among the rotator cuff, deltoid, glenoid labrum, and scapular muscle groups is distorted.

ETIOLOGY

The etiologic factors associated with rotator cuff disease are multiple, varied, and often combined. The analysis of shoulder action in the racket, throwing, and swimming sports demonstrates that many factors are occurring simultaneously. Biomechanical observations supporting this statement have been presented by several authors including Dillman[17] and Shapiro.[18] Jobe and Jobe[7] have demonstrated the activity of the supraspinatus during the acceleration and follow-through phases of the throwing motion. Fowler[19] observed fatigue and weakness of the rotator cuff and scapular muscle groups in swimmers. In view of these and other reports, it appears that a major if not the major etiologic factor in rotator cuff disease (tendinitis or tendinosis) is multiple overuse contractile overload (usually eccentric) of the rotator cuff (usually supraspinatus). From an anatomic view, the supraspinatus is a small muscle tendon unit in a key high-stress location. The basic etiologic factors of rotator cuff disease are outlined in Table 12-1.

MECHANISMS OF ROTATOR CUFF INJURY

The basic mechanical forces to which tendons are subjected are tension, compression, and shear. Analysis of sports activities, as well as activities of daily living suggests that the most prevalent mechanical force is tension overload secondary to intrinsic muscular contraction. Curwin and Stanish[20] have pointed out that eccentric contractions are more prevalent than concentric loading and multiple repetitions are probably a common cause of tendon overuse. These patterns of mechanical force are of course present in noncompartmentalized tendons (e.g., elbow extensor brevis, patellar, achilles, plantar fascia), as well as the compartmentalized rotator cuff (supraspinatus). The supraspinatus is a small, relatively weak muscle in a key location and is likely highly stressed by eccentric tensile overload in such sports as swimming, tennis, and throwing. Multiple occupational and living activities also take their toll.

TABLE 12-1
Etiologic Factors in Rotator Cuff Disease

I. Activity overuse
   A. Multiple repetitions (tension overload, usually eccentric)
   B. Muscle-tendon imbalances
      1. Strength
      2. Flexibility
   C. Glenohumeral instability (secondary impingement)
      1. Upward humeral migration
      2. Anterior-superior subluxation
   D. Acromioclavicular osteoarthritis
II. Age
   A. Physiologic
   B. Chronologic
III. Heredity
   A. Mechanical
      1. Acromial variant (primary impingement)
   B. Systemic factors
      1. Mesenchymal syndrome (predisposition to tendon disease)
      2. Other factors
         a. Estrogen deficiency
         b. ? gouty diathesis
         c. ? rheumatologic variants

The net result of tendon overuse results in rotator cuff disease. The histologic pattern of rotator cuff disease has a characteristic pattern of disorganized collagen, fibroblasts, and vascular elements without evidence of inflammatory cells. The term angiofibroblastic tendinosis has been coined by Nirschl[21] to identify these pathologic changes.

The pathoanatomic changes of angiofibroblastic tendinosis also occur commonly in the noncompartmentalized tendons (e.g., tennis elbow, patellar, achilles tendinitis, and plantar fasciitis). These tendons are also subjected to tension overload.

IMPINGEMENT: ALTERNATIVE CONCEPTS

It is evident that mechanical compression forces (impingement) also occur in and about the rotator cuff. The question is not whether they occur, but how, when, and why. In 1972, Neer[6] advanced the theory of primary impingement by hereditary acromial variance and subsequent coracoacromial arch stenosis, thereby causing rotator cuff disease by primary compression. For the majority of patients, however, this theory is highly suspect. The strongest evidence to support such a theory is the report by Bigliani[22] of an anatomic study on the acromion in cadaver specimens. This report suggested a beaked acromion (type 3 acromion) in 40 percent of specimens. Neer's original reported clinical series of full-thickness tears noted only 25 percent of patients with observable subacromial changes.[6] My surgical experience with full-thickness tears confirms Neer's observations of approximately 25 percent observable subacromial changes.[23,24] My surgical observations (arthroscopic), however, in partial-thickness rotator cuff cases (a younger, highly athletic population) reveal only 10 percent observable subacromial changes. The theory of primary impingement therefore comes under major challenge in that no clinical series reports clear, observable evidence of subacromial changes in over 25 percent of cases. Even in the Bigliani cadaver series the reported percentage was only 40 percent.[22] In addition, the presence of observable subacromial changes does not define the reason for their presence (e.g., primary hereditary variant vs. secondary reaction occurring as an end stage of rotator cuff disease).

PATHOANATOMIC CONSEQUENCES OF GLENOHUMERAL INSTABILITY

Review of the functional anatomy of the rotator cuff strongly supports the concept that a major function of the rotator cuff is to stabilize the glenohumeral joint by counteracting the forces of deltoid to migrate the humeral head upward when shoulder abduction is below 90°. Failure of the rotator cuff via fatigue and weakness of overuse is a highly plausible concept. Glenohumeral instability with either anterior-superior or superior migration is a likely consequence. A continuum of this instability has subsequent pathoanatomic consequences. In a review of 62 cases of arthroscopic patients who presented with partial-thickness rotator cuff disease, Guidi, Nirschl, and associates[16] noted a 92 percent alteration in the anterior-superior labrum. They have coined a name for this relationship, the SLIP (supraspinatus labrum instability pattern) lesion. They have further theorized the etiologic sequence of pathoanatomic damage as demonstrated in Table 12-2. This pathoetiologic model is a conceptual advancement of the model initially advanced by Nirschl in 1984.[23,24] The initial model advanced the concept of rotator cuff disease first and labrum distortion second. The present SLIP lesion model advances the concept that following fatigue and weakness, glenohumeral instability likely results in basically simultaneous damage to both the rotator cuff and the labrum.

TABLE 12-2
SLIP (Supraspinatus Labral Instability Pattern)

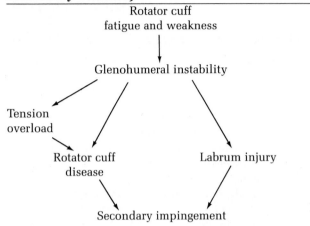

Bursitis—subacromial changes—progressive rotator cuff disease

SUPRASPINATUS LABRUM INSTABILITY PATTERN AND SECONDARY IMPINGEMENT

The evidence as noted is substantial to support the concept that rotator cuff failure (functional, pathoanatomic, or both) results in glenohumeral instability. The supraspinatus-labrum instability pattern (SLIP lesion) is an observable manifestation of this concept. The functional instability as noted by surgical observations (exam under anesthesia and arthroscopic exam) reveals that the humeral migration is usually anterior-superior or superior, although on occasion posterior-superior translation or combinations thereof do occur. Andrews[25] has suggested that instability patterns may also have a derogatory effect on the biceps attachment to the supraglenoid labral rim, especially in throwing athletes. This likely occurs at the time of forward humeral thrust at the interface of the cocking and the acceleration phases of throwing. Loss of normal biceps function would be anticipated to further magnify glenohumeral stability by loss of the humeral head depressor effect. Any form of superior humeral head migration can, of course, result in a space compromise of the coracoacromial arch. This arch stenosis can in turn result in secondary impingement of anatomic structures (bursa, coracoacromial ligament, rotator cuff, greater tuberosity of humeral head, and subacromion) in the arch. Reactive pathologic changes can certainly occur if the instability pattern persists in either fre-

TABLE 12-3

Secondary Impingement: Pathoanatomic Potential Changes in Coracoacromial Arch

I. Bursa
   A. Inflammation and swelling
   B. Fibrosis and thickening
II. Rotator cuff
   A. Partial erosion in critical zone
   B. Expansion of tendinosis plus fibrosis
   C. Full-thickness rupture
III. Coracoacromial ligament
   A. Inflammation and thickening
   B. Calcification at lateral insertion to acromion
   C. Rupture at lateral insertion
IV. Acromion
   A. Traction spur anteromedial corner (e.g., at insertion of coracoacromial ligament)
   B. Underside soft tissue degeneration (coracoacromial ligament, periosteum)
   C. Anterolateral and anteromedial reactive bony exostosis
V. Greater tuberosity
   A. Reactive exostosis
   B. Erosion

quency or intensity. The pathoanatomic alterations observed under these circumstances are outlined in Table 12-3.

There is very likely a progressive continuum of the pathoanatomic changes and wide variations in pathologic combinations that occur. End stage progressions of this process probably result in major full-thickness rupture, bony abutment of the humeral head (greater tuberosity) on the underside of the acromion, and ultimately rotator cuff arthropathy.

ROLE OF THE CORACOACROMIAL LIGAMENT

It is widely accepted that control of the humeral head is essential for normal shoulder function. Rotator cuff muscle strength and rotator cuff tendon health are vital to this function by providing dynamic control. It is likely that this important function has static passive backup support. The size, placement, and position of the coracoacromial ligament make it ideal for this function. Cadaver mechanical models also clearly demonstrate that the coracoacromial ligament is quite pliable and flexes in a cephalad direction with shoulder elevation.

This observation strongly suggests that the coracoacromial ligament does not act as a cutting edge, as is commonly thought. This finding further supports the concept that the ligament plays an important role in glenohumeral stability (Plate 21).

If, as I theorize, the coracoacromial ligament is an important backup control factor, aggressive surgical resection may be detrimental to the long-term normal balance and function of the glenohumeral joint, thereby potentially exaggerating rotator cuff disease and the pathoanatomic changes of secondary impingement. It is my opinion, therefore, that without clear observable evidence of pathologic change in the ligament (an expectation if impingement is occurring), aggressive resection is unnecessary and likely harmful. This position is supported by Watson,[26] who, like my surgical observations, has reported superior surgical results by sparing the coracoacromial ligament in association with rotator cuff surgery. Conversely, I observed no instances in which the results of rotator cuff surgery were compromised by failure to resect the coracoacromial ligament.

PRIMARY IMPINGEMENT

The theory of primary impingement of the rotator cuff with resultant rotator cuff disease was popularized by Neer's 1972 report.[6] Bigliani's 1984 report[22] of acromial morphology was thereafter also interpreted to support the concept of primary impingement. It should be noted that Neer's report was dedicated to patients with full rotator cuff rupture and Bigliani's study was on cadaveric specimens of elderly age.

It has been my observation that patients with arthroscopically confirmed partial-thickness rotator cuff disease rarely have beaked acromial morphology (type III Bigliani classification) or alteration in the coracoacromial ligament. It is clear on the basis of these observations that factors other than primary rotator cuff impingement are key to understanding the pathoetiology of rotator cuff disease, especially in the younger athletic population. It is my further observation that patients who present with full-thickness rotator cuff tears have an incidence of observable subacromial bony pathology or morphologic acromial change in 25 percent. This observation is consistent with Neer's 1972 report.[6] It should be noted as well that these changes are often not the changes of primary hereditary acromial beaking but rather represent coracoacromial ligament traction spurs and bony exostosis associated with acromioclavicular osteoarthritis. Thus these subacromial manifestations are better interpreted as secondary reactive changes. Regardless of etiology, these subacromial changes are capable of space compromise (coracoacromial arch stenosis) and impingement of the soft tissue structures of the arch. When these changes are present, they should be surgically addressed by limited acromioplasty and debridement.

ROTATOR CUFF PATHOLOGY

The basic pathologic changes in rotator cuff disease are best described as degenerative. These changes histologically are the same as observed in other areas of tendon overuse (e.g., tennis elbow, achilles, and patellar tendinosis) and the term angiofibroblastic tendinosis has been coined to identify this pathology.[21,27] The histologic presentation is a consistent identifiable pattern of disorganized vascular fibroblastic and collagen elements. Since there are no identifiable inflammatory cells in this basic pathologic change, the term tendinosis is substituted for tendinitis.

The thickness of the rotator cuff tendon varies, but on average a healthy tendon is 6 to 8 mm. The tendon thins some as it approaches its insertion site on the humeral head, especially the supraspinatus at the greater tuberosity. With age or tendon disease, the tendon may also thin.

The gross and infrastructure changes that occur with rotator cuff disease are located most often in the critical zone of the supraspinatus but also do occur in the infraspinatus and rarely in the teres minor. In partial-thickness disease, pathologic changes may occur on the intraarticular surface, intratendinous, bursal surface, or combinations thereof. Intraarticular surface and intratendinous changes are most common. In full-thickness tears, all three areas are involved (Plate 22).

In those cases where, in addition to tension, overload, impingement, and shear are etiologic factors other histologic changes may occur as companions to angiofibroblastic tendinosis. These changes include inflammation and fibrosis. Adjacent coracoacromial arch pathologic changes may also occur with secondary impingement including bursitis and bursal fibrosis, coracoacromial ligament inflammatory degeneration, as well as subacromial exostosis and traction spurs. Acromioclavicular osteoarthritis and exostosis may also occur as an independent but associated problem.

Rotator cuff disease with infrastructure and ultimately full-thickness failure presents in a variety of

horizontal, vertical, and full-penetration patterns. Full-thickness tears may span the spectrum of the small (e.g., 1 cm or less) to a full uncovering of the humeral head either by retraction of repairable cuff tissue or on occasion major dissolution of the rotator cuff.

TREATMENT OVERVIEW

The ultimate treatment protocol is, of course, dependent upon the pathologic presentation. In general, those shoulders that have not sustained permanent cuff damage but merely present as pain secondary to fatigue and weakness with perhaps an associated chemical inflammatory phase will respond nicely to conservative treatment. This includes a period of relative rest (1 to 2 weeks), anti-inflammatory medication, and a quality rehabilitation program. Most small partial-thickness (but permanently damaged) cuff tears will respond to a similar program.

The goal of rehabilitation is outlined in Table 12-4. The basic issue is not temporary pain control but a revitalization of degenerated and avascular unhealthy tissue. This includes a process of revascularization, collagen production, and ultimately collagen maturation. As a companion, the clinical manifestations of this biologic process are pain control in association with a restoration of strength, endurance, and flexibility.

In some instances, the partial-thickness degeneration proves refractory to the biologic goals of revitalization. Under these circumstances, an arthroscopic surgical approach with excisional debridement of the unhealthy and painful tissue may be the treatment of choice. Postoperative quality rehabilitation is a critical companion for complete success.

Some cases will present with additional pathologic problems such as instability, bursitis, coraco-

TABLE 12-4
Goals of Conservative Treatment Protocol

I. Enhance revitalization of tendinosis tissue
   A. Vascularization
   B. Fibroblastic infiltration
   C. Collagen production
   D. Collagen maturation

II. Enhance functional capacity
   A. Restoration of strength, endurance, and flexibility
   B. Restore glenohumeral functional stability

III. Control pain and inflammation
   A. Relative rest
   B. Anti-inflammatory medications

acromial arch stenosis, and acromioclavicular osteoarthritis. In these instances, these pathologic problems must also be addressed by arthroscopic techniques. In some instances, this could include labrum stabilization by biodegradable tack or multiple-suture transglenoid repair. On the other end of the spectrum (e.g., full-thickness rotator cuff tears), open surgical intervention is usually the treatment of choice followed by a quality rehabilitation program.

TREATMENT PROTOCOL PARTIAL-THICKNESS TEARS

Many shoulders in the relatively young athletic population present with partial-thickness permanent damage (e.g., degeneration and tears). If this damage, which is likely a combination of mechanical infrastructure distortion and avascular degenerative necrosis, is not too extensive, an opportunity for healing may be available by nonsurgical means. The manifestations of rotator cuff angiofibroblastic tendinosis are always accompanied by weakness not only of the rotator cuff muscles (e.g., supraspinatus, infraspinatus, and teres minor) but also of the scapular muscle groups (e.g., serratus anterior, rhomboids, trapezius, and levator scapulae). The goal of treatment is therefore to restore adequate strength, endurance, and flexibility to the above noted muscle groups. Restoration of normal muscle power in turn restores glenohumeral stability to normal provided other factors (e.g., labrum and ligamentous capsular deficiency) are not functionally compromised. In addition, the primary goal of the rehabilitative process is revascularization associated with collagen production and maturation as outlined in Table 12-4.

The best approach to rehabilitation encompasses resistance exercises in association with a flexibility program. Anti-inflammatory medications and relative rest are utilized to control pain, thereby allowing comfortable compliance with the rehabilitation process. It should be noted, however, that rest and anti-inflammatory medications do not strengthen or necessarily enhance revascularization.

SURGICAL INDICATIONS FOR PARTIAL-THICKNESS TEARS

The extent of damage in some partial-thickness rotator cuff tears may resist resolution by nonsurgical

TABLE 12-5

Surgical Indications for Partial-Thickness Rotator Cuff Tears

I. Failed conservative treatment
   A. Quality program (priority on rehabilitation exercise)
   B. Significant symptoms beyond 4 months
II. Unacceptable quality of life
   A. Unacceptable alteration of activity level
   B. Pain with or alteration of activities of daily living
   C. Rest or night pain
      1. Caution R/O other sources of pain (such as pulmonary tumor)
III. Clear evidence of permanent rotator cuff disease
   A. Clinical symptoms consistent with diagnosis
      1. Advanced pain phases (e.g., IV, V, VI, VII)—Nirschl classification
   B. Signs consistent with permanent rotator cuff disease
      1. Classical areas of tenderness
      2. Positive provocative signs
         a. Impingement
         b. Subluxation-relocation (Jobe)
         c. Leverage click (Nirschl)
         d. Resistance stress testing
         e. Weakness external rotation and abduction
         f. Atrophy (supraspinatus and infraspinatus)
         g. Atrophy scapular stabilizers (Kibler)
   C. Confirmatory imaging tests
      1. X-ray
      2. MRI
      3. Arthrogram
      4. CT arthrogram
IV. No extraordinary surgical risks

means. This is more likely the case in high-demand upper-extremity athletes such as racket, throwing, and swimming sport athletes. Prolonged attritional changes manifested by symptoms over a period of years also tend to be refractory to nonsurgical treatment. Under these circumstances, a surgical solution may be indicated. Specific surgical indications are outlined in Table 12-5.

It is my opinion and in practice that not all the indicators need be present and/or that all of the listed imaging tests be done. A typical situation is described for illustration in Table 12-7. In general, long-term observation has confirmed that pain phases as described in Table 12-6 are an extremely helpful tool in predicting a likely need for surgical intervention.

TABLE 12-6
Pain Phases (Nirschl Classification)

Phase	Symptoms
I	Pain and stiffness after activity Resolved within 48 h
II	Pain and stiffness after activity Lingers beyond 48 h Always dissipates with warm-up
III	Pain with activity beyond ADLs Pain does not cause an alteration of activity
IV	Pain with activity beyond ADLs Pain causes an alteration of activity
V	Pain with heavy ADLs and household chores (e.g., gardening, household cleaning)
VI	Pain with light ADLs (grooming, dressing, cleaning, etc.)
VII	Pain at rest including sleep disturbance

TABLE 12-7
Illustrative Typical Clinical Presentation for Surgical Indication Partial-Thickness Tear

I. Age 25–35 years

II. Active in overhead sports (e.g., 3 a week or more)

III. Pain refractory to quality rehab program for over 4 months. Pain phase 4 or greater.

IV. Clinical signs are consistent including
  A. Atrophy and weakness or rotator cuff and scapular muscle groups
  B. Classical areas of tenderness
  C. Positive provocative tests

V. Imaging
  A. X-rays (4 views) normal or evidence of
    1. AC osteoarthritis
    2. Cystic changes at greater tuberosity
    3. Y view generally normal
  B. MRI optional (e.g., not always done)
    1. Increased signal in supraspinatus
    2. Alteration anterior labrum on axial view

VI. Unacceptable quality of life
  Note: Patient must make this determination

TECHNICAL ASPECTS OF SURGERY
PARTIAL THICKNESS

With few exceptions the surgical approach to partial-thickness rotator cuff disease is arthroscopic. Although the beach chair position has some proponents,[28] in my observations, the lateral decubitus position with 10 to 15 lb traction is more versatile (especially if transglenoid suturing of the capsule becomes appropriate for major instability, which is always a surprise possibility). I rarely use more than two portals (e.g., posterior plus anterior over switching stick between the biceps and subscapularis tendons). These portals suffice for access to all aspects of the glenohumeral joint by switching the scope and instrumentation (e.g., scope posterior to anterior and vice versa for instrumentation) as indicated. Access to the coracoacromial arch is also easily accomplished utilizing the same two skin portals, but by redirecting into the arch (the anterior access just inferior to the coracoacromial ligament). Bursectomy, acromioplasty (when indicated), partial release of CA ligament when indicated, debridement of rotator cuff, and resection of the distal clavicle are all possible through these portals with relative ease once the learning curve has been mastered. For full resection of the distal clavicle and in most instances of partial-thickness rotator cuff surgery, the coracoacromial ligament is not resected or released. In these instances, for full access to the AC joint, the instrumentation (e.g., shavers and burrs) is reinserted superior to the coracoacromial ligament.

The extent and character of surgery for partial-thickness disease is, of course, dependent upon the pathoanatomy of the presentation including not only the cuff but also adjacent tissues. In many instances, combinations of pathoanatomic change are present and are outlined in Table 12-8. A typical presentation is, however, a tendinous change 3 mm in depth, 1.5 cm in diameter in the midsubstance and on the intraarticular side of the supraspinatus tendon (critical zone) extending to its insertion at the greater tuberosity. Anterior superior labrum degeneration without detachment indicative of instability (e.g., SLIP lesion) is a common companion. The biceps tendon, biceps attachment, coracoacromial ligament, and CA arch side rotator cuff are usually normal.

In the typical above noted presentation, the cuff and labrum are debrided with a shaver. It should be noted that the "Nirschl scratch test" as initially described for tennis elbow surgery is extremely helpful during this phase of the operation. The principle of the "scratch test" is that unhealthy tendinosis tissue is friable and peels off easily when challenged by a shaver or the scratching motion of the scalpel. Conversely, healthy tissue does not debride easily and it is therefore quite easy with operative experience to

TABLE 12-8
*Pathoanatomic Changes Commonly
Noted with Partial Thickness
Supraspinatus Tendinosis*

I. Rotator cuff
   A. Supraspinatus
      1. 90% articular surface and midsubstance
         tendon changes
      2. 10% bursal surface changes in association with
         articular side changes
   B. Infraspinatus
      1. 15% associated changes
II. Glenohumeral joint
   A. Labrum
      1. Alteration in 90% of cases
         a. Degeneration 80%
         b. Degeneration with detachment 20%
   B. Articular surfaces
      1. Alteration in 10% of cases (varying degrees of
         chondromalacia)
   C. Synovitis (10% of cases)
   D. Biceps changes or partial detachment (5%)
III. Coracoacromial arch
   A. Subacromion
      1. Traction spur, exostosis, or degeneration in
         10% of cases
   B. Coracoacromial ligament
      1. Degeneration in 5% of cases
   C. Bursitis (10% of cases)
   D. AC joint exostosis (10% of cases)
   E. Rotator cuff bursal side changes 10%
   F. Exostosis greater tuberosity 5% of cases

distinguish between unhealthy tissues and when the debridement is completed.

In those cases with extended and adjacent problems the pathoanatomy as presented is addressed. These needs could include debridement of tendons (e.g., infraspinatus and biceps), synovitis, osteoarthritis, and extensive areas of the labrum. Instability of the labrum might necessitate reattachment with a biodegradable tack and capsular deficiency might require transglenoid suturing. In partial-thickness rotator cuff disease coracoacromial changes are present only 10 percent of the time in my experience.[29,30] If in fact there is true pathoanatomic change in the coracoacromial arch, these issues are addressed as well. Under these circumstances, partial acromioplasty, partial bursectomy, resection of AC joint, partial release of coracoacromial ligament, resection of greater tuberosity osteophytes, or debridement of bursal side rotator cuff might be indicated (Plate 23).

SURGICAL TREATMENT FULL-THICKNESS ROTATOR CUFF TEARS

The surgical indications for full-thickness tears of the rotator cuff are similar to those of the partial-thickness group. In general, the patients are older and the dysfunction greater. Full-thickness rotator cuff tears can on occasion, however, demonstrate deceivingly good function. In these instances, the shoulder design, the ability of adjacent muscle tendon groups, and ligamentous capsular stability seem to compensate in spite of major anatomic deficiency. The norm, however, is significant weakness of abduction, or inability to initiate abduction in association with rest or night pain. In those cases of suspected full-thickness tear, I have found the arthrogram the most consistent as well as cost-effective imaging test. A positive test, of course, confirms the diagnosis. It should be noted that a negative arthrogram while being highly accurate in ruling out a full-thickness tear does not rule out significant rotator cuff (e.g., partial-thickness intrasubstance tendinosis) disease. Under the circumstances, confirmation by MRI or diagnostic arthroscopy is the best imaging approach.

As noted, some patients with full-thickness tears have unexpectedly good function. I have observed this even in patients with large tears (e.g., greater than 5-cm defects). Most cases with good function (e.g., full abduction, good power) have relatively small tears (e.g., less than 2 cm). In this group, conservative rehabilitation can be quite successful dependent upon activity level. If conservative treatment is implemented, the patient is always advised of the potential for expansion of the tear and increased mechanical dysfunction. However, this eventuality in my experience does not occur often. Conversely, it is highly likely that quality rehabilitation offers the opportunity for small tears to heal by sealing the torn tendon rim to the bare area of the humeral head (e.g., between the articular surface and greater tuberosity).

The usual indication for surgery in the good-function full-thickness tear group is unacceptable pain. This pain is often constant and present at rest and almost always disrupts activities of daily living. My surgical approach for this group of patients is outlined in Table 12-9. As with the partial-thickness group, wide variations in associated pathoanatomy may be present and should be addressed at the same time.

In those full-thickness tears with major functional deficits (e.g., major weakness with inability to

TABLE 12-9

Surgical Approach for Full-Thickness Rotator Cuff Tears with Abduction Function

I. Diagnostic arthroscopy
   A. Determine pathoanatomy
   B. Proceed to operative arthroscopy as indicated
II. Operative arthroscopy rotator cuff
   A. Tear less than 2 cm—no major retraction of cuff
     1. Debride rim of tear
     2. Burr bare area (e.g., between articular surface and greater tuberosity)
     3. Fix cuff with biodegradable tack for greater tuberosity
   B. Tear less than 2 cm—high-demand athlete
     1. Very stable cuff—operative arthroscopy
     2. Unstable cuff
       a. Open repair
       b. Deltoid mini-split incision
   C. Tear greater than 2 cm
     1. Open repair
     2. Deltoid mini-split incision
III. Operative arthroscopy, other structures as indicated
   A. Glenohumeral joint
     1. Labrum
     2. Capsule
     3. Articular surfaces
     4. Synovium
     5. Biceps
     6. Other capsulotendinous structures
   B. Coracoacromial arch
     1. Bursa
     2. Subacromion
     3. Acromioclavicular joint

TABLE 12-10

Technical Aspects of Open Repair Full-Thickness Rotator Cuff Tear

I. Manipulate to ensure full range of motion
II. Diagnostic arthroscopy
III. Operative arthroscopy as indicated
   A. Glenohumeral joint
     1. Remove loose fragments
     2. Debride
       a. Articular surfaces
       b. Labrum
       c. Synovium
       d. Biceps
     3. Operative repair
       a. Labrum
       b. Capsule
IV. Proceed to open repair
   A. Deltoid mini-split at acromioclavicular joint level
     Note: Do not release deltoid from acromion
   B. Do not do acromioplasty unless indicated (25%)
     1. Observable evidence of exostosis or arch compromise
     2. Minimal release (25% anterior edge) of coracoacromial ligament for exposure (30%)
   C. Resect AC joint if indicated (20%)
   D. Proceed with repair
     1. Sutures in bone or bone anchors
     2. Autogenous tendon patch graft (donor IT band) in frail repairs
   E. Irreparable tears
     1. Debride devitalized tissue
     2. Limited acromioplasty only as indicated
     3. Avoid heroic surgery (iatrogenic harm)
     4. Do not resect coracoacromial ligament

initiate normal abduction) the patient invariably proceeds with surgical intervention. Significant pain almost always accompanies a shoulder with this dysfunction. Although the diagnosis is obvious regarding the tear, companion pathoanatomy is often present and is best assessed by diagnostic arthroscopy. Anticipated open operative intervention is therefore preceded by diagnostic arthroscopy. On rare occasion, the rotator cuff lesion is less than expected and operative arthroscopic repair of the cuff suffices. Additional findings in the glenohumeral joint are common in the typical case and are addressed by operative arthroscopy at this time (e.g., loose bodies, chondromalacia, synovitis, labrum degeneration, or detachment and biceps alterations). Once arthroscopy is completed, the patient is rolled into a semi-beach-chair position and open surgery proceeds. The transition from arthroscopy to open

surgery positioning and draping rarely takes over 3 min.

The specifics of open operative technique[30] are outlined in Table 12-10. It should be noted that a deltoid mini-split incision is all that is needed. The deltoid is therefore not released from the acromion. In addition, the acromion is respected and a modified acromioplasty is done only if clearly observable pathoanatomic changes are present. This occurs as noted in only 25 percent of cases. For further clarification 75 percent of cases do not undergo an acromioplasty. In addition, the majority (90 percent) of cases do not demonstrate any abnormality of the coracoacromial ligament. It is unnecessary therefore to incise or resect the ligament in the majority of cases except for exposure. Under these circumstances (30 percent of cases) the anterior 25 percent edge of the ligament is released from the anteromedial aspect of the acromion.

The acromioclavicular joint demonstrates symptomatic osteoarthritic changes as an associated problem to full-thickness dysfunctional rotator cuff tears in 20 percent of cases. An open resection of the distal clavicle with removal of accompanying acromial spurs is undertaken in this circumstance. It should be noted that a significant segment of the coracoacromial ligament is often spared, even in these circumstances.

It has been my experience that most dysfunctional large tears (e.g., greater than 5 cm) are repairable. Frail repairs are reinforced by an iliotibial band autogenous tendon patch graft. In the large tears, the cuff tends to roll up and retract back to the infraspinatus and supraspinatus fossa. Calm methodical dissection is critical to clearly identify these tissue. Once found, the placement of no. 5 permanent suture aids a great deal in advancing the tissue back to an anatomic position. This process is greatly aided by full anesthesia relaxation. For reattachment, bony anchoring via suture through drill holes or bone anchors is critical for firm fixation. Ultimate function in major rotator tears is dependent upon the quality and healing potential of the repaired tissue.

On occasion, the rotator cuff tissue in large tears is simply absent (? chemical or avascular dissolution). This situation is more commonplace in such systemic problems as rheumatoid arthritis or cumulative overload. In these situations of an irreparable rotator cuff, the best treatment is debridement of all devitalized (e.g., painful) tissue including intraarticular glenohumeral synovitis and arthritic debris via arthroscopic approach. Heroic attempts to advance the subscapularis, infraspinatus, or autograft an intact biceps are fraught with major iatrogenic harm. An excision of the coracoacromial ligament is not recommended or perhaps better is condemned, as this approach removes the only remaining constraint to upward humeral migration and in my opinion is harmful. A limited acromioplasty in those instances where pathoanatomic exostosis is present is, however, indicated. Under no circumstance, in any open repair of the rotator cuff and especially in an irreparable presentation, should the deltoid be released from the acromion as part of the approach.[30]

DISCUSSION

The approaches articulated in this chapter reflect our expanded knowledge. More importantly, the noted concepts have major practical significance concerning patient care, especially for the higher-demand athletic population. A study reported by Bigliani and associates[31] in 1992 concerning return to tennis after full-thickness rotator cuff repair amplifies the point. The study citing patients operated upon utilizing the prior techniques of acromioplasty and an exposure encompassing deltoid release noted a return to varied levels of tennis on average at 18 months. In contradistinction, the techniques as cited in this chapter can be expected to return the majority of patients to tennis at a competitive level within 6 months.

The strides made in partial-thickness rotator cuff disease are even more dramatic. Chronic shoulder pain refractory to conservative care previously had no resolution other than an acceptance of lower activity. Now improved rehabilitation techniques and the availability of operative arthroscopy offer a significant opportunity to return patients to the level of pain-free activity enjoyed prior to injury or the onset of symptoms. These opportunities are enhanced by an improved understanding of the pathoanatomy and its etiology.

SUMMARY

The etiology, pathoanatomy, pathophysiology, and treatment of rotator cuff are discussed in detail. The theory of primary impingement is explored and challenged. Current surgical observations in association with expanding basic science information strongly support the concept that the major etiologic factors responsible for rotator cuff disease are tension overload secondary to fatigue, weakness, and vascular compromise of the rotator cuff in association with anterior-superior glenohumeral instability.

REFERENCES

1. Codman EA, Akerson I: The pathology associated with rupture of the supraspinatus tendon. *Ann Surg* 93:348–359, 1931.
2. Moseley H: *Ruptures of the Rotator Cuff.* Springfield, IL, Charles C Thomas, 1952.
3. McLaughlin H: Lesions of the musculo-tendonous cuff of the shoulder. *J Bone Joint Surg* (Am) 26:31–51, 1944.

4. De Palma A: *Surgery of the Shoulder*. Philadelphia, Lippincott, 1950.

5. Rathburn J, McNab J: The microvascular pattern of the rotator cuff. *J Bone Joint Surg (Am)* 52B:540, 1970.

6. Neer C: Anterior acromioplasty for the chronic impingement syndrome in the shoulder: A preliminary report. *J Bone Joint Surg (Am)* 54A:41, 1972.

7. Jobe F, Jobe C: Painful athletic injuries of the shoulder. *Clin Orthop* 173:117–124, 1983.

8. Inman J, Saunders J, Abbott L: Observations on the function of the shoulder joint. *J Bone Joint Surg (Am)* 26A:1, 1944.

9. Saha A: The classic mechanism of shoulder movements and a plea for recognition of "zero position" of the glenohumeral joint. *Clin Orthop* 173:3, 1983.

10. Sarrafin S: Gross and functional anatomy of the shoulders. *Clin Orthop* 173:11, 1983.

11. Hollingshead WH: *Anatomy for Surgeons: The Back and Limbs*. New York, Hoeber-Harper, 1958, vol 3.

12. Jobe F, Tibone J, Perry J, et al: An EMG analysis of the shoulder in throwing and pitching: A preliminary report. *Am J Sports Med* 1:3–5, 1983.

13. Scarpinato D, Bramwall J, Andrews J. Arthroscopic management of the throwing athlete's shoulder: Indications, techniques, and results. *Clin Sports Med* 10(4):913–927, October 1991.

14. Blatz D: Personal communications, San Francisco, 1984.

15. Kibler W, Chandler T, Pace B: Principles of rehabilitation after chronic tennis injuries. *Clin Sports Med* 11(3):661–671, July 1992.

16. Guidi E, Nirschl R: Supraspinatus labral instability pattern (slip lesions) in rotator cuff abnormality. Presented to American Orthopaedic Society for Sportsmedicine: Annual Meeting, Sun Valley, Idaho, 1993.

17. Dillman C: Biomechanical analysis of the shoulder in the tennis serve. Presented to the USTA National Conference on Tennis Medicine, Saddlebrook, FL, May 1, 1993.

18. Shapiro R: Biomechanical aspects of tennis. Presented to the Annual Meeting of the Society of Tennis Medicine and Science, Ponte Viedra, FL, Oct 12, 1992.

19. Fowler P: Swimming injuries to the rotator cuff. Instructional Course Lecture, American Academy of Orthopedic Surgery Annual Meeting, Las Vegas, NV, January 1985.

20. Curwin S, Stanish W: *Tendinitis: Its Etiology and Treatment*. Lexington, MA, Collamore Press, 1984.

21. Nirschl R: Muscle and tendon trauma: Tennis elbow, in Morrey B (ed): *The Elbow and Its Disorders*. Philadelphia, Saunders, 1985, pp 481–496.

22. Bigliani L, Morrison D, April E: The morphology of the acromion and its relationship to rotator cuff tears. *Orthop Trans* 10:216, 1986.

23. Nirschl R: Shoulder tendinitis. Presented to AAOS Symposium, Upper Extremity Injuries in Athletes, Washington, DC, Sept 17, 1984.

24. Nirschl R: Shoulder tendinitis, in Pettrone F (ed): *American Academy of Orthopaedic Surgeons, Symposium on Upper Extremity Injuries in Athletes*. St Louis, Mosby, 1986, chap 28, pp 222–337.

25. Andrews J, Broussard T, Carson W: Arthroscopy of the shoulder in the management of partial tears of the rotator cuff: A preliminary report. *Arthroscopy Related Surg* 162:117–122, 1985.

26. Watson M: Major ruptures of the rotator cuff: The results of surgical repair in 89 patients. *J Bone Joint Surg (Am)* 67B:618–624, 1985.

27. Nirschl R: Elbow tendinosis/tennis elbow. *Clin Sports Med* 11(4):851–870, 1992.

28. Skyhar M, Altchek D, Warren R, et al: Shoulder arthroscopy with the patient in the beach chair position. *Arthroscopy* 4(4):256–259, 1988.

29. Nirschl R: Rotator cuff tendinitis: Concepts of pathoetiology, in Barr J (ed): *Instr Course Lect* 38:439–445, 1989.

30. Nirschl R: Surgical treatment of rotator cuff tendinitis, in Barr J (ed): *Instr Course Lect* 38:446–461, 1989.

31. Bigiliani L, Kimmel J, McCann P, Wolfe I: Repair of rotator cuff tears in tennis players. *Am J Sports Med* 20(2):112–117, March–April 1992.

Injuries of the Acromioclavicular Joint Complex

Frank C. McCue III
William E. Nelson

The acromioclavicular joint and tissues surrounding the joint are frequently injured during athletic activities. This chapter describes anatomy of the acromioclavicular joint and its surrounding structures, a classification of injuries of the joint, and recommended treatment of these injuries.

The acromioclavicular (AC) joint is an osseous link between the upper extremity and the thorax. It is composed of the lateral end of the clavicle and the medial expansion of the acromion. These two bones are interconnected by the acromioclavicular ligament that spans the AC joint (Fig. 13-1). The ligament is in essence a capsule and surrounds the joint. This ligament provides stability for the joint in the anteroposterior as well as superior-inferior planes.

The joint is further stabilized by the coracoclavicular (CC) ligament which extends from the superior aspect of the coracoid to the inferior aspect of the clavicle. The CC ligament has two components: the conoid ligament that originates near the base of the coracoid and extends to the inferior surface of the clavicle, and the trapezoid ligament that passes upward from the middle of the coracoid process to its insertion under the clavicle, just medial to the AC joint. The two components of the coracoclavicular ligament provide AC joint stability in the superior-inferior plane. Additionally, the coracoclavicular ligament inhibits inferior-medial rotation of the scapula, including the attached acromion.

The coracoacromial ligament extends from the lateral third of the coracoid to the anterior margin of the acromion lateral to the facet of the AC joint. It joins two scapular processes, the coracoid and acromion; thus it adds no particular stability to the AC joint.

Although the acromioclavicular joint is a subcutaneous structure, the trapezius lies superior and posterior to the clavicle and inserts on the superior aspect of the lateral third of the clavicle as well as the superior margin of the scapular spine. This relationship occasionally leads to entrapment of the clavicle in the trapezius following disruption of the AC joint. The subclavius muscle lies between the clavicle and subclavian vessels and the adjoining brachial plexus.

The brachial plexus passes beneath the clavicle posterior and lateral to the subclavian vessels. Disruption of the AC joint rarely results in direct injury to the plexus, although the mechanism of injury to the joint may result in a stretching injury of the plexus.

MECHANISM OF INJURY

Injury to the acromioclavicular joint typically results from landing on the acromion during a fall or from a direct blow to the lateral shoulder. Inferiorly, and perhaps posteriorly, directed force sequentially stresses the acromioclavicular and then the coracoclavicular ligaments. If the stress induced by the force is excessive, the AC ligament is disrupted first, followed by the CC ligament. Ligamentous injuries occur frequently in athletic activities and are particularly common during the football season.

Fractures of the adjacent acromion and distal clavicle generally occur from direct impact. Fracture of the coracoid may result from avulsion at the origin of the short head of the biceps and coracobrachialis and pectoralis minor tendons or the coracoclavicular, coracoacromial, and coracohumeral ligaments. Alternatively, the coracoid may be fractured by the impact of a dislocated humeral head. Fractures of the acromioclavicular joint complex are not commonly seen in a sports medicine practice.

INJURY CLASSIFICATION

The majority of injuries to the acromioclavicular joint complex involve the ligaments surrounding the joint. Rockwood's system of classification is based upon displacement of the clavicle relative to the acromion. The amount of clavicular displacement indicates the extent of ligamentous injury.

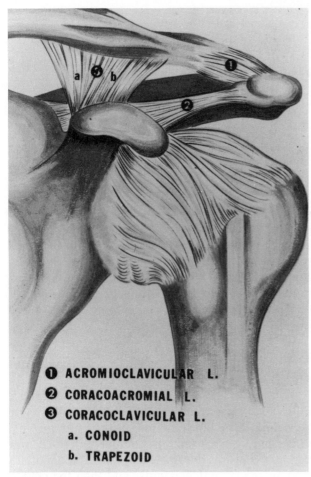

FIGURE 13-1
Anatomy of the acromioclavicular joint complex.

❶ ACROMIOCLAVICULAR L.
❷ CORACOACROMIAL L.
❸ CORACOCLAVICULAR L.
   a. CONOID
   b. TRAPEZOID

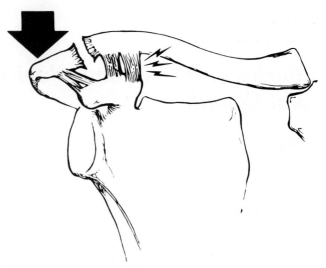

FIGURE 13-3
Type II AC injury. (*From Rockwood CA: Fractures in Adults. Philadelphia, Lippincott, 1991, with permission.*)

Type I AC injuries are characterized by the lack of clavicular displacement (Fig. 13-2). The force applied at the AC joint sprains the AC ligament but does not completely disrupt it. Thus the AC joint is tender but not deformed.

Mild prominence of the lateral clavicle indicative of AC subluxation is the clinical criterion for type II injuries (Fig. 13-3). The AC joint is widened and the acromion subluxes inferiorly as the AC ligament is completely disrupted. Thus the coracoclavicular distance is not increased.

Greater prominence of the lateral clavicle associated with dislocation of the AC joint indicates type III injury has occurred (Fig. 13-4). The CC ligaments

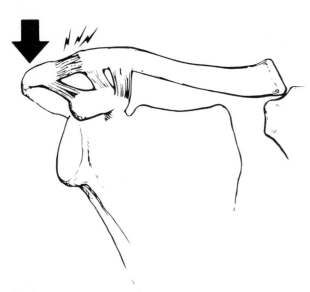

FIGURE 13-2
Type I AC injury. (*From Rockwood CA: Fractures in Adults. Philadelphia, Lippincott, 1991, with permission.*)

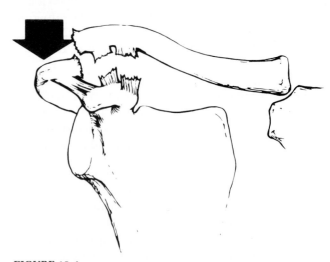

FIGURE 13-4
Type III AC injury. (*From Rockwood CA: Fractures in Adults. Philadelphia, Lippincott, 1991, with permission.*)

168

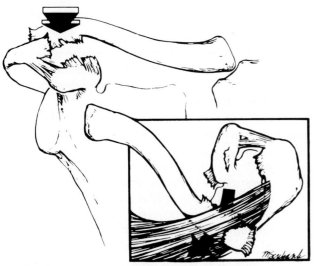

FIGURE 13-5
Type IV AC injury. (*From Rockwood CA: Fractures in Adults. Philadelphia, Lippincott, 1991, with permission.*)

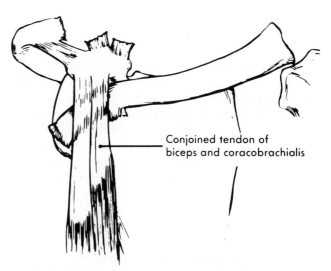

Conjoined tendon of biceps and coracobrachialis

FIGURE 13-7
Type VI AC injury. (*From Rockwood CA: Fractures in Adults. Philadelphia, Lippincott, 1991, with permission.*)

are disrupted, as well as the AC ligaments. (Rarely, the ligaments remain intact, while the periosteum of the clavicle splits, permitting the scapula to rotate inferiorly and medially.) The coracoclavicular distance is increased up to 100 percent.

Infrequently, clavicular prominence is observed at the posterior-lateral shoulder (Fig. 13-5). This deformity is indicative of a type IV injury. The AC and CC ligaments are disrupted, as is the clavicular portion of the deltoid origin. The lateral clavicle is displaced posteriorly into the trapezius.

Marked prominence of the lateral clavicle is associated with a type V AC injury (Fig. 13-6). The coracoclavicular distance is increased more than 100

percent. In addition to disruption of the AC and CC ligaments, the deltoid and trapezius are avulsed from the lateral clavicle.

Rarely, the lateral clavicle will not be prominent. Instead, a void will be observed medial to the acromion. Palpation of the shoulder will reveal displacement of the clavicle beneath the coracoid (Fig. 13-7). This relationship is indicative of a type VI injury. The AC and CC ligaments are disrupted. Patterson suggested inferiorly directed force applied to the clavicle while the scapula was retracted and the arm abducted might cause this type of AC injury.

FRACTURES

While the majority of athletic injuries of the acromioclavicular joint and its surround structures result in soft tissue damage, clavicular, acromial, and rarely, coracoid fractures can occur. Clavicle fractures tend to occur in the central third of the bone, probably because the boundary between the tubular and the flattened segments of the bone as well as the intersection of the anterior and posterior concave segments of the bone is located in the central third, providing a stress riser. Direct blows to the medial third probably occur less frequently, as the head and neck partially shield this area. Blows to the lateral clavicle may result in nondisplaced fractures that are stabilized by intact AC and CC ligaments, or displaced fractures that are associated with disruption of the CC ligaments. Distal clavicular fractures may be intraarticular. A direct blow to the acromion can result in a fracture, although AC ligamentous injury is much more likely. Forceful upward dislocation of

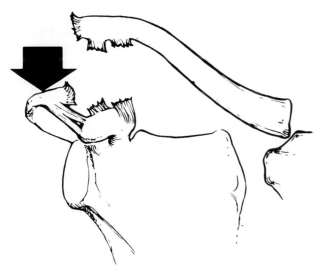

FIGURE 13-6
Type V AC injury. (*From Rockwood CA: Fractures in Adults. Philadelphia, Lippincott, 1991, with permission.*)

the humeral head may fracture the acromion, while medial dislocation of the humerus may fracture the coracoid. Coracoid impaction fractures are prone to occur at its base. Avulsions of the coracoid tend to occur closer to the end of the coracoid process where the biceps, coracobrachialis, and pectoralis-minor tendons, as well as the coracoclavicular, coracoacromial, and coracohumeral ligaments attach.

DIAGNOSIS

An athlete who sustains injury to the acromioclavicular joint or to the adjacent bones will complain of pain at the point of injury. Usually, a history of falling on the shoulder or receiving a blow to the shoulder will be reported. The athlete will typically deny upper extremity paresthesias or changes in sensibility. He or she may initially describe upper extremity weakness, but further questioning generally elucidates pain inhibition rather than paresis.

Physical examination begins with inspection of the shoulder. The contours of the injured and contralateral shoulders are compared. Often asymmetry is readily noticeable. Swelling may be present at the site of injury. The normal rounded contour of the shoulder is squared off, and the distal clavicle is prominent in cases of AC separation. In contrast, the silhouette of the lateral shoulder is normal in cases of clavicular fracture. Palpation of the sternoclavicular joint, clavicle, acromioclavicular joint, acromion, and coracoid process reveals tenderness, and often deformity, at the site of injury. Crepitus may be present with either fractures or AC separations. Pain with resisted elbow flexion and inspiration may indicate a coracoid fracture. Supraspinatus and infraspinatus weakness suggests entrapment of the suprascapular nerve that may be seen following coracoid fracture.

Sensibility to light touch provided by the axillary nerve should be assessed at the lateral shoulder over the deltoid, while radial, median, and ulnar sensibility are tested at the dorsal first web space and palmar tips of the index and little fingers, respectively. While the athlete will be reluctant to abduct the ipsilateral upper extremity, motor function of the axillary nerve can be evaluated by palpating the deltoid as the athlete only initiates abduction. As soon as deltoid contraction is palpated, the athlete is instructed to discontinue abduction. Wrist and digital flexion and extension provide ample checks of median and radial motor function. Palpating the first dorsal interosseous and abductor digitorum quinti

muscles during resisted abduction of the index and little fingers permits assessment of ulnar motor function. Palpating the radial pulse completes the neurovascular examination.

Usually the diagnosis can be made following a careful physical examination of the shoulder. However, confirmatory radiographic examination is appropriate. If the clinical diagnosis is AC injury, then an anteroposterior (AP) AC (not shoulder) view and either an axillary or scapular lateral view of the injured joint should be ordered. Additionally, an AP AC radiograph of the contralateral shoulder may be obtained for comparison. Weighted or stress views are uncomfortable for the patient and not generally necessary for athletes who have obvious AC disruption. However, bilateral views obtained with 10 lb of weight suspended from the athlete's wrists may discriminate type II and III injuries if the initial unweighted view does not demonstrate dislocation of the AC joint.

The AP radiographs should be inspected for widening of the AC joint, downward displacement of the acromion relative to the clavicle, or fracture of the distal clavicle or acromion. The distance between the inferior border of the clavicle and the superior margin of the coracoid should be observed. The normal CC distance is approximately 1 cm. The actual distance measured on the radiograph of the injured shoulder is not as helpful as the difference observed between the measured distances of the athlete's injured and normal shoulders. A difference exceeding 5 mm indicates disruption of the coracoclavicular ligaments, thus a type III AC injury. If the CC distance of the unweighted films does not differ by 5 mm, the CC ligaments may or may not be disrupted. Weighted films may then be obtained to separate type II and III injuries. Rarely, the AC joint is obviously dislocated, yet the measured coracoclavicular distance is normal. In this instance, a Stryker notch radiograph should be examined to confirm fracture of the coracoid.

If the clavicular fracture is suspected, then an AP clavicle view should be ordered so that the entire clavicle is visualized. Additionally, a lateral scapular view and perhaps a 45° cephalad view is indicated. Acromial and coracoid fractures can be diagnosed on axillary lateral and AP shoulder views.

TREATMENT

All AC injuries are treated acutely with application of ice over the injured joint and an oral analgesic medication. Although a shoulder sling can unload the joint and provide pain relief, many athletes are reluctant to wear the sling. Because the AC and CC ligaments are not disrupted in type I injuries, use of the sling is not essential. If the athlete has significant discomfort, a sling should be applied until the discomfort diminishes. Most type I injuries will not require a sling; those that do usually need a sling for only 1 or 2 days.

As soon as the acute pain subsides, shoulder range of motion and strengthening exercises may be initiated. Return to athletic activity is permitted when the athlete demonstrates full shoulder range of motion and normal shoulder flexion and abduction power. Return to athletics from type I injuries usually is possible in 1 to 2 weeks.

Type II AC injuries tend to be more painful; thus athletes with these injuries are more receptive to use of a shoulder sling during the phase of acute pain. Athletes typically discontinue the sling when the shoulder pain subsides, regardless of an arbitrary time frame that may be recommended to them. Generally, the sling is worn for 5 to 7 days, but it may be required for a longer period of time in some cases. Pain relief is provided initially by application of ice to the injured AC joint. Treatment with a narcotic medication is often appropriate initially. Nonnarcotic analgesics are indicated after the acute pain subsides (typically 2 to 3 days following injury).

Active shoulder range of motion exercises should be initiated when the acute pain has resolved. Shoulder abduction, forward flexion, and elevation are often limited because of injury to the trapezius and deltoid. Gentle exercise is begun within the pain-free range of motion. Ice may be applied to the shoulder during exercise to inhibit pain and muscle spasm. Isometric contraction is initiated at the beginning, halfway, and terminal pain-free range of each of the nine shoulder motions (forward flexion, backward extension, horizontal flexion, horizontal extension, abduction, adduction, external rotation, internal rotation, and elevation). If the athlete has a 90° arc of pain-free forward flexion, the isometric exercise for forward flexion is performed at 0, 45, and 90°. The athlete is instructed to resist only to the point of pain. When complete pain-free range of motion is achieved, heat packs and ultrasound prior to exercise are substituted for ice during exercise. Progressive resistive exercise is begun with free weights. As shoulder strength increases, lateral pulls, bent knee rowing, shoulder shrugs, dips, push-ups, pull-ups, and the military press are added. Sport-specific shoulder exercises are also added at this time.

When pain-free range of motion and symmetric shoulder strength are achieved, return to athletic participation is appropriate. Some athletes are ready to return in 2 weeks; most require 3 to 5 weeks of rehabilitation. Athletes who return to contact sports may benefit from protective padding over the AC joint. Shoulder pads with a high arch may be particularly useful for football players. Lacrosse shoulder pads can be modified to provide similar protection.

While most athletes with type II AC injuries return to play successfully following nonoperative treatment, a few have persistent pain at the subluxed AC joint. They may have radiographic signs of posttraumatic arthritis, but not necessarily (Fig. 13-8). These athletes may benefit from debridement of the AC joint and excision of 2 cm of the distal clavicle. A majority of athletes who undergo a distal clavicle excision are able to return to competitive athletics.

Clinical Case

An 18-year-old college football player who had a grade II+ AC separation in preseason football practice had been examined, and surgical repair of the AC joint was recommended. He was seen in consultation, and the pros and cons concerning open and closed treatment were discussed, along with the various indications and benefits of each. Also, the fact

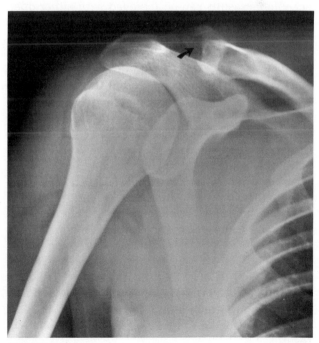

FIGURE 13-8
Calcification with AC ligament 1 year following type I AC injury.

that this is an area that individual orthopedists constantly debate as to the optimal treatment was discussed with the athlete. He opted for closed treatment. Soreness had abated in 10 days, and he returned to use and full activity 3 weeks postinjury, although he was protected with an AC pad and individualized shoulder pads at that time. He performed throughout the season without further injury, with the only residual being a moderately prominent AC joint compared with the normal side.

Commentary

This points out the fact that in the grade II injuries, even in those of a significant degree in which surgery may be advised in certain cases, conservative treatment will in many cases allow full and relatively safe return to activity, with the residual prominence not being a significant functional problem in most cases.

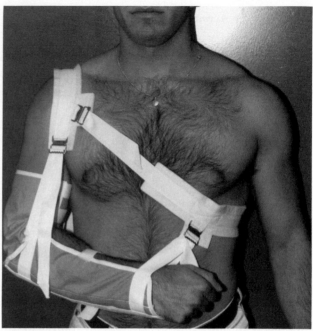

FIGURE 13-9
Kenny-Howard shoulder brace.

While consensus regarding treatment of acute type I and type II injuries has been achieved, operative vs. nonoperative treatment of acute type III injuries has been a matter of discussion. During the early 1970s, the majority opinion favored operative treatment of type III injuries. However, during the past two decades, many surgeons have documented successful nonoperative treatment. Recently, 72 percent of chairmen of orthopedic residency programs and 86 percent of athletic team surgeons indicated a preference for nonoperative treatment. Although acceptable results can be achieved with either operative or nonoperative treatment, a nonoperative approach eliminates the risk associated with anesthesia and essentially negates the risk of infection.

Many type III injuries can be successfully managed with a 3- to 5-week period of treatment with a Kenny-Howard shoulder brace (Fig. 13-9). Care must be taken to appropriately position the brace over the distal clavicle (rather than over the acromion). Additionally, the athlete should be advised to check the skin under the clavicular pad daily to limit injury to the skin from excess pressure. Gentle shoulder motion in the Kenny-Howard brace can be initiated at 3 weeks. Increased motion and strengthening are added at 5 to 6 weeks. The athlete is often ready to return to athletics at 8 to 10 weeks following injury. If treatment with a Kenny-Howard brace is selected, the athlete should be advised that some clavicular prominence is expected. Some athletes may be able to return to participation after a shorter period of bracing, but greater prominence of the clavicle might result.

Not all severe AC injuries are optimally treated nonoperatively. Type IV injuries may result in inter-

position of the trapezius that prevents closed reduction of the AC joint. Avulsion of the deltoid and trapezius associated with type V injuries may also result in soft tissue interposition that blocks closed reduction. The rare type VI injury, with subcoracoid clavicular entrapment, probably requires operative management.

When operative treatment is indicated, a vertical incision just medial to the AC joint promotes an adequate approach. If the clavicle is entrapped within the trapezius or beneath the coracoid, it can be grasped with a clamp and manipulated. The AC joint should be debrided. Then the joint can be reduced and the coracoclavicular ligament repaired with nonabsorbable suture. Although other authors have reported good results with temporary immobilization of the AC joint with a coracoclavicular screw, good results have also been achieved by supplementing the repaired coracoclavicular ligaments with a palmaris tendon graft placed over the clavicle and under the coracoid. Alternatively, a Dacron coracoclavicular loop can be used. The trapezius and deltoid should be repaired by suture to the clavicular and acromial periosteum. Postoperatively, the arm is placed in a sling for 2 weeks. Passive shoulder range of motion is then instituted. Pendulum exercise is usually begun 3 weeks after surgery, followed by active shoulder flexion and abduction at 6 weeks. Progressive resistive exercise generally commences 8 weeks following operative repair. Return to athletic activity is permitted when pain-free motion and normal shoulder power are regained.

Clinical Case

The patient was a 20-year-old wrestler who suffered a grade II-III AC separation while wrestling. As a heavyweight, his muscular structure made it difficult to ascertain any marked displacement clinically, and x-rays showed the clavicle at the upper edge of the acromion. This could be reduced subjectively, and an AC stabilizing brace was fitted and worn for 5 weeks. He got along well as far as pain and skin changes were concerned, and he appeared to be clinically stable on removal of the brace. However, when he returned to weight lifting over the ensuing 3-week period, a redislocation of the clavicle occurred, and at this time, surgery was carried out that revealed the dislocation with rupture of the ligaments and also avulsion of the deltoid and trapezial attachments to the clavicle, which were peeled back and actually prevented full reduction in the joint clinically.

Commentary

This points out the fact that even those who apparently respond well to closed treatment occasionally will need surgery. Those in whom this soft tissue obstruction can be ascertained at the time of the closed reduction require open reduction.

Nondisplaced distal clavicular fractures are treated in a sling until they are nontender. Shoulder motion exercises can then be instituted within the pain-free range of motion, which will progressively increase. Isometric exercise can also be undertaken within the pain-free range. When full pain-free motion has returned, resistive exercise can be initiated with light weight (such as 1 to 3 lb). The amount of weight is gradually increased. When the clavicle is nontender, full pain-free motion is demonstrated, and shoulder power is normal, the athlete can return to sports. Return from a nondisplaced distal clavicle fracture will likely take 4 to 6 weeks.

Displaced distal clavicle fractures probably are best treated by open reduction and internal fixation. The proximal fragment, which is usually displaced superiorly and posteriorly, can be pulled inferiorly and anteriorly. When the two clavicular fragments are opposed, Dacron tape or a tendon graft can be passed around the proximal fragment and under the coracoid. Alternatively, a medium-sized Steinman

pin can be passed laterally through the distal clavicle, AC joint, and acromion. Then the clavicle fracture is reduced and the pin is passed in retrograde fashion into the proximal clavicle. If a Steinman pin is used, it should always be bent at the lateral acromion to prevent migration. The clavicular periosteum and clavipectoral fascia should be repaired if possible. A shoulder sling should be worn for 6 weeks following clavicular fixation. At that time, if a fixation pin was used, it should be removed. Then a shoulder motion and strengthening program is instituted. When the athlete returns to play, the distal clavicle can be padded.

Intraarticular fractures that involve the AC joint may require secondary resection of the distal clavicle if persistent AC pain develops. In general, however, the distal fragment should be preserved if possible because the coracoclavicular ligaments will enhance acromioclavicular stability once the clavicle fracture has healed.

Most coracoid fractures can be treated with a sling until pain and tenderness have resolved. Widely displaced coracoid fractures may require internal fixation. If suprascapular nerve entrapment is present, early exploration may be more rewarding than late decompression.

Osteolysis of the distal clavicle may follow a specific injury to the AC complex or may result from repetitive trauma induced by weight training. Clinical examination of the involved clavicle may reveal AC tenderness, mild swelling, and pain with abduction and external rotation. Radiographs demonstrate osteoporosis and increased uptake is seen on the bone scan.

Elimination of push-ups, bench pressing, and shoulder dips may lead to resolution of pain. If pain persists, resection of the distal clavicle may permit return to athletic participation.

Clinical Case

A 22-year-old college lacrosse player had suffered a grade I injury to the AC joint with several recurrences. This was painful with use of the lacrosse stick, particularly in activities above the shoulder and across the chest that are necessary in handling the stick in play. X-rays showed osteolysis of the distal end of the clavicle, degenerative changes, and enlargement as well. He continued to play with subjective treatment throughout the year, including steroid injections, but a resection of the distal ¾ in of the clavicle was carried out for subjective needs at the end of the season.

Commentary
This case points out that grade I separations can lead to secondary surgery, particularly in those after which an overgrowth occurs causing impingement along with the joint damage and the need for secondary arthroplasty. This also occurs in some grade II or even grade III separations. Primary excision of the distal clavicle may be indicated in some grade II or III AC injuries if impingement is present at the AC joint when the clavicle is reduced. It is important to realize that osteolysis of the distal clavicle does occur in active individuals, particularly those involved in weight lifting. With time and subjective treatment, the majority of these will clear subjectively with symptomatic treatment without the need for surgical arthroplasty.

BIBLIOGRAPHY

Bannister GC, Wallace WA, Stubleferth PG, Hutson MA: The management of acute acromioclavicular dislocation. *J Bone Joint Surg (Am)* 71B:848–850, 1989.
Barrett GR, Ballard R: Recurrent posterior inferior dislocation of the acromioclavicular joint. *Contemp Orthop* 17:43–45, 1988.
Bergfeld JA, Andrish JT, Clancy WG: Evaluation of the acromioclavicular joint following first and second degree sprains. *Am J Sports Med* 6:153–159, 1978.
Cahill BR: Osteolysis of the distal part of the clavicle in male athletes. *J Bone Joint Surg (Am)* 64A:1053–1058, 1982.
Cook DA, Helner JP: Acromioclavicular joint injuries. *Orthop Rev* 19:510–516, 1990.
Cook FF, Tibone JE: The Mumford procedure in athletes. *Am J Sports Med* 16:97–100, 1988.
Cox JS: The fate of the acromioclavicular joint in athletic injuries. *Am J Sports Med* 9:50–53, 1981.
Cox JS: Current method of treatment of acromioclavicular joint dislocations. *Orthopedics* 15:1041–1044, 1992.
Deafenbaugh MK, Dugdale TW, Staeheli JW, Nielsen R: Non-operative treatment of Neer Type II distal clavicle fractures: A prospective study. *Contemp Orthop* 4:405–413, 1990.
Dias JJ, Steingold RF, Richardson RA, et al: The conservative treatment of acromioclavicular dislocation. *J Bone Joint Surg (Am)* 69B:719–722, 1987.
Fukuda K, Craig EV, An KN, et al: Biomechanical study of the ligamentous system of the acromioclavicular joint. *J Bone Joint Surg (Am)* 68A:434–440, 1986.
Galpin RD, Hawkins RJ, Grainger RW: A comparative analysis of operative versus non-operative treatment of Grade III acromioclavicular separations. *Clin Orthop* 193:150–155, 1985.
Gieck JH, Nelson WE: Injuries to the acromioclavicular joint—Mechanisms, diagnosis and treatment. *Athletic Training*, 22–28, 1979.
Glick JM, Milburn LJ, Haggerty JF, et al: Dislocation of the acromioclavicular joint: Follow-up study of 35 unreduced acromioclavicular dislocations. *Am J Sports Med* 6:263–270, 1979.
Kulund DN: *The Injured Athlete*. Philadelphia, Lippincott, 1982, pp 273–276.
Larsen E, Bjerg-Neilsen A, Christensen P: Conservative or surgical treatment of acromioclavicular dislocation: A prospective controlled randomized study. *J Bone Joint Surg (Am)* 68A:552–555, 1986.
Lavelle DG: Dislocations, in *Campbells Operative Orthopedics*, 8th ed. St Louis, Mosby, 1992, pp 1358–1364.
Neviaser RJ: Injuries to the clavicle and acromioclavicular joint. *Orthop Clin North Am* 18:433–438, 1987.
O'Donoghue DH: *Treatment of Injuries to Athletes*. Philadelphia, Saunders, 1976, pp 164–182.
Patterson WR: Inferior dislocation of the distal end of the clavicle. *J Bone Joint Surg (Am)* 49A:1184–1186, 1967.
Petersson CJ: Resection of the lateral end of the clavicle. *Acta Orthop Scand* 54:904–907, 1983.
Rockwood CA: Injuries to the acromioclavicular joint, in *Fractures in Adults*. Philadelphia, Lippincott, 1991, pp 1181–1251.
Taft TN, Wilson FC, Oglesby JW: Dislocation of the acromioclavicular joint: An end result study. *J Bone Joint Surg (Am)* 69A:1045–1051, 1987.
Walsh WM, Peterson DA, Shelton G, et al: Shoulder strength following acromioclavicular injury. *Am J Sports Med* 13:153–158, 1985.
Weaver JK, Dunn HK: Treatment of acromioclavicular injuries, especially complete acromioclavicular separation. *J Bone Joint Surg (Am)* 54A:1187–1194, 1972.

CHAPTER 14

Subacromial Arthroscopy

Raymond Thal
Richard B. Caspari

A thorough inspection of the subacromial space is an essential aspect of a complete arthroscopic evaluation of the shoulder. Important diagnostic information is obtained regarding the nature and extent of subacromial and rotator cuff pathology. Distinguishing features of primary and secondary impingement can be identified. This distinction is of particular importance in the throwing athlete. Arthroscopic subacromial decompression may be performed as indicated. When necessary, rotator cuff repair can then be performed using a mini-open deltoid splitting incision or a formal open approach.

ANATOMY AND PATHOGENESIS OF SUBACROMIAL IMPINGEMENT

The anatomy and pathogenesis of subacromial impingement and the anatomic rationale and technique for anterior acromioplasty have been described by Neer.[1] He showed that in the functional position of forward flexion, the supraspinatus tendon, the subacromial bursa, and occasionally the tendon of the long head of the biceps pass beneath the anterior edge of the acromion, the coracoacromial ligament, and at times the acromioclavicular joint. He defined three progressive stages of rotator cuff impingement. Stage I involves edema and hemorrhage of the rotator cuff and usually resolves with conservative treatment. Repeated inflammatory episodes may lead to the stage II changes of fibrosis and tendinitis. Stage III involves tearing of the rotator cuff and bone changes in the coracoacromial arch.[2]

Neer[1] also described the shape and slope of the acromion as important factors in the development of impingement syndrome. Bigliani[3] further classified acromial shape into three types based on the curvature of its undersurface as seen radiographically on a supraspinatus outlet view. A type I acromion is flat. Type II has a curved undersurface. A type III acromion is hooked. The incidence of rotator cuff pathology was noted to be higher in patients with a type II or III acromion. Rotator cuff disease was rarely observed in the presence of a type I acromion.[3]

Nirschl[4] described subacromial impingement as a secondary phenomenon. He reported that primary pathologic changes in the rotator cuff cause muscle weakness and imbalance with subsequent upward migration of the humeral head and impingement. The concept of muscle weakness is extremely important in the nonoperative and postoperative treatment of impingement syndrome. Strengthening the rotator cuff musculature can help limit abnormal upward displacement of the humeral head.[5,6]

SURGICAL GOALS

Anterior acromioplasty for decompression of the subacromial space has been well described in the literature.[1–3,5,7–18] The primary objectives, whether performed open or arthroscopically, are to debride the hypertrophic subacromial bursa, release the coracoacromial ligament, and resect the undersurface of the anterior acromion. Acromioclavicular joint debridement and/or distal clavicle resection may also be necessary. Neer notes that the "objective (of the anterior acromioplasty) is to render the undersurface (of the acromion) flat, without overhang."[2] The open technique describes resection of the curved undersurface of the acromion so that the remaining acromion is flat and in the plane of the posterior acromion[2] (Fig. 14-1). This essentially coverts a type II or III acromion to a type I acromion.

In recent years, developments have permitted these objectives to be achieved arthroscopically.[7–10,19–21] Arthroscopic acromioplasty offers certain advantages over the open procedure. Surgery performed arthroscopically requires less surgical dissection, resulting in less postoperative morbidity. The deltoid muscle fibers are left intact. Postoperative discomfort is moderate and can usually be controlled by oral analgesics. In most instances the procedure can be performed on an outpatient basis.

Glenohumeral joint evaluation allows for identification of any associated pathology, such as labral tears, lesions resulting from instability, partial tears of the biceps tendon, and partial-thickness tears of the undersurface of the rotator cuff. Impingement symptoms secondary to instability are common in the athlete's shoulder. Difficulty can be experienced in distinguishing primary and secondary impinge-

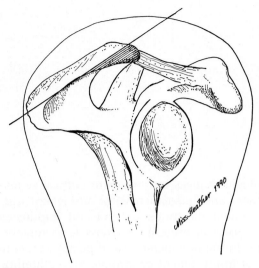

FIGURE 14-1
In a properly performed anterior acromioplasty, the curved undersurface of the anterior acromioplasty is resected so that the remaining acromion is flat and in the plane of the posterior acromion. (*After Neer, 1983.*)

ment on clinical ground alone. Treatment is very different, making this distinction quite important.

Subacromial decompression and acromioplasty is primarily indicated in patients with advanced stage II or III impingement syndrome who have failed conservative management. Subacromial decompression may be performed alone or in conjunction with rotator cuff repair, depending on the pathology and clinical circumstances. Conservative treatment includes rest, nonsteroidal anti-inflammatory medication, and occasional subacromial steroid injections. A structured rehabilitation program of rotator cuff stretching and strengthening is also essential.

OPERATIVE TECHNIQUE

Arthroscopic subacromial decompression can be performed with the patient in the lateral decubitus or the seated position. The seated position is more familiar for the surgeon accustomed to performing open shoulder procedures. It also allows for easier conversion to an open procedure using an anterior approach. We find glenohumeral arthroscopy to be more difficult in the seated position and therefore prefer the lateral decubitus position in most circumstances. The patient is tilted approximately 30° posterior, which positions the glenoid surface to be parallel to the floor. This also allows for easier access to the anterior aspect of the shoulder. Traction is applied to the patient's arm via a sterile, impervious stockinette and sterile rope. The arm should be placed in approximately 30° of abduction and 15° of forward flexion. Excessive arm abduction may inter-

fere with instrumentation through the lateral portal. Repair of the rotator cuff can be performed through an extension of the lateral portal to create a mini-open deltoid splitting incision. This is easily accomplished with the patient in the lateral decubitus position.

Glenohumeral Evaluation

Glenohumeral evaluation is performed using standard anterior and posterior portals. If instrumentation is required, an additional supraclavicular inflow portal or an arthroscopic pump with inflow through the arthroscope sheath may be used.

The glenohumeral joint is thoroughly examined, with particular attention given to the undersurface of the rotator cuff. Careful inspection of the glenohumeral ligaments and posterior aspects of the humeral head is also important to identify subtle glenohumeral instability, particularly in the throwing athlete.

Subacromial Bursoscopy

The arthroscope is removed from the glenohumeral joint and placed into the subacromial space. The same posterior skin incision may be used. The blunt trocar and arthroscope sheath are directed from the posterior portal anteriorly and superiorly toward the anterolateral corner of the acromion to enter the subacromial bursa (Fig. 14-2). Initial fluid distention is accomplished through the arthroscopic cannula. An in-to-out technique establishes the anterior portal. The arthroscope is advanced just lateral to the coracoacromial ligament and replaced by the sharp trocar. The trocar and arthroscopic sheath are then advanced to exit the previously established anterior skin incision. A second cannula is placed over the tip of the trocar and both cannulas are then brought

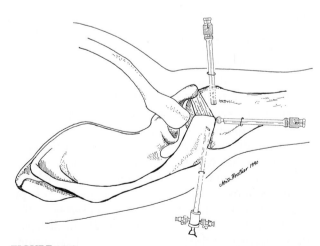

FIGURE 14-2
Portal placement and instrument location for evaluation of the subacromial space and coracoacromial ligament release.

into the bursa and separated. Inflow is now maintained through the anterior portal. One cubic centimeter of 1:1000 epinephrine solution is added to each 3-L bag of Ringer's lactate.

The subacromial space is lined by a thin membrane forming the bursal sac. Once the bursa is entered and distended, visualization is not difficult. Occasionally the arthroscope may be introduced within or between the bursal membrane and the acromion above or the rotator cuff below. If this occurs, the arthroscope should be removed and reinserted into the bursal space. Frequently there is a veil of bursal tissue within the posterior portion of the bursa. Resection of this tissue improves visualization and provides greater ease with instrumentation in the subacromial space.

The superior surface of the rotator cuff tendons, particularly the supraspinatus and infraspinatus, should be carefully examined. Internal and external rotation of the arm allows for a more thorough evaluation. The undersurface of the acromion and the coracoacromial ligament should also be examined. If an acromial hook is present (Fig. 14-3) or there is evidence of abrasion on the undersurface of the acromion (Plate 24), an acromioplasty is indicated. The abrasion on the undersurface of the acromion is usually located on the anterolateral aspect of the acromion. Patients with a prominent greater tuberosity, chronic bursitis, or occasionally, calcific tendinitis may also benefit from an acromioplasty.

Coracoacromial Ligament Release

A lateral portal is established approximately 2 to 3 cm distal to the anterolateral corner of the acromion (Fig. 14-2). It is important that this portal be in line

with the anterior margin of the acromion. The portal must be placed distal enough to allow instrumentation and visualization of the entire undersurface of the acromion, including the lateral border of the acromion, with the arthroscope in this lateral portal.

With the arthroscope in the posterior portal and a soft tissue shaver in the lateral portal, bursal tissue and loose soft tissue is removed from the acromion. A 4.5-mm round notchplasty burr is then used to lightly remove periosteum from the anterior edge of the acromion, exposing the margin of the acromion and the attachment of the coracoacromial ligament. Alternatively, the junction of the ligament and the anterior margin of the acromion can be identified with a spinal needle placed through the ligament and adjacent to the anterolateral corner of the acromion. The coracoacromial ligament is released by sectioning the anterior margin of the acromion with the burr, progressing from lateral to medial (Fig. 14-4). An approximately 4- to 5-mm width of bone (width of the burr) is removed. Bleeding is minimized with this technique because the coracoacromial ligament itself is not being cut; its bony attachment is being resected. An electrocautery or laser is rarely, if ever, needed. Care should be taken to detach the ligament completely but leave deltoid fibers intact (Plate 25).

Acromioplasty

The arthroscope is now switched to the lateral portal, and the burr is placed in the posterior portal for the acromioplasty (Fig. 14-5). The rotator cuff is again examined. Additional perspective is provided by viewing from this lateral portal. The cut edge of the anterior acromion is examined and the thickness is assessed. The shank of the cutter is rested against

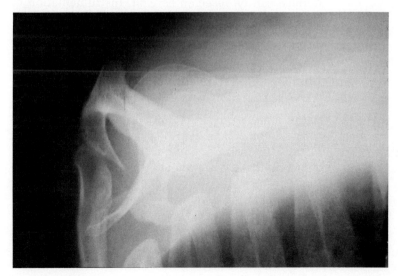

FIGURE 14-3
Radiographic demonstration of a large acromial hook.

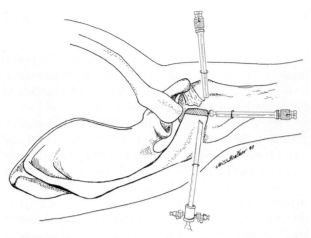

FIGURE 14-4
Coracoacromial ligament release is accomplished by sectioning the anterior margin of the acromion rather than cutting the ligament itself.

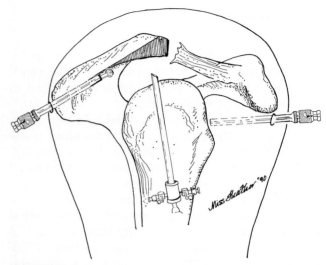

FIGURE 14-6
The tip of the burr is placed at the deepest point of the concavity of the acromion. Bone is resected by sweeping the cutter from lateral to medial and progressing anteriorly while maintaining the angle of the burr, using the angle of the posterior acromion as a guide.

the posterior lip of the acromion, which acts as a fulcrum. The tip of the burr is placed at the deepest point of the concavity of the acromion. Bone is resected by sweeping the cutter from lateral to medial and progressing anteriorly while maintaining the angle of the burr. The angle of the posterior acromion is the guide for the burr angle (Fig. 14-6 and Plate 26). In this way the acromion is tapered anteriorly while providing a smooth transition to normal bony cortex posteriorly. This technique eliminates the problem of determining the point at which enough bone has been resected. By following the angle provided by the posterior acromion, the appropriate amount of bone is automatically resected, resulting in a flat acromion (Fig. 14-6). The anterior edge of the acromion should now be tapered compared with its thickness, which was seen prior to acromioplasty.

The arthroscope is then returned to the posterior portal to view the contour of the undersurface of the

acromion from this perspective. The transition from normal bone to the area of the acromioplasty is inspected carefully. The resection area itself is also examined for irregularity.

Acromioclavicular Joint Examination and Debridement

The acromioclavicular joint is examined with the arthroscope in either the posterior or the lateral portal. Visualization and instrumentation of the acromioclavicular joint can be improved by externally depressing the clavicle while performing the viewing. Acromioclavicular joint debridement, osteophyte resection, or both is accomplished at this time. If indicated, the entire distal clavicle or only its undersurface can be resected as well. Instrumentation of the acromioclavicular joint and distal clavicle is best accomplished via the anterior portal.

Mini-Open Rotator Cuff Repair

Repair of some rotator cuff tears can be performed using a mini-open deltoid splitting incision. The torn rotator cuff is debrided back to healthy tissue with a motorized, end-cutting shaver or suction punch in the lateral portal and the arthroscope in the posterior portal. A trough is prepared in the greater tuberosity using a motorized burr and curette. Multiple sutures are arthroscopically placed in the rotator cuff using a suture passer. We prefer to place mattress sutures in the rotator cuff using a no. 2 nonabsorbable braided suture. This is accomplished ar-

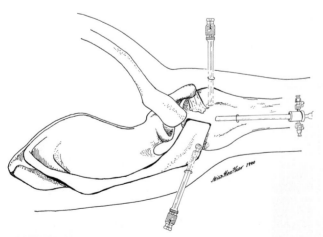

FIGURE 14-5
The acromioplasty is performed with the burr in the posterior portal and the arthroscope in the lateral portal.

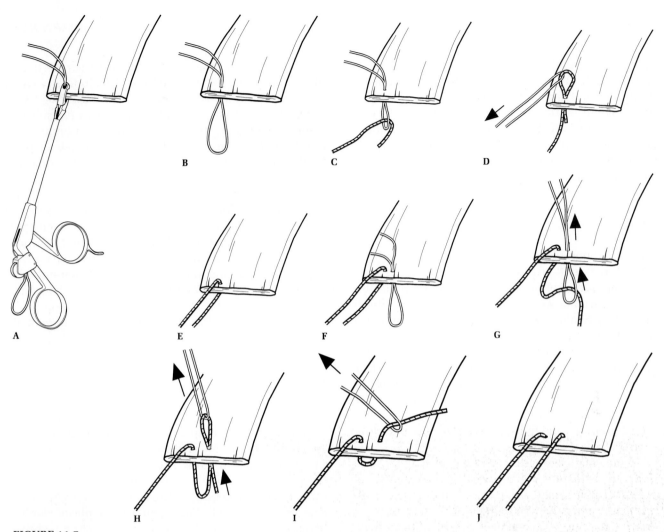

FIGURE 14-7

A–B. A suture loop is placed in the rotator cuff using the Shutt suture passer. This is accomplished by simultaneously placing both free ends of a 3-0 monofilament suture in the suture passer. As both free ends of the suture are passed through the rotator cuff, a suture loop is formed. *C–E.* This looped suture serves as a suture passer to pull a simple no. 2 nonabsorbable braided suture through the rotator cuff. *F.* A second looped suture is placed adjacent to the no. 2 nonabsorbable braided suture. *G–I.* The end of the braided suture that exits the inferior surface of the rotator cuff is threaded through the looped suture, outside the joint, and pulled through the rotator cuff, creating a mattress suture. *J.* Completed mattress suture.

throscopically using a looped suture passing technique[22] (Fig. 14-7) or the Concept suture shuttle. Traction is applied to the rotator cuff while mobilization above and below the rotator cuff is accomplished when necessary. The lateral portal is extended to create a small, deltoid splitting incision. Several bone tunnels are made extending from the trough through to the lateral aspect of the greater tuberosity. The sutures are brought through the tunnels and tied over a bone bridge after seating the tendon in the trough. The bone tunnels can be prepared using a variety of instruments. Our preference has been to use the Concept rotator cuff system designed by Snyder.[23]

POSTOPERATIVE CARE

Arthroscopic subacromial decompression without rotator cuff repair is an outpatient procedure. A sling is used for comfort and is discontinued as soon as tolerated, usually 1 to 2 days after surgery. A bulky compressive dressing is applied following surgery. This is removed on the second postoperative day, at which time showers are permitted. Band-Aid strips are then used until the portals are dry. Activities are advanced as tolerated. Heavy overhead activities and sports are gradually resumed after 6 weeks. Strenuous throwing and racket sports are avoided for 2 to 3 months. High-demand throwing athletes may re-

179

quire 4 to 6 months of rehabilitation before motion and strength are restored to allow throwing at the desired level. If a rotator cuff repair is performed, active range of motion is delayed to allow for healing of the rotator cuff. Early passive range of motion is encouraged. This is followed by a structured physical therapy program for range of motion, progressive strengthening, and stretching exercises.

RESULTS

Ellman[24] reported results in 82 consecutive patients who underwent arthroscopic subacromial decompression and acromioplasty with a 2- to 5-year follow-up. Patients were rated using the UCLA Shoulder Rating Scale. Satisfactory results were achieved in 89 percent of the 65 patients without full-thickness cuff tears. Of the 17 patients with full-thickness cuff tears, results were 65 percent satisfactory. Of the athletes evaluated, 87.5 percent were able to return to their preoperative sports activity following surgery. Similar results for arthroscopic subacromial decompression have been reported by other authors.[25,26,27]

Lucie et al.[26] reported results similar to those reported by Ellman.[24] When compared with a matched open acromioplasty group, the arthroscopic acromioplasty group had better results. The arthroscopy group had a shorter hospital stay, with surgery being performed as an outpatient or with a 23-h stay. They achieved an earlier return to function and an earlier range of motion, and required 2 weeks less physical therapy than the open group.

Burns et al.[27] reported a lower success rate in their athletic population than did Ellman. Overall, 65.5 percent of their patients returned to their previous level of activity. Nine collegiate athletes were evaluated in this study. Eight of these athletes were considered satisfactory by UCLA criteria. However, only five of these athletes (56 percent) were able to return to their previous sporting activity.

Hawkins et al.[28] reported on 112 consecutive arthroscopic subacromial decompressions and compared these results with a previously reported group of 108 open subacromial decompressions. Satisfactory results were achieved in 46 percent of the arthroscopy group. The open group achieved markedly better results, with an 87 percent satisfactory rate. Close evaluation of these data raises the important issues of proper surgical indications and proper surgical technique. Twelve patients who underwent arthroscopic subacromial decompression in this study "may not have actually had impingement syndrome"

based on the findings at the time of surgery. All 12 of these patients had unsatisfactory postoperative results. In addition, 10 patients in the unsatisfactory group obtained no relief from a preoperative subacromial Xylocaine injection. The diagnosis must be questioned in these patients as well. Nineteen patients underwent an open acromioplasty after a failed arthroscopic subacromial decompression. Eleven of these 19 patients obtained no relief from the open procedure. Assuming the open procedure was technically adequate, the preoperative diagnosis must again be questioned in these 11 patients. Intraoperative technical difficulty, which "may have prevented removal of enough bone from the acromion," was encountered in 8 cases. All 8 patients had unsatisfactory results. An inadequate acromioplasty was found in 14 of the 19 patients who underwent a subsequent open acromioplasty.[28]

CONCLUSION

Surgical indications are identical regardless of whether a subacromial decompression and acromioplasty is performed open or arthroscopically. Poor results can be expected if either procedure is performed for improper indications. Proper surgical technique is critical for a successful arthroscopic subacromial decompression. A well-done open acromioplasty would be expected to provide better results than a technically deficient arthroscopic procedure. Hawkins et al.[28] clearly demonstrate these points in their study.

Arthroscopic subacromial decompression is a technically demanding procedure. The control of bleeding and the determination of the amount of bone to resect are two commonly encountered technical difficulties. These problems are addressed in the described technique. We find this simplifies the procedure while providing more precise bone resection and contouring.

Precision in locating the anterior margin of the acromion is essential when using this technique for coracoacromial ligament resection. Using this landmark assures that the coracoacromial ligament is released at its bony attachment with resection of the appropriate amount of bone. Bleeding problems may be encountered if too little bone is resected and the ligament itself is divided. Excessive anterior acromionectomy risks leaving a bit of bone in the detached edge of the coracoacromial ligament in addition to removing more bone than necessary. Careful placement of the lateral portal in line with the anterior border of the acromion improves the accuracy of the coracoacromial ligament release. Early in the learning curve, spinal needles may help locate the anterior margin of the acromion. This becomes unnecessary as the surgeon develops more experience with the arthroscopic anatomy of the subacromial space.

Other techniques to address the problem of bleeding with coracoacromial ligament resection have been reported. Many advocate the use of epinephrine in the irrigation fluid as we have described.[7,21] Meyers[21] reports using a curette through the lateral portal to detach the ligament from the acromion in a subperiosteal fashion. Ellman[9] uses an electrosurgical knife to maintain hemostasis with coracoacromial ligament release. Recently, some surgeons have promoted the use of lasers for coracoacromial ligament release. We have found these unnecessary with our technique, thus eliminating the added inconvenience and expense of electrocautery or laser equipment. We occasionally use the arthroscopic pump with inflow through the arthroscope sheath. We do not consider the pump essential for control of bleeding, however, with this technique. The pump avoids the need for an anterior portal if inflow is achieved through the arthroscope sheath.

Attention to certain details is important when using this technique for acromioplasty. Because the posterior margin and slope of the posterior acromion are guides for the acromioplasty, the shank of the burr must remain in contact with the posterior lip of the acromion at all times. If the shank of the burr is lifted off the posterior lip of the acromion, the angle of resection becomes too acute and excessive acromion is removed (Fig. 14-8).

Complete medial to lateral sweeps must also be made with the burr to avoid leaving a ridge of bone at either margin. If the lateral portal has been established too far proximal, visualization of the entire lateral margin of the acromion is difficult with the arthroscope in the lateral portal. This technical pitfall may lead to incomplete resection of the lateral margin of the acromion.

Resection of an appropriate amount of bone and proper contouring of the acromion are important factors in a well-performed acromioplasty. Other authors have described using the burr or a probe to determine the depth of bone resected.[21] This is done by creating a pilot hole in the acromion of a measured depth. The acromioplasty is then performed by resecting the remainder of the anterior acromion to the depth of the pilot hole. The use of the acromioclavicular joint as a guide[7] can be inaccurate, particularly if osteophytes are present on the acromion or distal clavicle. The amount of bone that should be resected varies with patient size and acromial morphology. This technique automatically resects the appropriate amount of bone while efficiently contouring the acromion to the proper shape as described by Neer.[2]

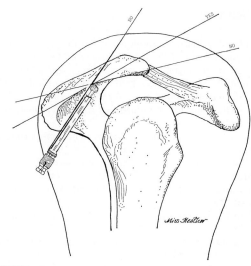

FIGURE 14-8
The shank of the burr must remain in contact with the posterior margin and slope of the acromion at all times to avoid error in the resection angle.

Rotator cuff repair using a mini-open deltoid splitting incision offers many advantages. Smaller, more cosmetic incisions are used. Since the deltoid is not detached from the acromion, postoperative rehabilitation is accelerated without concern for disruption of the repaired deltoid muscle fibers. Mini-open rotator cuff repair is technically quite demanding, however. Organization of the sutures must be maintained as they are placed arthroscopically. The security of the repair must not be compromised by the desire to complete the repair through a mini-open approach. A formal open repair should be used if satisfactory suture placement and/or fixation cannot be achieved with the mini-open approach. We have found small to moderate tears, which can be easily mobilized, to be best suited for repair using a mini-open approach.

Arthroscopy of the shoulder and subacromial space has greatly advanced our understanding of a variety of pathologic conditions of the shoulder. This is particularly true with regard to shoulder dysfunction in the throwing athlete. Therapeutic benefits can be realized when arthroscopic techniques are employed in the treatment of many of these conditions. The principles and goals of the open and arthroscopic procedures remain the same. As arthroscopic instrumentation and fixation devices continue to develop, more subacromial and rotator cuff surgery will be performed arthroscopically.

REFERENCES

1. Neer CS II: Anterior acromioplasty for the chronic impingement syndrome in the shoulder. A preliminary report. *J Bone Joint Surg (Am)* 54A:41–50, 1972.

2. Neer CS II: Impingement lesions. *Clin Orthop* 173:70–73, 1983.

3. Bigliani LV, Morrison DS, April CS: The morphology of the acromion and its relationship to rotator cuff tears. *Orthop Trans* 10:216–228, 1986.

4. Nirschl RP: Shoulder tendinitis, in *AAOS Symposium. Upper Extremity in Sports*. St Louis, Mosby, 1986, pp 322–337.

5. Kessel L, Watson M: The painful arc syndrome. Clinical classification as a guide to management. *J Bone Joint Surg (Am)* 59B:166–172, 1977.

6. Jobe FW, Jobe CM: Painful athletic injuries of the shoulder. *Clin Orthop* 173:117–124, 1983.

7. Andrews JR, Schemmel SP: Arthroscopic acromioplasty. *Surg Rounds Orthop* 49–50, 1989.

8. Caspari RB, Thal R: A technique for arthroscopic subacromial decompression. *Arthroscopy* 8(1):23–30, 1992.

9. Ellman H: Arthroscopic subacromial decompression: Analysis of one to three year results. *Arthroscopy* 3:173–181, 1987.

10. Gartsman GM: Arthroscopic acromioplasty for lesions of the rotator cuff. *J Bone Joint Surg (Am)* 72A:169–180, 1990.

11. Hawkins RJ, Abrams JS: Impingement syndrome in the absence of rotator cuff tear (stage 1 and 2). *Orthop Clin North Am* 18:373–382, 1987.

12. Hawkins RJ, Kennedy JC: Impingement syndrome in athletes. *Am J Sports Med* 8:151–158, 1980.

13. McShane RP et al: Conservative open anterior acromioplasty. *Clin Orthop* 223:137–144, 1987.

14. Neviaser TJ, Neviaser RJ, Neviaser JS, Neviaser JS: The four-in-one arthroplasty for the painful arc syndrome. *Clin Orthop* 163:107–112, 1982.

15. Post M, Cohen J: Impingement syndrome. A review of late stage II and early stage III lesions. *Clin Orthop* 207:126–132, 1986.

16. Raggio CL, Warren RF, Sculco T: Surgical treatment of impingement syndrome: 4 year follow-up. *Orthop Trans* 9:48–49, 1985.

17. Tibone JE, Jobe FW, Kerlan RK, et al: Shoulder impingement syndrome in athletes treated by an anterior acromioplasty. *Clin Orthop* 198:134–140, 1985.

18. Thorling J et al: Acromioplasty for impingement syndrome. *Acta Orthop Scand* 56:147–148, 1985.

19. Esch JC et al: Arthroscopic subacromial decompression: Results according to degree of rotator cuff tear. Presented at the annual meeting of the Arthroscopy Association of North America, Washington, DC, 1988.

20. Gartsman GM, Blair ME Jr, Noble PC, et al: Arthroscopic subacromial decompression. An anatomical study. *Am J Sports Med* 16:48–50, 1988.

21. Meyers JF: Arthroscopic management of impingement syndrome and rotator cuff tears. *Adv Sports Med Fitness* 2:243–260, 1989.

22. Thal R: A technique for arthroscopic mattress suture placement. *Arthroscopy* 9(5): 605–607, 1993.

23. Snyder SJ: The Concept rotator cuff repair system surgical technique brochure. 1991.

24. Ellman H: Arthroscopic acromioplasty, in *Operative Arthroscopy*. New York, Raven Press, 1991, p 555.

25. Paulos LE, Franklin JL: Arthroscopic shoulder decompression development and application. *Am J Sports Med* 18(3):235–244, 1990.

26. Lucie RS, Hardy PR, Hopkins RD: Comparison of arthroscopic anterior acromioplasty versus open acromioplasty for the treatment of subacromial impingement syndrome. Presented at the 11th annual meeting of the Arthroscopy Association of North America, Boston, MA, 1992.

27. Burns TP, Turba JE: Arthroscopic treatment of shoulder impingement in athletes. *Am J Sports Med* 20(1):13–16, 1992.

28. Hawkins R, Saddemi S, Moor J, et al: Arthroscopic subacromial decompression: A two-year to four-year follow-up study. Presented at the 11th annual meeting of the Arthroscopy Association of North America, Boston, MA, 1992.

CHAPTER 15

Shoulder Fractures in the Athlete

Edward V. Craig

INTRODUCTION

Fractures of the proximal humerus comprise 5 percent of all fractures. While these fractures are not uncommon, many of them occur in elderly, nonathletic patients having osteopenic bone. Thus the management is not entirely applicable to the management when these fractures occur in athletes. For instance, in the elderly population, these fractures often occur with minimal trauma. Thus, while the soft tissue around the shoulder is usually involved, the severity of the associated soft tissue trauma, and subsequent scarring and effects, are not as catastrophic as they may be when these fractures occur in young, athletic patients. In younger individuals, it usually takes much more energy to fracture the proximal humerus, and thus proximal humeral fractures in active, healthy, and athletic patients occur with more violent trauma, such as high-energy falls (skiing injuries) or during contact sports. Consequently, there is often a greater degree of associated soft tissue injury to surrounding cuff and deltoid, resulting in greater potential for scarring, compromise of motion and strength, and decreased athletic performance. For this reason, an argument can be made for more aggressive anatomic treatment of proximal humerus fractures in the athlete, in which the bone is much better suited for fixation methods, in order that rehabilitation may be begun soon after the injury, minimizing long-term adverse sequelae of the trauma. An additional factor is that higher-energy trauma in the athlete may be associated with other more serious soft tissue injuries, such as nerve and vascular pathology. While the incidence of proximal humeral fractures may be low in young athletes, the stakes are usually high; there is often a narrower margin for treatment error, so results may not be compromised, and thus prompt recognition and treatment are essential. Prompt recognition of these fractures, awareness of the associated injuries and potential complications, and restoration of anatomy offers the best chance of minimizing the impact of these adverse injuries on the athlete.

ANATOMIC CONSIDERATIONS

Several anatomic features related to the bone and soft tissue environment of the shoulder impact on these fractures when they occur in athletes. Concerning the bony anatomy of the shoulder girdle, it has long been recognized that when the proximal humerus fractures, it fractures along the lines of epiphyseal closure, thus producing identifiable segments that may be displaced by associated muscular attachments (Fig. 15-1). This pattern and degree of displacement have been the basis for the most common fracture classifications related to proximal humeral injuries, that of Neer and the A-O group. These classifications help us understand displacement patterns and resultant deformity. Neer recognized and made popular the idea that the deforming forces in proximal humeral fractures were the muscular attachments of the rotator cuff and pectoralis, tending to displace the fracture fragments in identifiable directions. It was recognized that these deforming forces should be neutralized before the fragments can be effectively reduced, in either a closed or an open fashion. The vast majority of fractures of the proximal humerus are either nondisplaced or minimally displaced. The displacement criteria utilized in the Neer classification help decision making in operative and nonoperative treatment. The displacement criteria of Neer (more than 1 cm displacement, more than 45° angulated) imply that if these criteria are not met, a fracture displaced less than this degree may be treated essentially the same as a nondisplaced fracture (Fig. 15-2). This management for minimally or nondisplaced fracture includes immobilization for comfort, followed, when early pain subsides, with initiation of isometric exercises to maintain muscle tone. When the acute pain subsides, early range of motion can be instituted, concentrating on forward elevation in the plane of the scapula, external rotation, and internal rotation. When union of the fracture occurs, more active and resistive exercises can be considered. This Neer fracture classification recognizes that with fractures

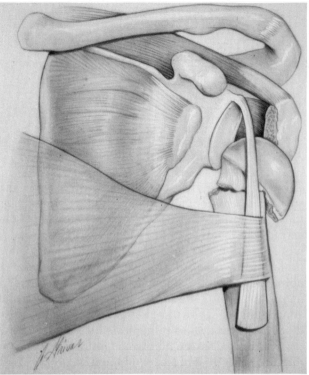

FIGURE 15-1
When the proximal humerus fractures, displacement is generally along the lines of the epiphysis. The lesser tuberosity is displaced by the subscapularis medially. The greater tuberosity, pulled by the supraspinatus, infraspinatus, and teres minor, may be displaced posteriorly, superiorly, or a combination of those two directions. The shaft is pulled medially by the pectoralis. The articular surface, often with some medial metaphyseal bone, may be free of all soft tissue attachments.

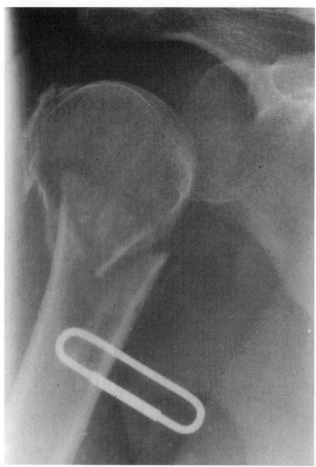

FIGURE 15-2
With the Neer classification, only those segments which are displaced are considered. In this fracture, although there is a fracture through the surgical neck and the greater tuberosity, none of these segments are significantly displaced from one another. This may be considered a one-part fracture without significant segment displacement.

involving the lesser tuberosity and the attached subscapularis, displacement occurs and the lesser tuberosity is displaced and pulled medially by the pull of the subscapularis. Subsequent malunion may thus limit internal rotation of the shoulder. The greater tuberosity, with its attachment site for supraspinatus, infraspinatus, and teres minor, is usually displaced in a more complex fashion. The greater tuberosity fragment, if displaced, is particularly problematic in the overhead athlete, where there is little tolerance for residual displacement of this fracture. The cuff tends to displace this fragment either superiorly or posteriorly, and both of these positions interfere with the overhead athlete. If the fragment is displaced predominantly by the pull of the infraspinatus and teres minor, the tuberosity displaces posteriorly, blocking external rotation and producing weakness of the attached external rotators. Likewise, if the greater tuberosity is displaced predominantly superiorly by the pull of the supraspinatus and becomes lodged in the subacromial space, there is some pure impediment to motion and strength because of the mechanical block in the subacromial space. This greater tuberosity displaced fracture is

probably the one that involves the greatest number of difficult treatment decisions in the athlete, as small degrees of displacement, otherwise well tolerated in a nonathletic population, can be extremely disabling for an athlete who relies on essentially normal strength, flexibility, and motion. In contrast to the tuberosity fractures, fractures through the surgical neck produce medial displacement of the humeral shaft, by the pull of the pectoralis major, latissimus dorsi, and teres major. If the surgical neck fracture is the only fracture present, the humeral head and detached tuberosities often remain in a relatively anatomic position, since the cuff attachments are undisturbed. The final fragment frequently involved in proximal humeral fractures is the articular segment of the humeral head, which has no soft tissue attachments. Because the displacement of this segment is usually very difficult to reduce anatomically, it is usually associated with interruption of blood supply to the humeral head, and it is often

184

among the most devastating of any injuries to the athlete.

The second common classification of proximal humeral fractures is the A-O classification. This classification places greater emphasis on the humeral head blood supply; it is more complicated and has more subgroups but may give a more accurate definition of the risk of humeral head necrosis. Thus, to effectively treat an athlete with proximal humeral fracture, an understanding of the muscle attachments around the proximal humerus is critical, because this not only explains the displacement pattern of the fracture but also gives an idea of adequacy of the blood supply of the humeral head.

This blood supply is another critical anatomic factor that must be considered in treating proximal humeral fractures. While the humeral head blood supply arises from the axillary artery as both anterior and posterior humeral circumflex vessels, the main blood supply from the humeral head is provided by the arcuate artery, a continuation of the ascending branch of the anterior humeral circumflex artery. This artery courses superiorly to enter the bone in the intertubercular groove, sending branches to both lesser and greater tuberosities and to a large segment of the humeral head (Fig. 15-3). This branch has the potential to be disrupted by any fracture involving greater and lesser tuberosities or anatomic and surgical neck and is also frequently disrupted by extensive soft tissue dissection in the course of surgical

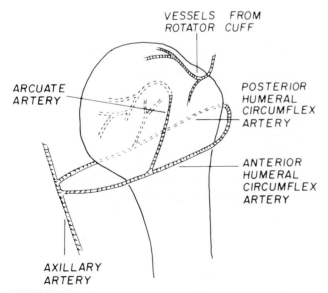

FIGURE 15-3
The blood supply of the proximal humerus arises from both posterior and anterior humeral circumflex arteries. The predominant nutrient vessel for the proximal humerus is the arcuate artery, a branch of the anterior humeral circumflex artery.

approaches to proximal humeral fractures. It is well recognized that extensive dissection during a surgical approach for internal fixation of a proximal humeral fracture may disrupt the blood supply of the humeral head, leading to secondary avascular necrosis, a sequela that may be devastating in the young athlete.

An understanding of relevant neurovascular anatomy is also critical in treating these fractures. The incidence of nerve injuries in proximal humeral fractures ranges from 5 to 30 percent. These nerve injuries are usually associated with violent trauma, such as occurs with fracture dislocations. The brachial plexus is medial to the coracoid process of the scapula. While severe stretch injuries to the brachial plexus certainly can occur with violent trauma associated with fracture, the most common nerve injury is to the axillary nerve, which leaves the plexus in the posterior cord at the level of the axilla, courses 3 to 5 mm medial to the musculotendinous junction of the subscapularis, and is in close proximity to the inferior capsule before emerging in the quadrilateral space. After emerging from the quadrilateral space, it ennervates the deltoid muscle and teres minor and sends a sensory branch to the upper lateral arm. This nerve is frequently at risk with anterior fracture dislocations of the proximal humerus. While an uncommon injury, the resultant paralysis of the deltoid muscle in a young athlete is disastrous.

Serious vascular injuries associated with proximal humeral fractures in athletes are unusual. As with most vascular injuries, they most commonly occur in older patients whose arteries have less elasticity, resulting in potentially devastating injuries. Early diagnosis of these vascular injuries is critical. Most frequently involving the axillary artery, the clues to vascular injury are an expanding axillary hematoma or absent distal pulses. However, since collateral circulation may initially mask the extent of the injury, a high degree of awareness of the vascular anatomy around the shoulder girdle should be present. Diagnostic modalities such as Doppler ultrasound or arteriogram are useful to further evaluate the patency of major vessels in the shoulder girdle adjacent to fractures of the proximal humerus.

MECHANISM OF INJURY

Fractures of the proximal humerus in athletes most commonly occur via a number of common mechanisms. Direct trauma, that is, a blow directly to the anterior or anterolateral shoulder, typically occurs with a fall directly on the lateral aspect of the shoulder. Alternatively, indirect trauma via a fall on an outstretched hand can transmit enough force to fracture the proximal humerus. In older patients this commonly occurs during a fall from a standing height, as compromised bone quality is an important predisposing factor in fracture production. Since the athlete usually has better-quality bone, falls, when they occur, usually are more violent and from a greater distance. Arm position is also related to the development and pattern of fracture. With the arm in the abducted position, the greater tuberosity may lock against the acromion as the athlete falls. Further rotation of the humerus may produce a severe rotatory torque, resulting in either humeral fracture or a glenohumeral dislocation, or both.

Of course, fractures may also be produced by violent muscular contraction, such as occurs with electroconvulsive therapy or grand mal seizure activity. Most commonly these are posterior fractures and fracture dislocations since the combined forces produced by the internal rotators of the humerus are so much greater than those of the external rotators. However, anterior fracture dislocations may also occur during seizure activity, and associated cuff and tuberosity damage is common.

Pathologic fractures, while thought of more as occurring in the infirm, can also occur in the proximal humerus of athletes and should be a consideration when a fracture occurs in an athlete with relatively minor trauma. Bone cysts and tumors, not infrequently located in the proximal humerus, may be responsible for pathologic fractures of the proximal humerus in athletes involved in overhead sports and thus should be ruled out if a fracture occurs in an overhead athlete during relatively routine maneuvers, such as an overhead throw or a tennis serve.

CLINICAL AND RADIOGRAPHIC EVALUATION

Because the bony anatomy of the humerus is so well protected by soft tissues of the rotator cuff and deltoid, fractures of the proximal humerus may be initially overlooked, and high-quality x-rays are essential as part of the initial evaluation. Clinically, the athlete with a humeral fracture presents by splinting the arm adjacent to the chest. Any move of the shoulder is painful, and the athlete is usually unwilling to contract the shoulder girdle muscles, a fact that may simulate an associated nerve injury. Ecchymosis, frequently accompanying proximal humeral fractures, may not be evident for 24 to 48 h. Crepitus in the area of the pathology is common. Specific point ten-

derness over the greater tuberosity commonly occurs with displaced and nondisplaced fractures involving the greater tuberosity. Associated bony injuries may also occur, depending on the degree of trauma, and consideration should be given for associated cervical spine, clavicle, rib cage, and scapula injuries.

Careful neurovascular examination is essential prior to fracture reduction or manipulation. With the arm splinted or in a sling, it is usually possible to feel a contraction of the deltoid (axillary nerve) or biceps (musculocutaneous nerve). Simple firing of the muscle is enough to test the nerve integrity. Distal pulses should be evaluated and care taken to observe the area of proximal humerus for expanding hematoma. If the initial neurologic and vascular examinations are unremarkable, the athlete can then be scheduled for radiologic studies.

X-RAY EVALUATION

Optimum treatment of fractures in the athlete depends upon precise definition of the extent of injury. In fractures of the proximal humerus this mandates proper radiographic evaluation so that the position of the humeral head relative to the glenoid, the humeral head relative to the tuberosities and shaft, and tuberosities relative to their usual anatomic position are able to be determined. Thus, x-rays in at least two planes are mandatory. The usual minimum radiographic series in acute shoulder trauma is the trauma series, which adds an axillary view to the previous mentioned anteroposterior (AP) and lateral.

The true AP of the glenohumeral joint angles the cassette beam approximately 40° from the perpendicular line to the chest. This produces a radiograph that is a true AP through the glenohumeral joint (Fig. 15-4). This x-ray gives the most important information about the position of the humeral head relative to the shaft, and the superior-inferior position of the greater tuberosity relative to the humeral head. In addition, it may provide information about the humeral head relative to the glenoid. Additional scapular, clavicular, or rib injuries are often identified on this view (Figs. 15-8 and 15-9). The true lateral of the glenohumeral joint provides further information relative to the degree of angulation of the humeral shaft relative to the humeral head and gives an excellent view of the anterior-posterior displacement of the greater tuberosity relative to the head (Fig. 15-5). The axillary view is the best view for identification of the location of the humeral head relative to the glenoid (Fig. 15-6). It has been estimated that 60 to 70 percent of posterior dislocations of the humerus are

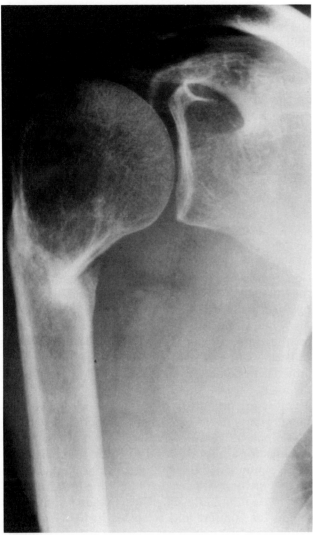

FIGURE 15-4
A true AP of the proximal humerus gives a view through the glenohumeral joint and the relative position of the tuberosities and the head segment to the shaft.

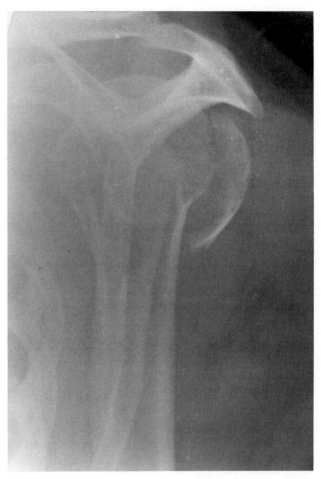

FIGURE 15-5
A true scapula lateral, in addition to identifying the humeral head relative to the glenoid fossa (in the center of the scapula Y), is also useful for the extent of posterior displacement of the greater tuberosity, as seen in this x-ray.

missed by the initial examiner; however, this would probably not be so if the axillary x-ray were routinely obtained and interpreted correctly on each patient with acute shoulder trauma. The axillary view also gives further information of the position of both lesser and greater tuberosities relative to the shaft and the humeral head.

The trauma series is usually easily obtained with a minimum of discomfort to the athlete. The x-rays can be taken with the patient either in or out of a sling, and with the patient standing, sitting, or supine. While the axillary view does require some abduction of an acutely painful arm, a minimal amount of arm abduction (20°) is usually required for an x-ray to be positioned in the axilla in order to obtain this axillary view.

Absolute accuracy regarding the position of the greater and lesser tuberosities is difficult when using

plain radiographs, and a computed tomography (CT) scan can be an invaluable adjunct to the initial evaluation. Since any degree of tuberosity malunion is often very poorly tolerated by the athlete, it is important for precise initial localization of the tuberosity segments. While less critical in the nonathletic population, which may tolerate slight degrees of nonanatomic tuberosity reduction, it seems logical to routinely utilize the CT scan for precise definition of the tuberosities in the athlete (Fig. 15-7). An additional valuable role for CT scan is in the evaluation of fracture dislocations, since it will precisely define the presence and extent of any fragments or fractures of the glenoid associated with the dislocation. With more complex fractures of the proximal humerus, three-dimensional reconstruction may be considered for better understanding of the image of the fracture.

Many fractures and fracture dislocations are characterized by disorders or disruptions of the rotator cuff. If there is a question of the integrity of the rotator cuff, based on either fracture pattern or clin-

187

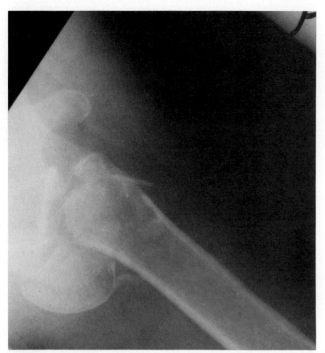

FIGURE 15-6
An axillary view is the best view to identify the humeral head relative to the glenoid fossa, as seen in this posterior fracture dislocation.

has the advantage of being able to image precisely the rotator cuff, provide good information about fracture anatomy, and provide some information about the potential for vascular disruption of the blood supply of the humeral head.

DISPLACEMENT CRITERIA

The vast majority of fractures of the proximal humerus are either nondisplaced or minimally displaced. Two common classifications have been useful for the analysis of proximal humeral fractures. In the classification of Neer, the one most commonly used, there are displacement criteria generally recognized to help the decision making in operative and nonoperative treatment. In addition, this classification gives a practical guide to the treatment of these fractures based on the location of the deforming forces of the muscle.

The AL classification places greater emphasis on the humeral head blood supply, is more complicated, and has more subgroups but may give a more accurate definition of the risk of humeral head necrosis.

It is important to recognize that in the displacement criteria of Neer (more than 1 cm displacement, more than 45° angulation) management may be the same as for a nondisplaced fracture. It appears that these patients will do well in considering these fractures together. Management includes, for nondisplaced or minimally displaced fractures, immobilization for comfort and when early pain subsides, initiation of isometric exercises to maintain muscle

ical examination, further soft tissue imaging may be necessary. While ultrasound and arthrogram have been utilized in the literature to determine cuff integrity, it is probably more logical in fractures of the proximal humerus to utilize the magnetic resonance imaging (MRI) scan. The MRI scan, while not able to give as precise bony anatomic detail as the CT scan,

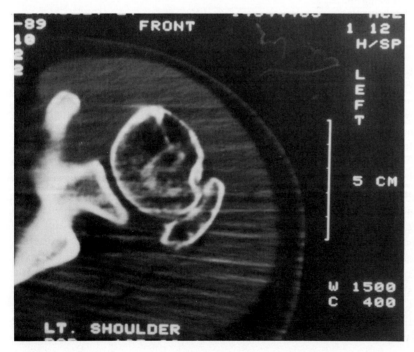

FIGURE 15-7
A CT scan gives more precise information about the position of the tuberosities relative to the head. Here is seen a posteriorly displaced greater tuberosity segment and the donor site from which it originated.

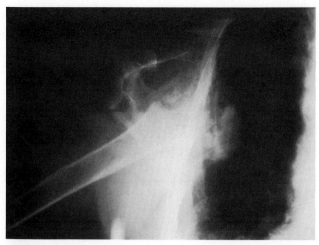

FIGURE 15-8
With multiple trauma, an AP view of the shoulder can often include additional information. Here is seen medial displacement of the humeral shaft and what appears to be a bony density inside the rib cage.

tone. When the acute pain subsides, early range of motion can be instituted concentrating on forward elevation in the plane of the scapula, external rotation, and internal rotation. When union of the fracture occurs, more active and then resistive exercises can be considered.

If the fracture has been nondisplaced, a return to sports of any type would appear to be practical when the fracture has healed and when there is enough motion and muscle tone to protect the athlete. Return to predominantly lower extremity in cutting sports can occur before a return to sports using the involved extremity, as there may be a long delay in the achievement of normal range of motion and strength of the extremity, even with nondisplaced fractures.

FRACTURES OF THE SURGICAL NECK

While these fractures are the most common of all proximal humeral fractures, the vast majority are undisplaced. If these fractures are nondisplaced or show minimal displacement, the athlete may be treated functionally, with a sling for comfort, followed by early rehabilitation. The patient can be examined 7 to 10 days following injury, and once the greater tuberosity is felt to move as a unit with the shaft, gentle range of motion exercise with Codman circular rotations, forward elevation with a pulley, and external and internal rotation can be begun. Because the rotator cuff is intact in these fractures, isometric exercises may begin for the cuff and deltoid

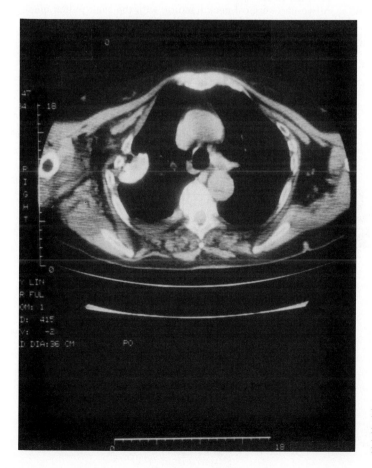

FIGURE 15-9
A CT scan identifies this bone density as the humeral head, which has been dislocated inside the thorax in this multitrauma patient.

immediately, as these exercises may minimize the muscle atrophy associated with inferior subluxation of the humerus commonly seen. Displacement may occur if vigorous rehabilitation is begun too early before the fracture is sticky. In addition, excessively aggressive exercises designed to produce range of motion may contribute to the development of nonunion in some patients.

Fractures of the surgical neck may be accompanied by extension of the fracture line into one or both tuberosities. If the tuberosity extension does not result in significant replacement of the tuberosity, the fracture lines in the tuberosities may be ignored. This fracture may present as impacted, varus angulation, with or without subtuberous comminution. Despite the fact that the rotator cuff is not pulling directly on the fracture fragment, the head not infrequently appears to be somewhat abducted, often as a result of a spike of bone impaled in the deep fascia of the deltoid.

When displaced, the head fragment usually remains anatomic, while the shaft displaces medially and anteriorly by the pull of the pectoralis major (Fig. 15-10). For many years it was suggested that elevation of the extremity and immobilization in the overhead position should be used to reduce and hold the fracture; however, this maneuver actually may exaggerate the pull of the pectoralis major muscle, which must be relaxed if closed reduction is to be effective. This fracture may be accompanied by a dislocation of the humeral head out of the glenoid fossa.

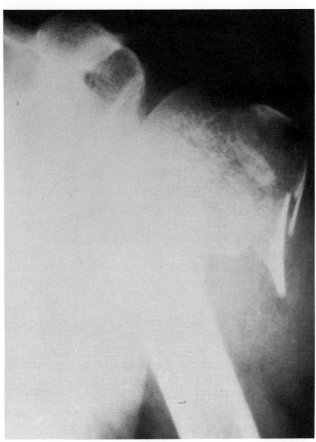

FIGURE 15-10
A two-part surgical neck fracture, with the shaft pulled medially by the pull of the pectoralis. The humeral head generally stays in relatively anatomic position. Intact tuberosities maintain blood supply to the humeral head.

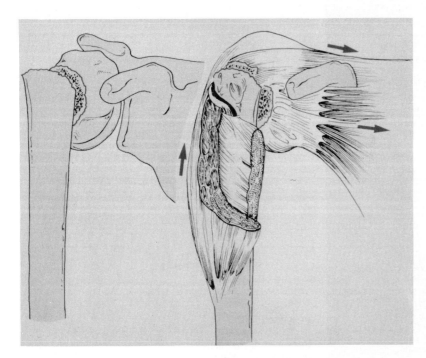

FIGURE 15-11
With two-part displacement, if closed reduction is impossible, it is often due to interposition of the biceps tendon or capsule between the fracture fragments.

If the dislocation is anterior, this may be associated with brachial plexus injury, and careful neurovascular examination should be performed.

The treatment of this fracture depends on the anatomic characteristics of the fracture, the extent of displacement of the fragments, the extent of comminution, and the age, demands, needs, and expectations of the athlete. If the fracture is displaced or significantly angulated, closed reduction should be attempted. This is performed after relaxing the pull of the pectoralis major by bringing the arm into slight adduction, so the shaft can be brought under the humeral head. As this is accomplished, the shaft can be impacted into the humeral head. If displacement exists and closed reduction is unsuccessful, this is usually secondary to soft tissue interposition by biceps, subscapularis, or capsule, and open reduction and removal of the interposed tissue should be combined with internal fixation (Fig. 15-11). An impacted and significantly angulated fracture may also be disimpacted and reduced. This significantly varus malunion, especially if combined with anterior angulation, may limit forward elevation to an unacceptable degree in an overhead athlete.

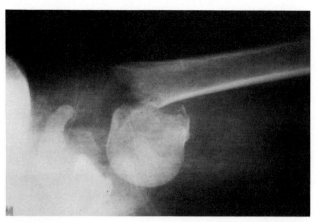

FIGURE 15-13
An axillary view shows the degree of displacement and angulation.

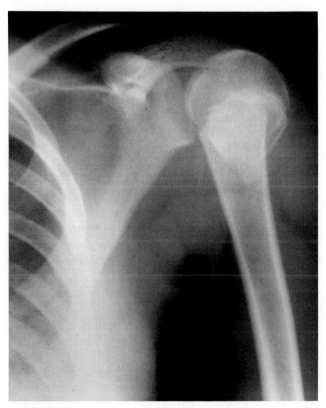

FIGURE 15-12
A two-part surgical neck fracture in a teen-age student. An AP view shows the position of the humeral head relative to the glenoid.

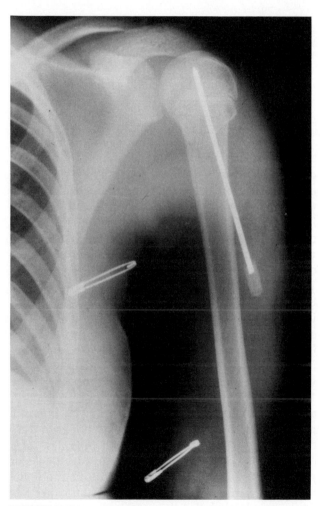

FIGURE 15-14
For two-part surgical neck fractures, especially in young adults in whom there is adequate bone stock, percutaneous pin fixation is often helpful. Care should be taken regarding the insertion site of the pin, and assurance obtained that the pin does not protrude through the articular surface of the humeral head.

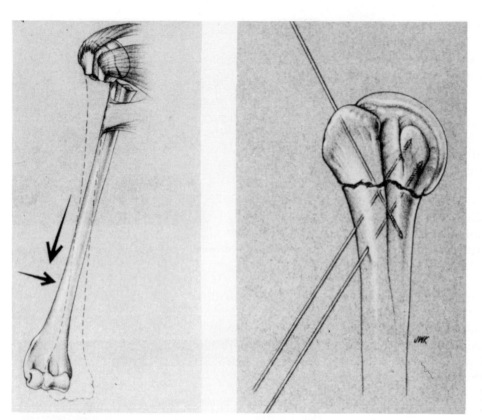

FIGURE 15-15
While one or two pins can be angled infralateral to supramedial, an additional pin is often helpful angled from the greater tuberosity down into the shaft, to prevent rotatory displacement.

Not infrequently, reduction may be obtained after traction but may be lost as the traction is decreased. In this situation, the options include adding external fixation following reduction, closed reduction percutaneous pin fixation, and open reduction internal fixation. My preference in the athlete, because of the generally good bone stock, is for closed reduction and percutaneous pin fixation under fluoroscopic control (Figs. 15-12, 15-13, and 15-14). Two AO threaded-tip pins are drilled with power from the lateral aspect of the deltoid insertion proximally into the humeral head. Another pin originates superiorly in the greater tuberosity and extends inferiorly to the shaft, adding further fixation and minimizing the potential for rotatory displacement, which may exist if a single pin is utilized (Fig. 15-15). However the technique of closed reduction and percutaneous pin fixation is achieved, there is potential for rotatory or angular malunion, pin tractinfection, and migration of smooth pins. Use of a cannulated screw may offer the same advantages of percutaneous fixation without some of the problems inherent in utilizing K wires. When the fracture has adequately healed, the pins are removed and motion is initiated.

Open reduction and internal fixation offers the advantages of precise restoration of anatomy and the ability to provide stable enough internal fixation so that early motion may be begun more aggressively,

minimizing potential for motion-impeding fracture healing. The most common indications for open reduction internal fixation in the athlete include multiple trauma, an irreducible neck fracture, a fracture that is reducible but unable to be held, or a patient whose age, level of compliance, bone quality, or medical condition precludes the use of closed reduction and percutaneous pin fixation.

Many methods have been described for open reduction internal fixation of surgical neck fractures, including intramedullary rods and intramedullary nails, tension bands, plates, screws, staples, wire, and combinations of these. Whatever the type of fixation used, the goal of open reduction internal fixation is to provide the athlete with stable enough internal fixation to allow early rehabilitation to begin without fracture displacement. The methods currently most popular for open reduction internal fixation have been tension band, intramedullary rod fixation, or side plate and screws. In most young athletes, a side plate and screws may be quite a good option; however, many patients with this fracture have some element of osteopenic bone, and it may be difficult to obtain secure internal fixation with a plate and screws. In addition, if a plate and screws is selected, care must be taken not to excessively strip soft tissue during the surgical approach, as this may interfere with the ascending branch of the anterior humeral circumflex vessel, contributing to the environment that may exist for development of late avascular necrosis.

SHOULDER FRACTURES

My preference for operative treatment of shoulder fractures is to utilize a tension band for dynamic compression of the fracture, with or without the additional translational stability provided with intramedullary fixation. For the tension band, a heavy nonabsorbable (No. 5 Tevdek) suture or wire is utilized (Fig. 15-16). While there have been many kinds of intramedullary devices, the two most common are Rush rods or Ender's nails, either of which may be modified with a proximal hole, through which a heavy suture may be passed to augment fixation.

For the surgical technique, the athlete is in a beach chair position near the side of the operating table, to permit arm extension off the operating table so an intramedullary rod may be passed antegrade. The surgical approach is via a long deltopectoral incision (in those patients in whom intramedullary fixation alone might be considered, a deltoid splint may be adequate). A 14- or 16-gauge spinal needle or angiocath may be helpful to pass the suture through the rotator cuff and tuberosity. Care is taken not to extensively strip the soft tissue and periosteum, particularly in the region of the biceps and rotator cuff insertion, thus avoiding injury to the anterior humeral circumflex vessels and arcuate artery, which

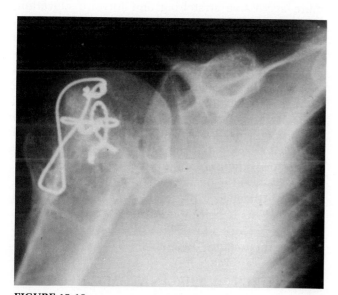

FIGURE 15-16
A two-part displacement is usually adequately fixed with a tension band from the cuff-tuberosity junction to the shaft of the humerus. Either heavy nonabsorbable suture or wire is useful for fixation.

supplies the bulk of the vascularity to the humeral head. Once the fracture is exposed, any soft tissue interposed between fracture fragments is removed. Since this is most frequently the biceps tendon, the biceps may be located medial to the pectoralis major insertion and traced proximally to its position between the fracture fragments. Anterior capsule, anterior cuff tissue, or deltoid fascia may also be interposed between the fracture fragments. Once all soft tissue is removed, the fracture fragments are realigned and plan for fixation is made.

In the young athlete, there is ordinarily satisfactory enough bone quality and thick enough rotator cuff tendon so that secure internal fixation can be obtained with tension band technique alone, without the addition of intramedullary fixation. If the tension band is to be utilized alone, once the soft tissue is removed from the fracture and the fracture site cleared of fibers or clot, two drill holes are made in the greater tuberosity. A heavy nonabsorbable suture is passed through one of the greater tuberosity drill holes, through the supraspinatus at the juncture of the tendon and greater tuberosity, and then back through the second drill hole in the tuberosity. Likewise, drill holes are made in the humeral shaft, an equal distance from the fracture site as the drill holes in the tuberosity, and the suture is crisscrossed before being passed through the drill holes in the shaft of the humerus. A second heavy nonabsorbable suture is added in the same fashion, securing shaft and tuberosity head fragments. The fracture is reduced and the heavy sutures are tightened and tied, effecting compression at the fracture site. If the tension band technique is to be utilized alone without intramedullary fixation, the arm is carefully brought into forward elevation and rotated internally and externally to make certain that satisfactory stability of the fracture is present to permit early range of motion (Fig. 15-17).

An alternate method of fixing this fracture has been described, in which Rush rods or Ender's nails have been modified to contain a superior hole through which the tension band sutures are passed. Putting the suture through the superior holes in the rod permits deeper placement of the rod in the cortical bone of the proximal humerus than would ordinarily be permitted if the rod were to be placed over the suture utilized for the tension band. If this technique is utilized, two drill holes are placed for the rods at the juncture between the articular surface of the humeral head and the greater tuberosity. The rotator cuff is not detached from the head. Utilizing A-O or Deschamp suture pass, the nonabsorbable No. 5 suture is passed down one entry point and out

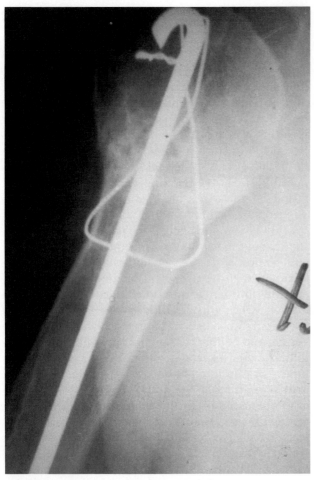

FIGURE 15-17
An intramedullary rod (in this case, a Rush rod) can be added for additional translational stability.

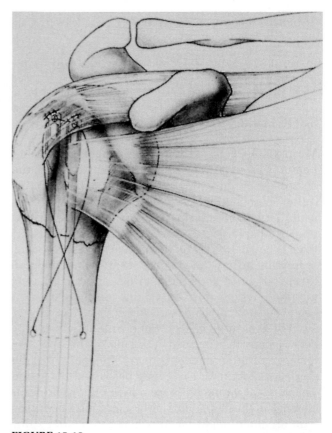

FIGURE 15-18
Technique for open reduction internal fixation of a displaced surgical neck fracture. A Rush rod or Ender's rod may be modified with a proximal hole through which the tension band may be threaded. This allows the rod to be buried farther within the humerus than would ordinarily be possible, minimizing late hardware prominence that may necessitate rod removal.

another. Each end is then passed through a superior drill hole in each one of two intramedullary rods. The rods are then placed in the drill holes that have been made for them and then passed distally across the fracture site. Each end of the protruding sutures is then crisscrossed, and passed through drill holes in the humeral shaft an equal distance from the fracture as the entry point of the rods. A second set of sutures can also be passed in the second hole of the rod to augment the fracture fixation. Once the rods are passed distal to the fracture, the fracture is reduced, the rods passed to the greatest depth possible, and then the tension band tied over the lateral aspect of the fracture site (Fig. 15-18). This fixation is usually secure enough to permit early range of motion, but the fracture stability must be tested in the position of elevation and internal and external rotation. The wound is closed over a drain, a sling and swath is applied, and early motion is permitted, depending on the degree of security of fracture fixation. Union usually occurs within 6 weeks, and the exercise program can be advanced to more active exercises and

more aggressive stretching and forward elevation, external rotation, and internal rotation. Because this fracture does not involve disruption of tuberosities and rotator cuff, quite rapid progression of active exercises can be permitted.

While late sequelae of this fracture may include stiffness, malunion, or nonunion, avascular necrosis typically does not occur, since the blood supply to the humeral head is maintained through the intact tuberosity segments. The most common complication of this fracture, nonunion of the surgical neck, more commonly occurs when nonoperative treatment is utilized as initial management of a displaced fracture. This is particularly true if a hanging cast is employed, since the weight of the cast may act to distract the fracture fragments.

FRACTURES OF THE ANATOMIC NECK

These fractures are extremely rare, so there is little long-term experience to guide us in the ideal way to manage them. Nevertheless, because of their location, there are numerous challenges and difficult treatment decisions. This fracture may initially be difficult to recognize if it is not displaced. It is not infrequently associated with fractures of one or more tuberosities. The location of the fracture line at the anatomic neck is such that the blood supply to the humeral head is disrupted, and the risk of late avascular necrosis is quite high. In addition, because of lack of soft tissue attachment to the articular surface to help control the segment, because the head segment is usually quite small, and because it is frequently angulated or rotated within the shoulder capsule, closed reduction of this fracture is usually impossible.

In the young athletically active patient, despite the risk of avascular necrosis, it is worthwhile to attempt an open reduction and internal fixation. It is, however, important to treat this fracture promptly by whatever means utilized, since delay in reduction probably contributes to the likelihood of late avascular necrosis (Figs. 15-19 to 15-23).

The usual surgical approach to this fracture is through a long deltopectoral incision. The coracoid muscles are retracted without osteotomy of the coracoid process. Entrance to the joint is via division of the subscapularis and the interior capsule, approxi-

mately 1 cm from the insertion of the lesser tuberosity. Medially extending the incision along the rotator interval will permit retraction of the subscapularis muscle and permit full inspection of the joint. Loose debris is removed and the fracture pattern and extent of the damage to the humeral head are analyzed. If the humeral head articular surface is in good condition, full external rotation makes the donor site of this fracture fully visible and an attempt may be made to reattach the displaced humeral head to the intact tuberosity shaft segment. Fixation may be considered with either a screw, Steinmann pin, or Kirschner wire, from the greater and lesser tuberosity into the head. The purchase on the humeral head segment is often difficult, as the humeral head is typically a very small fragment. Once fixed, the humeral head should be examined by full external rotation of the humerus to ensure that articular penetration has not occurred. If pin fixation is utilized, the pins may be removed at approximately 6 to 8 weeks postoperatively. If the screws are utilized, they are best left in place unless the head begins to fragment or collapse or there is evidence of screw penetration in the articular cartilage. It must be remembered that follow-up x-rays of this fracture are critical. Onset of avascular necrosis may be delayed. If avascular ne-

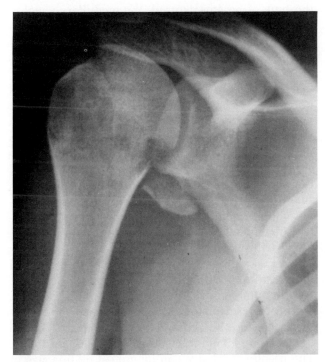

FIGURE 15-19
Anatomic neck fracture in a 15-year-old. This fracture line was initially overlooked because of the displaced lesser tuberosity, metaphyseal, and articular surface piece.

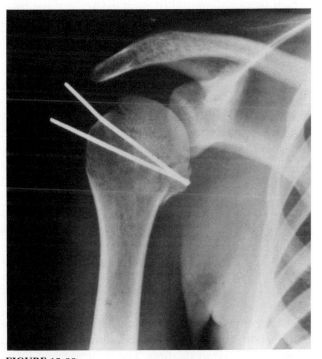

FIGURE 15-20
An open reduction internal fixation of the medial metaphyseal lesser tuberosity segment appears anatomic.

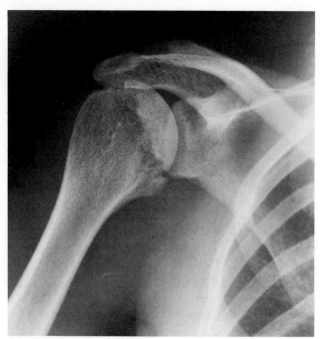

FIGURE 15-21
Four months later, while there is healing of the fracture site, it is clear that there has been a fracture through the anatomic neck, with probable nonunion. The vascularity of the head segment is in question.

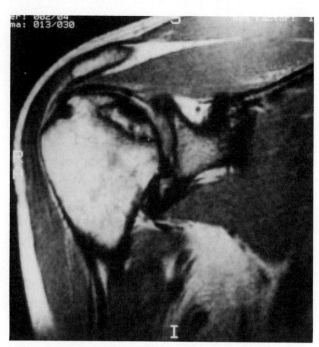

FIGURE 15-22
An MRI scan of the patient, indicating avascular necrosis of the humeral head.

crosis develops and if it is associated with collapse of the humeral head or hardware penetration into the humeral head articular cartilage, then wear on the glenoid can also occur, often leading to subsequent destruction of the glenoid, necessitating resurfacing of that structure as well.

If tenuous internal fixation exists, or if the head is fragmented or comminuted, even if this occurs in an athlete, it is probably better to proceed with primary prosthetic arthroplasty. Certainly, in older patients or recreational athletes, because of the high incidence of avascular necrosis in this fracture, primary prosthetic arthroplasty is probably a better initial choice of treatment. This bypasses the potential problems caused by collapse of the humeral head, internal fixation penetration, and severe scarring around the shoulder girdle that may compromise a late prosthetic arthroplasty. Because the tuberosities and rotator cuff are not interfered with in this fracture, and only the subscapularis is divided for entry into the joint, rapid and aggressive rehabilitation, consisting initially of range of motion and then proceeding to strengthening exercises, can be initiated in 24 h of surgery, thus minimizing the potential for stiffness, weakness, and delay in return to the athlete's sport.

If primary prosthetic arthroplasty is chosen, the surgical approach is similar to that utilized for open reduction internal fixation. The deltopectoral interval is entered, without detachment of either the pec-

toralis tendon or the deltoid origin or insertion. The coracoid muscles are retracted, and the joint entered by a direct incision through the subscapularis. The humeral head segment is removed, the joint is irrigated, and the glenoid is examined. Depending on the type of prosthesis used, the medullary canal of the humerus is reamed and prepared, and a trial implant is seated. Correct sizing of the implant depends on the humeral prosthetic system utilized. There is ordinarily a variability of stem thicknesses, stem length, and humeral head sizes. Both modular and nonmodular systems can be utilized for the humeral head, and both cemented and uncemented stems can be decided upon. In general, whatever the system utilized, the top of the humeral head should be positioned relative to the tuberosity, so that the top of the prosthesis protrudes approximately 2 to 3 mm superior to the top of the greater tuberosity. Likewise, the version of the humeral head should be approximately 40 to 45° of retroversion. With most humeral arthroplasty systems, the fin of the prosthesis can act as a guide to the amount of retroversion of the prosthesis. With the fin just lateral (posterior) to the bicipital groove, the prosthetic head will be placed in retroversion. In most instances, the prosthesis can be utilized without cement, and in the younger patient or athlete, this is probably desirable. The precise head size can be judged by this size of the head fragment, which has been removed. If this is not possible, owing to extreme comminution or

196

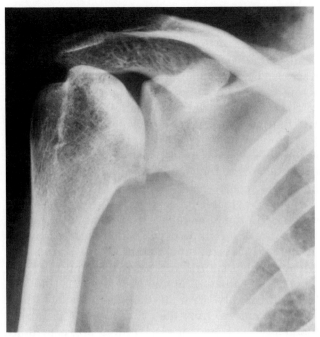

FIGURE 15-23
Two years later, there is collapse and deformity of the humeral head. The patient required arthroplasty of the shoulder at age 16.

the difficulty with measurement, the largest head size that will ensure both stability of the implant and ability to close the rotator cuff around it should be employed. Once the prosthesis has been inserted, the subscapularis is then closed anatomically to the point of its division, and the wound is closed in layers over a drain. Range of motion is generally begun within the first 24 h after surgery, and the only muscle requiring protection is the subscapularis. It is thus usually possible to begin isometric exercises at 2 to 3 weeks postoperatively and progressive resistive exercises once the subscapularis has healed. Active internal rotation is avoided for 10 to 12 weeks. It is particularly important to protect the repaired subscapularis in the throwing athlete. Return to throwing sports is not permitted until range of motion is near normal, strength in both internal and external rotation is near normal, and endurance of the cuff is tested and found to be satisfactory.

FRACTURES INVOLVING
THE TUBEROSITIES

Fractures involving the tuberosities in athletes are among the most problematic. The tuberosities serve as attachment sites for the rotator cuff, and thus fractures involving these tuberosities are invariably associated with damage to the cuff tendons as an integral part of the injury. Tuberosity fractures may occur

in isolation or as part of more complex three- and four-part fractures. They not infrequently are associated with dislocations of the head and shaft of the humerus. Finally, small degrees of tuberosity displacement, because they must move with the attached rotator cuff in the relatively small confines of the subacromial space, may have a great impact on the athlete's ability to return to sport. Because of this, the usual 1 cm displacement criterion in the Neer classification for closed vs. open reduction treatment probably should be reassessed in the athlete who has a tuberosity fracture. This is particularly true if the fracture involves the greater tuberosity, as a small amount of superior displacement may lead to considerable disability from impingement of the rotator cuff. Because this type of impingement, secondary to tuberosity displacement, does not involve primarily any abnormality of the bony acromion or acromioclavicular joint, it has been termed nonoutlet, or secondary, impingement. However, the effect on the athlete in terms of pain symptoms and rotator cuff dysfunction is the same. Because of this nonoutlet impingement, late bony procedures aimed at enlarging the subacromial space, such as an anterior acromioplasty, are usually unsuccessful without anatomically repositioning the greater tuberosity to its original position. Because of late problems associated with malunion or nonunion of displaced tuberosity fractures, I favor aggressive restoration of anatomy in the athletic population.

ISOLATED LESSER
TUBEROSITY FRACTURES

If the lesser tuberosity fracture is minimally displaced, it may be treated as with all nondisplaced fractures (Fig. 15-24). However, if displacement occurs, it is the pull of the subscapularis that is the deforming force and thus responsible for final lesser tuberosity position. The displacement produced by the subscapularis must thus be considered, whether for closed or open reduction of this fracture. Because this fracture involves neither the surgical neck of the humerus nor the greater tuberosity, significant interruption of the blood supply to the humeral head does not occur, and avascular necrosis is not a problem with an isolated lesser tuberosity fracture.

Lesser tuberosity displacement occurs both with and without dislocation of the humeral head. If humeral head dislocation accompanies an isolated lesser tuberosity fracture, it is most frequently a posterior dislocation. Isolated lesser tuberosity fractures without dislocations are unusual and result from bony avulsion by the subscapularis tendon. The size of the fragment is highly variable and may include a

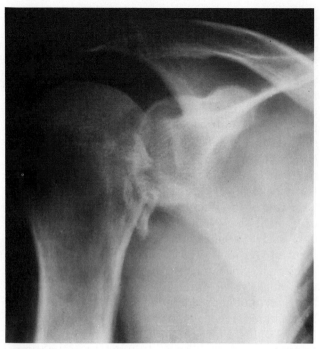

FIGURE 15-24
If the lesser tuberosity fraction is isolated and near anatomic, little residual deformity or dysfunction exists. However, many of these are associated with a posterior dislocation.

segment of the articular surface. The displaced fracture fragment may be confused with calcific tendinitis of the subscapularis. Unlike the greater tuberosity fracture, the displacement of which may cause significant problems in the subacromial space, the displacement of the lesser tuberosity is medial and does not ordinarily affect use of the arm in the abduction or elevated position. However, if the fragment is large or is severely displaced, it may block or interfere with internal rotation, and this certainly may be a problem in the overhead athlete.

Treatment of an isolated lesser tuberosity fracture in the athlete depends upon many factors, including arm dominance, type of sport, and individual goals and demands. If the displacement is minimal, the arm can be immobilized in internal rotation, as the surrounding soft tissue attachments of the subscapularis to the rest of the cuff and shaft ordinarily permit the fragment to be well approximated with the arm in internal rotation. A sling may be utilized for comfort, with rapid progression of exercises as the level of comfort improves.

If the fragment is large, if it is significantly displaced, or if it is the dominant arm in a throwing or overhead athlete, strong consideration should be given for operative restoration of the lesser tuberosity fragment. The surgical approach is via deltopectoral incision, leaving the coracoid muscles attached to the coracoid process and without detachment of the coracoid process. Care is taken to minimize the

extent of dissection in this anterior surgical approach, as disruption of the arcuate artery branch may compromise the vascular supply of the humeral head. Of the several types of fixation utilized for this fracture, heavy nonabsorbable suture or use of a screw and washer have been the most popular. If the fragment is comminuted or small, it may be excised, and the subscapularis and capsule directly repaired to the tuberosity donor site. If it is large, a heavy nonabsorbable suture is used to anatomically replace the lesser tuberosity fragment to the donor site. Two drill holes are made from the donor site to emerge through the greater tuberosity, and two drill holes are made in the humeral shaft adjacent to the donor site of the lesser tuberosity. An angiocath may be used to pass sutures through these holes. Four heavy nonabsorbable sutures are passed around the fragment at the juncture of the subscapularis and the lesser tuberosity. Two of these sutures are then passed to emerge from the drill holes in the greater tuberosity, and two of the sutures are passed to emerge from the drill holes in the humeral shaft. The lesser tuberosity segment, once repaired anatomically, is fixed to the greater tuberosity, bicipital groove area, and the shaft of the humerus. Prior to fixation of the lesser tuberosity segment, the omnipresent rent in the rotator interval is closed with nonabsorbable suture, as this takes tension off the

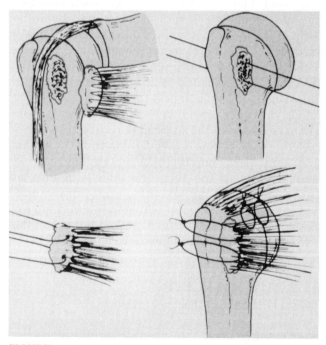

FIGURE 15-25
With significant displacement of an isolated lesser tuberosity fracture, open reduction and internal fixation is wise. A heavy nonabsorbable suture from the displaced segment emerging through the area of the greater tuberosity is passed. Early closure of the rotator interval defect takes tension off the lesser tuberosity, making repair less troublesome.

198

lesser tuberosity segment and makes the repair easier (Fig. 15-25). Early range of motion is initiated, but resistive exercises are not permitted until radiographic signs of healing of the fracture site are evident.

LESSER TUBEROSITY FRACTURE DISLOCATIONS

Lesser tuberosity fractures associated with posterior dislocations of the humeral head are more common than isolated lesser tuberosity avulsion fractures. Because these usually involve more severe trauma and more significant displacement, nerve injuries may accompany these fracture dislocations. In addition, these fractures are not infrequently associated with minimally or nondisplaced surgical neck fractures, which may complicate attempts at closed reduction. As with all posterior dislocations, the lesser tuberosity fracture dislocation may be missed by the initial examiner unless high-quality x-rays are obtained at the time of injury. Because of the potential for associated nerve injuries, careful clinical neurovascular checks should be performed on the patient. In addition, high-quality imaging studies are particularly helpful. A CT scan not only identifies precisely the position of the lesser tuberosity but can identify the extent of the impression defect in the humeral head and any associated glenoid fractures that may have occurred at the time of the dislocation.

Reduction of the humeral head dislocation can usually be successfully accomplished closed, if the patient is seen within the first 2 weeks of injury. Under general anesthesia or regional block, the arm is brought into forward flexion and slight adduction and traction. Gentle pressure is applied from posterior to anterior to relocate the humeral head back into the glenoid fossa. However, once the humeral head is relocated, closed treatment of the lesser tuberosity fracture may be somewhat difficult. As with isolated lesser tuberosity fractures, the lesser tuberosity fragment is better apposed with the arm in internal rotation. On the other hand, as with most posterior dislocations, there may be associated posterior capsular disruption, which is usually treated most effectively with the arm in slight external rotation. Thus my preference is to immobilize the arm in approximately 10 to 20° of external rotation after relocation of the humeral head. In this position, the lesser tuberosity fragment can be radiographically evaluated to determine its precise position. If it is reasonably apposed to the head and shaft, it may be

left alone. If it is significantly displaced with the arm in external rotation, it should be treated like any displaced isolated lesser tuberosity fracture, with open reduction and internal fixation, depending on the age of the patient, the size of the fragment, the amount of articular surface involved, or the particular needs or desires of the athlete.

A more difficult treatment challenge occurs when the lesser tuberosity fracture dislocation is associated with a minimally displaced or nondisplaced fracture of the surgical neck. In this athlete, closed reduction by adducting the arm across the chest may displace the neck fracture, thus turning a two-part fracture dislocation into a more complicated three-part fracture. If lesser tuberosity fracture dislocation is accompanied by a surgical neck fracture, it is probably wisest to do an immediate open relocation of the humeral head. This is done by a deltopectoral approach. Several sutures are placed around the lesser tuberosity and subscapularis and these can be retracted. The humeral head is usually easily disengaged from its locked position posterior to the glenoid by placing a blunt retractor between the humeral head and the glenoid and by gently levering the humeral head off the posterior glenoid rim. After relocation of the humeral head in external rotation, the lesser tuberosity segment and the attached subscapularis can be anatomically repaired via heavy nonabsorbable sutures.

GREATER TUBEROSITY FRACTURES AND FRACTURE DISLOCATIONS

Isolated fractures involving the greater tuberosity are not uncommon and in fact occur with such frequency in the skiing population that they have been termed the "skier's fracture." With an isolated fracture of the greater tuberosity, the blood supply to the humeral head via the anterior humeral circumflex vessels and soft tissue attachments remains quite good, and avascular necrosis does not occur. The extent of displacement, position of displacement, and size of the bone fragment are all highly variable. The fracture is also highly variable in its presentation, as greater tuberosity fractures may occur with or without dislocations. Because the supraspinatus, infraspinatus, and teres minor insert on the greater tuberosity, this fracture is invariably associated with injury and disruption of the rotator cuff. To a variable degree, any or all of the individual facets for cuff insertion may be involved in this fracture, making the amount of bone seen radiographically highly variable. The fragments may be displaced not at all, to a minimal degree, or to a marked degree, and variable degrees of comminution may exist. When seen with a shoulder dislocation, the humeral head and shaft are dislocated anteriorly (Fig. 15-26). In a young and athletic patient, these may or may not be associated with a Bankart lesion and may lead to some of the same problems of instability recurrence that can occur in any athletic population. Late untoward sequelae of this fracture are frequent and problematic and depend on the adequacy of the restoration of the anatomy and the successful treatment of associated soft tissue injury to the rotator cuff. Because of the associated problems caused by persistent displacement of the greater tuberosity segment within the confines of the subacromial space, an argument can certainly be made for aggressively restoring the precise anatomy of this fracture. It is probable that with this fracture, above all others, the "1 cm displacement" rule, as a general guide for closed vs. open reduction of this fracture, may not be applicable. Lesser degrees of displacement are often associated with marked impairment of function, particularly in the young, athletic individual who requires normal flexibility, range of motion, and strength.

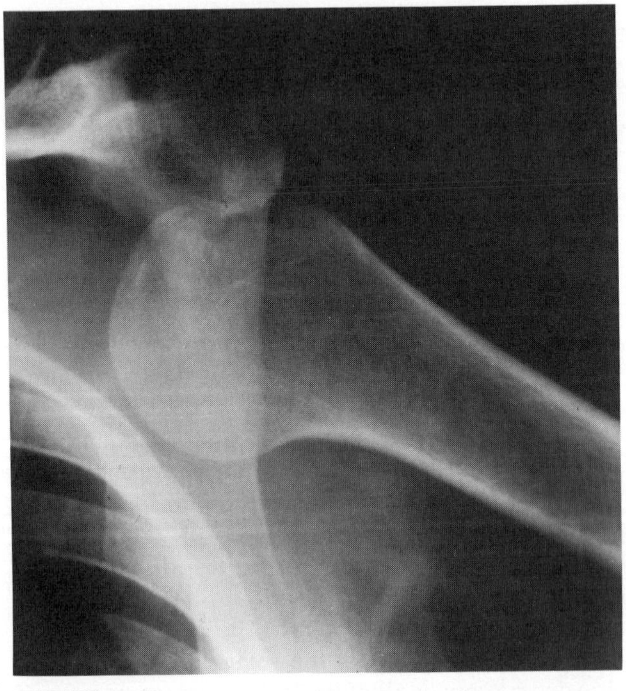

ISOLATED GREATER TUBEROSITY FRACTURES WITHOUT DISLOCATION

A displaced fracture may present in a highly variable fashion. Variations in size and location produce variation in radiographic appearance. For instance, a small greater tuberosity fragment in the subacromial space may be confused with calcific tendinitis (Fig. 15-27). In addition, a relatively small avulsion fragment of the greater tuberosity may be associated with a much more severe rotator cuff tear than would be inferred by the size of the greater tuberosity fragment alone.

The two most common locations of the displaced tuberosity segment are superior and posterior. The superior displacement is produced predominantly by the pull of the supraspinatus and infraspinatus tendons and may be seen above the humeral head in the subacromial space. Failure to correct this distortion of the subacromial space anatomy caused by this displaced tuberosity invariably leads to limitations in elevation and abduction and a me-

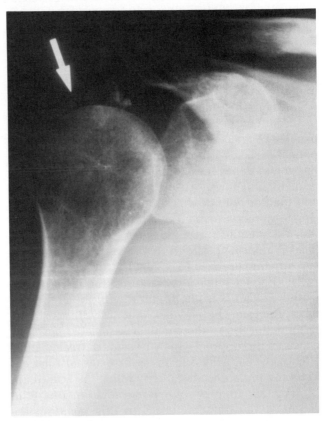

FIGURE 15-26
A two-part anterior fracture dislocation. The greater tuberosity is left behind in the glenoid fossa. Relocation of the humeral head often repositions the tuberosity in its anatomic position.

FIGURE 15-27
Displacement of the greater tuberosity in the subacromial space, particularly if the bone is somewhat osteopenic, may mimic soft tissue calcification in the rotator cuff and confuse the clinician.

chanical block to these motions by the fracture fragment. Pain and weakness occur because of the abnormal position of the tuberosity and cuff. If the position of the fracture fragment appears to be predominantly posterior, it is the pull of the teres minor and infraspinatus that is the main deforming force (Fig. 15-28). The precise degree of posterior displacement of the fracture may be difficult to judge on plain radiographs, and there is a clear-cut role for CT scan to demonstrate not only the precise position of the fracture fragment but also its distance from the donor site.

An isolated greater tuberosity fracture without displacement may be treated like all fractures without displacement. If there is displacement of the greater tuberosity segment, the clinician should carefully assess the position and degree of displacement and attempt to determine the impact of that fixed amount of tuberosity displacement on the individual athlete. There is little argument that significant displacement of the greater tuberosity superiorly or posteriorly cannot be accepted (Fig. 15-29). However, occasionally the tuberosity segment will appear to be an "open-book" type of fracture, with a gapping of the anterior cortex of the greater tuberosity and no gap of the posterior cortex of the greater tuberosity. Since this results in neither superior displacement with subsequent late impingement nor posterior displacement with its subsequent block to external rotation, the "open-book" type of fracture can usually be treated nonoperatively.

Small degrees of posterior displacement of the tuberosity are probably better tolerated than small degrees of superior displacement (Fig. 15-30). Because of the limited space under the coracoacromial arch, any superior displacement more than 3 to 5 mm should probably be considered for open reduction and anatomic relocation of the greater tuberosity to its donor site. As when this fracture is operatively treated acutely, it is usually not difficult to restore anatomy and may be done through a small deltoid split incision. Some surgeons have advocated treating the displaced greater tuberosity segment closed, requiring maintenance of the arm in the awkward position of either abduction or external rotation, which rarely results in anatomic repositioning of the tuberosity segment. Some have suggested applica-

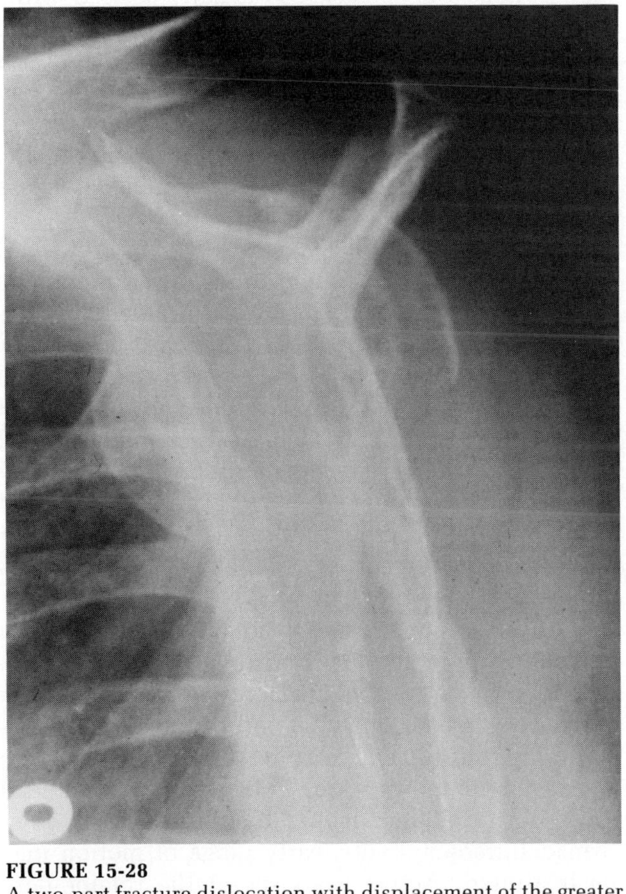

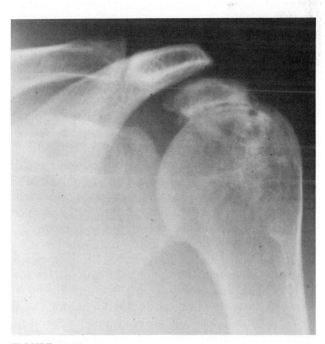

FIGURE 15-28
A two-part fracture dislocation with displacement of the greater tuberosity. The position of the greater tuberosity is determined by the pull of the rotator cuff and is often posterior to the humeral head.

FIGURE 15-29
If the greater tuberosity is pulled superiorly and heals in that position, there is limitation of motion and diminished function because of the mechanical block in the subacromial space and the shortened position of the rotator cuff.

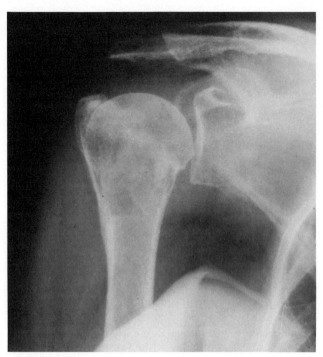

FIGURE 15-30
An AP view of the shoulder gives little information about the extent of posterior displacement of the greater tuberosity. While mild degrees of posterior displacement may be well tolerated, superior displacement compromises the subacromial area and may markedly interfere with function in the overhead athlete. Near anatomic restoration of a displaced greater tuberosity is prudent, as late probable secondary malunions are inadequately handled by an acromioplasty alone.

tion of an external fixator to manipulate the greater tuberosity segment into place and hold the position. However, while this may be possible, it is not infrequent that these methods of closed reduction often lead to compromise in the anatomic position of the greater tuberosity, a problem in the overhead athlete. Displaced greater tuberosity fractures have been known to displace late, and x-rays should be checked at intervals to make certain that delayed displacement has not occurred.

In my opinion, greater tuberosity fractures should be aggressively treated in the overhead athlete with anatomic restoration. If the fracture is to be treated operatively, the surgical approach is via an anterior or anterosuperior surgical approach, with a split in the deltoid muscle, taking care not to split the deltoid farther than 5 cm for fear of injury to the terminal branches of the axillary nerve. Blunt retractors may be placed beneath the deltoid, giving exposure of the hemorrhagic bursa and fracture fragments. Clot should be cleared out of the donor site, the fibrinous and hemorrhagic material removed, and the fragment identified. There is invariably a tear in the rotator cuff associated with this fracture. If the fracture fragment of bone involves predominantly the facet for the supraspinatus insertion, the tear in the

cuff is usually in the rotator interval between the supraspinatus and subscapularis. If the fragment of bone involves the facets of infraspinatus or teres minor, the more posterior facets than that for the supraspinatus, the soft tissue component of the injury is usually tendinous disruption of the supraspinatus as well as a rent in the rotator interval. The pattern, location, and type of tear in the rotator cuff associated with the fracture displacement must be carefully analyzed in order to plan an anatomic repair.

In most instances, the greater tuberosity piece may be anatomically reduced to its donor site and fixed well with either nonabsorbable suture or screw (with or without washer). If heavy nonabsorbable (No. 5 Tevdek) suture is to be utilized, drill holes are made in the greater tuberosity, if this is a solid piece of bone. Concomitant drill holes are also made in the bicipital groove lesser tuberosity area and in the shaft of the humerus, so the greater tuberosity fragment can be anatomically restored and fixed, both to the shaft of the humerus and to the lesser tuberosity–bicipital groove piece. If there is any question about the adequacy of the greater tuberosity piece, the nonabsorbable suture can be passed at the juncture of the rotator cuff and greater tuberosity, and the tuberosity manipulated into place. It is usually easiest, while putting traction on the greater tuberosity segment, to repair the rent in the rotator interval or rotator cuff before putting the greater tuberosity back to its anatomic position, as closing the rotator cuff at the rotator interval takes tension off the fracture site, making anatomic restoration of the tuberosity less troublesome.

If the surgeon elects to utilize a screw and washer, it is wiser to angle the screw through the greater tuberosity, aiming it in an inframedial direction so it can engage the medial cortex of the humerus. This gives more secure purchase of the greater tuberosity piece than if the screw is directed up into the cancellous bone of the humeral head, and also minimizes the risk of penetration of the humeral head with hardware. It has, however, been reported that a prominent screw in the area of the greater tuberosity may lead to late problems in the subacromial space, requiring hardware removal.

Addition of an anterior acromioplasty, while a consideration in an older person, is usually not necessary in the young athlete. However, sacrifice of the coracoacromial ligament as part of the surgical procedure is routine. Once the fracture has been fixed, the arm is immobilized in a sling and swath, and if the security of the fracture fixation has been confirmed intraoperatively, early range of motion may be instituted. Active exercises of the rotator cuff, however, should be avoided until there is radiographic union of the greater tuberosity.

GREATER TUBEROSITY FRACTURES WITH DISLOCATION

Greater tuberosity fractures in association with anterior dislocations occur more frequently than fractures occurring without dislocation. As with most anterior dislocations, two-part greater tuberosity fracture dislocations are not uncommonly associated with nerve injuries, particularly involving the axillary and musculocutaneous nerves, and nerve function must be tested in any athlete, both before and after relocation of the humeral head. When this fracture accompanies a glenohumeral dislocation, the position of the fracture fragment is variable. In some instances it may appear to "be left behind" as the humeral head dislocates anteriorly, implying a significant soft tissue disruption and rent in the rotator interval (Fig. 15-31). In addition, the periosteal soft tissue envelope is usually disrupted, making this fragment extremely unstable and contributing to the potential for displacement as the humeral head is relocated. Alternatively, there may be a small fragment of the greater tuberosity that seems to accompany the humeral head as it dislocates. This is a deceptive injury and may signify a more significant tear of the rotator cuff, with the insertion of the cuff simply avulsing a small fragment of teres minor facet as the humeral head dislocates.

In many instances, closed reduction of the humeral head results in adequate restoration of the greater tuberosity to its anatomic position. If so, the tuberosity may be treated as with any nondisplaced fracture. The mechanism of reduction is as with any anterior dislocation, with traction and countertraction, followed by maintenance in some internal rotation. If the greater tuberosity is displaced posteriorly or superiorly following reduction, consideration should be given for operative restoration of the greater tuberosity segment to its anatomic position.

Once the shoulder has been relocated, if the greater tuberosity position is anatomic, recurrent dislocation or residual symptoms of instability are unusual. However, when these fractures occur in young athletes, they may be accompanied by a Bankart lesion. While historically recurrence is unusual, if dislocation occurs with a greater tuberosity fracture and if operative restoration of the greater tuberosity segment is considered in the young athlete, the anterior glenoid labrum complex can be inspected through the rent in the rotator interval by putting traction on the humeral head and retracting the greater tuberosity segment posteriorly. If a Bankart lesion is indeed seen incidentally at that time, consideration should be given to suturing this Bankart lesion at the time of greater tuberosity fixation.

I have found it possible to place one or two sutures through this Bankart lesion via the exposure obtained through the rent in the rotator interval without the need for subscapularis division, as is ordinarily necessary for a Bankart repair.

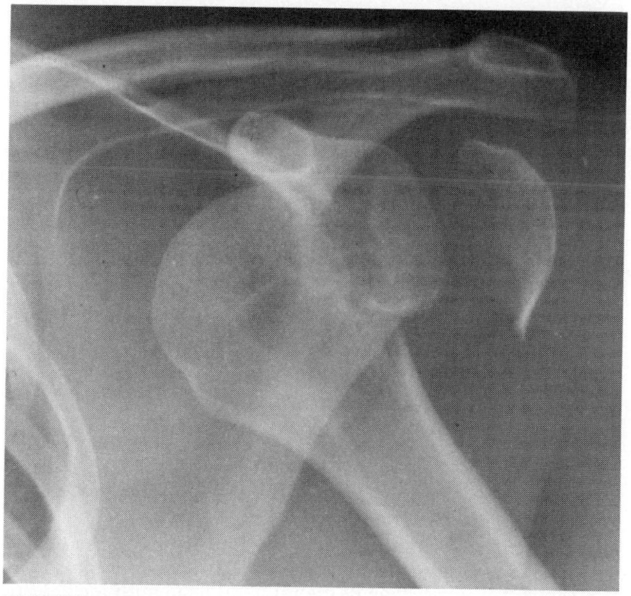

FIGURE 15-31
A two-part greater tuberosity fracture dislocation, with a large greater tuberosity segment.

LATE SEQUELAE OF UNREDUCED GREATER TUBEROSITY

There are approximately 4 to 5 mm of space between the superior surface of the supraspinatus and the coracoacromial arch as the arm is elevated overhead. Displacement of the greater tuberosity via fracture can significantly alter the position of the cuff and tuberosity so that the relationship between the coracoacromial arch and cuff is dramatically altered. With significant superior displacement, abduction of the arm both actively and passively is limited by impingement of the superiorly displaced greater tuberosity. The clinical hallmark of a superior malunion of the greater tuberosity is inability to externally rotate when the arm is in the abducted position, as the greater tuberosity mechanically blocks motion in this position.

The pain and disability produced by an ununited or malunited greater tuberosity cannot be adequately addressed by a bony decompression of the acromion, and restoration of the normal greater tuberosity relationship and length of the rotator cuff is necessary. If the greater tuberosity has been retracted for a lengthy period of time, restoration of its original position is technically difficult and requires extensive capsular releases, mobilization of the greater tuberosity piece and attached supraspinatus, preparation of a bed for the greater tuberosity segment, and secure internal fixation of the piece. Indeed, the difference between the technical ease of acutely restoring the anatomy in this fracture with the difficulty of doing a late reconstruction to reposition the tuberosity is such that these fractures are best treated aggressively acutely.

Malunion of the greater tuberosity retracted posteriorly is even more technically difficult and challenging (Figs. 15-32 and 15-33). The retracted external rotators shorten and scar to the posterior capsule. The tuberosity piece frequently heals via callus to the posterior humeral shaft and even may heal to the posterior rim of glenoid itself. Clinical presentation of this includes marked external rotation weakness. As the arm is externally rotated, there is a mechanical block to external rotation produced by the greater tuberosity, which may mechanically lever the humeral head out of the glenoid, causing the unusual

symptom complex. If the injury has been associated with a previous anterior dislocation, significant posterior malunion can begin to lever the humeral head out, causing the unusual symptom complex of sense of anterior instability with mechanical limitation of external rotation as the humeral head is levered out of the socket.

Late treatment for a posterior malunion of the greater tuberosity usually consists of extensive lysis of intraarticular and extraarticular adhesions and a great deal of difficulty in mobilization and repositioning of the greater tuberosity segment (Figs. 15-34 and 15-35). This segment usually needs to be osteotomized and carefully separated from the associated callus, taking care to protect the axillary nerve adjacent to the inferior capsule. In addition, extensive posterior and superior capsular releases are ordinarily needed for mobilization of the piece and attached rotator cuff, which may be in a fixed and shortened position. Preparation of the donor site is necessary, but the precise position of the tuberosity on the donor site may be difficult to determine if treatment is delayed. External rotation of the arm may be necessary to adequately position the greater tuberosity segment back to its anatomic position. As noted previously, this injury may be accompanied by the pres-

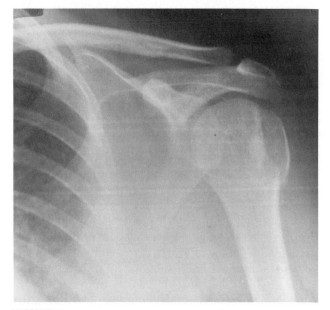

FIGURE 15-32
An AP x-ray following reduction. While the greater tuberosity appears to be satisfactory from a superior-inferior position, it is difficult to tell the extent of posterior displacement. There is a suggestion of a residual donor deficit and nonanatomic position of the greater tuberosity.

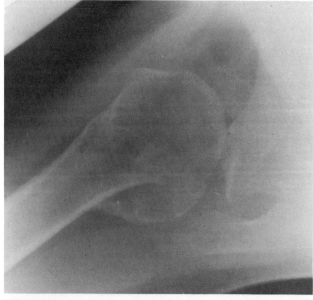

FIGURE 15-33
The axillary view shows that the greater tuberosity has healed with marked posterior displacement. External rotation of the arm can result in levering of the humeral head anteriorly, leading to residual or recurrent instability. Osteotomy to reposition the greater tuberosity is difficult but mandatory.

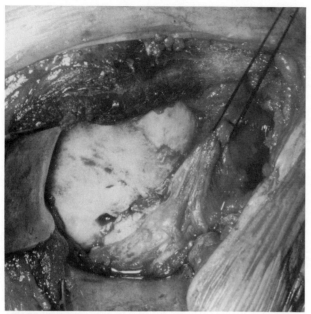

FIGURE 15-34
Intraoperative photograph. Greater tuberosity has retracted and healed to the posterior humerus, resulting in obvious defect over the humeral head. The suture identifies the supraspinatus insertors onto the greater tuberosity. This malunion makes the rotator cuff ineffective, because of its shortened posterior position.

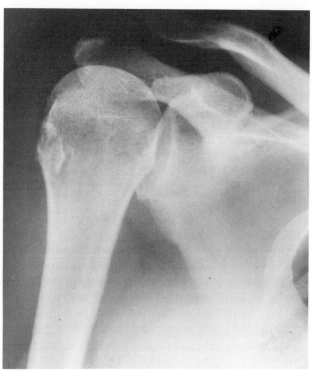

FIGURE 15-36
Plain radiograph following relocation of an acute traumatic two-part anterior fracture dislocation. The teres minor facet is repositioned anatomically, but continued dysfunction, weakness, and pain exist.

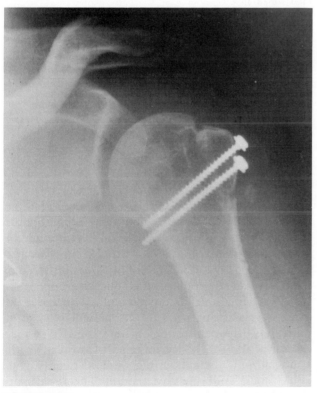

FIGURE 15-35
Osteotomy and internal fixation of the greater tuberosity segment to its anatomic position.

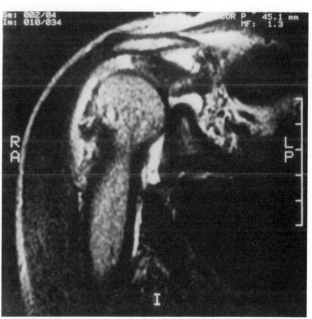

FIGURE 15-37
An MRI scan indicating the full extent of the injury. The teres minor facet is the only bony lesion present. However, there is extensive disruption of the rotator cuff. The supraspinatus and infraspinatus have been torn, and the bony facet has been avulsed by the teres minor.

ence of a Bankart lesion, and failure to recognize this associated Bankart lesion may prove problematic if an extreme position of external rotation is needed to position the greater tuberosity back to its anatomic site. There is thus the potential of redislocation of the humeral head during or after the tuberosity repair if the Bankart lesion is left unrepaired (Figs. 15-36 and 15-37).

THREE-PART FRACTURES AND FRACTURE DISLOCATIONS

These fractures are unusual in young patients; but, when they occur, they are high-energy fractures associated with significant soft tissue trauma. The complex pattern of displacement, and the associated soft tissue injuries, make treatment difficult. These fractures include the three-part greater tuberosity fractures and fracture dislocations and three-part lesser tuberosity fractures and fracture dislocations.

In three-part greater tuberosity fracture, there is a fracture through both the surgical neck and the greater tuberosity segment (Fig. 15-38). The greater tuberosity is displaced superiorly or posteriorly by the pull of the external rotators and in fact may come to lie under the acromion, making retrieval by any closed method impossible. The lesser tuberosity remains with the head segment, ordinarily maintaining its blood supply. However, a fracture through the surgical neck destabilizes the head tuberosity segment, so the humeral head is rotated by the intact lesser tuberosity. The articular surface, therefore, is rotated inward by the intact lesser tuberosity, and the subscapularis faces posteriorly. Additionally, the shaft is pulled medially by the pectoralis major, adding to the difficulty of closed reduction. In addition, complicating treatment, the long head of biceps is often caught between the fracture segments. This complex displacement pattern, with significant displacement of the greater tuberosity and complex rotatory displacement of the humeral head, makes accurate closed reduction extremely difficult, if not impossible. In addition, with three-part fractures, the tuberosity displacement is pathognomonic of a rotator cuff tear.

In a three-part lesser tuberosity fracture, it is the greater tuberosity segment which is intact and remains with the humeral head to provide blood supply. The lesser tuberosity is fractured and displaced medially by the pull of the subscapularis. Because it is a fracture through the surgical neck, destabilizing the humeral head segment, the intact greater tuberosity rotates the articular surface anteriorly. While the fracture and displacement patterns are complex, the intact tuberosity in each of these fracture types

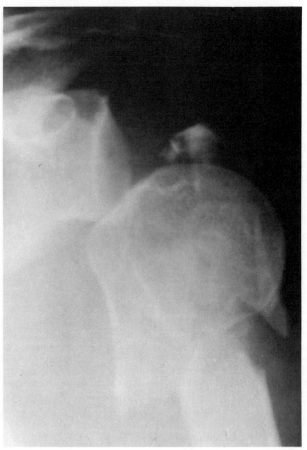

FIGURE 15-38
A three-part greater tuberosity fracture. The greater tuberosity is pulled superiorly by the supra- and infraspinatus. The intact lesser tuberosity rotates the articular surface in a posterior direction. The fracture through the surgical neck destabilizes the humeral head tuberosity segment, making closed reduction impossible. The lesser tuberosity probably maintains satisfactory blood supply to the humeral head, making the risk of avascular necrosis less likely.

usually is enough to maintain the blood supply and hence humeral head viability. However, in some patients, whether because there is inadequate blood supply via the remaining tuberosity, there is unrecognized fracture through the remaining tuberosity, or in some instances, an operative reduction has stripped the remaining blood supply, late avascular necrosis may occur. Because of this possibility, some have advocated primary prosthetic arthroplasty for three-part fractures in the patient at high risk for avascular necrosis, such as the patient who is elderly, has osteopenic bone, or has extensive comminution of the tuberosity fragment. However, in the young athletic patient, with good bone quality, good bone stock, and healthy tendons, every attempt should be made to retain the articular surface of the humeral head and reconstruct the displaced tuberosities and soft tissue around it.

206

The results of closed treatment of this fracture have been extremely unfavorable in the literature, and because of this and the difficulty in achieving any accurate closed reduction, my preference is to immediately proceed to an open reduction internal fixation of any three-part fracture.

These three-part fractures can also be associated with shoulder dislocations and, if so, are termed three-part fracture dislocations. If the greater tuberosity is fractured, the humeral head usually is dislocated anteriorly along with the intact lesser tuberosity. If the lesser tuberosity is fractured, the humeral head dislocation is posterior. I believe the trauma involved in a closed reduction in this complex fracture is such that it may well interrupt any remaining blood supply. Therefore, the less traumatic approach to relocation of this fracture is an open relocation, where the head can gently be pried from its dislocated position back into the glenoid fossa. Care must be taken with an anterior fracture dislocation to respect the proximity of the brachial plexus and axillary artery and, with posterior displacement, to respect the location of both axillary and suprascapular nerves. Once the humeral head is relocated in the glenoid fossa, operative internal fixation can proceed, as with a three-part fracture without an associated dislocation.

The surgical plan is to first reduce the tuberosities to one another, aligning them in the correct position with the articular surface of the humeral head and then reducing the tuberosities to the shaft of the humerus. The fracture is approached by a deltopectoral interval. Because exposure may be difficult, a portion of the deltoid insertion or pectoralis insertion may be divided for better exposure. The biceps tendon is the guide to the fracture anatomy. It is usually intact and, if so, can be found just medial to the pectoralis tendon. By following the biceps tendons superiorly, the location of the greater tuberosity segment with the attached external rotators can be found posterior to the biceps tendon (Fig. 15-39). Likewise, the lesser tuberosity with the attached subscapularis is usually anterior to the biceps tendon. The debris can be removed from the glenohumeral joint and the fracture anatomy, extent of comminution, health of the humeral head, and position of the fracture fragments identified. The tuberosity segment that is displaced is identified and several stay sutures are placed through the tuberosity tendon junction so that the fragment can be manipulated into place.

While many methods of fixation are described for three-part fractures, the most helpful is found to be a wiring to bring the tuberosities to one another and to the shafts and intramedullary fixation to help control translation. This technique, utilizing either

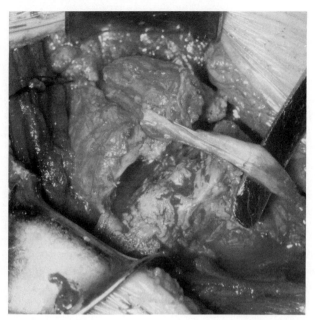

FIGURE 15-39
The surgical approach to three-part fracture is via a long deltopectoral incision. The biceps tendon is found distally and followed proximally. The biceps tendon is a useful guide to the location of the fractured tuberosity segments.

nonabsorbable suture (No. 5 Tevdek) or wire fixation, requires initially the reduction of the tuberosities to the head segment. Two 14-gauge culpotomy needles are used, with the stylet passed through subscapularis and lesser tuberosity, then through the head segment and out the greater tuberosity and supraspinatus tendon (Fig. 15-40). The rotational deformity of the head is then reduced. Two drill holes

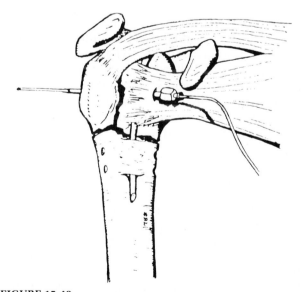

FIGURE 15-40
A culpotomy needle can be utilized to reduce the lesser and greater tuberosities to one another prior to securing the tuberosity construct to the shaft of the humerus.

207

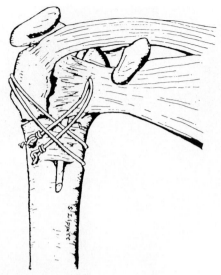

FIGURE 15-41
Open reduction internal fixation of a three-part fracture entails first securing the lesser and greater tuberosities to one another and then utilizing the tension band technique to secure the tuberosities to the shaft of the humerus.

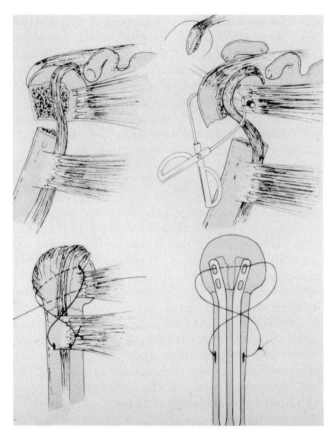

FIGURE 15-42
Open reduction internal fixation of three-part greater tuberosity fracture. These sequential internal fixation steps initially bring lesser and greater tuberosity segments to one another, and then secure these to the shaft of the humerus. Intramedullary fixation can be added to assure translational stability.

distal to the shaft are then made below both lesser and greater tuberosities. The 20-gauge needles are used to pass the suture through these drill holes as well. The tuberosities are first reduced to one another and then the construct is reduced to the shaft of the humerus, and the sutures or wire are crisscrossed over the lateral aspect of the fracture site, securing the fixation. A second wire or suture is then utilized as well (Figs. 15-41 and 15-42). Finally, the rotator interval is repaired. Stability must be checked intraoperatively so that the surgeon can know how aggressively to pursue the postoperative rehabilitation.

Consideration should also be given to utilizing intramedullary fixation such as a Rush rod to augment translational stability. Whatever means of internal fixation is utilized, care must be taken during the dissection to avoid stripping the soft tissues excessively, maximizing the chances that the remaining intact tuberosity will in fact maintain the viability of the humeral head.

FOUR-PART FRACTURES

Fortunately, four-part displacement is rare in the young athlete. These fractures tend to be seen in patients who are older, with osteopenic bone. This fracture represents the most difficult problem of all. Both tuberosities and attached cuff are displaced from each other and from the shaft. The shaft is pulled medially by the pull of the pectoralis. The articular surface, usually free of any soft tissue attach-

ments, may be crushed or comminuted and may be free-floating or dislocated, either anteriorly, posteriorly, inferiorly, or laterally. There is invariably a longitudinal rent in the rotator cuff between greater tuberosity and lesser tuberosity segments. In some patients, the tuberosity fragments may be joined to each other via the bicipital groove, but these segments still are separated from the shaft and from the articular surface of the humeral head, thus behaving like a true four-part fracture. The head fragment, often widely displaced, is devoid of blood supply and the incidence of avascular necrosis is reported to be high (Figs. 15-43 and 15-44). In addition, the extensive bony and soft tissue damage often has accompanying nerve injury, may include vascular injury, and may lead to the late development of heterotopic ossification, especially in association with humeral head dislocation.

A variant of this fracture has been described in which the head segment is impacted into valgus, while the tuberosities, though fractured, are not widely displaced. This fracture probably does not

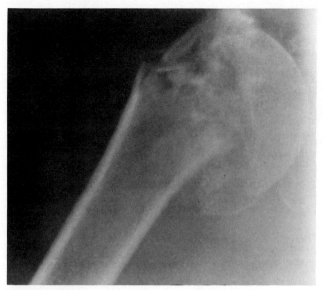

FIGURE 15-43
A four-part fracture of the humerus, which was treated nonoperatively. An initial x-ray is seen.

have the high incidence of associated avascular necrosis that four-part displacement fractures have.

Because of the tuberosity and head displacement and the extent of soft tissue damage, treatment of this fracture is extremely difficult (Fig. 15-45). Closed reduction has been associated with extremely poor results because of the inability to restore the anatomy and the marked amount of subsequent fracture deformity. Comminution of the articular sur-

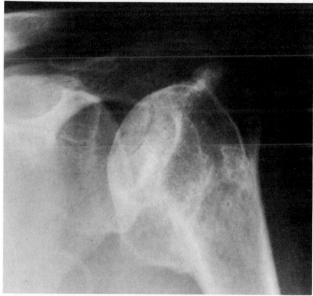

FIGURE 15-44
Three years later, there is a healing of the tuberosity segments, although the greater tuberosity is malunited superiorly. There also appears to be avascular necrosis of the articular surface segment.

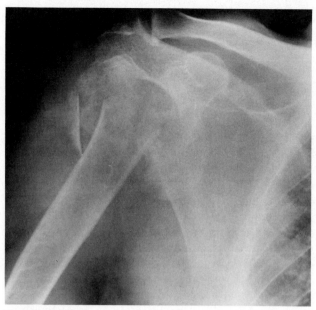

FIGURE 15-45
A four-part anterior fracture dislocation. The humeral head is dislocated from the glenoid fossa and is in the subcoracoid position. The lesser and greater tuberosities are fractured and separated from one another. The articular surface has no soft tissue attachments to bring satisfactory blood supply.

faces, devascularization of fragments, and difficulty in achieving stable fixation make open reduction internal fixation difficult as well, and thus many have suggested a primary prosthetic arthroplasty with reconstruction of the tuberosities around the implant. This may give the best chance of achieving immediate fracture stability, permitting early motion and return to activity. In the young athlete, especially with high demands, the role of prosthetic arthroplasty is less clear. However, there is little disagreement that in the older patient in whom the fracture is most commonly seen, operative treatment should initially consist of primary prosthetic arthroplasty.

In the athletic patient, especially one who is younger, attempts should be made for an open reduction internal fixation. In these younger patients, bone stock is usually better and fixation of the tuberosity and head segment may be possible. The articular surface, although small and extremely unstable, is usually not the thin "eggshell" fragment so frequently seen in older patients with this fracture. In addition, there may be some inferior capsular tissue remaining with the head, since the head often is in continuity with some of the medial metaphyseal bone when it fractures. Nevertheless, attempts at internal fixation have led to mixed results, with hardware complications, avascular necrosis, and nonunion all being clear risks if one attempts to treat this fracture by preserving the humeral head. Nevertheless, all things considered, an attempt should be

209

made to perform some type of limited internal fixation with screws or sutures in the young athletic population.

If open reduction internal fixation is attempted, the surgical approach is similar to that for a three-part fracture, with a long deltopectoral incision. The long head of biceps is isolated and followed proximally, leading the surgeon to the rotator interval and location of the tuberosities on either side of the tendon. Stay sutures are placed in the lesser tuberosity, which is retracted with the subscapularis. The condition of the humeral head is assessed, and the humeral head is manipulated into place relative to the greater tuberosity and shaft. In addition, the critically important greater tuberosity segment with all of the external rotators and supraspinatus is assessed in terms of its ability to maintain internal fixation. An attempt is first made to assemble the humeral head and greater tuberosity to the shaft via pins or screws. If the bone is of sufficient quality to hold these important fragments together, greater and lesser tuberosities may be repaired to each other and to the

shaft of the humerus via the same tension band techniques used with other fractures. While an intramedullary rod may be considered to add some element of translational stability, the usual insertion site for the rod, the sulcus between the articular surface of the humeral head and greater tuberosity, is, by definition, fractured, so it may be impossible to add an intramedullary rod unless it is placed directly through the articular surface of the humeral head. Once the fracture is reduced and fixed, it should be assessed for stability. If it is clear that the fracture fragments are not able to be held reasonably securely, attempts at open reduction internal fixation with preservation of the humeral head can be discontinued, and primary prosthetic arthroplasty can then be performed (Figs. 15-46 and 15-47).

Primary prosthetic arthroplasty is probably best saved for a middle-aged or older recreational, non-contact athlete. The younger, contact sport athlete, who desires to remain active, is probably not a good

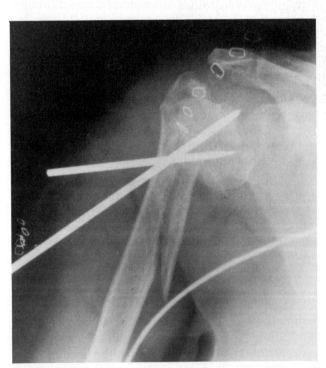

FIGURE 15-46
A four-part fracture with displacement. An attempt has been made to secure the displaced segments with limited internal fixation. Unfortunately, there is often inadequate bone stock to permit secure purchase with limited internal fixation, and the immediate postoperative film shows not only penetration of the articular surface with Steinmann pins but also little fracture stability and malposition of the humeral head relative to the greater tuberosity segment.

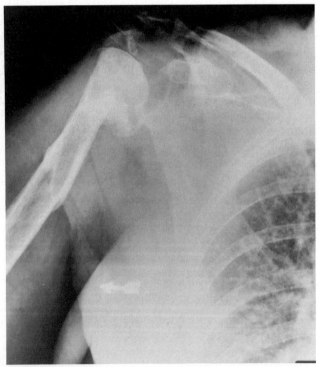

FIGURE 15-47
Not surprisingly, given initial healing, there is nonunion of the greater tuberosity and attached rotator cuff located in the subacromial space. There is callus formation inferior to the neck of the humerus. Stiffness and pain have resulted, necessitating a late total shoulder replacement. Compromise on fracture stability is often necessary with limited internal fixation of four-part fractures, and it is often impossible to begin early range of motion necessary for a good result. A primary prosthetic arthroplasty is probably a better choice in this situation.

candidate for primary prosthetic arthroplasty. On the other hand, if a four-part fracture is present in this very vigorous athletic population, there is probably no ideal treatment that can assure the athlete eventual motion, strength, and function of the involved shoulder.

The surgical technique for primary prosthetic arthroplasty has become well established. A long deltopectoral incision is made without detachment of the proximal deltoid, though a small amount of distal deltoid incision and superior pectoralis major tendinous insertion may be considered. The biceps tendon is utilized as a guide to the fracture fragments and the individual rotator cuff tendons are followed proximally. The biceps tendon should not be excised or divided, as this serves as a guide not only to the tuberosities but to the proper tension in the soft tissues around the prosthesis. The displaced greater tuberosity with the attached tendons and lesser tuberosity with the attached subscapularis are identified and tagged with a stay suture. The humeral head segment is assessed, and if it is elected to proceed with the prosthesis, the humeral head segments are removed and the humeral head can be saved for bone graft. The humeral shaft should be prepared for prosthetic insertion, the precise method depending on the type of prosthesis involved. Because of the loss of rotational stability associated with greater and lesser tuberosity fractures, it is often necessary to use methyl methacrylate cement to ensure fixation of the humeral stem. The trial prosthesis is adjusted for proper degree of retroversion (approximately 40° retroversion) and proper depth of the stem within the shaft of the humerus. This is a critical portion of the procedure, as inserting the prosthesis too deeply will make the soft tissue envelope quite lax, potentially leading to prosthetic instability. On the other hand, if the soft tissue envelope is too taut, the prosthesis may ride high in the glenoid, leading to superior glenoid wear, limited motion, and prosthetic impingement against the acromion. The biceps tendon can be utilized as a guide to the proper depth of insertion. With the tuberosities assembled around the implant, the implant is set proud enough so that there is stability anteriorly and posteriorly, and inferior translation of approximately one-half of the glenoid is permitted. There is usually a gap between the inferior surface of the prosthesis and the medial metaphyseal bone of 1 cm or less. The proper head size or stem size is selected, based on the ability to reconstruct the tuberosities around the implant.

Two sutures are passed through the greater tuberosity or the cuff-tuberosity junction, and two sutures are passed through the lesser tuberosity or the tuberosity-cuff junction. These are the sutures that will be secured to the fins of the prosthesis. In addition, several drill holes are made in the shaft of the humerus and sutures passed through the shaft of the humerus to emerge from the fracture site, so that these sutures can be passed through the tuberosity as well, securing the tuberosities to the shaft. The prosthetic replacement is ordinarily cemented into place in the proper depth and version. Initially, the greater tuberosity is secured to the fin of the prosthesis and to the shaft of the humerus and bone graft is added at the tuberosity shaft juncture (Fig. 15-48). Secondarily, the lesser tuberosity is secured to the fin of the prosthesis and the shaft of the humerus with bone graft added (Fig. 15-49). The greater tuberosity is usually assembled first to the prosthesis, because this, with its attendant supraspinatus, infraspinatus, and teres minors, clearly represents the critical part of the operation. If tuberosity shaft union occurs, ordinarily the functional results of prosthetic replacement are quite good. If greater tuberosity nonunion occurs, the disability of the nonfunctioning rotator cuff attached to the tuberosity is

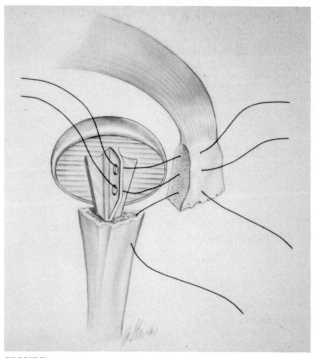

FIGURE 15-48
For prosthetic replacement in four-part fractures, the initial maneuver is to secure the greater tuberosity, with its important supraspinatus and external rotators, to the prosthesis and to the shaft of the humerus.

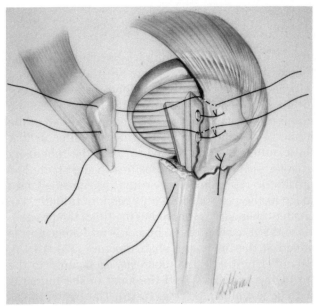

FIGURE 15-49
Following secure fixation of the greater tuberosity to the prosthesis and the shaft, the lesser tuberosity is then secured to the remaining bone and prosthesis.

great. Following the prosthetic insertion, the rotator interval is then closed, with nonabsorbable suture, the prosthesis is once again tested for stability and for security of the tuberosity fixation, and the wound is closed in layers over a drain (Fig. 15-50). Initially, only passive motion is permitted, with active motion

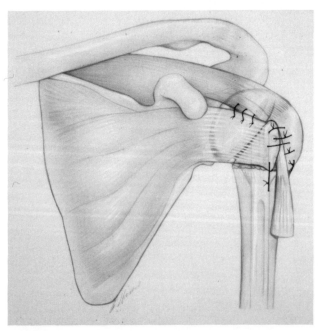

FIGURE 15-50
The completed prosthetic implant for a four-part fracture including closure of the rotator interval and security of the tuberosity segments both to the prosthesis and to the shaft of the humerus.

not permitted until there are radiographic signs of union of the tuberosities to the shaft.

COMPLICATIONS OF FRACTURES IN ATHLETES

Many of the complications associated with proximal humerus fractures in athletes have been described. Nerve injuries, whether as isolated injuries or as larger injury to the brachial plexus, are not uncommon and reflect a degree of soft tissue damage with high-energy trauma. In young patients, associated plexus stretch injuries often result in some element of recovery, though recovery may not be complete. Nevertheless consideration should be given for exploration of complete nerve lesions where there is no improvement in function at 3 months after injury.

Vascular injuries are uncommon but are potentially devastating when they occur. The elderly appear to be at high risk because of the decreased elasticity of the blood vessels. Early diagnosis of these injuries is important, and clues include an expanding axillary hematoma and absent radial pulses. Nevertheless, it is critical to recognize that collateral circulation may mask an injury, and there should be a high degree of clinical suspicion. It may be necessary to assess vascular patency with either Doppler or arteriographic studies at the time. If there is a vascular injury that requires surgical treatment, expeditious fracture fixation should be achieved first before vascular reconstruction.

Avascular necrosis, a devastating complication if it occurs in the young patient or the athlete, is most commonly seen with anatomic neck fractures and displaced four-part fractures of the proximal humerus. While this may occur with three-part fractures of the proximal humerus in older patients, there is usually adequate blood supply remaining if three-part fractures occur in the younger patient to avoid potential development of late avascular necrosis. The extent of vascularity of the humeral head may be assessed by a variety of means. While not all avascular necrosis is symptomatic in the proximal humerus, the symptomatic or progressive avascular necrosis, which is unresponsive to nonoperative treatment, is usually treated with prosthetic arthroplasty.

Heterotopic ossification is an often discussed complication of proximal humeral fractures. However, the overall incidence of heterotopic ossification with proximal humeral fractures is uncommon. Heterotopic ossification is most often associated with fracture dislocations and may be associated with surgical treatment, especially that surgical treatment which is delayed past 10 to 14 days. However, even heterotopic ossification, if it develops, may not cause a significant loss of function. The treatment of this complication depends on the level of symptoms. If the symptoms warrant surgical treatment, excision is desirable but should be delayed until the heterotopic bone is "cold." Excision may be difficult, particularly in the inferior aspect and around the brachial plexus. Neurovascular structures indeed are at risk during any excision of heterotopic ossification.

Perhaps the most common complication of proximal humeral fractures is residual stiffness. This occurs to a greater or lesser degree in almost all fractures of the proximal humerus, although it tends to be less of a problem in the younger athlete than in the aging athlete. The degree of residual stiffness depends on several factors. In addition to age, these factors include the severity of the initial injury, particularly the extent of soft tissue injury, the duration of immobilization, how early rehabilitation is begun, and the residual anatomic position of the fracture fragments.

As the cause is often multifactorial, the treatment of shoulder stiffness following fracture needs to be addressed in a variety of ways. Among the options include continuing ongoing rehabilitation, surgical release of adhesions, or changing and repositioning of the fracture fragments if malunited. It is probably, however, not prudent to consider manipulation under anesthesia for stiffness that has occurred as a result of fracture, as refracture of the proximal humerus is a significant risk with manipulation.

Malunion can occur with any fracture of the proximal humerus, because either the initial accepted reduction was less than anatomic, or anatomic reduction that was achieved was later lost. The symptoms of malunion are highly variable and fracture-dependent. The most common symptoms, however, are reduced motion and pain. The treatment of malunion of the proximal humerus depends on the level of symptoms, the precise symptoms, and how distorted the anatomy is. When the athlete presents with some degree of malunion and symptomatic stiffness, it is always worth an attempt at further stretching and rehabilitation if the problem is predominantly one of stiffness. For tuberosity malunion that is symptomatic, osteotomy and fixation are usually required. As discussed previously, subacromial decompression alone is usually ineffective for pain and stiffness caused by malunited greater tuberosity. For malunion associated with joint incongruity, arthroplasty, with or without tuberosity osteotomy, is usually the treatment of choice.

While nonunion may occur with any fracture of the proximal humerus, the most common fracture leading to nonunion is the two-part surgical neck fracture. This is fortunately more often a problem in the aging patient than in the young athlete. The causes of nonunion of the neck are most often soft tissue interposition and include either capsular or biceps tendon interposition. The treatment for nonunion of the surgical neck is highly dependent on the quality of the bone, age of the patient, the functional demands of the patient, and the status of the joint. Open reduction internal fixation with bone grafting is an effective course of treatment but may require immobilization if the fixation is not secure. If this is the case, a second operation may be required for removal of the internal fixation and lysis of adhesions. However, if a surgical neck nonunion occurs and the quality of bone is poor, there are multiple fracture lines, or there is associated degenerative joint disease, especially if the patient is elderly, a prosthetic replacement of the humerus with or without glenoid replacement should probably be considered.

REHABILITATION FOLLOWING HUMERAL FRACTURE

The athlete is interested in beginning the process of rehabilitation as quickly as possible following the fracture about the shoulder. For any one athlete, the time course is highly variable and involves timing decisions about initiation of exercises, rapidity of progression, and in particular, return to sport. The timing always depends on the age of the athlete, the dominance of the arm, whether the athlete is predominantly a lower- or upper-extremity competitor, the level at which the athlete participates, and the rapidity with which the athlete needs to be able to return to competition.

In general, with fractures of the proximal humerus, the earlier that rehabilitation is begun, the less likelihood exists that stiffness, the complication that impacts most adversely on the overhead athlete, will result. On the other hand, too early and too vigorous an initiation of range of motion risks displacement of the fracture fragments and subsequent malunion or nonunion.

A rehabilitation of the fracture itself may proceed independent of an overall conditioning program of the athlete. As soon as the initial soreness of the fracture subsides enough that general movement of the body is more comfortable, the athlete may continue to maintain an overall conditioning program, with use of such lower-extremity devices as a stationary bike or Stairmaster. Running can be initiated while still in a protective sling, as soon as the pain in the shoulder is such that impact with the ground is not painful.

If the fracture is either nondisplaced or has been reduced by a closed method, the specific rehabilitation of the fracture may be begun when the initial soreness of the fracture subsides. When early healing of the fracture has occurred enough for the fracture to be "sticky," gentle motion and flexibility exercises are begun. The clinical test for early fracture stability is to place one hand on the greater and lesser tuberosity while the other hand rotates the humerus at the elbow. If, during internal and external rotation of the humerus, the tuberosities can be felt to move with the shaft of the humerus, enough fracture stability exists for initiation of range of motion. The first exercise begun is the Codman circular exercise, in which the arm is dangled with the elbow bent at 90° as the patient bends at the waist, rotating the arm in a clockwise and counterclockwise direction and swinging the arm medially and laterally in flexion and extension. Gravity aids to bring the arm away from the side of the body, so that the athlete does not need to use active muscle power to raise the arm up. Therefore, the greater amount of flexion at the waist that the athlete can achieve, the more that gravity is able to assist in bringing the arm away from the side of the body. The next motion worked on is forward elevation in the scapula plane by using a standing overhead pulley, with the noninjured arm used to motor the injured arm. Exactly when this exercise is added is variable, but usually this may be begun within the first 10 to 14 days following fracture of the proximal humerus that has been treated closed. The arm should be moved in the plane of the scapula, as raising the arm in the purely frontal plane puts tension on the greater tuberosity if this has been fractured. In addition, movement of the arm in the purely abducted or lateral plane is usually difficult and painful soon after injury. Bringing the arm up in the plane of the scapula usually allows the most flexibility while maintaining the tuberosities in a more neutral position. The most difficult motion to regain is external rotation. However, this also is a critical motion to achieve, as external rotation is necessary for full use of the arm above shoulder level. Initially, external rotation may be added with the athlete supine, bending the elbow at 90° with approximately 10 to 15° of abduction, and the elbow resting on a pad or towel. A stick, cane, or golf club can be held

in the uninjured arm and be used to gradually rotate the injured arm into external rotation.

Prior to any stretching exercises, pretreating the athlete with either anti-inflammatory or pain medication is useful, and additional modalities, such as a TENS or electrical stimulation, often are helpful in achieving muscle relaxation, so that the productivity of the exercise period may be maximized. Brief periods of stretching exercise frequently throughout the day are ordinarily more effective than a long aggressive period of stretching.

This technique of frequent short periods of stretching exercises to restore flexibility following the fracture continues through the weeks and months following the shoulder injury. The intent of these exercises is to restore full mobility and flexibility, while at the same time protecting the fracture and minimizing the muscle pull on fragments that might have been initially displaced. While ideally the goal of stretching therapy is to restore the normal motion of the shoulder as compared with the uninjured arm, it is important to remember that both arms may not have had equal motion prior to the time of the injury. For instance, the amount of external rotation in the dominant arm of a thrower is often greater under normal circumstances than in the contralateral arm.

The second phase of exercises begins by having some maximal isometrics, as initial stages of restoring the muscle tone, strength, and endurance are begun. It is important to concentrate on each muscle of the shoulder girdle, to maintain balance and control of the glenohumeral and scapulothoracic musculature. Muscle imbalance produces an inefficient and incomplete rehabilitation and sets the athlete up for reinjury after fracture healing. It is wisest to titrate the resistance during isometric exercises and to save significant resistance for the time when there are radiographic signs of healing of the fracture.

Each muscle group should be addressed in turn, including the internal and external rotators, the adductors and abductors, anterior, posterior, and middle deltoid, biceps and triceps, and all of the scapular stabilizer and motor muscles. The isometric exercises can also be performed 4 to 5 times a day and follow a period of stretching. The stretching is important prior to the isometric exercises, so that the amount of lost motion can be minimized and the joint is loosened up in preparation for the strengthening sessions. Isotonic strengthening exercises are ordinarily begun at approximately 8 to 10 weeks from the time of injury, initially utilizing resistive rubber bands, such as Theraband, and adding free weights soon after. In general, these exercises are most effective if performed slowly and with the arm below shoulder level. Fatigue aching during the time of these exercises and immediately afterward is not uncommon and diminishes as the endurance of the muscle groups increases.

Since many athletes quickly become bored or frustrated with pure isotonic exercises, at approximately 3 to 3 1/2 months, isokinetic training can be introduced. This permits the shoulder to be exercised at both slow and vast velocities, the slow speeds helpful in minimizing residual strength deficits, high speeds restoring the muscle endurance. Initially these exercises are also begun with the arm below shoulder level, in a more comfortable arc, but especially in the overhead athlete, these are later performed at and above shoulder level in an effort to duplicate the sports-specific motion of the shoulder. Additional free weights or machinery may be utilized as the strength of the athlete improves.

During this period of shoulder strengthening, the strength and motion is often such as to allow participation in limited sports activities. The athlete must be carefully monitored and the level of participation in the sport adjusted as need be. When range of motion is 90 percent of normal and strength is 80 to 90 percent of normal, the athlete may be allowed to return to full activity. Obviously, the athlete engaging in predominantly lower-extremity sports is usually able to return sooner than the overhead athlete. It must be remembered, however, that premature return, especially if there are limitations of range of motion, strength, or endurance, risks reinjury of the fractured shoulder or, more frequently, different injury, as the athlete compensates for the fractured extremity.

At the time of return to athletic competition, consideration should be given for some protective equipment, but the need for this depends on the type of sport involved and the position and degree of involvement of the athlete. In contact sports, since the shoulder is a frequently injured part, during a fall or during person-to-person contact, some type of shoulder pad is useful to protect the middle and lateral portions of the clavicle, the rotator cuff, and the proximal humerus. Properly fitting shoulder pads should allow as much mobility as possible, and padding is often utilized around and below the standard shoulder pad as a means of additional protection during contact.

FRACTURES OF THE CLAVICLE

Fractures of the clavicle in athletes are becoming increasingly common with the increasing popularity of contact sports. These fractures are usually not difficult to recognize and usually unite uneventfully with many different treatment methods. Nevertheless, the frequency with which clavicular injuries are seen and the difficulty of managing the early and late complications of these fractures attest to their importance. The clavicle is the most common fracture site in childhood, and it is estimated that 1 out of 20 fractures involves the clavicle. Fractures of the clavicle may constitute as much as 44 percent of shoulder girdle injuries.

Although clavicular fractures have been classified by fracture configuration, the usual classification is by location of the fracture. The Craig classification of clavicular fractures (Fig. 15-51) is as follows:

Group 1.   Fracture of the middle third
Group 2.   Fracture of the distal third
    Type 1.   Minimal displacement (interligamentous)
    Type 2.   Displaced secondary to a fracture medial to the coracoclavicular ligaments
        A.   Conoid and trapezoid attached
        B.   Conoid torn, trapezoid attached
    Type 3.   Fractures of the articular surface
    Type 4.   Ligaments intact to the periosteum (children), with displacement of the proximal fragment
    Type 5.   Comminuted, with ligaments attached neither proximally nor distally but to an inferior comminuted fragment
Group 3.   Fracture of the proximal third
    Type 1.   Minimal displacement
    Type 2.   Displaced (ligaments ruptured)
    Type 3.   Intraarticular
    Type 4.   Epiphyseal separation (children and young adults)
    Type 5.   Comminuted

FIGURE 15-51
The Craig classification of clavicular fractures.

The incidence of clavicular fractures in adults appears to be increasing, owing to a number of factors, including the increase in popularity of contact sports and the occurrence of many more high-velocity vehicular injuries. The mechanism of injury may be direct or indirect. In athletes, these fractures may result from a fall on the outstretched hand, a fall or blow on the point of the shoulder, or less commonly, a direct blow to the clavicle itself, as in stick sports like lacrosse and hockey.

CLINICAL AND RADIOGRAPHIC FINDINGS

Because of the characteristic clinical presentation in the athlete, displaced fractures of the clavicle present little difficulty with diagnosis if the patient is seen soon after injury. There is usually a clear-cut history of some type of trauma, and clinical deformity is obvious if the proximal fragment is displaced upward and backward and, on some occasions, tenting the skin. The involved arm droops forward and downward, and the patient usually presents splinting the involved extremity at this side, since any movement elicits pain. Examination of the patient reveals tenderness directly over the fracture site. There may be ecchymosis and the patient may angle ahead toward the injury, trying to relax the flow of the pectoralis on the fragment. Nondisplaced fractures or isolated fracture of the articular surface may not cause deformity and may be overlooked unless they are sought for radiographically.

There may be associated skeletal injuries with clavicular fractures, such as sternoclavicular and acromioclavicular joint separations, head and neck injuries, and rib fractures. With more severe trauma, injuries to the lung and pleura, or vascular and brachial plexus injuries are not uncommon (Figs. 15-52 to 15-54).

While in most instances of clavicular shaft fractures, the diagnosis is not in doubt because of the clinical deformity, to obtain an accurate evaluation of the fragment position, two projections of the clavicle are typically utilized, an anteroposterior view and a 45° cephalic tilt view. An anteroposterior x-ray view can include the upper third of the humerus, the shoulder girdle, and the upper lung fields, so that associated shoulder and lung injuries may be identified. For fractures of the distal clavicle, which may be particularly difficult, standard x-rays may not reveal the extent of the injury. A cephalic tilt view may be helpful to assess the area of the distal third of the clavicle.

TREATMENT

As early as the late 1920s, more than 200 different treatment methods had been described for fractures of the clavicle. In general, excellent results have

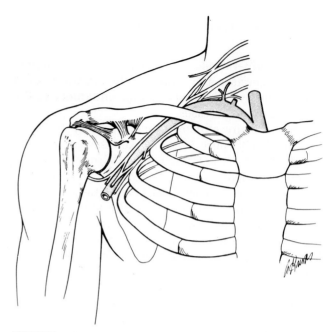

FIGURE 15-52
The location of the brachial plexus and vascular structures just posterior to the clavicle place these at risk by either fracture fragment or late callus formation.

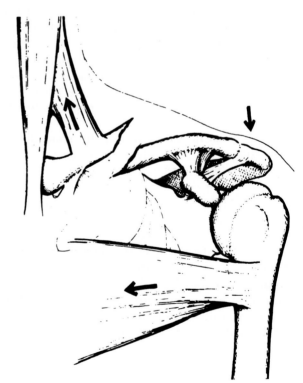

FIGURE 15-53
The displacement of a midshift clavicle fracture. The shoulder girdle sags inferiorly and medially, and the medial segment is pulled superiorly by the pull of the sternocleidomastoid.

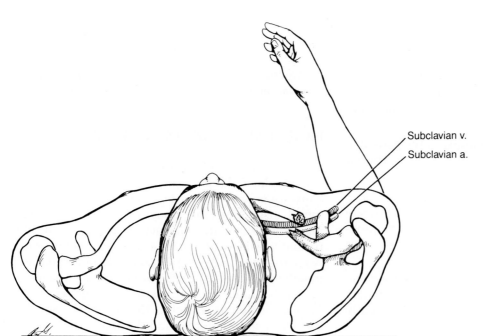

FIGURE 15-54
Proximity of the subclavian vein and artery to the fracture fragments with a midshift clavicle fracture.

been reported with nonoperative treatment of these fractures. However, the exact method of treatment of the fractured clavicle depends on several factors, including age and the medical condition of the patient, the location of the fracture, associated injuries, and in the athlete, the type of sport and the ability of the athlete to be away from the involved sport while healing occurs.

In general, the goal of treatment is to achieve healing of the bone with minimal deformity, minimal loss of function, and minimal morbidity. The main principles of nonoperative treatment historically have included bracing of the shoulder girdle to raise the outer fragment upward, outward, and backward, depressing the inner fragment, and to enable the ipsilateral elbow and hand to be used, so that associated problems with immobilization can be avoided. In general, while fractures in the child are quite easy to treat and heal quite rapidly with minimal immobilization, fractures in the adult are more difficult to treat, since the quality of bone and periosteum is different and the associated soft tissue and bony injury is often greater. In addition, the potential for healing is less than in adults and the incidence of nonunion has been reported to be approximately 5 percent. In general, while a wide range of treatment methods have been outlined for clavicular fractures, my preference is for a commercially available figure-of-8 splint following closed reduction. To reduce the clavicle, the patient is seated on a stool with a surgeon behind; after meticulous preparation, the area of fracture and fracture hematoma is infiltrated with Xylocaine. The knee is placed between the scapulae,

the outer edges of the shoulder are held securely, and the shoulders are pulled upward, outward, and backward. The fracture may then be manipulated into place. The commercially available figure-of-8 is preferable to a more rigid and cumbersome immobilization, such as a plastic spica cast. In addition, the figure-of-8 bandage has the advantage of leaving both hands and elbows free. A sling may be added to the figure-of-8 to provide additional support for the arm and to make sleeping more comfortable. In general, immobilization is maintained for 6 to 8 weeks.

Although rotation of the arm at the side in any direction and to any extent is permitted early, the active use of the arm at chest level and above is not permitted until clinical union occurs. If refracture occurs during the treatment period, continued immobilization is probably appropriate. Athletics are not permitted until 6 weeks after clinical and radiographic union, because of the risk of refracture. At 6 weeks after injury, the patient is taken out of the figure-of-8 dressing and placed in a sling for an additional 3 weeks for added protection, while isometric and mobilization exercises are begun.

In general, the indications for open reduction internal fixation of acute clavicular fractures of the athlete include the following.

1. Neurovascular injury or compromise that is progressive or that fails to reverse with closed reduction of the fracture.

2. Severe displacement caused by comminution with resulting angulation and tenting of the skin

217

severe enough to threaten its integrity and that fails to respond to closed reduction.

3. An open fracture that requires operative debridement.

4. Multiple trauma, when mobility of the patient is desirable and closed methods of immobilization are impractical or impossible.

5. Type 2 distal clavicular fractures.

6. Factors that render the patient unable to tolerate closed immobilization, such as neurologic problems of parkinsonism, seizure disorder, or other neurovascular problems.

7. The very rare patient for whom the cosmetic lump over the healed clavicle is intolerable and who is willing to exchange this for potentially equally noncosmetic surgical scar and the possibility of a nonunion.

8. A floating shoulder, that is, a fracture through the clavicle and an unstable associated scapular fracture. Primary internal fixation of the clavicle usually stabilizes the floating shoulder, making the patient more comfortable and aiding rehabilitation.

If surgery for fractured clavicle is to be undertaken, the choices have historically tended to be between plate fixation and intramedullary fixation. My preference for acute fractures is for intramedullary fixation for the following reasons:

1. There is less exposure of the fracture and therefore a smaller skin incision.

2. Little periosteal stripping is needed.

3. Late removal of hardware is less problematic.

4. No screw holes are made to act as a potential area of weakness of the bone.

5. A useful internal fixation intramedullary device is a Knowles pin, with a hub that is large enough to prevent pin migration and which is easily palpable beneath the skin when removal is desired. The threaded distal under the pin also helps to prevent migration. To insert this pin, the patient is placed in a "beach chair" position; a small horizontal incision is made at the level of the fracture, which is then exposed. The fracture is reduced and held with towel clips. The Knowles pin is then drilled from lateral to medial, entering the clavicle in the posterolateral aspect of the acromion, avoiding the acromioclavicular joint, if possible. It is then directed toward a medial fragment of the clavicle and down the intramedullary portion of the fragment. When any acute

fracture is added, my preference is to add bone graft acutely because of the risk of nonunion.

FRACTURES OF DISTAL CLAVICLE

These fractures are not uncommon and can mimic acromioclavicular joint separations. Some may have a history of poor healing and late complications. For type 1 distal clavicular fractures, in which the ligaments are intact, displacement is minimal, and the patient may be treated with a sling for comfort, early isometric exercises, and discontinuation of the immobilization as symptoms permit. Type 2 distal clavicular fractures are difficult to treat nonoperatively. Immobilization is difficult, the fragments are distracted by muscle forces and the weight of the arm, and the proximal fragment is unstable. It is this fracture that mimics the acromioclavicular separation. Although closed treatment has been successful, union is often delayed and shoulder stiffness may add to the morbidity. A nonunion has been reported in the literature to occur with type 2 distal clavicle fractures.

My usual treatment method for type 2 distal clavicular fractures is as follows. I examine the athlete. I examine the distal clavicle area of the athlete. If on clinical examination there appears to be good bone-to-bone contact, as evidenced by bone-to-bone crepitation, which the athlete can feel, I believe an attempt at closed treatment is helpful with the arm in a sling. If there is no bone-to-bone crepitus or wide separation on the x-rays, I believe consideration should be given for open reduction internal fixation. Although there have been a variety of treatment methods for operative fixation of this, my preference is an open intramedullary fixation, utilizing a Knowles pin. It must be remembered that with this fracture, the coracoclavicular ligaments are usually attached to the distal fragment, with the proximal fragment pulled upward by the contraction of the trapezius. Therefore, a fracture union can be achieved, and the acromioclavicular joint and clavicle are made stable. The surgical technique is as follows. With the patient in the "beach chair" position and the head turned away from the side of the fracture, a small vertical incision is made at the fracture site. The deltotrapezius interval is split horizontally and the fracture site exposed. A heavy nonabsorbable suture or piece of Mersilene tape can be placed around the coracoid process and proximal clavicular segment to aid in the security of the reduction. This is passed prior to the reduction of the fracture. In general, prior to reduction of the fracture, a Knowles pin is drilled from the posterolateral aspect of the acromion, emerging from the medullary canal of the distal clavicle segment. Once the pin is seen and the subacromial space is palpated to make certain that the pin has not violated it, the fracture is reduced; the reduction may be maintained with towel clips and the Knowles pin is advanced through the intramedullary canal of the proximal clavicular fragment. The nonabsorbable suture, or tape from the coracoid to the clavicle, is then securely tied for added fixation. The patient is placed in a sling and swath postoperatively, and isometric exercises are begun in the early postoperative period. The Knowles pin is removed after radiographic signs of early fracture healing (6 weeks).

Type 3 fractures of the distal clavicle are often not recognized acutely. If they do appear acutely, if they are unstable, or when they appear to be an extension of a type 2 injury into the joint, they can be treated as a type 2 injury. If late symptomatic degeneration of the acromioclavicular joint occurs, owing to this intraarticular fracture, the distal 2 cm of clavicle can be excised at a later time.

Rehabilitation following the clavicular fractures of the athletes is usually not problematic. Since the injury does not involve the glenohumeral joint or typically the subacromial space, long-term sequelae of stiffness and attendant reduction in range of motion and strength of the rotator cuff and deltoid are extremely unusual. Therefore, the prime consideration should be given to healing of the bony clavicular healing. If healing, the patient may be immobilized for a long period of time without fear of the shoulder's becoming stiff, if this is an isolated injury. Therefore, maximum protection of the fracture should be the goal of treatment. When the fracture is clinically united, range of motion can ordinarily be begun and rapidly advanced with minimal diminution of shoulder mobility. Isometric exercises can be begun while the patient is in the sling and the clavicle is being protected. In general, resistive exercises are begun with the arm below shoulder level within the first 3 weeks following injury. Range of motion and strengthening exercises above shoulder level are not permitted until clavicular healing has occurred. In those patients who may have been treated operatively, exercises with the arm above shoulder level are not permitted until the intramedullary fixation is removed. Both the therapist and patient work together, using passive exercises (either therapist alone, or utilizing the patient's uninvolved arm) to stretch the injured shoulder in forward elevation, external rotation, and internal rotation. Thus the initiation of range of motion has as its aim minimal residual stiffness that may impact on the ability of the athlete to perform a sport. While ideally these exercises could be performed in a pain-free fashion, the athlete must recognize that stretching exercises in subacutely injured tissue is uncomfortable, but the pain is more likely to feel like tightness or stretching pain rather than acute sharp pain of fracture. It is usually quite helpful before doing stretching exercises to apply heat to the shoulder for 10 or 15 min to relax some of the muscle and augment the blood flow to the area. Following clavicular fractures, the same late program of strength-increasing and sports-specific endurance rehabilitation is done as is typically done for any fracture of the proximal humerus.

CHAPTER 16

Management of Frozen Shoulder and Calcific Tendinitis

Mehrdad M. Malek
Gregory C. Fanelli
Dana R. Verch

Frozen shoulder and calcific tendinitis are both painful conditions of the shoulder that can cause significant disability. Although these conditions are not commonly seen in the young athlete, the older athlete may be predisposed to these injuries.

This chapter discusses the management of frozen shoulder and calcific tendinitis. We discuss etiologic predispositions and causation, review the history and physical exam findings, and outline the current treatment options. The chapter is divided into two parts. The first part addresses frozen shoulder and the second addresses calcific tendinitis.

FROZEN SHOULDER

Frozen shoulder describes a clinical syndrome in which the patient has a restricted range of both active and passive glenohumeral motion for which no other cause can be identified.

The etiology of frozen shoulder is unknown and is more a diagnosis of exclusion. There can be an overlap of symptom complexes, and frozen shoulder may coexist with other types of shoulder pathology.

Frozen shoulder can be separated into two groups, primary frozen shoulder and secondary frozen shoulder.[18] Patients with a negative history and physical exam with respect to their decreased range of shoulder motion are classified as primary frozen shoulder. Secondary frozen shoulder occurs in patients who develop decreased shoulder range of motion after a traumatic episode.

The diagnosis of frozen shoulder is made when progressive shoulder pain and stiffness occur in a patient and no other cause of the symptoms can be found.[21] There appears to be no consensus among authors as to how much shoulder motion loss constitutes frozen shoulder.[6,14,24,27,28,31] Murnaghan diagnosed frozen shoulder in patients with a typical history who have less than 30° of external rotation, forward elevation less than 130°, and combined abduction of less than 120°. We feel that functional loss of motion is more important than absolute numbers, and make the diagnosis of frozen shoulder when there is 50 percent loss of shoulder motion compared with the normal side coupled with the appropriate history.

The pathomechanics of frozen shoulder are not well understood. A relationship to myofascial pain syndrome, trigger pains, and autoimmune disease has been proposed.[15,33] There are several predisposing factors related to frozen shoulder; these are outlined in Table 16-1. These predisposing factors must be looked for in the history and physical exam, and appropriately corrected.

The physical examination should include careful examination of the cervical spine, thoracic spine, trunk, shoulder, upper extremity, and chest. The shoulder range of motion as recommended by the American Society of Shoulder and Elbow Surgeons should include measurement of:

1. Active and passive forward elevation, angle between arm and thorax, patient supine
2. Passive external rotation, arm by side, elbow 90°, angle between forearm and sagittal plane
3. Active internal rotation, arm behind back, tip of thumb to highest spinous process
4. Active abduction, angle between arm and trunk
5. Independent glenohumeral motion

Patients with primary frozen shoulder will typically go through three phases:

I. *Painful phase* occurs insidiously and may last several months.

II. *Stiffening phase* follows with progressive loss of external and internal rotation, and abduction. This phase may last 4 to 12 months.

III. *Thawing phase* gradually occurs over 6 to 9 months with progressive and gradual resumption of functional shoulder range of motion and decreasing pain.

TABLE 16-1
Predisposing Factors in Frozen Shoulder

Immobilization	Thyroid disorders
Middle age	Intrathoracic disorders
Diabetes mellitus	Intracranial pathology
Trauma	Personality disorder
Cervical disk disease	

Patients with secondary frozen shoulder present with symptom onset after a specific initiating event. The specific cause of the secondary frozen shoulder must be identified and corrected. The differential diagnosis is outlined in Table 16-2.

The duration of symptoms is unpredictable. Traditional studies indicate frozen shoulder is a self-limiting condition lasting 12 to 18 months.[11,12,18,35] Other investigations indicate that most patients never regain all of their shoulder motion and that symptoms may last longer than 18 months. Early presentation and dominant arm are good prognostic indications.[1,13]

Diagnostic studies used to evaluate frozen shoulder include blood work, radiographs, bone scan, arthrography, and arthroscopy. Routine blood work should be performed to rule out diabetes mellitus, thyroid disorders, infection, and collagen vascular disease that may be causing secondary frozen shoulder.

AP and lateral radiographs taken in the plane of the scapula plus an outlet view to evaluate acromial

TABLE 16-2
Differential Diagnosis of Frozen Shoulder

Trauma	Bone
Fractures	Neoplasm
Dislocation (especially	AVN
posterior)	Metabolic bone disease
Hemarthrosis	Infection
Soft tissue	C-spine
Rotator cuff injury	Nerve compression
Biceps tendon	Neoplasm
Bursitis	Infection
RSD	Intrathoracic disorders
Fibrosites	Abdominal disorders
Neoplasm	Psychogenic
Nerve entrapment	Primary frozen shoulder
Thoracic outlet	
Polymyalgia	
rheumatica	
Joints	
Degenerative	
metabolic	
Septic arthritis	
Neoplasm	

morphology are the minimum views necessary to evaluate the shoulder. These radiographs are usually normal with the exception of mild osteopenia in chronic cases, and some mild degenerative changes.[2,30]

Bone scans with technetium (99m pertechnetate) show increased uptake in frozen shoulder patients; however, there seems to be no association between the bone scan findings and the duration of symptoms, the initial severity of disease, arthrographic findings, or the eventual recovery.[2]

Arthrography typically but not in all cases shows decreased joint volume, irregular joint outline, and variable filling of the biceps tendon sheath.[22] The shoulder joint volume is reduced to less than 10 to 12 mL with variable lack of filling of the axillary fold and subscapular bursa. (Fig. 16-1A,B).[22]

Neviaser[21,23] defined four stages of arthroscopic changes in adhesive capsulitis:

Stage 1 A mild reddened synovitis

Stage 2 Acute synovitis with adhesions of the dependent folds of the synovial lining (Plates 27 and 28)

Stage 3 Adhesion maturation

Stage 4 Chronic capsular adhesions

The goals of treatment of frozen shoulder are to decrease pain, restore motion, and increase function of the shoulder. Treatment of secondary frozen shoulder consists of diagnosis and appropriate treatment of the pathology causing the secondary frozen shoulder. This is followed by gradual and progressive mobilization of the shoulder.

Treatment of primary frozen shoulder is somewhat more challenging. This treatment can be divided into operative and nonoperative categories. Nonoperative treatment consists of decreasing pain and restoring mobility and is dependent on the stage of frozen shoulder the patient presents to the physician. We prefer nonsteroidal anti-inflammatory agents or mild analgesics for pain control. This is followed by progressive mobilization techniques in physical or occupational therapy. If necessary, modalities are used to assist the mobilization exercise program. Occasionally a subacromial space or glenohumeral space injection of steroid and local anesthetic will enhance the patient's tolerance to physical therapy. When mobility is returning, a shoulder muscle group strengthening program is initiated.

Stellate ganglion blocks have not proved to be effective in our patients and we have discontinued

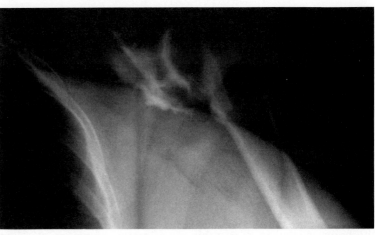

B

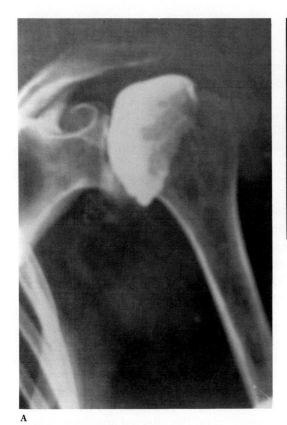

A

FIGURE 16-1
A. Arthrogram of a normal shoulder with smooth joint outline and no filling of the biceps tendon sheath.   B. Arthrogram of a shoulder with decreased range of motion (frozen shoulder) and joint volume, irregular joint outline, and some filling of the biceps tendon sheath.

the usage. We have no experience with oral corticosteroids, prolonged traction, radiotherapy, or distention arthrography.

When physical therapy has been ineffective or fails to progress, manipulation of the shoulder under general or regional anesthesia may be considered. Since there is risk of fracture and other complications with this treatment, we utilize this very cautiously.

At this time our preferred method for treatment of refractory frozen shoulder when nonoperative measures have failed is arthroscopic capsular release with controlled shoulder manipulation under general anesthesia. This gives in one series better results than manipulation alone, and we believe the controlled capsular release decreases the risk of fracture in the osteopenic bone around the shoulder.[25]

We outline the timing of our frozen shoulder treatment as follows: When the patient presents for the initial office visit a careful history and physical is performed. The diagnosis is made of primary vs. secondary frozen shoulder. It is critical to rule out cervical spine disease, chest disease, and primary shoulder pathology. When evaluation of the cervical spine and chest is normal, plain x-rays and an arthrogram of the shoulder are ordered.

The plain radiographs are to rule out bony pathology, and the arthrogram is used to rule out rotator cuff tear as well as to visualize the contracted shoulder joint capsule.

Physical or occupational therapy is started after the first office visit, and the patient is scheduled for return clinical evaluation in 6 weeks. Therapy includes the use of modalities such as heat, ultrasound, and message of trigger points to increase soft tissue extensibility. This is followed by a gentle passive and active range of motion exercises.

Nonsteroidal anti-inflammatory agents are used to relieve mild pain if it is present. Also, if pain is a problem, a transcutaneous electrical nerve stimulation (TENS) unit and/or subacromial and glenohumeral steroid injections can be used to augment physical therapy.

The patient is examined again after 6 weeks of therapy to assess progress. Therapy is continued for 6 months. If the patient has made no significant improvement after 6 months of therapy, consideration is then given to manipulation of the shoulder under anesthesia with arthroscopic capsular release. This usually occurs when a plateau is reached after at least 6 months of therapy.

After range of motion has been achieved to functional levels, progressive strength training is instituted. Care must be taken to avoid inducing an overuse syndrome by instituting strength training before range of motion is restored.

223

CALCIFIC TENDINITIS

Calcific tendinitis is another cause of shoulder pain and disability of unknown etiology. In this disease, reactive calcification occurs in the rotator cuff tendons followed by spontaneous resorption over time with subsequent tendon healing. The painful stage of the disease occurs during calcium resorption with no or mild pain during calcium deposition.[19,34]

The calcification occurs entirely within the tendon substance and not at the tendon insertion into the bone as seen in dystrophic calcification associated with joint degeneration (Fig. 16-2). Microangiographic studies indicate that there may be areas of anatomic and transient hypoperfusion in the rotator cuff tendons leading to zones of tissue hypoxia. This may be related to intratendinous calcium deposition.[29]

Calcific tendinitis occurs most frequently in middle age, and females are affected more often than males.[3,4,17,34] The right shoulder is affected more often than the left.[9] Occupation seems to play a role in calcific tendinitis, with increased incidence occurring in sedentary occupations.[9] There seems to be no relationship to any generalized disease process.[34] And there seems to be no correlation between tendon tears and calcific tendinitis,[20] or trauma and calcific tendinitis.[34] Several classifications have been proposed but do not seem to be useful in clinical management since they fail to consider the cyclic nature of the disease.[3,4,8]

The pathology of calcific tendinitis consists of calcific deposits within the substance of the rotator cuff tendons. It has been proposed that calcific tendinitis may result from a wear-and-tear effect or age-related degeneration in the rotator cuff tendons.[5,7] There is no conclusive evidence to support these theories, especially since this is a self-healing disease entity. Uhthoff[33] proposes the calcification is mediated by cells in a viable environment and proposes three distinct shapes for evaluation of the disease:

1. Precalcific.
2. Calcific.
3. Postcalcific. It is not known what triggers the fibrocartilaginous transformation in the first place, but hypoxia and genetic susceptibility have been proposed.[7,32]

The acute, or painful, phase follows the chronic, or indolent, phase of calcifying tendinitis. During initial intratendinous calcium deposition, there is little if any pain. When pain exists, it often radiates to the area of the deltoid insertion. The range of motion may be decreased by pain, and the patient may not be able to sleep on the affected shoulder. When the calcium deposit is large enough, a painful arc impingement type of clinical picture may be present.

The acute phase when resorption is occurring is characterized by intense and excruciating pain. This causes the patient to lock and splint the affected extremity to keep the shoulder from moving. There seems to be no associated subacromial bursitis, and it is postulated that the edema and the proliferation of cells and vessels causes an increased intratendinous pressure that is the cause of pain rather than a bursitis.[34]

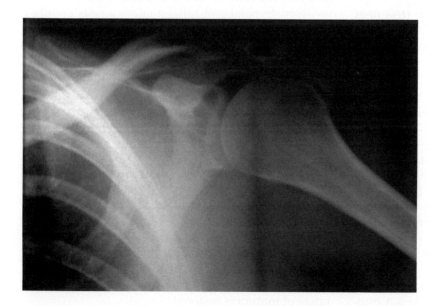

FIGURE 16-2
Calcific tendinitis. A mature case of calcific tendinitis within rotator cuff tendons.

Radiographic studies that are most helpful are AP shoulder films with the humerus in neutral, internal, and external rotation. Deposits in the supraspinatus are best seen on the neutral view, while those in the infraspinatus and teres minor are seen on internal rotation, and those in the subscapularis in external rotation. An outlet view will show the relationship of the deposit to the acromial arch, and indicate possible impingement. Axillary view, CT, MRI, xerogram, bursograms, and arthrograms are not indicated for initial workup. It is important to note that the calcium deposits in calcific tendinitis are localized inside the rotator cuff tendon and not in continuity with or extending into the bone. This must be clearly distinguished from stippled calcifications seen at the tendon insertion in cases of arthropathies.[34]

There are two types of radiologic manifestations of the calcific tendon deposits. One has a fluffy, poorly defined appearance and is usually encountered in acute cases undergoing the resorptive phase. The second is a more uniform density with a well-defined periphery, and presents during the chronic or formative phase.

Screening laboratory values should include calcium, phosphorus, alkaline phosphatase, white blood cell count, erythrocyte sedimentation rate, glucose, uric acid, and iron. These values are normal in primary calcific tendinitis. The possibility of autoimmune disease has been presented by some authors.[32]

The differential diagnosis is between calcifying tendinitis and dystrophic calcification. The latter is part of a degenerative process that includes acromioclavicular arthritis, glenohumeral arthritis, and rotator cuff tear. The calcification is stippled and is located at the tendon insertion into the bone. Primary calcific tendinitis has intratendinous calcium deposits and is not associated with the other degenerative changes.

Treatment of calcific tendinitis consists of either operative or nonoperative methods. The treatment goal is relief of pain and restoration of shoulder function. Nonoperative therapy options include physical therapy, nonsteroidal anti-inflammatory drugs or mild analgesics, needling of the lesion, and radiation therapy. Operative treatment includes arthroscopic or open surgical debridement of the intratendinous calcific deposit.

Our initial approach to calcific tendinitis is nonoperative. We use physical therapy to decrease the muscle spasm and to maintain range of motion. Modalities as well as the exercise program are used at our therapist's judgment based on the individual response of each patient to treatment. Mild analgesics

or nonsteroidal anti-inflammatory agents are also employed.

Injection of the subacromial space with local anesthetic and steroid has had no lasting effect. We have had no experience with needling of the lesions; however, other authors report good results most of the time.[16,26]

Our surgical indications include recurrent attacks for 1 to 2 years, multiple failed injections, and dense deposits over 1 cm in size. We prefer the arthroscopic technique described by Ellman for our procedure.[10] The patient is positioned as for shoulder arthroscopy in the lateral or beach chair position. The glenohumeral joint is inspected, and if a questionable area is seen this is marked with a suture marker. The arthroscope is then placed in the subacromial space and the bursa is debrided. The rotator cuff is inspected and the calcific deposit localized with spinal needle probing. Some authors use C-arm enhancement to help localize the deposits.[36] Multiple penetrations are used to express the calcium deposits from the rotator cuff tendon. If necessary, the rotator cuff tendon can be incised in line with its fibers to help with localization. The calcium is then removed with a curette and suction shaver debridement. The coracoacromial ligament is released. If the patient has a hooked type 3 acromion, an acromioplasty is performed. Using this technique, Ellman reports 94 percent satisfactory results.[10] Postoperatively activity is increased as tolerated and range of motion exercises are used to prevent postoperative adhesions.

SUMMARY

Frozen shoulder and calcific tendinitis are two distinct clinical entities that should not be mistaken for one. They are much less common in young athletic individuals than in the older or middle-aged group. Each presents with different stages of development, and diagnosis is by exclusion. Trauma may play a role in each group but is not a mandatory precedent. Treatment generally is nonoperative; however, the chronic and nonattached case may require arthroscopic or surgical intervention.

ACKNOWLEDGMENT

This manuscript was supported in part by the National Knee Research and Education Foundation. We thank Cindy Smallwood for her help in the preparation of this manuscript.

REFERENCES

1. Binder AI, Bulger DY, Hazleman DL, Roberts S: Frozen shoulder: A long term prospective study. *Ann Rheum Dis* 43:361–364, 1984.

2. Binder AI, Bulgen DY, Hazleman BL, et al: Frozen shoulder: An arthroscopic and radionuclear scan assessment. *Ann Rheum Dis* 43:365–369, 1984.

3. Bosworth BM: Calcium deposits in the shoulder and subacromial bursitis: A survey of 12,122 shoulders. *JAMA* 116:2477–2482, 1941.

4. Bosworth BM: Examination of the shoulder for calcium deposits. *J Bone Joint Surg (Am)* 23:567–577, 1941.

5. Brewer BJ: Aging of the rotator cuff. *Am J Sports Med* 7:102–110, 1979.

6. Brockner FE, Nye CJS: A prospective study of adhesive capsulitis of the shoulder in a high risk population. *Q J Med* 198:191–204, 1981.

7. Codman EA: *The Shoulder.* Boston, MA, Thomas Todd, 1934.

8. DePalma AF: *Surgery of the Shoulder,* 2d ed. Philadelphia, Lippincott, 1973.

9. DePalma AF, Kruper JS: Long term study of shoulder joints affected with and treated for calcific tendinitis. *Clin Orthop* 20:61–72, 1961.

10. Ellman H: *Arthroscopic Management of Calcific Tendinitis.* Monterey, CA, Arthroscopy Association of North America, November 1992.

11. Grey RG: The natural history of idiopathic frozen shoulder. *J Bone Joint Surg (Am)* 60:564, 1978.

12. Haggart GE, Digman RJ, Sullivan TS: Management of the frozen shoulder. *JAMA* 161:1219–1222, 1956.

13. Hazleman BL: The Painful Stiff Shoulder. *Rheumatol Rehabil* 11:413–421, 1972.

14. Kay N: The clinical diagnosis and management of frozen shoulders. *Practitioner* 225:164–172, 1981.

15. Kessel L: *Clinical Disorders of the Shoulder.* New York, Churchill Livingstone, 1982, p 82.

16. Lapidus PW: Infiltration therapy of acute tendinitis with calcification. *Surg Gynecol Obstet* 76:715–725, 1943.

17. Lippman RK: Observations concerning the calcific cuff deposits. *Clin Orthop* 20:49–60, 1961.

18. Lundberg BJ: The frozen shoulder. *Acta Orthop Scand* 119(suppl):1–59, 1969.

19. McLaughlin HL: Lesions of the musculotendinous cuff of the shoulder III. Observations on the pathology, course, and treatment of calcific deposits. *Ann Surg* 124:354–362, 1946.

20. Murnaghan JB: Frozen shoulder, in *The Shoulder.* Philadelphia, Saunders, 1990.

21. Neviaser JS: Arthrography of the shoulder joint. *J Bone Joint Surg (Am)* 44:1321–1330, 1962.

22. Neviaser TJ: Arthroscopy of the Shoulder. *Orthop Clin North Am* 18(3):361–372, 1987.

23. Neviaser RJ: Painful conditions affecting the shoulder. *Clin Orthop* 173:63–69, 1983.

24. Ogilvie-Harris DJ, Wiley AM: Arthroscopic surgery of the shoulder. *J Bone Joint Surg (Am)* 68:201–207, 1986.

25. Patterson RL, Darrack W: Treatment of acute bursitis by needle irrigation. *J Bone Joint Surg (Am)* 19:993–1002, 1937.

26. Quigley TB: Checkrein shoulder, a type of frozen shoulder. *N Engl J Med* 250:188–192, 1954.

27. Quigley TB: Indications for manipulation and corticosteroids in the treatment of stiff shoulders. *Surg Clin North Am* 43:1715–1720, 1969.

28. Rathbun JB, Macnab J: Microvascular pattern of the rotator cuff. *J Bone Joint Surg (Am)* 52B:540–553, 1970.

29. Resnick D: Shoulder pain. *Orthop Clin North Am* 14(1):81–97, 1983.

30. Rizk TE, Christopher RP, Pinals RS, et al: Adhesive capsulitis (frozen shoulder): A new approach to its management. *Arch Phys Med Rehabil* 64:29–33, 1983.

31. Sengar DPS, McKendry RJ, Uhthoff HK: Increased frequency of HLA-AI in calcifying tendinitis. *Tissue Antigens.* 29:173–174, 1987.

32. Travell JG, Simmons DG: Myofascial pain and dysfunction, in *Trigger Point Manual.* Baltimore, MD, Williams & Wilkins, 1983, pp 410–424.

33. Uhthoff HK, Sarkar K: Calcifying tendonitis, in *The Shoulder.* Philadelphia, Saunders, 1990.

34. Watson-Jones R: Simple treatment of stiff shoulders. *J Bone Joint Surg (Am)* 45:207, 1963.

35. Weber SC: *Technique and Results of Arthroscopic Treatment of Calcific Tendonitis of the Rotator Cuff Using Fluoroscopic Localization.* Arthroscopy Association of North America, April 1991.

CHAPTER 17

Neurologic Problems in the Athlete's Shoulder

John J. Kelly

INTRODUCTION

To the weekend athlete who participates in activities such as softball, tennis, and touch football, shoulder injuries are common. Usually, these are relatively simple to diagnose and treat since they typically affect soft tissues and respond to analgesics and rest. Occasionally, they are more severe and persistent with considerable pain and immobility. When this happens, unless there is a clear-cut orthopedic explanation, the question of neurologic involvement is often raised.

Neurologic involvement can be difficult to diagnose in these patients. For one thing, when in severe pain during the acute stages of the injury, these patients can be very difficult to examine. Focal atrophy, which is the hallmark of involvement of motor nerves, is less reliable in the shoulder since pain and disuse alone without neurologic involvement can produce considerable atrophy. In addition, sensory loss and reflex change, which stamp more distal limb syndromes as neurologic, are often missing with neurologic shoulder injuries. For these reasons, patients in whom neurologic involvement is suspected are often referred to physicians with special expertise in this field, and they often require detailed electrodiagnostic studies of shoulder nerve and muscle function.

It is important to diagnose these conditions early, since undetected neurologic involvement in a shoulder injury can lead to severe morbidity and delayed recovery. Thus it is incumbent on the physician seeing these patients early to evaluate them carefully for neurologic involvement. This chapter will outline an approach to these patients and discuss some of the common shoulder neurologic syndromes.

NEUROLOGIC CONDITIONS AFFECTING THE SHOULDER

Neurologic shoulder injury usually refers to damage to nerves and nerve roots. Myopathies, neuromuscular junction, and anterior horn cell disorders can cause profound weakness and atrophy but are chronic disorders that rarely affect one shoulder, and the diagnosis is usually clear from evaluating other areas of the musculoskeletal system.

Disorders that affect nerves and nerve roots almost invariably produce pain at the site of primary injury, probably owing to damage to the small nerves that supply the connective tissue of the nerve itself, the "nervi nervorum." This provides a valuable clue to the locus of the injury. In addition to local pain, discomfort is felt distally in the distribution of the nerve, particularly if it has a prominent dermatomal component. This pain can be of several types. Shooting pain, for instance, is common and is often associated with intermittent compression of the nerve. Constant pain with burning and aching features is usually associated with chronic compression and axonal damage. The distribution of the pain can be a valuable clue to the involved nerve, but more helpful is the distribution of sensory symptoms and sensory loss. Muscle involvement with weakness, atrophy, and reflex loss is also a valuable clue to identification of specific nerve or root injuries but is sometimes difficult to evaluate clinically during acute injuries.

Evaluation of these patients is, of course, greatly aided by laboratory studies, which will be discussed in more detail below in reference to individual syndromes. Plain x-rays and CT of the shoulder and cervical spine are mainly useful to show bony changes such as fractures, dislocations, spurs, and foraminal narrowing. MRI of the brachial plexus and cervical spine is most useful in demonstrating predominantly soft tissue abnormalities such as tumors and disk and spinal cord abnormalities. With the improvement of MRI technique, cervical myelography is now performed infrequently for cervical problems.

Careful electrodiagnostic evaluation, consisting of nerve conduction studies and needle EMG (referred to collectively as EMG from this point on), is of equal importance in the evaluation of the difficult shoulder problem. In entrapment neuropathies, nerve conduction studies are of paramount importance, provided the electromyographer can stimulate above and below the site of compression. This is particularly useful for the major named peripheral nerves of the arm but not so suitable for the brachial plexus and not possible for the nerve roots. For these loci of injury, needle EMG is most suitable for diagnosis. Differentiation of brachial plexus from nerve root damage can, however, be challenging on occasion. Accurate localization rests on a combination of nerve conduction study results (particularly the sensory studies) and the finding of denervation in the paraspinal muscles. The latter suggests that the process is affecting the motor nerve proximal to the neural foramen since the branch to the paraspinal muscles exits from the spinal nerve root immediately after it leaves the foramen. Conversely, sparing of the paraspinal muscles with clear-cut and marked distal denervation suggests a plexus location for the nerve injury.

Specific Syndromes

RADICULOPATHY

Cervical nerve root compression syndromes (radiculopathies) are common and generally fairly straightforward in their diagnosis. Symptoms may start with little or no trauma and evolve over several days to weeks. Almost all patients will complain of neck and limb pain with exacerbation of both in certain critical head positions. The neck pain tends to be in the root of the neck and radiates into the ipsilateral trapezius and sometimes into the medial scapular region of the upper back. The more distal distribution of the pain and numbness (if it occurs) with head movement (and sometimes with cough or strain) is important in the recognition of the involved root (Table 17-1). In addition, the pattern of reflex loss and muscle weakness is an important determinant of root involvement. Demonstration of sensory loss, however, is often difficult despite sensory symptoms since there is considerable overlap of the dermato-

mal distribution of adjacent roots. Even complete sectioning of individual roots at surgery can result in no demonstrable sensory loss. On the other hand, this clinical clue can help to differentiate nerve root from peripheral nerve lesions, where the innervation patterns are much more autonomous and sensory loss easy to demonstrate. An important clue to diagnosis is the provocation of classical root pain by flexing the patient's head toward the ipsilateral shoulder (Spurling's sign). The patient's head is flexed sharply toward the side of shoulder or arm pain radiation. In a positive test, the patient feels sharp pain into the ipsilateral trapezius and often down the arm in the distribution of the affected root. Occasionally, if the examiner is lucky, the patient may even feel transient numbness in the distribution of the root. If not effective, a sharp blow on top of the flexed head can often provoke typical root distribution symptoms. Relief then can be obtained by providing manual upward traction on the patient's head. This should be contrasted to the "reverse Spurling's sign" where pain is felt on the side opposite head flexion, usually in the trapezius muscle. This indicates muscle spasm and is typically seen in muscle overcontraction states such as tension myalgia and postwhiplash syndromes.

Laboratory studies are often essential in securing the diagnosis and planning management. Plain cervical spine films are now less commonly obtained but are still valuable in assessing bony integrity and the foramina. Plain films and CT are also useful in recognizing bony spurs that may be encroaching on the nerve roots or spinal cord. MRI is, however, the most useful test. This should be obtained if the diagnosis is uncertain and if surgery is contemplated. In young athletes, MRI typically shows a disk herniation encroaching on the affected root (Fig. 17-1). In older athletes, cervical spondylosis, bony spurs, and foraminal stenosis more commonly affect the nerve roots (Fig. 17-2). EMG has a

TABLE 17-1
Radiculopathies

Root	Frequency, %	Pain Distribution	Sensory Loss	Weakness	Reflexes
C5	<5	Shoulder	Outer arm	Delt, bic	BJ, BRJ
C6	10	Outer arm	Outer arm, thumb	Delt, bic, pronator	BJ, BRJ
C7	60	Midarm	Digits 2–4	Tric, pron, finger ext	TJ
C8	20	Inner arm	Digits 4–5	Hand	Finger flex
T1	<5	Inner arm	Digit 5	Hand	None

Reflexes: BJ = biceps jerk; BRJ = brachioradialis jerk; TJ = triceps jerk.

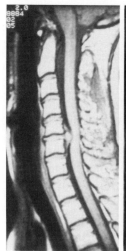
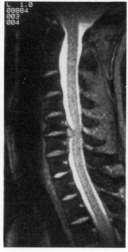
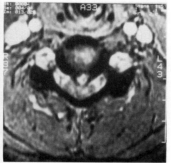

FIGURE 17-1
MRI of the cervical spine, showing a soft disk compressing the spinal cord. The advantage of MRI over other imaging studies is apparent here because it shows the nature of the anatomic defect and shows the state of the underlying spinal cord. In this patient, the midline disk does not affect the cervical roots but would be expected to cause a cervical myelopathy.

more limited role in cervical radiculopathy than in the other disorders discussed below. Acutely, within the first 2 to 3 weeks after the onset of symptoms, the EMG is of limited usefulness, unless the examiner needs to exclude a peripheral nerve entrapment. During this period, the typical changes of denervation (positive waves and fibrillation potentials) are absent since they take about 3 weeks to develop after a nerve is sectioned. After the initial 3 weeks, the EMG is most useful and shows acute denervation in the appropriate myotome distribution of the involved root, including the paraspinal muscles, thereby indicating that the pathologic process is intraspinal. Nerve conduction studies are typically normal even in the face of severe radiculopathy unless there is also peripheral nerve entrapment, not an uncommon occurrence. Because of the need for delay, EMG is indicated only when the diagnosis is unclear or peripheral nerve or plexus involvement needs to be excluded.

Management is almost always conservative in these patients. Pain relief with nonsteroidal anti-inflammatory drugs and intermittent cervical traction usually leads to rapid reduction of discomfort with more gradual recovery of the neurologic deficit. The appropriate point to refer for surgical decompression is controversial. Most patients can be managed without surgery but patients who have large disk protrusions affecting the appropriate root with marked weakness and pain, especially if the pain is not rapidly improved by conservative management, should probably undergo early decompression. The results are usually excellent, and most patients can resume their recreational athletic pursuits after a suitable interval.

Case Study

The patient was a 25-year-old lawyer who played rugby on weekends. After one weekend game, he had stiffness in the left side of his

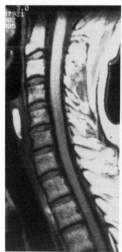
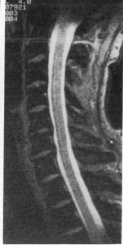
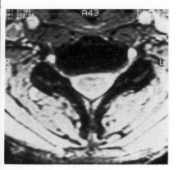

FIGURE 17-2
This MRI shows a minor defect at C5-6 on the sagittal sections, but the horizontal sections show foraminal narrowing at the C5-6 interspace on the right due to bony overgrowth and osteophytes, the cause of the patient's C6 cervical radiculopathy.

neck. During that night, the discomfort became worse and pain radiated into his shoulder and slightly down the outside of his left arm. Symptoms were made worse by turning the head to the left. Later that day, at work, he noted intermittent numbness of the middle digit of the left hand, and he felt some weakness of the left arm when he picked up his 2-year-old son that evening. The next day, the pain was much worse, the numbness became more intense, and he consulted his sports medicine physician. On examination, he held his neck stiffly, and flexion to the left provoked pain in the root of the neck and into the left trapezius. Muscle strength testing disclosed moderate weakness of the left triceps and pronator teres. The left triceps reflex was absent. Despite numbness of digits 2 and 3 of the left hand, no sensory deficit could be demonstrated. Cervical spine radiographs were normal and EMG to exclude radial neuropathy was normal. MRI showed a herniated disk at the C6-7 interspace with entrapment of the C7 nerve root, which appeared swollen. He was treated with nonsteroidal anti-inflammatory drugs and intermittent cervical traction with rapid resolution of pain and more gradual return of muscle strength over the next few weeks.

Comment

This is a fairly typical case history for an acute cervical radiculopathy in a young athlete. Onset of symptoms was gradual over 48 h, and Spurling's sign and other physical findings pointed to a C7 radiculopathy. This was confirmed by the MRI. Neither the MRI nor the EMG was, strictly speaking, necessary from a diagnostic standpoint. Management was appropriate. This patient responded quickly and there was no need to consider surgical therapy. Patients with persistent pain and weakness, especially if moderate to severe and in the dominant limb, are a much greater problem. Even with adequate root decompression, muscle weakness resolves slowly over weeks to months and therefore cannot be used to judge adequacy of therapy in the acute stages. Persistent radicular pain, however, suggests unrelieved root compression and, in the face of at least moderate neurologic deficit, I am more inclined to recommend early surgical intervention in patients with pain unrelieved by cervical traction.

A rare but devastating radicular syndrome is *root avulsion*. This disorder usually requires severe and sudden distraction of the head and shoulder with traction on the cervical roots. It can also selectively affect the lower cervical root when forceful abduction is applied to the arm, such as dragging a heavy patient. These are often associated with plexus injury as well, but the root injury determines the prognosis. These patients have a paralyzed and lifeless flail arm. There is no sensation in the arm from shoulder down and the arm is useless. The arm invariably develops secondary trophic changes with swelling and other vasomotor changes. In addition, owing to its insensate state, the limb is prone to injury and infection. Most patients keep the arm firmly strapped to their side. Careful laboratory evaluation is important early for prognostic purposes. Cervical spine x-rays, CT scan, and MRI are usually negative. The cervical myelogram characteristically shows outpouchings of the arachnoid (pseudomeningocele) where the root has been torn out of the subarachnoid space and lack of evidence of the cervical roots. The EMG shows denervation potentials (fibrillations and positive waves) in the paraspinal muscles, thereby suggesting that the injury is intraspinal. Nerve conduction studies show the peculiar combination of absent motor responses in the limb with preserved sensory responses. The latter occurs because the sensory neuron lies in the dorsal root ganglion that is distal to the site of avulsion; thus the distal axon is intact and able to conduct normally despite its disconnection from the spinal cord. The motor axon, however, is separated from its cell body, which lies in the spinal cord; thus the distal axon totally degenerates. If it can be proved that the roots are avulsed, recovery is deemed hopeless given current technology. These patients usually have proximal limb amputations.

PLEXOPATHY

Acute plexopathies are much more difficult to evaluate than radiculopathies or entrapment neuropathies owing to the complexity of the brachial plexus (Fig. 17-3, Table 17-2). Fortunately, these are less common injuries in the recreational age group. *Traumatic* plexopathies are usually obvious. Acute neurologic deficit is associated with fractures of the clavicle or shoulder and/or soft tissue injury. Tumors of the apex of the lung (*Pancoast syndrome*) can infiltrate the lower trunk of the plexus and present with pain in the supraclavicular area and down the inside of the arm, numbness in the C8,T1 dermatomes (digit 5 and hypothenar eminence), weakness of the intrin-

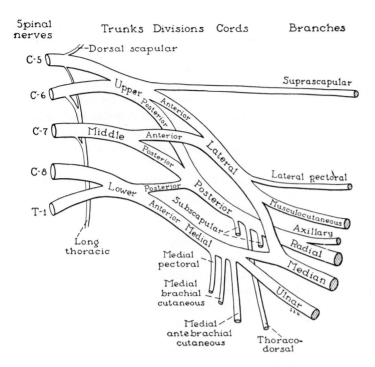

Spinal nerves   Trunks   Divisions   Cords   Branches

FIGURE 17-3
This figure shows the complexity of the brachial plexus. However, for practical clinical purposes, most of the time the plexus can be divided into three main functional divisions (see Table 17-2).

sic hand muscles, and Horner's syndrome. Diagnosis is made by CT or MRI of the chest.

Thoracic Outlet Syndrome (TOS)

This is a controversial syndrome that is grossly overdiagnosed. Patients mistakenly diagnosed with TOS typically have pain in the shoulder area or proximal arm with arm and hand use and with elevation of the arm over the head. They may have numbness or weakness of the hand as well. Most of these patients have other problems ranging from cervical radiculopathies to myofascial pain syndromes of the shoulder. Unequivocal neurogenic TOS occurs but is quite rare. With use of the arm, these patients have reproducible pain and numbness in digits 4 and 5 of the hand with variable degrees of weakness and atrophy of the intrinsic hand muscles (especially those of the thenar eminence). These symptoms are brought on by abducting the affected limb

over the head or by downward traction on the arm, and the symptoms are relieved by the neutral position. There is a poor correlation between the presence of vascular signs of thoracic outlet (i.e., Adson's sign) and neurologic involvement. In addition, most studies have shown a poor correlation with the presence of cervical ribs although most patients will have rudimentary cervical ribs. Patients with the suspected TOS should be carefully evaluated by a physician familiar with its presentation (and skeptical of its frequency). Imaging studies of the plexus and cervical spine to look for cervical ribs and exclude other cause, such as Pancoast tumors, should be performed. Careful EMG of the shoulder and limb is important to exclude cervical radiculopathy and peripheral entrapment neuropathies. Surgery (first rib resection or section of the myofascial band between the rudimentary cervical rib and first rib) should be carried out only in severe, unequivocal cases since it is rarely necessary and carries a high morbidity. These patients can often be managed by a program of physical therapy and exercises designed to change posture.

Brachial Plexitis (Parsonnage-Turner Syndrome)

This disorder is by far the commonest of the brachial plexopathies and usually affects young athletes. It is generally thought to be immunologically mediated and, like most of these diseases, can be triggered by a variety of events including trauma as well as viral illnesses, surgery, and immunization. Often, however, there is no antecedent event. When triggered by trauma, there can be considerable confusion as to

TABLE 17-2
Brachial Plexus Simplified

Plexus Part	Motor Deficit	Sensory Deficit
Upper	Shoulder abduction, elbow flexion	Shoulder, radial forearm, and thumb
Lower	Hand	Digits 4 and 5, ulnar forearm
Posterior	Deltoid, elbow flex, wrist and finger extension	Dorsum of forearm and hand

whether or not the trauma caused the disorder. The onset is almost invariably sudden and dramatic. Patients are often awakened from sleep with severe pain in the shoulder region, so severe that narcotics are usually required. The severe pain persists for days to weeks (sometimes months). The pain is usually constant and localized deep within the shoulder area. It is not, as a rule, exacerbated by cough, strain, or head movements, which helps to exclude radiculopathy. Occasionally, the pain radiates into the arm in a radicular or peripheral nerve distribution, but this is rare. Because of the severe pain, it is often impossible to examine these patients acutely. As the pain begins to remit, it becomes obvious that there is marked weakness, and atrophy rapidly appears in affected muscles. Although termed a plexopathy, the disorder is more a mononeuropathy multiplex of the plexus. Typically, there is relatively selective involvement of combinations of the long thoracic, axillary, musculocutaneous, and suprascapular nerves, in descending order of frequency. Rarely, more distal forearm nerves are affected including the anterior and posterior interossei, the radial, median, and ulnar. Occasionally, the opposite shoulder girdle is affected, sometimes with a delay of several weeks to months. The process runs its course over weeks to months; then the patient stabilizes and begins to improve. A good recovery is the rule, and generally a young patient has an 85 to 90 percent chance of a satisfactory recovery although it may take a year or longer. Physical therapy is important during the recovery phase. Imaging studies of the plexus and cervical spine are helpful early to exclude structural lesions. Fortunately, most of these patients are relatively young; therefore, the imaging studies are usually negative. EMG is the most helpful test, although it usually requires a wait of about 3 weeks from onset before the diagnostic changes are fully developed. The EMG confirms that the process is extraspinal and that the individual nerves deriving from the plexus are affected. EMG is especially useful in evaluating muscles that are difficult to examine, such as the serratus anterior or supraspinatus. Affected muscles show marked denervation. This syndrome is especially a diagnostic problem when it affects a single nerve, such as the long thoracic (see below) or posterior interosseous.

Case Study

The patient was a 33-year-old banker who was awakened during the night after a vigorous day of tennis (not unusual for him) with severe pain in the right shoulder. The pain was intense and located in the region of the supraclavicular fossa and scapula. It was constant but made worse by moving the arm. He could not get back to sleep despite using some acetaminophen with codeine that he had left over from an ankle sprain. The next morning, he called his orthopedist for an evaluation. On exam later that morning, he was red-eyed and clearly in severe pain. He held the arm rigidly against his chest, and other than a rudimentary examination, nothing other than tenderness in the supraclavicular fossa could be found. X-rays of the shoulder region were normal. The pain gradually eased over the next few days and the patient was able to move his arm more freely. However, he noted that he had trouble raising his arm above the horizontal plane and had trouble gripping a key. On repeat exam 2 weeks later, he had full passive range of motion of his shoulder. Reflexes were intact, as was sensation. He had weakness of shoulder abduction and flexion and of flexion of the distal phalanges of the thumb and digits 2 and 3. In addition, his scapula was noted to wing on shoulder flexion. Cervical spine x-rays were normal. An EMG showed normal motor and sensory conduction studies. Needle EMG, however, showed denervation of the deltoid, the serratus anterior, and the flexor digitorum profundus (median head) and the flexor pollicis longus. He was treated with physical therapy and gradually (over months) made a complete recovery.

Comment

The history is typical in that the pain frequently starts at night, often after a day of unaccustomed exertion, and wakens the patient from sleep. It is very severe and usually restricted to the shoulder region. It is constant and does not have the positional qualities of cervical radiculopathy. The weakness that develops is typically patchy and not explainable by one contiguous lesion of the plexus, and imaging studies are negative. EMG is the most useful test as it can document the nonanatomical, patchy, somewhat mononeuropathy pattern of acute denervation typically seen in these patients. As in this patient, most of these patients do very well, although full recovery may take a year or more.

Zingers (Stingers, Burners)

These are severe shoulder and arm pains suffered by athletes participating in contact sports. The pain is provoked by sharp, sudden distraction of the head to the opposite side, as in making a tackle or blocking in football. The athlete feels sudden, severe pain that radiates from the shoulder down the arm to the hand. There is often an associated transient numbness and paralysis of the arm. The whole episode resolves over seconds to several minutes, and there is generally no persisting deficit. Once the episode occurs, the athlete seems to be more susceptible to further episodes with much less severe trauma. The exact pathomechanism of zingers is not clear since there are no published reports of EMG studies in these patients. They likely represent traction on the brachial plexus or cervical roots. Since the roots are the most vulnerable of the two to traction, they likely bear the brunt of the damage. Zingers are generally benign but should be taken seriously, since recurrent episodes can result in chronic nerve damage and the cervical roots are unusually susceptible to traction injury. Rest and proper padding can help. The neck must be padded so that the head cannot be severely and suddenly distracted to either side. Modern equipment with neck roll collars and padding can usually accomplish this task. Patients who develop persistent symptoms and neurologic deficit should be prohibited from further contact until the symptoms and findings resolve and then only allowed to play with careful supervision and padding.

Case Study

A 20-year-old college fullback began to experience "zingers" for the first time in midseason. These would occur particularly after blocking the defensive end on sweeps or making a tackle with his shoulder. He would feel a sudden, severe, sickening pain from his shoulder down his left arm. The pain would immobilize him. The arm would be limp and numb for several seconds, and he had to hold it with the other arm. Then the numbness would begin to resolve and the mobility would slowly return. Within 2 to 3 min, the arm would be back to normal except for persistent aching in the shoulder. Over the next 2 weeks, the episodes became more frequent and were provoked by successively less severe contact, and he began to develop some persistent numbness in his left hand. The trainer then intervened and he was placed in a neck roll collar. This completely relieved the symptoms, and he was able to resume contact without difficulty.

Comment

This is a typical case history. These injuries are very common and can result in prolonged disability unless detected and treated early in their course. Generally speaking, neurodiagnostic studies are not necessary in these patients unless there are atypical features or unless a fixed deficit develops.

ENTRAPMENT NEUROPATHY

These are also relatively uncommon lesions but can be easily overlooked. The following is a description of the most common syndromes (Table 17-3).

Spinal Accessory

The most common cause of this syndrome is a stab wound or lymph node biopsy or other surgery in the posterior triangle of the neck, lateral to the edge of the sternocleidomastoid, before the nerve innervates the trapezius muscle. Abnormal pressure due to an improperly fitting backpack in that area, for example, can also damage the nerve. Patients are often misdiagnosed with rotator cuff injuries and the like. They complain of pain in the shoulder with arm abduction and inability to abduct the arm beyond 90 percent. Standard examination reveals little, but careful observation from the back discloses that the upper trapezius is atrophied and that the medial-superior portion of the scapula wings when the arm is fully abducted. The pain, scapular winging, and abduction limitation are caused by the inability of the trapezius to stabilize the scapula when the arm is fully abducted. EMG is helpful in confirming the di-

TABLE 17-3
Mononeuropathies

Nerve	Muscle	Motor Deficit	Sensory Deficit
Long thoracic	Serratus ant.	Arm flexion	None
Suprascapular	Supra- and infraspinatus	Arm internal rotation	None
Axillary	Deltoid	Arm abduction	Deltoid insertion
Accessory	Trapezius	Arm abduction	None
Musculocutaneous	Biceps br.	Elbow flexion	Radial volar forearm

agnosis. Operative repair is necessary when the nerve has been fully transected, which can be established by EMG.

Long Thoracic

This nerve can be injured by vigorous movements of the arm and upper body (shoveling, chopping trees). It is also commonly affected, often in isolation, in the brachial plexitis syndrome. These patients complain of pain on flexing the fully extended arm on the shoulder because of inability of the serratus anterior to fixate the scapula. They have great difficulty working with their arm in the horizontal position or above. Unless the examiner is familiar with this disorder and carefully evaluates shoulder mechanics during a full range of mobility, this diagnosis can be easily missed. Many of these patients have also been treated for other conditions before the correct diagnosis was reached. The history is often helpful, but the classical finding is inability to fully flex the extended arm on the shoulder despite seemingly normal bulk and strength in component shoulder muscles and normal joint mobility. The examiner should stand behind the patient and observe as the patient slowly raises and lowers the arm through the full range of flexion. As the arm approaches the horizontal, the inferior medial border of the scapula begins to wing and the patient has difficulty raising the arm any farther. The winging can also be brought out by having the patient push forward against a wall with the affected arm horizontally outstretched (Fig. 17-4). The examiner can then confirm the finding by applying manual pressure on the scapula from behind, which allows the patient to fully flex the arm on the shoulder without pain, a motion impossible to perform without the examiner's assistance. Although the clinical picture is often diagnostic, EMG is useful in confirming the diagnosis and determining the severity of the nerve lesion. If the nerve is completely degenerated and there has been no clinical improvement in over a year, the prognosis is poor and consideration for surgical fixation of the scapula should be given. If the nerve is only partially damaged, physical therapy and continued waiting are in order. Surgical fixation of the scapula to the posterior ribs greatly aids arm flexion and should be considered in those patients who are greatly disabled owing to involvement of the dominant arm.

Case Study

The patient was a 42-year-old salesman who had spent the previous weekend working in his yard. This had consisted mostly of landscaping, and he had to shovel and move a large pile of topsoil. That evening, he developed some aching in his shoulder and scapula region that persisted over the next few

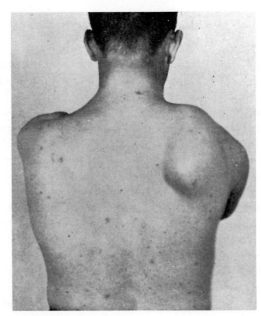

FIGURE 17-4
Isolated long thoracic nerve palsy with winging of the scapula due to weakness of the serratus anterior. This is a disabling condition and is often missed unless the back is inspected during the full range of shoulder motion. Characteristically, the inferior medial angle of the scapula pops out and wings dramatically when the fully extended arm is flexed past 90° on the shoulder.

days. The next morning, he found that he had difficulty shaving and brushing his teeth because he could not raise his right arm to his face and the attempt to do so was associated with pain in the shoulder region. Several days later, he saw his orthopedist, who found his exam to be normal except for weakness of arm flexion. He ordered an EMG, which was normal, and scheduled an arthrogram to look for a rotator cuff tear. The next day, the patient called in a panic. His precocious 12-year-old daughter had noticed that when he tried to shave, his left shoulder blade stuck way out. The orthopedist examined him once again and indeed found that the child was correct. With forward flexion of the arm, there was marked winging of the scapula. He was treated with physical therapy and gradually made a complete recovery.

Comment

This case demonstrates the ease with which this diagnosis can be missed and the severe disability that can result from this lesion. The EMG was negative in this case. This can happen because the study is done too soon (before the denervation changes have developed) or because the muscle is not studied, since study of the serratus anterior is not routine and is somewhat difficult to do. In addition, the true nature of the lesion is open to question. This could have been a stretch injury or a restricted form of brachial plexitis. At any rate, these patients generally do quite well with conservative measures, and exploration of the nerve is almost never warranted.

Suprascapular

These neuropathies are quite rare. Unless part of the brachial plexitis syndrome, they are usually due to entrapment at the suprascapular notch. This may follow blunt trauma to the shoulder or may occur spontaneously. Patients often have pain in the medial posterior shoulder region, or they may be pain-free. The true hallmark is selective atrophy of the supra- and infraspinatus muscles with difficulty abducting and externally rotating the arm. EMG is useful to detect the selective involvement of these muscles, thereby excluding radiculopathies and plexopathies. Occasionally, there may be a delay in conduction across the suprascapular notch. If severe and progressive, these patients should be treated surgically with excision of the suprascapular ligament. However, in some cases, the nerve lesion may be in an area other than the suprascapular notch. Patients with entrapment of the nerve at the splenoglenoid notch have been reported, and in pathologic specimens, it has been shown that violent shoulder motions, such as baseball pitching, put stress on the nerve at multiple sites and may be due to vascular injury due to stretch with secondary nerve injury. In patients with splenoglenoid notch entrapment, pain is generally absent (since pain fibers exit the nerve proximal to the notch) and patients present with relatively asymptomatic weakness and atrophy of the infraspinatus muscle, which is relatively asymptomatic, even in world-class athletes. EMG is essential in these patients to localize the process.

Axillary

Damage to the axillary nerve is usually caused by trauma or brachial plexitis. Traumatic causes include dislocation of the shoulder or fracture of the neck of the humerus. The axillary nerve can also be stretched by blunt trauma to the shoulder. The resultant deficit is wasting and weakness of the deltoid muscle with marked impairment of shoulder abduction. In addition, sensory loss occurs in a small area over the insertion of the deltoid into the humerus. EMG is useful in confirming the mononeuropathy nature of the injury and in predicting outcome. If the nerve is only partially damaged and some of its fibers are still conducting, the outlook is good and full recovery generally occurs within a few months. If the muscle is completely denervated, the patient should be followed for several months. If there is clinical or EMG evidence of reinnervation after about 4 months, the patient should continue to be treated conservatively. If not, the nerve should be explored and reanastomosed. In either case, the patient usually makes a satisfactory recovery, since the distance for regeneration of the nerve is short.

Musculocutaneous

This uncommon mononeuropathy can follow shoulder dislocation or sudden violent movements of the arm, especially extension of the forearm with presumed stretching of the nerve. It can also be a rare manifestation of the brachial plexitis syndrome, although it almost never occurs as an isolated incident. Patients with this neuropathy have marked weakness of elbow flexion, especially with the forearm fully supinated, and sensory loss over the radial aspect of the volar forearm. Rupture of the biceps tendon can be confused with this disorder but can be distinguished by the physical features and the lack of sensory loss. If in doubt, EMG is helpful. Treatment follows the same principles listed above for the axillary nerve.

CONCLUSIONS

As our society becomes increasingly active, larger numbers of patients will be presenting with shoulder injuries due to weekend or casual athletic pursuits. The vast majority of these will not have neurologic involvement and will not require the services of a physician knowledgeable about peripheral nerve injuries. However, for the difficult or unusual case, it is important that those who manage these patients, including sports medicine physicians and orthopedists, be familiar with these disorders, since if they are missed early, patients do poorly and morbidity is increased. Unfortunately, the majority of physicians caring for these patients have limited training in peripheral nerve disease. In addition, EMG studies, which are often essential in diagnosis, management, and prognosis, are frequently poorly done and either not helpful or actually incorrect, deflecting the clinician even further from the correct diagnosis. Patients with subtle but important nerve lesions are often missed, leading in some cases to inappropriate surgery. Thus physicians who see large numbers of these patients should identify a physician knowledgeable in these areas and able to carry out adequate clinical evaluations and electrodiagnostic studies when needed.

CHAPTER 18

Shoulder Pain—Medical Causation

Donald Knowlan

INTRODUCTION

The late great baseball mogul Branch Rickey was fond of saying, "Luck is the residue of design!" In approaching the problem of shoulder pain, the clinician might keep this thought in mind.

Shoulder pain is one of the more frequent complaints that a patient will present to a primary care physician. In considering the etiologic possibilities, it is obvious that traumatic and musculoskeletal considerations should be the first thought of the physician, but prudent clinicians will briefly review in their minds the many other possible causes for shoulder pain. By doing so, they may uncover a treatable cause for the complaint.

Shoulder pain is usually caused by local musculoskeletal disorders related to trauma or overuse. It can also be caused by problems originating in adjacent structures, be part of general systemic disorder, or even be referred pain from distant internal organs.

In this chapter I selectively highlight certain aspects of these "nonorthopedic" conditions to broaden the diagnostic considerations.

A general outline of the medical causes of shoulder pain is listed below.

Medical Causes of Shoulder Pain

1. Local
   A. Injury—tear—rotator cuff
   B. Tendinitis—calcific (rotator cuff) biceps
   C. Infections—joint
   D. Impingement syndromes
   E. Adhesive capsulitis
2. Referred from local structures
   A. Spinal cord
      1. Tumor
      2. Disk
      3. Arthritis
      4. Intrinsic disease
   B. Compression syndrome—thoracic outlet syndromes
      1. Cervical rib
      2. Scalene anticus syndromes
      3. Brachial plexus involvement
      4. Costoclavicular compression
   C. Venous Occlusive disease

   D. Shoulder-hand syndrome (reflex sympathetic dystrophy)
3. Part of a systemic condition
   A. Osteoarthritis
   B. Rheumatoid arthritis
   C. Crystal-induced arthritis
      1. Gout
      2. Pseudogout
   D. Polymyalgia rheumatica
   E. Seronegative spondyloarthropathies (Reiter syndrome and other disorders)
   F. Bacteremia—endocarditis, gonococcal
   G. Lyme disease
   H. Neoplasm—hematologic
   I. Amyloid
   J. Hemoglobinopathies
4. Referred from internal organs
   A. Cardiac
      1. Coronary artery disease—angina
      2. Pericarditis—friction rub
      3. Aortic aneurysm
   B. Pulmonary
      1. Upper lobe lesion—Pancoast tumor
      2. Diaphragmatic irritation
         a. Pneumonia
         b. Embolism
         c. Effusion, etc.
   C. Gastrointestinal
      1. Esophagus
      2. Liver
      3. Gallbladder
   D. Spleen—Kehr's sign
   E. Subphrenic disease
      1. Ruptured viscus
      2. Abscess

LOCAL CAUSES

Injuries to the shoulder, both acute and chronic, are discussed elsewhere. Obviously, the primary care physician should make this evaluation and refer the patient when indicated.

Two more common medical causes of monoarticular disease are infectious arthritis and crystal-induced arthritis. If a septic joint is suspected, it is appropriate to tap the joint diagnostically before beginning therapy, observing the rheumatologic aphorism—"A monoarticular arthritis is septic until proven otherwise!" In general, one should tap every monoarticular arthritis for diagnosis and to rule out infection.

When crystal-induced arthritis involves the shoulder, it is important to know that these disorders rarely involve the shoulder joint alone. When the shoulder is involved in these conditions, it is usually part of a rarer generalized multiple joint manifestation of the disorders. If the diagnosis is not known, there may be easier joints to tap (knee, elbow, etc.). On the x-ray of the shoulder, the linear calcification of pseudogout can be seen. The shoulder is more frequently involved in pseudogout (larger joints) than in true gout.

REFERRED PAIN FROM ADJACENT STRUCTURES

Neurologic disorders (discussed elsewhere in this text) originating in the spinal cord, such as disks, tumors, and arthritis, can cause shoulder pain. The pattern of the pain suggests its origin. The pain is felt in the shoulder (C4, C5, C6 nerve dermatome) and may be most severe there but is associated with pain of lesser or greater degree in the neck. Later the pain may radiate distally along the upper extremity dermatome distribution (C5–T1). Physical findings are usually noted upon examination of the neck.

Compression Syndromes Compression syndromes involving the shoulder are secondary to many different area etiologies (congenital, traumatic, and overuse, etc.) and result in a variety of patterns of discomfort and disability for which individuals seek medical attention. The presentation may have a neurologic, arterial, and/or venous pattern depending on the location of the compression area.

Since neurologic disorders are discussed elsewhere in this text, I should only point out that the pattern of neurologic involvement with this syndrome follows the pattern of the well-localized nerve distribution of the upper extremity. Neurologic pain in the upper extremity tends to be intermittent, sharp, and radiating. So one may have shoulder pain with a specific radicular pain pattern that depends upon the nerve involved.

Compression syndromes involving the upper extremity comprise a group of syndromes that interfere with the passage of neck and mediastinal vascular structures and nerves into the axillary area and upper extremity and are classified broadly under the name "thoracic outlet syndrome."

ARTERIAL COMPRESSION SYNDROMES

The causes of vascular compression are multiple. It can be of congenital or traumatic origin. It can be caused by unusual positional changes such as carrying suitcases, sleeping with the arms extended over the head, or using heavy back packs, as in the military or recreational hikers. It is also seen in individuals with overuse syndromes involving the upper extremities with throwing motions as in pitching.

In arterial compression there are points that are most vulnerable to the syndrome: first, as the artery passes through the scalenus triangle between the scalenus muscles or as it passes between the first rib (or cervical rib) and clavicle (the costoclavicular area) and finally, as it passes through the subcoracoid space near the pectoralis muscle. The compression may involve bones (first rib, cervical rib, clavicle, spine, or scapular) or muscles, the subclavian, scalenus group, or pectoralis group or both. Movements of the shoulder may aggravate the compression.

The history is helpful in the diagnosis of upper extremity vascular compression. The patient may complain of fatigue with exercise, athletes with throwing. Endurance is limited and velocity reduced. A pitcher loses speed each inning, notes diminished velocity, and cannot pitch as long. He complains the arm is "heavy and swollen," although it is not. The pain is dull and aching in contrast to neurologic pain, which is sharp and radicular. The pain of vascular compression is related to effort and relieved by rest and dependency.

The physical examination holds the real clues. There may be a difference in blood pressure recordings between the upper extremities, often greater than 20 mmHg. Nuber et al.[1] describe 13 athletes with arterial compression in the upper extremity and all but one had a diminished radial pulse. Bruits are commonly heard in the involved extremity, especially when in a position of function. The bruits are heard in the supraclavicular, infraclavicular, or axillary areas.

Certain maneuvers are helpful in the diagnosis. Elevating the chin while extending the neck or rotating the head laterally while holding a deep inspiration will diminish the radial pulse on the affected side (Adson maneuver). One may also hyperabduct the affected extremity (raising the arms fully above the head) and externally rotating the hands and again observing for changes in intensity of the radial pulse on the affected side.

Pulse differences, delayed arterial filling of the hand (Allen's test), cool hands and fingers, arterial necrosis of hands and fingers, Raynaud's phenomenon (unilaterally), cold hands, and cold sensitivity especially on one side may also be clues to the diagnosis of arterial compression syndrome originating near the shoulder. Further diagnostic tests are required to confirm and localize the diagnosis. X-rays of the chest, shoulder, and neck are necessary. Nerve conduction studies may be indicated. Doppler studies may be helpful but are not conclusive. They may help in localizing the area of obstruction. Arteriograms are more conclusive, but even these must be performed in a position of function to maximize their value. MRI angiograms are now replacing routine arteriogram as a safer procedure.

Treatment depends upon the etiology and location of the lesion. It is prudent to begin with a conservative regime. A period of nonoperative rehabilitation should be tried directed toward strengthening and positioning of the neck muscles, particularly when a specific cause is not found despite extensive diagnostic tests. A careful history should be combined with therapy directed to avoiding aggravating positions and the strengthening of different muscle groups to maintain proper balance. At times, even correction of an obvious defect, such as a cervical rib, is not always curative. A conservative and careful personally designed rehabilitative program is a good initial approach even in an athlete.

VENOUS OCCLUSIVE DISEASE OF THE UPPER EXTREMITY

Signs and symptoms of upper extremity venous occlusive disease are rarely the result of thoracic outlet syndrome but more commonly the result of the "de novo" appearance of a venous clot within the deep veins (subclavian-auxiliary system) of the upper extremity. It is as common in the athlete and nonathlete population. It was initially felt to be related to extremes in effort ("effort syndrome"), such as weight lifting, and occurs in that situation today. New etiologies have been uncovered and include trauma, catheters, hypercoagulable states, neoplasms, vasculitides and cocaine and IV drug use. Initially felt to be benign with a pulmonary embolism risk of zero, Horattas et al.[2] recently reported a 12.6 percent incidence of pulmonary embolism in this group of patients.

The clinical picture in the athlete is fairly constant. There are usually two forms of presentation; the first and more common is that of the acute onset of a dull, constant, annoying type of pain in the axillary and shoulder area with minimal upper arm radiation, the slow development of moderate swelling of the extremity, and the later appearance of superficial venous pattern in the arm and shoulder.

The second pattern of presentation is a much slower semiacute onset of swelling of the upper extremity and venous pattern formation over a period of several weeks, with a slowly increasing intensity of an intermittent dull, aching axillary and upper arm pain and discomfort.

The usual noninvasive diagnostic tests such as Doppler flow techniques, plethysmography, and radionucleotide tests can be helpful but are less effective in the diagnosis of upper extremity venous occlusive disorders than in lower extremity venous problems. Venography remains the definitive test, although the MRI venogram may become the ultimate test of choice.

Treatment approaches over the years have varied, and for many years, the treatment choice was no treatment. In view of the potential for pulmonary emboli, a 3- to 5-day course of heparin therapy followed by a variable period of oral coumadin therapy is recommended. Attention should be directed toward eliminating any certain compression causing anatomic structures such as cervical ribs. A search for underlying systemic disorders such as collagen vascular disease, hypercoagulable states, and neoplasms is in order. Modification of position factors (sleep patterns, etc.) and changes in lifting techniques may be beneficial. Stretching techniques may be beneficial as they may reduce the effects of compression.

There is some evidence to suggest the clots in the upper extremity continue to extend rather than to throw emboli, and consideration should be given to ligation of these vessels to prevent future catastrophic events.

The concepts and approach to this disorder are changing and the frequency increasing, so that therapeutic decisions require constant review.

SHOULDER AND HAND SYNDROME (REFLEX SYMPATHETIC DYSTROPHY SYNDROME)

This disorder of unknown etiology usually follows trauma to neck, shoulder, or upper extremity, myocardial infarction, or cerebral vascular disease and is associated with conditions known to involve long periods of nonuse of the upper extremity. It presents with shoulder pain and often pain in the wrist and/or hand, with swelling of the wrist and hand, and is accompanied by vasomotor instability (Raynaud's phenomenon). It is often extremely disabling, results in long-term atrophy, and "burns out" months after onset. Minor variations of this disorder are now more common.

The best treatment is early mobilization and activity with emphasis on the shoulder area. Once it is evident that the shoulder-hand syndrome is present, intense physiotherapy is the best approach.

Fortunately, this painful and disabling disorder is less common today, with the emphasis on early ambulation and activity.

SYSTEMIC CAUSES OF SHOULDER PAIN

Common arthritides may involve the shoulder, but rarely is it the only joint involved in such conditions.

Rheumatoid arthritis is the commonest cause of inflammatory involvement of the shoulder joint in susceptible individuals (young women, age 25 to 45). It is rarely an isolated finding. The diagnostic clinical features of the disease are long present when the shoulder is involved, and the diagnosis should be apparent.

Osteoarthritis is the commonest chronic arthritis that affects the acromioclavicular joint and may be an overuse-related event or be posttraumatic in origin. It may occur simply as a "wear and tear" phenomenon. It is recognized clinically by localized tenderness, and the pain is aggravated by elevation of the arm above the shoulder and by lying on the shoulder during sleep. Conservative physical therapy with nonsteroidal anti-inflammatory drugs begins therapy with local injection to follow in the more resistant cases.

Osteoarthritis involving the glenohumeral joint causes a nonlocalizing "toothache"-like pain that is aggravated by motion and may be associated with muscle atrophy and contractions. Crepitation on physical examination is a feature. Treatment consists of intense physiotherapy and pain-relieving measures.

The crystal-induced arthritis involving the shoulder has been mentioned. The diagnosis does not present a problem. In gout, the shoulder is involved only in the rarer form of polyarticular arthritis. A diagnosis can be made by taping the most accessible joint and looking for the diagnostic crystals under polarized light. A similar statement can be made about the syndrome "pseudogout" with its calcium pyrophosphate crystals seen under the polarizing light of the microscope when examining joint fluid. In addition, the linear calcification seen in this con-

dition may be present in the x-ray examination of the shoulder.

The seronegative spondyloarthropathies (Reiter syndrome, psoriatic arthritis, and the enteropathic arthritis) may involve the shoulder during their course. Since these are illnesses of the young, an appreciation of the clinical course of these conditions is helpful in reaching a proper diagnosis. This is illustrated by the following case report.

Case Report
A 24-year-old white male professional football player reported to the trainer during summer camp in late July, complaining of acute onset of fever, chills, and diarrhea that became bloody. Campylobacteria was detected in the stool cultures and he was given a course of erythromycin. He became asymptomatic. Three weeks later he complained of pain in the right jaw and sought dental help. Two weeks later a dull ache appeared with slight decrease range of motion in the right shoulder. Three weeks later (6 weeks after onset of symptoms) in early September, he awoke with a swollen, painful, slightly tender right knee, but denied injury. A tap revealed an exudate with 75,000 WBC, an increase in protein, but no blood and no organism. A bone scan revealed lesions in the jaw, shoulder, knee, and left ankle, which later flared. He was found to be positive for HLA B27 antigen. A diagnosis of postgastrointestinal infection Reiter syndrome was made. He was given a course of indocin (150 to 200 mg per day) with improvement but was unable to play until December, when all his joint involvement (including the left ankle, which flared in October) spontaneously cleared.

This is a fairly typical course for Reiter syndrome, in my experience. It is the commonest form of arthritis in the young athlete. It is often missed because we see the condition in a single phase of its natural course, "a snapshot single-frame view of a motion picture reel."

This illness follows a gastrointestinal infection (acute bacterial *Salmonella, Shigella, Yersinia,* or *Campylobacter* and/or a genital urinary infection (nonspecific urethritis or prostatitis secondary to the *Chlamydia* organism) occurring in a genetically susceptible individual and is an immunologically reactive response. The knee is the commonest joint involved, but the ankle, elbow, wrist, hip, and shoulder may be involved in sequence as it was in this individual. Few athletes can participate in athletic activities during the active phase of the illness, which lasts from 6 weeks to 3 months, and up to 6 months. It may become chronic, limiting long-term participation, or exacerbate and remit over the years with or without a stimulus.

Achilles tendinitis and plantar fasciitis are common presentations of this disorder, and during the course of the illness, acute conjunctivitis, iriditis, and painless rashes of the mucous membranes of the mouth and penile area are seen. A diastolic murmur of the aortic valve has been described.

It is important to recognize its frequency in the young and its natural history in order to properly rehabilitate the athlete. The clue in a more recent case I've seen was a bilateral conjunctivitis. Physicians who evaluate athletes should be familiar with its chronic course and its tendency to exacerbate and remit.

Psoriatic arthritis is another arthritic condition involving large joints that is present with the classic psoriatic rash. The arthritis has a number of patterns. There may be back pain, peripheral joint, or migratory large joint involvement. The rash is the clue.

In the arthritis associated with the inflammatory gastrointestinal diseases, regional ileitis and ulcerative colitis, the gastrointestinal symptoms are almost always present first, so the etiology can be suspected. The arthritis in these conditions can have a variety of presentations, including the commoner back (sacroiliac) discomfort; a generalized arthralgia with a limited arthritis; a rheumatoid-like disorder (hands and feet); large multiple migrating joint disease, or more rarely large-joint monoarticular disease (knee, hip, shoulder, or elbow).

The important point here is that any arthritic disorder or pattern of arthritis seen in individuals with these disorders should be suspected of being part of the pattern of the general disease, be it psoriasis or inflammatory bowel disease.

Lyme disease is a typical spirochetal illness with three phases. The first phase is the rash (erythremia chronica migrans) with its hyperemic and central clearing, following a tick bite. The ticks carry the spirochete to the human from the deer. It is associated with a "flu-like" illness of 7 to 10 days; 2 to 6 weeks later phase II appears with either cardiac or neurological symptoms. The cardiac presentation characteristically involves the A.V. node with varying degrees of block. The neurologic involvement is sometimes diffuse and variable, often confusing, with multiple presentations of one or many parts of the nervous system, including any area of the brain, cranial nerves, spinal cord, or motor or sensory systems.

In the third phase (6 months to 2 years later) there is a subacute migratory polyarthritis involving large joints, usually the knee, but also the elbow, ankle, hip, and shoulder, with pain, swelling, slight redness, and an inflammatory exudative nonbacterial fluid aspiration. The diagnosis is made from the clinical picture and the slow resolving IgG antibody titer during the arthritic or late phase of the illness. The tick (*Borrelia burgdorferi*) DNA can now be detected with polymerase chain reaction in the synovial fluid of the involved joint in patients with Lyme arthritis.[6]

Certain malignancies, especially hematological disorders, i.e., acute leukemia, may present with single large-joint involvement as part of a migratory arthritis. The shoulder joint is commonly involved in this rare presentation of these disorders. The pain is usually out of proportion to the objective findings. There have been reports of the joint findings appearing days or even a few weeks before the hematological evidence of disease.

Among individuals with hematological disorders, none has a more interesting musculoskeletal presentation than those with disorders of hemoglobin (Hb) synthesis or structure, known as the hemoglobinopathies. The most well-known of these disorders, classified according to their abnormal electrophoretic patterns, is sickle cell disease (S-S), in which a single amino acid substitution in the normal hemoglobin protein is responsible for the hemolytic process and clinical presentation. Numerous genotypes of the sickling syndrome other than Hb S-S have been described. Classifications depend upon the abnormal amino acid substituted in the hemoglobin protein and are named accordingly sickle C, D, E, etc., with combinations of all these types also occurring.

When joint pain occurs in individuals with hemoglobinopathies, there are several possible causes including local infection or thrombus with avascular necrosis. A more generalized, vague discomfort is seen in sickle cell trait. Any time one suspects avascular necrosis involving the hip or shoulder (the two commonest joints involved), a search for an underlying hemoglobinopathy should be made. Aseptic necrosis occurs in 20 to 68 percent of patients with the hemoglobinopathy S-C disease and in 4 to 12 percent of individuals with the hemoglobinopathy S-S disease. Arthritis involving the shoulder joint should always raise the possibility of a hematological disorder.

SHOULDER PAIN REFERRED FROM INTERNAL ORGANS

Shoulder pain can be a reflection of pathology in an internal organ. This is the result of many factors but particularly due to the fact that the phrenic nerve (C3, C4, C5), the sole motor nerve to the diaphragm, forms in the neck and traverses the inner thoracic cavity on its route to the diaphragm. Its sensory fibers (C3, C4, C5) supply sensation to the lower posterior neck and shoulder area. Any stimulation of the phrenic nerve will transmit back to the cord and its sensory distribution along the C3, C4, and C5 dermatomes.

During the routine physical examination, referred pain can be suspected when the examiner can find no area of tenderness and the patient can complete the normal range of motion for the shoulder joint.

The Heart Of all the organs that refer pain to the shoulder, none is more important to consider as a source than the heart and the presence of underlying coronary artery disease. Despite a huge assortment of diagnostic tools the history remains the focus of the diagnosis for this condition.

Case Report

A 54-year-old physician, a long-term jogger, began to notice a dull, aching pain in the left shoulder while jogging that disappeared when he rested. The pain became more intense, with earlier onset and longer period for relief. A visit to his friend, an orthopedist, resulted in a trial of nsaids and then a cortisone injection, without relief. Six months after the onset, he collapsed and expired while running. At autopsy, he had extensive three-vessel coronary artery disease with occlusions.

The key to the diagnosis of coronary artery disease is a high level of suspicion and a thorough history with particular emphasis on the character of the pain. Although in over 90 percent of patients with coronary disease, there is a lower substernal component, in 5 to 10 percent the pain is located in one of the common radiation sites, the jaw, shoulder, elbow, wrist, arm, teeth, or face. When it is located in a radiation site, at times a vague minimal substernal discomfort is present on careful questioning.

The pain of coronary disease when isolated to the shoulder (almost always the left) is dull and heavy, never sharp, and is unrelated to the range of motion of the shoulder. It is usually precipitated by exercise, cold weather, heavy meals, and emotional upset. It is relieved in a few minutes by rest when brought on by exercise. Coronary pain always lasts for minutes, and not seconds, as in musculoskeletal disorders, or days, as in depressive disorders. Nitroglycerin, a therapeutic agent, can be used diagnostically. It will relieve the pain of angina in 1 to 3 min. It can be used prophylactically if one takes it before the exercise to see if it controls the pain.

Coronary artery disease should be suspected in an individual over 40 with onset of shoulder pain with exercise, who has a normal physical examination, and in whom the pain is relieved with rest.

The diagnosis once suspected can be further confirmed by the use of nitroglycerin diagnostically and prophylactically. One can obtain an electrocardiogram during pain and also obtain an exercise stress test that reproduces the pain to help further substantiate the diagnosis.

Pulmonary Referral Pathology, particularly tumors, at the pleural apex or superior sulcus (Pancoast tumors) may invade the local area and commonly present as shoulder pain. Demaziere and Wiley[3] describe three young (below 40) patients presenting with severe shoulder pain with a frozen shoulder felt to be local, who later were discovered to have locally primary invasive neoplasms that were detected only after a period of persistent pain and an unresponsive frozen shoulder.

Disease states such as pleural effusions, lower-lobe pneumonia, and pulmonary emboli commonly present with referred pain to the local shoulder secondary to diaphragmatic irritation. A simple chest film can be a very rewarding diagnostic test in a patient with a puzzling problem of chest pain.

Subdiaphragmatic Source of Shoulder Pain Pathologic organs that lie below the diaphragm may cause shoulder pain through diaphragmatic irritation and referable sensation to the phrenic nerve sensory distribution of C3, C4, C5.

Pain in the left shoulder may be the earliest clue to disease of the spleen. The classic Kehr's sign (pain in the left shoulder with rupture of the spleen) has been devalued by many but not by Lowenfels,[4] who modified its use with elevation of the foot of the bed, combined with gentle pressure to stimulate the phrenic nerve and produce a positive sign in nine of ten patients with ruptured spleens. Minor abdominal trauma with subsequent left shoulder pain a week or two later is a variant of this sign.

Dilatation of the stomach and/or left colon ("the splenic flexure syndrome") may cause shoulder pain but is accompanied by left anterior discomfort as well. Gastric ulcers adjacent to the diaphragm have been reported presenting as shoulder pain.[5]

Perforations of abdominal organs with pneumoperitoneum and air under the diaphragm may produce shoulder pain, often with a negative general examination. A chest film will be helpful here.

Gallbladder disease may refer pain to the right shoulder, but it is usually the liver with a rapidly expanding capsule secondary to abscesses or tumor that may irritate the diaphragm and refer pain to the right shoulder.

REFERENCES

1. Nuber GW, McCarthy WJ, Yao JS, et al: Arterial Abnormalities of the Shoulder in Athletes. *Am J Sports Med* 18(5):514–591, 1990.
2. Horattas MC, Wright DJ, Fenton AH, et al: Changing concepts of deep venous thrombosis of the upper extremity—Report of a series and review of the literature. *Surgery* September 1988, 561–567.
3. Demaziere A, Wiley AM: Primary chest wall tumor appearing as frozen shoulder, review and care presentation. *J Rheumatol* 18:911–914, 1991.
4. Lowenfels AB: Kehr's sign—A neglected aid in rupture of the spleen. *N Engl J Med* 274(18):1019–1049, 1966.
5. Valenzuela GA, Mittal RK, Shaffer HA, Hanks J: Shoulder pain: An unusual presentation gastric ulcer. *South Med J* 82:1446–1447, November 1989.
6. Nacton JJ et al: Detection of *Borrelia burgdorferi* DNA by polymerase chain reaction in the synovial fluid from patients with Lyme arthritis. *New Engl J Med* 330(46):229–234, 1994.

BIBLIOGRAPHY

Bathon JM: Shoulder pain, in *Principles of Ambulatory Medicine*, 3d ed. Baltimore, Williams & Wilkins, 1991, chap 63, pp 799–806.
Thornhill TS: Shoulder pain, in Kelly WN, Harris EA, Ruddy S, Sledge CB: *Textbook of Rheumatology*, 4th ed. Philadelphia, Saunders, 1993, chap 26, pp 417–440.
Kozin F: Painful shoulder and reflex sympathetic dystrophy syndrome, in McCarty D, Koopman WJ (eds): *Arthritis and Allied Conditions*, 12th ed. Philadelphia, Lea and Febiger, 1993, chap 99, pp 1643–1676.

CHAPTER 19

Shoulder Rehabilitation—Rotator Cuff Disease

Janet Sobel

The shoulder is the most versatile joint in the human body, and as such it must balance a perfectly coordinated interplay of stability and mobility. In meeting the demands of sports and daily activities, the shoulder is likely to undergo changes that lead to overuse damage. In fact, the instability–rotator cuff disease–impingement continuum as described by Jobe[33] is the most common overuse injury in the upper body. Through application of prehabilitation principles in athletes participating in overhead sports, we can often prevent the onset of rotator cuff disease. In those who present to us with the disease already in progress, effective conservative management can often resolve it. Where surgery is necessary, comprehensive rehabilitation is essential to the athlete returning to fullest functional potential. This chapter surveys the factors relevant to rotator cuff disease and then reviews the current knowledge on rehabilitation of rotator cuff disease.

ANATOMIC AND BIOMECHANICAL CONSIDERATIONS

The shoulder complex is made up of five joints whose coordinated actions result in efficient and accurate use of the arm: the sternoclavicular; acromioclavicular; scapulothoracic, suprahumeral or humerocoracoclavicular joint (the coracoacromial arch, subacromial bursa, and the humerus); and the glenohumeral joint. With essentially no inherent stability from the glenohumeral joint surfaces, the stability must be provided for by soft tissues. The capsule-ligamentous complex provides static stability, while dynamic stability is created by the many interacting muscles.

In the upper body's kinetic chain, the shoulder joint complex is the link between the trunk and the arm. With contributions from the acromioclavicular and sternoclavicular joints, the coordinated interactions of the glenohumeral and scapulothoracic joints create mobility without compromising stability. Any disturbance of this delicate balance can result in injury. Morrey and An describe the variety of ways in which the muscles act to dynamically stabilize the joint: through passive muscle tension; moving the joint, which results in tightening the ligamentous constraints; creating a barrier effect (e.g., subscapularis); and compressing the joint surfaces (the rotator cuff).[39] These muscles can be divided into four groups based on their origins and insertions:[16,35]

1. Scapulohumeral: supraspinatus, infraspinatus, teres minor and subscapularis, teres major, deltoid, coracobrachialis
2. Axioscapular (scapula to spine): trapezii, levator scapula, rhomboids major and minor, and serratus anterior
3. Axiohumeral: latissimus dorsi, pectoralis major
4. Scapuloradial and scapuloulnar: biceps and triceps

Table 19-1 reviews each of the muscles, and their function.

In addition to their independent roles in movement at the glenohumeral joint, the muscles of the rotator cuff act together to dynamically stabilize the joint. Thus the muscles must simultaneously stabilize and mobilize! The major role of the supraspinatus is to compress the humeral head against the glenoid, providing a fulcrum for elevation of the arm; 97 percent of its contractile force is directed toward glenohumeral joint compression.[66] The supraspinatus accounts for 50 percent of the torque output in humeral elevation up to 90°.[29,32] Howell[28] found that the supraspinatus and deltoid are equally responsible for producing torque about the shoulder in flexion and scapular plane elevation, or scaption (Perry, 1990). The subscapularis, infraspinatus, and teres minor act together to pull the humeral head down to the lower, wider portion of the glenoid in elevation. This rolling down, or "caudal glide," is critical to normal function of the shoulder joint complex and injury prevention. According to Saha, if a healthy relationship exists, locking of the greater tuberosity against the acromion never occurs in active elevation due to this or caudal glide of the humeral head in the glenoid.[57] The interactions of the deltoid and rotator cuff create one of the force couples at the shoulder

TABLE 19-1

Muscles and Their Functions[34]

Muscle	Function	Comments
Supraspinatus	Stabilizes humeral head in glenoid Abducts shoulder	Best manual muscle tests: "Empty can"; prone horizontal abduction at 100° with full external rotation
Infraspinatus	Stabilizes humeral head in glenoid Externally rotates	
Teres minor	As infraspinatus	
Subscapularis	Internally rotates Stabilizes humeral head in glenoid	
Teres major	Extends, adducts, internally rotates	Tightness limits scapular rotation for full humeral elevation
Deltoid	Anterior: flexes, internally rotates Medial: abducts Posterior: extends, externally rotates	
Coracobrachialis	Flexes, adducts shoulder	
Trapezius	Anterior: elevates and upwardly rotates scapula; stabilizes for scapular adduction Medial: adducts scapula, stabilizes for upward rotation Lower: depresses and upwardly rotates scapula, stabilizes for scapular adduction	Best manual muscle test for middle trapezius: Prone horizontal abduction at 90° with full external rotation For lower trapezius: Prone, arms overhead with elbows straight, full external rotation
Levator scapula	Scapular adduction, elevation and downward rotation	
Rhomboids	Scapular adduction, elevation and downward rotation	
Serratus anterior	Abducts, upwardly rotates scapula; stabilizes medial border of scapula against thorax	Weakness results in winging of the medial border of the scapula
Latissimus dorsi	Extends, adducts, internally rotates	
Pectoralis major	Adducts, internally rotates Upper: flexes, internally rotates, horizontally adducts to opposite shoulder Lower: horizontally adducts to opposite hip	
Pectoralis minor	Pulls coracoid anterior and caudally, tilting scapula anteriorly	Pectoralis minor: tightness may cause pressure on the underlying cords of the brachial plexes and axillary vessels, and/or may limit full shoulder flexion

joint complex, whose balanced interactions are essential to normal mechanics. A force couple is the application of combined forces to produce a specific type of rotation or movement.[18,25] The combined actions of the upper and lower trapezius rotate the scapula around the acromioclavicular center of rotation, depressing the vertebral border and elevating the glenoid fossa.[25,61] It is noteworthy that lower trapezius weakness is a common finding in patients with rotator cuff dysfunction. The trapezius and serratus anterior act as a force couple in holding the scapula against the thorax, thus preventing winging; and in tracking the scapula anteriorly, laterally, and superiorly for upward rotation of the glenoid fossa.[13] The serratus anterior, trapezii, and rhomboids stabilize the scapula to the thorax. Along with the rotator cuff muscles, the biceps and triceps each has a stabilizing role at the glenohumeral joint. The biceps dynamically prevents upward humeral head subluxation, and the triceps prevents subluxation downward.[41]

Additional Considerations

Age and hereditary factors must be taken into consideration in treating the athletic individual's shoulder. Since people of all ages are participating in sports more and more, degenerative and age-related changes are relevant. These may begin as early as the second decade in the acromioclavicular joint, eventually leading to acromial and acromioclavicular joint spurs that may cause narrowing of the supraspinatus outlet.[29] Shoulder range of motion decreases with age owing to mechanical stresses, osteoarthritis, and altered scapular position.[10] Finally, degeneration of the rotator cuff itself is at least partly related to the aging process. Petersson found that in 27 untraumatized, asymptomatic shoulders in patients 55 to 85 years old, 13 had partial or full rotator cuff tears.[50] De Palma had similar findings.[14] Although aging of the rotator cuff is a chronologic process, its pace and intensity are largely affected by the demands placed upon it and its physiologic ability to handle these demands. In approaching a patient's rotator cuff problem, age clearly is a significant factor. In working with the older athlete, it is essential to consider the degenerative factors of aging, e.g., subacromial space compromise, decreased vascularity, spurs and arthritic changes, alteration in the quality of the capsule, rotator cuff degeneration, and slower healing times.[59] In the younger athlete's shoulder restoring the mobility-stability balance is the critical concern. Factors in the problem may well include faulty sport mechanics, training errors, and strength-flexibility imbalances.

Sports Considerations   Rotator cuff disease is common to several sports. A study by Scovazzo et al.[58] found shoulder problems in 66 percent of elite swimmers, 57 percent of professional baseball players, 44 percent of college volleyball players, 29 percent of college javelin throwers, and 7 percent of pro golfers. We have found rotator cuff tears to be the second most common overuse problem in recreational and professional tennis players. In each sport, factors may include excessive repetition rate and motion extremes, training intensity, technique faults and biomechanical flaws, and force generated. Psychosocial pressure and rigorous schedules often overpower physical warnings. The shoulder is the

link in the kinetic chain between the lower body, the trunk, and the arm. As it is fairly far along the kinetic chain, it is subject to overload by technique faults in previous links. Thus compromised lower body mechanics and/or flexibility or strength deficits earlier in the kinetic chain can also contribute to shoulder overload in its effort to compensate.

Impingement Syndrome and Its Role in Rotator Cuff Disease

In order to effectively rehabilitate the shoulder, it would be ideal to understand the pathologic processes involved. Impingement syndrome has often been used as a catchall term to describe the factors involved at the shoulder. Recently, several authors have described what seem to be the major factors, and we appreciate that impingement syndrome and rotator cuff disease are not equatable. There is currently considerable discussion as to the cause-and-effect relationships that exist among these factors.[4,19,33,43,45,68] Early concepts, largely based on shoulders in patients over 40 where disruptions in the size of the subacromial space (e.g., spurs, osteophytes, coracoacromial ligament thickening) were common, described a primary impingement of the rotator cuff in the coracoacromial arch in which there is a wearing down of the rotator cuff against the anterior acromion simply from overhead movements.[42] In 1984, Nirschl introduced the concept of a secondary impingement process in the younger population, in which the rotator cuff tendons are subjected to tensile overload from intrinsic muscle contraction, especially eccentric, and excessive shear forces.[47] At the same time, glenohumeral instability (from heredity, trauma, or overload) with labrum deficiency, common to overhead sports, contributes to more rotator cuff overload, with resultant fatigue, weakening avascularity, and pathologic changes within the cuff, dysfunction, and altered shoulder mechanics. The rotator cuff fails in its role, and leads to a secondary impingement syndrome with bony changes, coracoacromial arch compromise, and joint dysfunction.[45] Clark and Sidles noted that, since at least half the capsular surface receives an insertion of fibers from the rotator cuff, some of the tension generated by the cuff may be distributed to the capsule. Tears in the rotator cuff, then, will alter the anatomy of the capsule.[12] Jobe introduced the concept of athletic shoulder dysfunction as a continuum of instability and impingement: Overuse stretches and breaks down the static stabilizers, allowing anterior humeral head subluxation, and disrupts the balanced interaction of the rotator cuff and scapular stabilizers as they try to provide stability.[33]

Pathoanatomic factors have also been implicated by some as major factors in shoulder problems. These include anatomic variations in the shape of the acromion,[4,29] shape of the coracoid,[22] and slope of the shoulder.[29] Hereditary factors that might affect injury potential include "mesenchymal syndrome" as described by Nirschl,[45] in which a systemic constitutional factor results in multiple sites of tendon pain and alteration. Calcific deposits in the tendon are not uncommon in the over-40 athlete. Apparently there is no relationship between the size of the deposit and the symptoms,[49] and thus its effect on rehabilitation potential does not seem to be significant. Adhesive capsulitis, or frozen shoulder, occurs most commonly in 40- to 60-year-olds. Nobuhara studied 2027 patients with limited shoulder motion and found 32 percent with degenerative rotator cuff disease.[48] It has been our experience that in patients with both adhesive capsulitis and rotator cuff disease, it is critical that restoration of rotator cuff strength be addressed before or with regaining full shoulder motion, but certainly not after.

Treatment Focus

The core of creating normal shoulder function is in reestablishing the constant interplay of stability and mobility among all the players in the shoulder joint complex. Dysfunction and/or structural alterations of any of these will most likely set off a chain of events leading ultimately to its failure in meeting the demand of sport and often of daily living. Unfortunately, it is often the sports and daily activities themselves that create these stresses and imbalances. If continued performance is to be expected, these imbalances must be identified and corrected. Shoulder dysfunction in the young athlete, then, may be initiated by instability, rotator cuff weakness, flexibility, and strength imbalances; changes under the coracoacromial arch; and/or ligamentous inadequacy.

Principles of Treatment

- The ligaments are the static stabilizers of the shoulder but are often injured in sports participation. Their dysfunction in repeated throwing will allow excessive humeral head translation, resulting in possible impingement of the rotator cuff in the coracoacromial arch. With stretching of the capsule and ligaments, their effectiveness decreases and the rotator cuff and scapular rotators become overloaded in trying to compensate.[33] A

tight posterior capsule may result in forcing the humeral head upward against the undersurface of the acromion in forward flexion.[29,38]

- The rotator cuff muscles are the dynamic stabilizers, centering and holding the humeral head in the glenoid, positioning the joint effectively, and forming a barrier resisting translation. Each sport induces certain imbalances that may in and of themselves promote injury. The nature of most overhead sports creates an overloading of the posterior cuff muscles and overdevelopment of the anterior cuff. At the same time, excessive external rotation motion is needed for maximum performance and internal rotation motion diminishes significantly. Chandler et al.[11] found significant tightness of the tennis player's internal rotation and proposed that this might cause a vicious cycle of microtrauma to the tight muscles, instabilities, further imbalances, and injury. Flexibility and strength deficits throughout the kinetic chain, previous injury with inadequate rehabilitation, day-to-day posturally induced imbalances, and poor cardiovascular conditioning also play roles. Among professional tennis players, we have found significant weakness in the rotator cuff and scapular stabilizers, often before the player complains of pain or is aware of a problem. Loss of dynamic stabilization from these sport-induced imbalances and further muscle deterioration ensues. They fatigue earlier and an intrinsic tension overload results, developing into a vicious cycle of pathologic changes, decreased efficiency, superior humeral head migration, and impingement.[47] In an isokinetic study, Falkel et al. found that swimmers with shoulder pain have lower external to internal rotator endurance (42 percent) than swimmers without pain (56 percent) and nonswimmers (67 percent). They concluded that once the imbalance of external rotation: internal rotation falls below 50 percent, the swimmer's stroke mechanics are altered and further problems ensue.[18] This may also be an issue in throwing and racket sports.

- Changes under the coracoacromial arch. With progression of rotator cuff disease, the subacromial bursa becomes involved and the normally gliding surfaces become thickened and adherent with chronic cuff irritation and another vicious cycle. Eventually degenerative changes in the acromioclavicular joint, e.g., spurs or osteophytes, add to the cycle. Guidi and Nirschl's algorithm summarizes the interactions very effectively (Fig. 19-1).

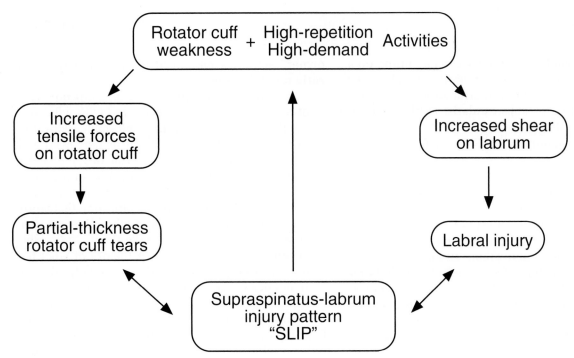

FIGURE 19-1
Algorithm of factors in rotator cuff disease.[24]

Extrinsic factors that will alter mechanics and enter into the cycle include:

- Cervical problems: Spondylolysis, cervical strain, or C5-C6 nerve root irritation will result in weakening of the spinati as well as spasms of the upper trapezius and levator scapula.

- Poor posture, a common problem in the recreational athlete who spends considerable time at a desk or computer, will result in functional dorsal kyphosis, weakening of the scapular rotators and retractors, and tightening of the anterior shoulder structures.

- Serratus anterior palsy from long thoracic nerve paralysis (e.g., in weight lifters) will result in failure of the scapular placement mechanism, winging, and instability.

- Suprascapular nerve injury (not uncommon in weight lifters, baseball players, volleyball players, and photographers) from compression may result in infraspinatus atrophy and dysfunction.[6,54]

- Thoracic outlet syndrome and vascular lesions have been found in baseball pitchers owing to hypertrophy of the pectoralis minor and scalenus, humeral hypertrophy, and glenohumeral subluxation.[49] Any effective rehabilitation program will address itself ultimately to identifying and correcting or minimizing all the factors involved in each patient.

Conservative Treatment of Rotator Cuff Disease

SUBJECTIVE EVALUATION

Developing an effective treatment plan for rotator cuff disease begins with a thorough subjective evaluation. We begin with asking the patient about the current problem, then working outward to the history and other issues.

Is this your dominant arm? For all activities and sports?

How did the problem start? Often with rotator cuff disease, the patient will describe a several-month history of minor awareness of something wrong, then a sudden increase in symptoms with an overhead activity.

What caused you to seek out medical attention? What is the primary complaint? This may be pain and/or weakness and/or instability and/or loss of motion. Catching and crepitus are usually a secondary complaint. Night pain or pain that interferes with their sport is often what spurs patients to seek medical attention.

When does it hurt? Common complaints include:

- Night pain, especially with lying on the involved side, common with rotator cuff disease.

- Pain with the arm overhead, especially against resistance, or in driving with the hand atop the wheel.

249

- Pain with arm behind the back, e.g., putting on a coat or reaching to the back of the car. This may suggest weakness of the anterior-superior capsule, supraspinatus, or subscapularis, as they are all stressed in this position.
- Pain with arm out to side (e.g., reaching for parking ticket).

Pain Intensity   A visual analog scale is helpful, in which patients identify the pain intensity on a 0 to 10 line scale in daily activities (A), sports (S), and at rest (R). Using the pain phases, they also identify their current level of pain (Table 19-2).

Where does it hurt? Often the worst pain is referred to the deltoid tubercle. If pain is experienced below the elbow, it is likely that the problem is more than rotator cuff disease. The patient may describe acromioclavicular joint pain or anterior, middle, or posterior shoulder pain.

Sports   What sports do patients participate in and how has this affected their participation? They may complain of a "dead arm" feeling in overhead sports, indicative of a labral injury; pain on bench press and/or pushups (where the arm is extended, externally rotated, and abducted) is stressing the anterior-superior capsule and middle glenohumeral ligament. Many tennis players will complain of pain in the serve or high backhand volley. Baseball and tennis players and swimmers often complain of early fatigue with rotator cuff dysfunction. Very importantly, has there been any recent change in equipment, technique, or playing intensity? This is often a precursor to injury.

Lifestyle and ADLs   It is essential to know other activities in which the patient participates that may factor into the problem. Extensive cooking, heavy outdoor work or house cleaning, and "Harry homeowner" activities may need to be curtailed during early rehabilitation.

How long has this problem been going on? What treatments have you undergone and with what success? Patients are often uncomfortable with this subject for fear of being disloyal or perceived as a "doctor shopper." It is often the role of the physical therapist to put them at ease with this. In my experience, a number of patients are undergoing a variety of treatments at once (including chiropractic manipulations, acupuncture, and even other physical therapy) so that it is critical to make them comfortable with informing the therapist. A history of what has or has not been successful will also be helpful in effectively designing a course of treatment.

Cortisone Injections?   Although the deleterious effects of cortisone (e.g., compromised healing potential, possible weakening of tissue, and predisposition to further injury) are well known, many patients present with a history of multiple cortisone shots. Many a physician will resort to trying physical therapy once a series of cortisone shots hasn't "worked." This is probably one of the great frustrations of physical therapists, as we are already at a disadvantage because the quality of the tissue has likely been compromised. Ellman, Hanker, and Bayer reported that multiple cortisone injections have been associated with a less favorable postoperative result in full-thickness rotator cuff tears.[17] Watson found a direct correlation between the number of preoperative injections and the quality of the rotator cuff tissue at the time of repair.[65] Kennedy and Willis, in a study on the effect of steroid injections on the rabbit's achilles tendons, found the normal tendon to substantially weaken for up to 14 days after injection. They attributed this to cellular necrosis.[35] It has been this author's experience that, among patients with similar symptoms, those with multiple injections do not progress as well as those without injections. Several authors found no significant difference in pain in patients injected with cortisone vs. placebo or in injected vs. physical therapy, acupuncture, or nsaids.[3,62,67]

Past History   Any previous shoulder problems? What sports did the patient participate in? Other significant injuries? These may predispose the patient to shoulder injury in sports. Were they rehabilitated?

Relevant Medical History   Are there any other joint or medical problems? Attention should be paid to cervical and elbow problems.

TABLE 19-2
Nirschl's Pain Phases[45]

Phase 1: Mild pain after activity, resolves withn 24 h

Phase 2: Pain after activity, resolves with warm-up

Phase 3: Pain on activity that does not affect exercise activity

Phase 4: Pain on activity that does affect exercise activity

Phase 5: Pain caused by the activities of daily living

Phase 6: Constant pain (usually dull and aching) that does not disturb sleep

Phase 7: Dull, aching pain that does disturb sleep

Medications   What is the patient taking for this problem? Has it been effective and are they taking it as prescribed?

Are you getting better, worse, or neither at this time?

Additional Tests   Has the patient had x-rays, MRIs, or arthrograms?

Further Information   Does the patient have any specific goals, time deadlines, or sport commitments that need to be addressed? Is there any other information that the therapist should know?

OBJECTIVE EXAMINATION

Observation

The objective examination begins during the subjective evaluation, during which the therapist can observe the patient's overall posture. The head forward, protracted shoulders posture is extremely common. The resultant stretch-weakening of the scapular stabilizers, tightening of the anterior shoulder and chest, and compromise of the subacromial space sets the shoulder up for sport injury. Any deformities in the body alignment, scoliosis or kyphosis, or differences in the scapular positions is noted. In observing the scapula, several factors should be noted:

"*Scapular slide,*" as described by Kibler,[36] in which the spine to scapula distance on the involved side is more than 0.5 cm greater than on the uninvolved side. This indicates weakness of the scapular stabilizers.

Scapular winging: If the serratus is weak, the scapula will migrate proximally and the inferior an-

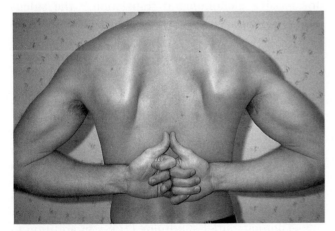

FIGURE 19-2
Scapular winging. Left: Medial border. Right: Inferior angle.

gle moves medially. Trapezius weakness results in downward scapular migration and lateral drifting of the inferior angle (Fig. 19-2).

Muscle atrophy: Wasting of the supraspinatus or infraspinatus, often evident as compared with the nondominant side or excessive prominence of the scapular spine, probably indicates rotator cuff disease, but suprascapular nerve entrapment or C5-C6 nerve root compression should be considered.[26] The medial scapular muscles and posterior shoulder muscles are also observed. Further observation should include swelling, skin changes, or bulging of the biceps.

Palpation   The sternoclavicular joint and acromioclavicular joint are palpated for tenderness, swelling, or malalignment. The greater tuberosity and supraspinatus insertion (arm extended, hand behind back) and the biceps groove are palpated. Posteriorly there may be tenderness at the levator scapula insertion or in the quadrangular space.

Clearing Tests of the Neck   This involves active and passive range of motion in all planes, including Spurling's test (compression on the neck in lateral flexion with rotation to stress the facet joints and put pressure on the nerve root), distraction with the neck in slight flexion, and compression on the extended neck.

Active Range of Motion   This is observed with attention to differences between the involved and uninvolved sides. Patients are asked to report pain and "crunching," catching, or clicking as they go through the movements. Hypomobility of the sternoclavicular and acromioclavicular joints can be assessed by placing a finger in the supraclavicular groove as the patient elevates the arm. Normal movement will push the finger out of the groove.[29] In observing scapulothoracic movement, it is helpful for the therapist to place the web space of the hand at the inferior angle of the scapular and thumb along the lateral edge. Crepitus or snapping may be noted at the superior medial aspect of the scapula. Lagging of the scapula may indicate weakness of the scapular rotators. The scapulohumeral rhythm should be observed in flexion, abduction, and scaption. The "shrug sign," or abnormal elevation of the scapula during active elevation, indicates significant rotator cuff dysfunction.[29] Lowering the arm from 120 to 70° places maximum tension on the rotator cuff,[65] and patients will often complain of pain here. Actively, functional internal rotation can be assessed with reaching the hand behind the low back: The thumb should reach at least to T8 (Fig. 19-3). Overhead the hand should reach down to approximately T4. Rotator cuff or labral tears may cause a catching pain and jerky glenohumeral rhythm.[26]

Passive Range of Motion In addition to measurement of all cardinal plane motions, this should include the passive accessory movements, for hyper- or hypomobility, ideally of all the shoulder complex joints but at least of the glenohumeral joint. This includes caudal, anterior, posterior, and lateral glides and posterior shear (at 90° flexion). With abnormal range of motion, the end-feel shoulder should be noted. Crepitation may be noted at any of the joints. A tight posterior capsule shoulder should be noted, as it may be a factor in anterior instability. It is helpful to test for generalized joint laxity by checking finger and elbow motion. For example, elbow hyperextension and ease of touching the thumb to the volar forearm indicates an individual with generalized ligamentous laxity who is predisposed to instability.

Strength Manual muscle testing of all the muscles of the shoulder joint complex is indicated. Table 19-3 is a summary of the tests we have found most useful. In addition to manual muscle tests, isokinetic testing may be indicated based on the individual's needs and pain level. We rarely test isokinetically initially, as the information is of questionable value.

SPECIAL TESTS

Impingement tests: A variety of impingement tests have been described (Neer,[42] Hawkins and Kennedy,[27] the coracoid impingement test[22]). However,

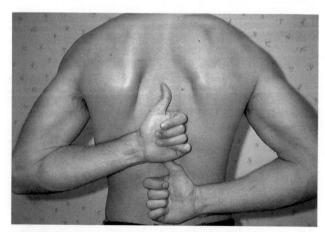

FIGURE 19-3
Loss of motion: Functional internal rotation.

TABLE 19-3

Manual Strength Tests for Rotator Cuff Disease

Sitting or standing
  Scaption with internal rotation ("empty can")
  Scaption with external rotation
  Grip strength
  Elbow flexion
Prone
  Horizontal abduction at 100° with external rotation
  Horizontal abduction at 90° with neutral rotation
  Chicken wings (elbow bent, arm extended, adducted, and externally rotated)
  Extension with external rotation
  Extension, adduction, internal rotation with elbows bent, hands on small of back (test scapular adduction and downward rotation)
  Overhead lift, elbows straight
  External rotation
  Internal rotation

with a good history, the contribution of the physical therapist performing these tests is questionable at best. Chances are the physician has already done it, and the therapist is likely recreating the pain and irritation. Furthermore, even if the test is positive it is not actually informative—putting pressure on any inflamed tissue will certainly cause pain. These tests do little if anything in guiding the treatment plan and are not, in this author's experience, generally warranted in the therapist's exam.

Acromioclavicular joint compression, by putting overpressure on the arm horizontally adducted across the chest, will cause pain with acromioclavicular joint arthritis.[69]

Stability tests include the load and shift test for passive glenohumeral translation,[26] the sulcus sign,[26] apprehension tests, and others as described in Chap. 20.

Drop arm test: The arm is passively flexed beyond 120° and slowly lowered. If the patient is unable to, if the arm suddenly drops or he or she shrugs the shoulder, this indicates major rotator cuff weakness (Fig. 19-4).

Biceps tests include Speed's sign (pain along the biceps groove with resisting flexion on the arm with elbow extended and forearm supinated); Yergason's sign (pain with resisted supination at 90° elbow flexion); and Ludington's test (with hand atop head, the biceps is forcefully contracted (Fig. 19-5).[18]

Thoracic outlet syndrome (TOS): in addition to the many tests for TOS, Leffert described one in which the arms are abducted above 90° and then the

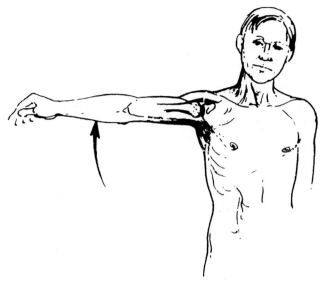

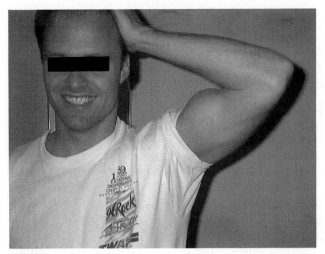

FIGURE 19-5
Ludington's test.

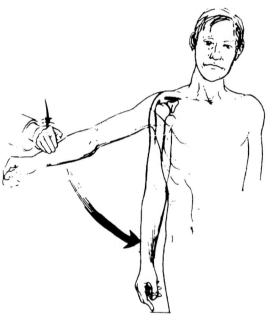

FIGURE 19-4
Drop arm test.

REHABILITATION

Watson observed that, "whether athletic or not, almost all patients want to consider themselves quick healers and the athlete, more than anyone, must confront the time barrier of physiological healing and recovery."[65] Keeping this in mind and working through this with each patient is a critical component throughout rehabilitation.

Overview

Once examination findings are put together, a treatment plan is designed for dual purposes: (1) So that patients can have a sense of what they are going to experience, how much will be expected of them in terms of time, pain, lifestyle and sport modifications, and when they can expect results. Input from patients as to their needs and willingness to make the

patient rapidly flexes and extends the fingers. A positive test includes fatigue or cramping of the forearm muscles within 20 s and/or pallor or decreased pulse in the involved arm (Fig. 19-6).[69]

Overall Fitness   Often, an athletic patient will present with a variety of problems or a history of one injury after another, complaining that "I feel like I'm falling apart." In this type of situation, or when there are no obvious factors causing the shoulder injury, a thorough evaluation of the overall fitness level is indicated. Old injuries and lower body imbalances should be assessed at some point throughout the rehabilitation program.

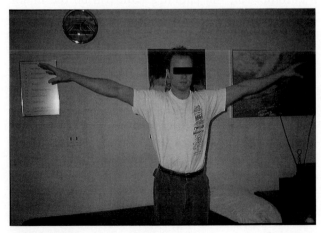

FIGURE 19-6
Leffert's test for thoracic outlet syndrome (TOS).

253

necessary commitment will allow the therapist and patient the greatest chance for success. (2) To establish a framework from which there will be numerous modifications along the way based on the patient's signs and symptoms. At this point, patients must be advised that this is only a base, and their input with respect to pain, progressing too fast or too slowly with exercises that are too easy or too hard is critical information. In this author's experience, rehabilitation of rotator cuff disease with instability should *not* at any time recreate pain, unless there is also a frozen shoulder.

The major pathologic considerations in establishing a rehabilitation program are: is there a full or partial tear; is the injury chronic or acute; is there instability; is there a frozen shoulder?

The goal with a partial tear will be to restore full normal function. A shoulder with a full tear can be rehabilitated but the patient must be aware that the restoration of function will be somewhat limited. In a study by Itoi and Tabata of 320 shoulders with full-thickness rotator cuff tears (average age 63 years with range 28 to 53), 124 were treated conservatively with rest, medications, and exercise. Pain, motion, strength, and function were graded. They found that the most effective aspect of the four in conservative treatment was pain relief. Also, the two factors of greatest prognostic value were preserved active range of motion and muscle strength. Pain severity was not a factor. Based on this, they concluded that better results of conservative treatment can be expected in patients with preserved motion and strength, regardless of pain intensity. Long-term results (6 years) were less satisfactory than short-term.[30]

With an acute injury, greater emphasis must first be placed on quieting the pain and inflammation with attention to soft tissue healing timetables. With a chronic tear, the patient's pain can be the major guide to progression. Where there is instability, modification of the motion arcs is critical to avoid overloading the anterior structures. With adhesive capsulitis, both issues must be addressed. The initial phase is geared toward controlling pain and inflammation while maintaining overall fitness and conditioning, correcting postural maladaptations, total arm strengthening without stressing the shoulder joint complex, early exercise, and active rest. Absolute rest is absolutely contraindicated, as it deconditions tissues, encourages atrophy, decreases vascular supply, and is detrimental to the healing process. Fyfe and Stanish[20] reported on the mechanical and chemical changes in tendon that result from immobilization. Patients are advised to maintain as high an activity level as possible while avoiding abusive overload. This means: (1) avoiding anything that reproduces the pain for which they sought attention and (2) avoiding positions and activities that compromise the healing tissue, e.g., sleeping or lying on the involved side, overhead work, activities with the arm abducted, activities that involve twisting the arm (e.g., cooking, washing floors or windows, using screwdrivers). (3) They can participate in sports with modifications to avoid further tissue injury. For example, weight lifting without bench presses, pushups (or avoiding just the hyperextended position and using a wide grip), overhead press, and pulldown until the rotator cuff can stabilize more effectively; tennis ground strokes only; swimming breaststroke. If passive range of motion is limited, efforts should be made to restore it early. Joint mobilization of accessory movements is indicated to achieve full motion, e.g., caudal glide for full elevation, anterior glide for full external rotation with abduction, posterior glide if flexion and internal rotation are limited, and lateral glide for all glenohumeral movements.[16] The amplitudes and planes of motion are progressed as tolerated. Isometrics, protected-range rotator cuff strengthening, and exercises to strengthen the scapular stabilizers can be initiated in the submaximal, nonpainful ranges of motion and effort. The purpose of this early exercise is to enhance tissue oxygenation and nutrition.

We have found heat and high-voltage electrical stimulation before exercise and ice afterward to be the most effective of all the modalities in the early phases. During this period, most patients are seen twice a week. Twenty-five minutes of electrical stimulation to comfort with moist heat is symptomatically helpful to most patients. If after three to four sessions the patient feels it is not, it may be discontinued or ultrasound added.

All the modalities are discussed in depth later in the chapter. Often the patient is on an antiinflammatory medication. If tolerated well, we have found these effective initially in the rehabilitation program to control pain and inflammation, allowing an early start on exercise. Since we have found that a shoulder that had several cortisone injections is a greater rehabilitation challenge, it is our great preference when possible to see a patient before injections. If the pain is too great and limits all efforts at exercise, an injection may be helpful to allow the rehabilitation effort to proceed. In our experience its necessity is not common.

Progression from the initial phase is based on the patient's pain and exercise tolerance. The goal of the second phase, which overlaps with the initial phase, is to restore the healthy normal dynamic interplay of the shoulder joint complex. While several authors stress the importance of regaining full range of motion in the initial phase,[36,68] we do not consider full motion a prerequisite to progressing to this stage. However, at this time it does become essential in order to allow the motion needed for functional strengthening. Strength criteria for progressing to this stage include the patient's ability to tolerate 3 lb with the rotator cuff foundation exercises (Fig. 19-7) and scapular stabilizer strengthening. Heat and electrical stimulation modalities are used only as needed. Ice is used after exercises as long as any pain or signs of inflammation persist. Full-motion exercises are initiated here as described in Table 19-4. Emphasis is placed on restoring the synchronous muscle interactions using PNF diagonals (Table 19-5) to engage the neuromuscular balance of all the force couple components. Agility and cardiovascular work that doesn't stress the healing tissue is appropriate in this period.

TABLE 19-4
Full Shoulder Isotonic Program

These are added once the patient is able to tolerate well 3 lb with each of the foundation exercises

Shrugs
Military press
Scaption with external rotation
Diagonal 2 flexion-extension
(D1 if instability)
Bent row
Dips
Horizontal front and side lift
Straight arm push-ups wall to chair to floor
Prone overhead lifts
Prone horizontal abduction: at 100° with external rotation; at 90° with external rotation; and in neutral rotation
Prone extension with external rotation
Supine flexion-extension

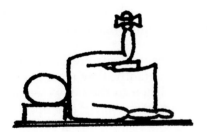

Side Lying External Rotation
(30 repetitions)

A

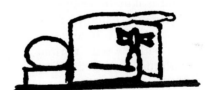

Side Lying Internal Rotation
(30 repetitions)

B

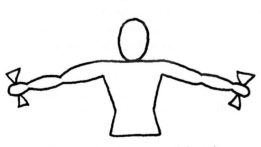

Empty Can (15 repetitions)

C

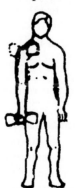

Biceps Curl (15 repetitions)

D

FIGURE 19-7
Foundation exercises to restore rotator cuff integrity. *A.* Side lying external rotation (30 repetitions). *B.* Side lying internal rotation (30 repetitions). *C.* Empty can (15 repetitions). *D.* Biceps curl (15 repetitions).

TABLE 19-5
PNF Diagonals[37]

	D1 flexion	D1 extension	D2 flexion	D2 extension
Scapular components	Elevation, protraction, upward rotation	Depression, retraction, downward rotation	Elevation, retraction, upward rotation	Depression, protraction, downward rotation
Shoulder components	Flexion, adduction, external rotation	Extension, abduction, internal rotation	Flexion, abduction, external rotation	Extension, adduction, internal rotation
Scapular muscles	Serratus	Levator rhomboids	Trapezii (all)	Pectoralis minor
Scapular components	Pectoralis major, anterior deltoid, biceps, coracobrachialis	Teres major, latissimus dorsi, triceps, posterior deltoid	Supraspinatus, teres minor, infraspinatus, middle deltoid	Subscapularis, pectoralis major

D1 flexion: flexion-adduction-external rotation
D1 extension: extension-abduction-internal rotation
D2 flexion: flexion-abduction-external rotation
D2 extension: extension-adduction-internal rotation

The third phase of rehabilitation prepares the patient for return to sport. Criteria for progression to this stage usually include absence of medications and modalities (except ice), full pain-free range of motion, and dynamic strength balance restoration as documented on manual and isokinetic testing. A study by Warner et al.[64] compared external rotation:internal rotation (ER:IR) work and torque ratios at 90° per s and 180° per s in patients with normal shoulders, impingement syndrome, and instability. In both torque and work, ER:IR was 65 to 75 percent in normal patients, 50 percent in impingement, and 100 percent in instabilities. They concluded that impingement is associated with posterior capsule tightness and relative weakness of the external rotators; and instability is associated with excessive external rotation motion and relative weakness of the internal rotators. Our criteria for sports return include:

- Full pain-free range of motion in the ranges demanded by the sport.
- ER:IR peak torque and work outputs 65 to 75 percent with the dominant arm 10 to 20 percent stronger than the nondominant. In a lean individual ER peak torque should approximate 14 to 16 percent body weight and IR 20 percent. All these criteria are not absolutely essential but the ER:IR work ratio is. Great attention should be paid to the shape of the output curve, as normal output with an abnormal curve is unacceptable (Fig. 19-8).
- Normal muscle tests of scaption, Centinela supraspinatus test ("empty can"), lower trapezius strength test (Fig. 19-9),[34] and Blackburn's supraspinatus test (prone horizontal abduction with external rotation) (Fig. 19-10).[7]
- Phase 2 or lower pain in activities of daily living.
- Attention to good postural alignment.

Once these are achieved, patients are prepared for sports return. Most importantly, they must have developed the ability to listen to the body's warning signals and to respond immediately and appropriately. It is the therapist's responsibility to educate patients fully in this respect throughout the rehabilitation program. They should be comfortable with using the pain phases or another objective interpretation of pain to help with this. Additional education is needed to make patients aware of their sports deficiencies with respect to promoting specific strength and flexibility imbalances at the shoulder and with respect to overall fitness.

Sport return is undertaken gradually and methodically, controlling the variables of duration, frequency, and intensity. The athlete starts out with limited participation time (approximately one-fourth to one-third normal) and participates no more frequently than on alternate days. The environment must be noncompetitive so that the most stressful strokes or motions can be avoided. One of the variables is progressed with each session so that injurious factors can be identified. If there is any question as to the athlete's sports technique or equipment being a factor in injury, it must be addressed before competitive participation. The therapist can either

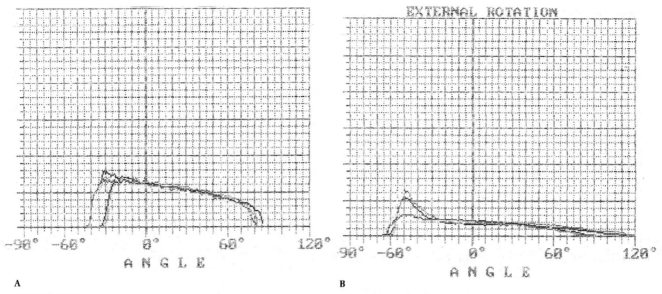

A　　　　　　　　　　　　　　　　　　　**B**

FIGURE 19-8
Isokinetic external rotation curves. *A.* Normal shape.　*B.* Abnormal shape.

work with the patient or refer the patient to a qualified professional with whom there will be good communication. Rehabilitation exercises should be maintained throughout the return to sport, and until the athlete is back fully and is asymptomatic for at least 3 months. They can then gradually be weaned off, but the athlete should check strength and motion periodically.

In patients with frozen shoulder, both rotator cuff and scapular muscle strength and motion restoration must be balanced. In stretching, abduction should be avoided, as the humeral head cannot glide inferiorly and iatrogenically induced impingement

syndrome is likely. Stretching may include PNF principles of hold-relax and contract-relax,[37] passive prolonged stretches, repeated brief stretches, dynamic stretching, and mobilization. It is noteworthy that, in a study by Nicholson, during which he compared patients doing active stretching only with those doing active and mobilizations, he found that only passive abduction was significantly better in the mobilization group and that no significant difference in pain scores was found in the two groups.[44] Once reasonable range of flexion (150°) and external rotation (65°) are achieved, greatest emphasis should be placed on rotator cuff strengthening while contin-

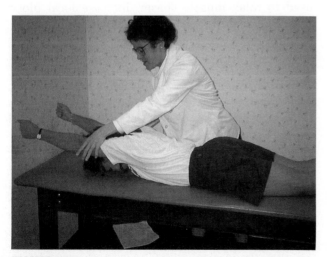

FIGURE 19-9
Manual muscle test for lower trapezius strength.

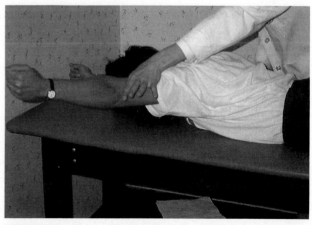

FIGURE 19-10
Prone muscle test for supraspinatus strength.

257

uing to work toward greater motion. In patients with neck involvement, the neck area must be addressed also.

We use physical therapy modalities to create the environment wherein exercise can be tolerated as early and full as possible, as exercise is the key to restoration of function. However, as the modalities are an important aspect of all conservative rehabilitation programs, it is appropriate to review the current thinking on them:

Modalities

Heat has been found to have the following effects:

1. Vasodilation, increased oxygenation and nutrient supply, increased metabolic rate
2. Increased extensibility of collagen tissue through changes in its vasoelastic properties
3. Analgesia by acting on the free nerve endings, increasing the pain threshold
4. Decreased muscle spasm through lessened muscle spindle activity[55]

Thus the heat modalities can be effective to decrease pain and stiffness, muscle spasm, and contracture, and increase metabolism and range of motion.

Ultrasound transmits high-frequency sound waves through the skin (using a coupling gel) to the deeper tissues.[2] It has both thermal effects as described above and nonthermal effects due to the vibration of molecules. These include increased cell membrane permeability and ionic transport[55] with absorption of excess calcium and adhesions.[2] According to Rivenburgh,[55] it stimulates fibroblastic activity in the synthesis of reparative tissue. However, no direct anti-inflammatory effects of ultrasound have been documented. Ultrasound is the deepest heating of all modalities, capable of penetrating more than 2 cm. A study by Binder and associates in which patients with tennis elbow were treated with ultrasound vs. a placebo found that 63 percent of the ultrasound patients improved with respect to pain and strength as compared with 11 percent of the placebo group.[5]

We have sometimes found ultrasound useful before exercise for its thermal effects and to make the tissue more susceptible to remodeling by tensile forces.

Phonophoresis uses ultrasound to deliver therapeutic levels of topically applied medications to the inflamed tissues. The more common anti-inflammatory medications used are cortisol, dexamethasone, and salicylates. Studies by Griffin and associates, Kleinkort and Wood, and Moll found phonophoresis more effective than ultrasound or placebo with a variety of conditions. However, the specific diagnosis is unknown.[29] As phonophoresis is often used with a steroid, great caution should be used by the therapist in view of the effects of steroids in lessening collagen and ground substance production and decreasing the tensile strength or tendon. It is this author's opinion that the potential risks far outweigh the benefits, especially in those patients with a history of multiple injections. Among patients we see with a history of treatment elsewhere, never has one reported a significant improvement with phonophoresis where other modalities failed.

Cold decreases temperature up to 4 cm deep.[55] It is effective in vasoconstriction, decreased inflammation and swelling, decreased pain by blocking the sensory impulses through decreased nerve conduction velocity, and decreased muscle spasms through inhibition of the stretch reflex.[55] We have found 20 min of ice following exercise throughout the rehabilitation program to be effective. Any of the ice forms (commercial or homemade) are valuable, but convenience and ease of use unquestionably improve patient compliance.

Transverse friction massage in which the tissue is massaged deeply across its fibers is promoted by many to enhance circulation, reduce excessive scar formation, and realign scar.[36] This author finds no place for it at the shoulder in that it generally is extremely painful and many patients who have received it describe a distinct worsening of symptoms. Finally there is no scientific research to substantiate its value.

High-voltage electric stimulation (HVES) uses a short-pulse, high-duration monophasic waveform to deliver electric current deep into the tissues. It is used to relax muscle spasm, increase local blood flow, reduce edema, and decrease pain through endorphin release.[1,52] Although there is little scientific research to support its effectiveness, we have found it to be of great value clinically in controlling pain, increasing mobility, and improving exercise tolerance. It can also be effective postoperatively to prevent or decrease neuromuscular disassociation and disuse atrophy, and for muscle reeducation.

Iontophoresis uses electric stimulation to deliver medications to deep tissue. Since it is based on galvanic current passing between bipolar electrodes, it must use medication with ionic components, as compared with phonophoresis, which drives whole molecules. It penetrates to only approximately 1 cm, so that its depth of penetration is considerably less than that of phonophoresis.[2] We have not found iontophoresis useful in our treatment of rotator cuff disease, largely in view of the same concerns expressed above with phonophoresis.

Therapeutic Exercise

The exercise program is the key element of rotator cuff disease rehabilitation. Modalities are used primarily to facilitate fullest possible exercise program adherence. Thus the average patient gets three to six sessions of heat and electrical stimulation, exercise, and ice afterward in addition to a home exercise program. After the first few weeks (or sooner if indicated) the heat and stimulation are discontinued unless they seem necessary.

The available strengthening modes are:

Isometrics, which strengthen without joint stresses. Progression variables are intensity, duration, and motion range.

Isotonics, a fixed-weight resistance exercise that offers concentric and eccentric loading. Progression variables are weight, repetitions, sets, and ranges of motion. This may employ free weights or weight machines.

Isokinetics, a fixed-speed variable-resistance exercise that accommodates to the patient's output throughout the motion. Progression variables are intensity of effort, speed, and duration.

Rubber tubing, a highly convenient exercise form that offers an infinite number of exercises and offers greatest resistance at the motion extremes. Progression variables are repetitions, range of motion, and resistance intensity.

Proprioceptive neuromuscular facilitation (PNF) places specific demands on the neuromuscular mechanism by stimulating the proprioceptors to elicit a desired response.[37] Each of the two diagonals creates a movement pattern of facilitation, working the muscles from their fully lengthened to shortened positions. These motions can be applied manually or with any of the above resistance forms.

Flexibility exercises are used early to regain normal motion arcs. Later, flexibility exercises are recommended after strengthening. Their purpose is to overcome the sport-induced imbalances, prevent injury during sport participation, create a motion range throughout which strengthening will be done, and allow the motion needed for good sport form. Static and dynamic stretches each play a role. Stretching is desirable only with specific goals and with an ongoing strengthening program throughout the motion extremes.

EMG studies by Jobe, Pink, Perry, Townsend, and Moseley[40,51,61] have addressed the effectiveness of a number of exercises on each of the rotator cuff

and scapular muscles. Table 19-6 lists many of the muscles and the exercises that benefit them most. Moseley, Jobe, Pink, et al.[40] found that the most important exercises for the scapular muscles are scaption, row, push-ups with a "plus," and press-ups (dips).

Townsend, Jobe, Pink, et al. studied 17 exercises and found the ones most important for the rotator cuff were scaption with internal rotation (the "empty can") for the anterior and middle deltoid, subscapularis, and supraspinatus; and forward flexion and horizontal abduction with external rotation for the infraspinatus and teres minor. They found greatest supraspinatus activity in the military press.[6] Blackburn, McLeod, White, et al. found highest supraspinatus activity on prone horizontal abduction at 100° with external rotation. They found this to also be valuable for the infraspinatus and teres minor.[7]

The program we have found to be most effective is described fully in Appendix A. However, the critical feature of any rehabilitation program is individualization. Absolute attention must be focused on adapting the program to the individual, and away from adapting the patient to the program. The progression of exercise is based on the patient's tolerance to the previous level. Learning to use body signals for activity modification will be the key to future overuse injury prevention. It is the overlapping of exercise forms that we have found most efficient, effective, and interesting for the patient, thus allowing fuller compliance. Closed kinetic chain exercises, e.g., straight arm push-ups, dips, chin-ups, pull-ups, hand walking on a stairmaster, BAPS, or treadmill, may be indicated. Normal, pain-free motion and strength are the basis for beginning sport-specific activities. A number of studies indicate isokinetic norms at the shoulder to include ER:IR of approximately 2:3 or 3:4.[15,31] Sport-specific movements such as easy ball toss or slow golf swing are progressively graduated. Plyometrics with a medicine ball (such as across the body throwing, overhead throws) help tremendously in the transition to sport. See Appendix B for a return to tennis program.

As noted by Watson, conservative treatment is the athlete's best chance of return to sport.[65] However, if the conservative approach fails, several surgical approaches are available.

Prehabilitation

Athletes involved in baseball, tennis, swimming, golf, weight lifting, and volleyball are highly vulnerable to rotator cuff disease. Often weakness exists before clinical symptoms present. For such athletes, a

TABLE 19-6
Beneficial Exercises for the Muscles of the Shoulder Joint Complex

Muscle	Exercises
Supraspinatus	Scaption with internal rotation ("empty can") Scaption with external rotation Military press Flexion Prone 100° horizontal abduction with external rotation D2 flexion
Infraspinatus and teres minor	Airplanes (prone horizontal abduction with external rotation) External rotation Flexion Prone extension with external rotation D2 flexion
Teres major	Dips D1 extension
Subscapularis	Scaption with internal rotation Military press D2 extension
Serratus anterior	Push-up Bench press with a plus D1 flexion
Latissimus dorsi	Chin-ups Pull-downs Dips D1 extension
Trapezius	Upper: Shrugs Middle: Prone horizontal abduction at 90° with external rotation, elbow straight Lower: Prone overhead lifts D2 flexion
Deltoid	Anterior: Flexion Scaption Middle: Abduction Scaption Posterior: Extension Prone horizontal abduction with arm in neutral and external rotation
Rhomboids	Row Prone horizontal abduction D1 extension

prehabilitation exercise program is greatly beneficial. The following eight strengtheners combined with posterior capsule stretching would be effective:

1. Scaption with internal rotation ("empty can")
2. Side lying external rotation
3. Biceps curls
4. Prone overhead lifts
5. Prone horizontal abduction with external rotation
6. Diagonal 2 flexion-extension
7. Straight arm push-ups or bench press
8. Military press

Stretches should include:

1. Horizontal adduction
2. Towel stretch
3. Overhead stretch
4. Anterior chest stretch if needed
5. Others as needed based on tests

SURGERY AND POSTOPERATIVE REHABILITATION

Several authors have recommended criteria for surgery with full-thickness tears to include at least 6 months of conservative treatment with no change in pain or an unsatisfactory plateau.[9,42,46] Obvious acute ruptures are generally repaired promptly. A study by Gazielly on 40 patients with rotator cuff tears concluded that it is beneficial, when surgery is recommended, for the patient to get preoperative therapy for 1 month. This facilitates full shoulder motion recovery, increases patient familiarity with the postoperative program and exercises, and establishes the therapist-patient relationship.[21]

For partial-thickness tears 3 to 6 months of quality conservative care is recommended to attempt resolution of the problem. The concepts include revascularization and recollaginization of necrotic tendinosis tissue with restoration of strength, endurance, and flexibility. Failure to achieve these goals is reflected clinically by persistence of pain and/or weakness. Of the many possible surgeries, certain issues are most important to the therapist who will be working with the patient. In order to work toward achieving the patient's fullest possible restorative potential, the therapist should consider the following.

Repair of Torn Rotator Cuff

Partial-thickness tears (involving only superficial, middle, or deep fibers) are much more common and the surgeon may or may not recommend surgical correction. Since the patient's quality of life is the final determinant, the ultimate decision for surgery is made by the patient. Full-thickness tears (extending from the articular surface to the bursal surface) will vary in size, which somewhat determines the type of repair (soft tissue repair or repair into bone). In a massive tear with considerable tissue retraction and/or very poor tendon quality, the surgeon may have done a tendon transfer or patch graft or may have found repair impossible. Extremely retracted tissue or tissue of poor quality may make for a more tenuous repair; thus more cautious rehabilitation is indicated. Some surgeons may use an abduction splint, after which the therapist must take extreme caution to avoid compromising the repair.

Decompression

This is designed to free up the subacromial space and generally involves removing about one-third of the undersurface of the anterior acromion. Resection of the coracoacromial ligament, excision of the outer end of the clavicle, and debridement of the bursa are options that may affect the postoperative course. The most critical rehabilitation issue is whether the deltoid was released at the time of exposure.

Arthroscopic vs. Open Surgery

Rehabilitation will be quicker after arthroscopy largely because there may not be disruption of the deltoid. Several authors recommend strongly against detaching the deltoid from the acromion because they find it unnecessary and unworthy of the increased risk of pain and its delaying effect on rehabilitation.[29,46]

Instability

Glenohumeral instability is a common companion to partial-thickness rotator cuff tendinitis. If a labral tear was present and restoration of labral stability was undertaken, the postoperative rehabilitation is modified (see Chap. 20).

Other more obvious factors to the therapist include patient age, lifestyle needs, and history of injections. A study of factors influencing the postoperative outcome considered the size of the tear, amount of retraction, preoperative cortisone injections and preoperative strength of external rotation, and abduction to affect postoperative results.[29] The postoperative rehabilitation and the technique specifics are totally dependent upon the above. The surgeon's experience and technique plus the quality of tissue add additional critical dimensions to the rehabilitation process and the ultimate outcome. Table 19-7 reviews surgical considerations in rehabilitation.

Postoperative Rehabilitation

Postoperative arthroscopic decompression rehabilitation can begin with immediate passive range of motion, using a sling for comfort and progressing to active motion as soon as the patient is able. Resisted exercises can begin at about 3 weeks and full functional return can be expected in 6 weeks to 3 months postoperatively. Open decompression, in which the deltoid was detached and reattached, necessitates a much slower process. It is recommended that active abduction and external rotation are avoided until about 3 to 4 weeks postoperatively and resisted deltoid strengthening held off until 6 to 12 weeks. Open decompression with a deltoid split allows a timetable more like the arthroscopic one, but somewhat more gingerly. See Appendix D for rehab specifics.

TABLE 19-7
Surgical Factors in Rehabilitation

1. Arthroscopy glenohumeral
   a. Number of portals (two or more)
   b. Adequate removal osteophytic spurs (glenohumeral)
   c. Glenoid rim burring
   d. Capsulolabral suturing or biodegradable staples
2. Arthroscopy coracoacromial arch
   a. Two portals or more
   b. Excessive bleeding
   c. Major bursectomy
   d. Acromioplasty
   e. Excision coracoacromial ligament
3. Open surgical approach
   a. Deltoid mini-split or deltoid release
   b. Major acromioplasty or mini-acromioplasty (Nirschl)
   c. AC resection
4. Open repair rotator cuff
   a. Size of tear
   b. Retraction—fibrosis of rotator cuff
   c. Direction and pattern of tear
   d. Quality of tendon
   e. Suture technique (soft tissue and/or into bone)
   f. Direction suture lines
   g. Supportive autogenous tendon graft

After repair of a full-thickness tear, rehabilitation begins with early (approximately 1 to 2 days postoperative) passive motion. The extent of allowable motion may be limited by the surgeon. A sling is generally worn for 1 to 2 weeks. Active exercise may begin at approximately 1 week except for external rotation and abduction. Active abduction can begin at approximately 2 to 4 weeks postoperative and resisted at 4 to 8 weeks. Close communication between the surgeon and therapist is essential, as the surgeon must determine the progression based on the size of the defect, adequacy of the repair, and other healing restraints. The patient should be advised that a perfectly smooth postoperative course is uncommon, and the ups and downs as well as considerable pain are no cause for concern as to the outcome. For 6 to 10 weeks, clicking, catching, and referred pain to the deltoid tuberosity are common and are not a long-term problem. A massive tear that was not repaired can begin active exercise as early as the patient can tolerate unless the deltoid was detached. If there was a labrum tear and sutured repair, a delay in rehabilitation may be indicated and again must be directed by the surgeon. The overall rehabilitation program postoperatively follows the same principles as conservative treatment and is detailed in Appendix C.

A number of studies evaluating postoperative outcome report a high degree of pain relief.[22,53,60] Strength results varied, with external rotation approximately 70 to 90 percent and abduction 70 to 80 percent.[8,23,38] In most cases, strength continues to progress well beyond 6 months postoperatively, and full strength was usually achieved at 1 year.[8,23,63] None of these studies describe the postoperative rehabilitation or if indeed there was any, so it is difficult to draw any conclusions as to the role of or ideal course of therapy.

The goal of any program, whether conservative or surgical, for rotator cuff disease is to restore the integrity of the tissue and the dynamic functional biomechanics of the shoulder joint complex so that it can perform maximally in maintaining its ideally balanced stability-mobility interplay. Any factors that affect this interplay, whether ligamentous, structural, or muscular, must be addressed for long-term success. With these factors considered, good patient education and compliance make continued full sport involvement realistic. No doubt as we improve our knowledge the rehabilitation programs will continue to improve. Much of our future knowledge will likely come from scientific research as well as sensitivity to patient response to current treatment programs.

APPENDIX A: PROGRAM FOR CONSERVATIVE TREATMENT OF ROTATOR CUFF DISEASE

I. Initial phase (usually 3 to 6 weeks): Reduce inflammation, restore rotator cuff integrity
   A. Heat, electrical stimulation 2 times a week for 2 to 3 weeks followed by gym program:
      1. UBE (Fig. 19-11)
      2. Pulleys for internal-external rotation (active assisted if needed); shrugs; biceps
      3. Weight machines: row to neutral; scapular protraction on chest press (straight arm press) (Fig. 19-12); lateral pull-down front; triceps.
      4. Mobilization and stretching as needed
      5. Ice after exercise
   B. Daily home exercise program: No weight to start, progress once able to tolerate two to three consecutive sessions at that level. Emphasize absolute adherence to proper form and hand positioning in exercises.
      1. Warm-up before exercise
      2. Foundation exercises: Side lying rotations of 30 to 50 repetitions each (depending on patient's athletic demands); biceps and scaption with internal rotations of 10 to 15 repetitions each
      3. Flexibility of tight areas, e.g., posterior and inferior shoulder. Three repetitions of 20-s holds
      4. Ice after exercise
   C. Avoid abuse in ADLs and sport, e.g., avoid side lying on involved side, overhead lifting, and horizontal abduction above 80° beyond neutral and shoulder twisting movements. Avoid overhead movements in sport. Avoid any activity that reproduces the pain for which the patient sought treatment. Emphasize correct postural alignment at all times.
   D. Medications per physician
   E. Overall fitness program and strengthening arm as needed

Note: All time frameworks are extremely variable. Each program is highly individualized. The primary basis for progression is the patient's readiness based on signs and symptoms. The exercises themselves may also be altered to accommodate each patient's needs and tolerance.

Criteria for advancement: Able to tolerate all foundation exercises with 3 lb; no night pain. If, with careful monitoring and specific modifications based on individual tolerance, they simply cannot accomplish this, patients may need to recheck with the doctor for consideration of cortisone injection, other tests, and reevaluation. If the shoulder is injected with cortisone we generally hold on therapy for 10 days after injection. The patient does range of motion and ice during this period.

II. Intermediate phase: Rehabilitation exercise program (bringing tissue to normal)
   A. Modalities and medications as needed
   B. Exercises in gym:
      1. UBE
      2. Isokinetic external rotation—internal rotation in modified neutral or scapular plane. Begin with submaximal effort, midrange, midspeed exercise. Progress each variable at a time until working full effort, full range of motion, full velocity spectrum from 60 to 300°/s with 10- to 15-s bouts
      3. Pulleys as above, eliminating external rotation–internal rotation and adding PNF diagonals
      4. Weight machines: sets and repetitions depending on patient's needs. Usually 1 to 3 sets of 10 to 15 repetitions: lateral pull-down front and back, row, straight arm presses, shrugs, biceps, triceps. Emphasize precontraction of scapular stabilizers with all overhead movements (Fig. 19-13)
      5. Mobilization and stretching as indicated
      6. Ice after exercise
   C. Home exercise program: 2 to 3 times a week
      1. Warm-up
      2. Foundation exercises with 3 to 5 lb: side lying internal rotation; side lying external rotation; scaption with internal rotation
      3. Full rehabilitation program: prone overhead lifts; prone horizontal abduction at 100° with external rotation, at 90° with external rotation and in neutral rotation; prone extension with external rotation; military press; D2 PNF diagonal; scaption with external rotation; biceps; triceps french curl

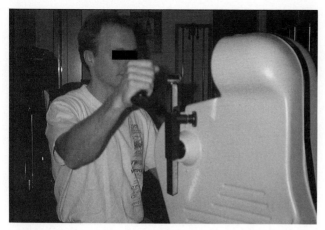

FIGURE 19-11
UBE.

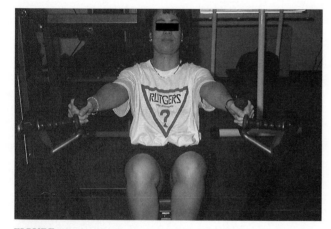

FIGURE 19-12
Straight arm press.

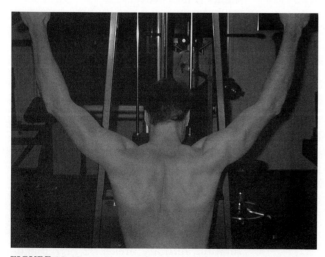

FIGURE 19-13
Lateral pulldown with precontraction of scapular stabilizers.

4. Isoflex or tubing on alternate days: scaption with external rotation–internal rotation, PNF diagonals; internal rotation and external rotation; extension with external rotation; shoulder pinch; shoulder shrug; flexion; horizontal abduction at shoulder and waist heights

5. Stretching as indicated

6. Ice after exercise

D. Fitness programs: agility, speed; rehabilitation of old injuries elsewhere, total arm strength

E. Continue precautions of phase I, emphasize postural correction through day

F. Criteria for advancement: Nirschl's phase 2 pain; full pain-free range of motion; normal pain-free manual muscle test of scaption, prone overhead lift, prone horizontal abduction; external rotation:internal rotation peak torque and work 65 to 75 percent at 60°/s; dominant arm at least equal to non-dominant; no need for medication or modalities except ice; ability to listen and respond to body's signals

Note: Depending on patient's accessibility, the program may be modified as to frequency of physical therapy, isotonics, isoflex. Where patients are able, they alternate physical therapy, isotonics, and isoflex, doing each 2 times a week. Where patients are unable to get physical therapy, isoflex and isotonics are alternated, 3 times a week each. In patients who need more rest or need to continue sports participation, the isoflex may be eliminated, thus exercising 2 to 4 times a week.

III. Advanced phase: Preparation for return to sport
   A. Gym workout
      1. UBE with attention to sport needs, e.g., sprints, endurance
      2. Isokinetic external rotation–internal rotation with high-speed endurance bouts of 45 s and sports-specific programs
      3. Pulleys for sport-specific movements
      4. Weight machines as in phase II
      5. Neuromuscular reeducation: e.g., BAPS, Stairmaster
   B. Home exercises as in phase II progressing weights
   C. Neuromuscular reeducation: 2 to 3 times a week
      1. Sport-specific plyometrics with medicine ball

264

2. Surgical tubing, reproducing the needs of the sport
3. Reproduce the sport movements without a ball (e.g., golf swing, tennis strokes, throwing motions). Working with a pro or trainer, and reviewing equipment is indicated at this time

IV. Return to sport
   A. Use guidelines specific to sport
   B. Methodically progress variables, each on its own:
      1. Duration (15 to 20 min to start)
      2. Types of motion, e.g., in tennis, avoid overheads and serves at first, progressing to all strokes
      3. Frequency. Every other day for 1 to 2 weeks then 2 days on, 1 day off, then progressing to full schedule. Swimmers must avoid days with double practices.
      4. Intensity. The patient needs to play in an absolutely noncompetitive environment until all other variables have been fully progressed

APPENDIX B: RETURN TO TENNIS GUIDELINES

1. These are *only* guidelines and serve as a basis for modification in response to the patient's signs and symptoms. Each schedule must be *individualized* based on the nature and duration of the problem as well as the athlete's needs.

2. Ice shoulder for at least 15 min within 30 min after play.

3. Each day of play must be followed by a day of rest. Once fully returned, the player can play 2 days on, 1 day off for 2 weeks, then 3 days on, 1 day off, etc.

Day
1: 20 min FH groundstrokes
3: 30 min FH, BH groundstrokes
5: 45 min FH, BH groundstrokes
7: 45 min groundstrokes, FV and BV
9: 1 h groundstrokes, FV and BV
11: 1 h GS, FV, BV, easy OH
13: 1 h GS, FV, BV, OH
15: 1 h, add easy S
17: Full schedule

Key to abbreviations:
FH: Forehand
BH: Backhand
GS: Groundstrokes
FV: Forehand volley

BV: Backhand volley
OH: Overhead
S: Serves

Return to golf and to baseball schedules is outlined, in Middleton K, Courson R, Young R, Andrews JR: *Preventive and Rehabilitative Exercises for the Shoulder and Elbow*. Birmingham, AL, American Sports Medicine Institute, 1989.

APPENDIX C: PROTOCOL FOR POSTOPERATIVE ROTATOR CUFF REPAIR

I. Preoperatively
   A. Attempt to strengthen with foundation exercises
   B. Attempt to regain full motion
   C. Patient education
      1. Overview of postoperative course
      2. Use of sling and frequent use of ice
      3. Pain expectations
         a. Expect pain similar to preoperative pain for 6 weeks to 3 months postoperatively.
         b. Expect catching, clicking, and pain around deltoid for up to 6 weeks.

II. Postoperatively
   A. Immediate days 1 to 4 or 1 to 7 depending on physician, quality of repair, and patient's response
      1. Sling full time for 1 to 3 days, then gradually wean. Keep arm supported often on arm of chair during weaning.
      2. Modalities as needed. Heat, electrical stimulation, ice.
      3. Range of motion
         a. Pendulum
         b. Low-intensity mobilizations
         c. Passive flexion, external rotation, abduction
         d. Active assisted motion with bar or pulley for flexion, rotation as permitted
      4. Scapular isometrics, shrugs
      5. Isometrics all shoulder motions
      6. Cervical range of motion and strengthening, elbow and hand motion
   B. Early rehabilitation: Motion. 1 to 6 weeks
      1. Weeks 1 to 3:
         a. Continue exercises and modalities as in first week.
         b. Active shoulder flexion. If unable, muscle stimulation over supraspinatus with active effort is helpful.
         c. Begin UBE.
      2. Weeks 3 to 6:
         a. Begin active abduction and external rotation (depending on repair)
         b. Achieve 90 to 100 percent motion all planes, passive and active

      c. Wean off modalities except ice
      d. Begin arm strengthening with isotonics (elbow, forearm) and grip strengthening
      e. UBE, row, pulley for shrugs, biceps
      f. Continue joint mobilization as needed
      3. Advance to next level once 90 percent to full active motion is achieved, and patient has minor pain
   C. Intermediate rehabilitation: Strengthening. Weeks 6 to 10
      1. Modalities only if needed.
      2. Home exercises: Begin isotonic rotator cuff foundation exercises to 3 lb. Once comfortable with 3 lb, add full isotonics program as outlined in conservative care intermediate phase.
      3. In gym: UBE, row, straight arm presses, pulleys as above and adding internal and external rotations. Once able to do 10 lb, begin isokinetic external rotation–internal rotation.
      4. Joint mobilization as needed. Advance to next phase when patient has full active and passive motion; dominant arm is at least 80 percent of nondominant arm.
   D. Advanced rehabilitation: Full strength, motion, endurance, 10 weeks to 3 or 4 months
      1. Discontinue modalities except ice
      2. UBE
      3. Isotonic strengthening all motions
      4. Add isoflex or surgical tubing
      5. Isokinetic high-speed endurance bouts and slow-speed strengthening bouts

   Advance to next phase when dominant arm is 10 to 20 percent stronger than nondominant, external rotation to body weight is 14 to 16 percent; internal rotation to body weight is 18 to 20 percent; external rotation:internal rotation work and peak torque is 66 to 75 percent.

   E. Functional progression: 3 or 4 months to 6 months
      1. Continue strength, endurance, and flexibility
      2. Follow preparation for return to sport as outlined in conservative care
   F. Return to sport: 6 to 9 months
      1. Continue strengthening and flexibility
      2. Follow guidelines of conservative care

All exercises and time frames are subject to change by surgeon's guidelines based on quality of repair and patient's response.

APPENDIX D: PROTOCOL FOR POSTARTHROSCOPIC ARCH DECOMPRESSION AND DEBRIDEMENT

I. Preoperatively
   A. Attempt to restore strength and full range of motion within patient's pain limitations
   B. Instruct in postoperative pendulum, isotonic, and flexibility exercises
   C. Instruct in use of ice 3 to 5 times a day postoperatively
   D. Use of sling days 1 to 3 postoperatively
II. Postoperatively
   A. Immediate: Days 1 to 4
      1. Modalities for pain and inflammation control
      2. Passive range of motion all motions 3 to 5 times a day
      3. Active-assisted range of motion with pulley, bar 3 to 5 times a day
      4. Ice
   B. Early rehabilitation: days 4 to 10 postoperatively
      1. Continue modalities, passive and active assisted motion (2 to 3 times a day)
      2. UBE
      3. Active motion all planes
      4. Row, shrugs, biceps on pulley
      5. Rotator cuff foundation exercises to 3 lb
   C. Intermediate rehabilitation: day 10 to 3 weeks
      1. Wean off modalities except ice (after exercise)
      2. Continue stretching 1 to 2 times a day
      3. Gym program:
         a. UBE
         b. Pulleys: External rotation–internal rotation, upright row, PNF diagonals, shrugs, biceps
         c. Weight machines: row, straight arm press, lateral pull-down front and back, triceps, emphasize scapular stabilization
      4. Home program
         a. Warm-up before exercise
         b. Foundation exercises
         c. Full isotonic program as outlined in conservative approach
   D. Advance rehabilitation: 3 to 6 weeks
      1. Continue stretching once a day
      2. Sport-specific isokinetics. Strength should be within normal limits.
      3. Isoflex or rubber tubing
      4. Isotonics as above, increasing weights
   E. Preparation for sport return weeks 6 to 9
   F. Return to sport weeks 9 to 12

REFERENCES

1. Alon G, De Domenico G: High voltage stimulation: An integrated approach to clinical electrotherapy. Chattanooga, Chattanooga Corp, 1987.
2. Antich TJ: The principles of ultrasonic driving. *J Orthop Sports Phys Ther* 4:99–102, 1982.
3. Berry H, Fernades L, Bloom B, et al: Clinical study comparing acupuncture, physiotherapy, injection and oral anti-inflammatory therapy in shoulder cuff lesions. *Curr Med Res Opin* 7:121–126, 1980.
4. Bigliani LU, Morrison DS, April DW: The morphology of the acromion and its relationship to rotator cuff tears. *Orthop Trans* 10:216, 1986.
5. Binder A, Hodge G, Greenwood AM, et al: Is therapeutic ultrasound effective in treating soft tissues lesions? *Br Med J* 290:512–514, 1985.
6. Black KP, Lombardo JA: Suprascapular nerve injuries with isolated paralysis of the infraspinnatus. *Am J Sports Med* 18:3, 1990.
7. Blackburn TA, McLeod WD, White B, et al: EMG analysis of posterior rotator cuff exercises. *Athl Training* 25:40–45, 1990.
8. Brems JJ: Rotator cuff tear: Evaluation and treatment. *Orthopedics* 11:69–82, 1988.
9. Burns TP, Turba JE: Arthroscopic treatment of shoulder impingement in athletes. *Am J Sports Med* 20:1, 1992.
10. Calliet R: *Shoulder Pain.* Philadelphia, Davis, 1982.
11. Chandler TJ, Kibler WB, Uhl TL, et al: Flexibility comparisons of junior elite tennis players to other athletes. *Am J Sports Med* 18:2(134–136), 1990.
12. Clark J, Sidles JA, Matsen FA: The relationship of the glenohumeral joint capsule to the rotator cuff. *Clin Orthop* 254:29–34, 1990.

13. Codman EA: *The Shoulder.* Boston, Thomas Todd, 1934.

14. DePalma AF, Gallery G, Bennett CA: Variational anatomy and degenerative lesions of the shoulder joint in Blount WP (ed): *AAOS Instructional Course Lectures VI*, Ann Arbor, Edwards, 1949, pp 255–281.

15. Ellenbecker TS: A total arm strength isokinetic profile of highly skilled tennis players and its relation to functional performance measurement. *Isoks Exerc Sci* 1:1,9–21, 1991.

16. Ellenbecker TS, Derscheid GL: Rehabilitation of overuse injuries of the shoulder. *Clin Sports Med* 8:3,583–604, July 1989.

17. Ellman H, Hanker G, Bayer M: Repair of the rotator cuff: End-result study of factors influencing reconstruction. *J Bone Joint Surg (Am)* 68A:1136–1144, 1986.

18. Falkel JE, Murphy TC, Malone TR: *Shoulder Injuries: Sports Injury Management.* Baltimore, Williams & Wilkins, 1988, vol 1, p 2.

19. Fu FH, Havner CD, Klein AH: Shoulder impingement syndrome. *Clin Orthop* 269:162–173, August 1991.

20. Fyfe I, Stanish WD: The use of eccentric training and stretching in the treatment and prevention of tendon injuries. *Clin Sports Med* 11:3,601–623, July 1992.

21. Gazielly DG: Preoperative management and rehabilitation of rotator cuff tears, in Post, Melvin, Morrey, et al (eds): *Surgery of the Shoulder.* St Louis, Mosby, 1990, pp 234–237.

22. Gerber C, Terrier F, Ganz R: The role of the coracoid process in the chronic impingement syndrome. *J Bone Joint Surg (Am)* 67B:703–708, 1985.

23. Gore DR, Murray MP, Sepic SB, Gardner GM: Shoulder muscle strength and range of motion following surgical repair of full thickness rotator cuff tears. *J Bone Joint Surg (Am)* 68A:266–272, February 1986.

24. Guidi E, Nirschl RP: unpublished data, December 1992.

25. Halbach JW, Tank RT: The shoulder, in Gould JG, Davies GJ (eds): *Orthopaedic and Sports Physical Therapy.* St Louis, Mosby, 1985, chap 21, pp 497–517.

26. Hawkins RJ, Bokor DJ: Clinical evaluation of shoulder problems, in Rockwood CA, Matsen FA (eds): *The Shoulder.* Philadelphia, Saunders, 1990, chap 4, pp 149–177.

27. Hawkins RJ, Kennedy JC: Impingement syndrome in athletes. *Am J Sports Med* 8:151–158, 1980.

28. Howell SM, Imobertsteg AM, Seger DH, Marone PJ: Clarification of the role of the supraspinatus muscle in shoulder function. *J Bone Joint Surg (Am)* 68A:3,398–404, March 1986.

29. Iannoti JP (ed): *Rotator Cuff Disorders*, AAOS Monograph Series. Park Ridge, American Academy of Orthopaedic Surgeons, 1992.

30. Itoi E, Tabata S: Conservative treatment of rotator cuff tears. *Clin Orthop* 275:165–173, February 1992.

31. Ivey FM, Calhoun JH, Rusche K, et al: Normal values for isokinetic testing of shoulder strength. *Med Sci Sports Exerc* 16:127, 1984 (abstr).

32. Jarvolm U, Palmerud G, Herberts P, et al: Intramuscular pressure and electromyography in the supraspinatus muscle at shoulder abduction. *Clin Orthop* 245:102–109, August 1989.

33. Jobe FW, Kvitne RS: Shoulder pain in the overhand or throwing athlete: The relationship of anterior instability and rotator cuff impingement. *Orthop Rev* 18:963, 1989.

34. Kendall FP, McCreary E: *Muscles: Their Testing and Function*, 3d ed. Baltimore, Williams & Wilkins, 1983.

35. Kennedy JC, Willis RB: The effects of local steroid injections on tendons: A biomechanical and microscopic correlative study. *Am J Sports Med* 4:11–21, 1976.

36. Kibler WB, Chandler TJ, Pace BK: Principles of rehabilitation after chronic tendon injuries. *Clin Sports Med* 11:3,661–624, July 1992.

37. Knott M, Voss DE: *Proprioceptive Neuromuscular Facilitation*, 2d ed. New York, Harper & Row, 1968.

38. Matsen FA, Arntz CT: Rotator cuff tendon failure, in Rockwood CA, Matsen FA (eds): *The Shoulder.* Philadelphia, Saunders, 1990, chap 16, pp 647–677.

39. Morrey BF, An K: Biomechanics of the shoulder, in Rockwood CA, Matsen FA (eds): *The Shoulder.* Philadelphia, Saunders, 1990, chap 6, pp 208–245.

40. Moseley JB, Jobe FW, Pink M, et al: EMG analysis of the scapular rotator muscles during a shoulder rehabilitation program. *Am J Sports Med*, 1991.

41. Murphy T: Instructional course notes, in *Combined Topics: Clinical Management of Inflammatory Shoulder Dysfunction.* Williamsburg, December 1992.

42. Neer CS II: Impingement lesions. *Clin Orthop* 173:70–77, 1983.

43. Neviaser TJ, Neviaser R: Observations on impingement. *Clin Orthop* 60, May 1990.

44. Nicholson GC: The effects of passive joints mobilization on pain and hypomobility associated with adhesive capsulitis of the shoulder. *J Orthop Sports Phys Ther* 6:238–246, 1985.

45. Nirschl RP: Rotator cuff tendinitis: Basic concepts of pathoetiology, in Barr JS (ed): *Instr Course Lect* 38:439–445, 1989.

46. Nirschl RP: Rotator cuff surgery, in Barr JS (ed): *Instr Course Lect* 38:447–462, 1989.

47. Nirschl RP: Shoulder tendinitis in Pettrone FA (ed): *AAOS Symposium on the Upper Extremity in Athletes.* St Louis, Mosby, 1984, pp 234–257.

48. Nobuhara K, Sugiyama D, Ikeda H, Makiura M: Contracture of the shoulder. *Clin Orthop* 254:105–110, May 1990.

49. Norris TR: History and physical examination of the shoulder, in Nicholas JA, Hershman EB (eds): *The Upper Extremity in Sports Medicine.* St Louis, Mosby, 1990, chap 3, pp 41–90.

50. Petersson G: Rupture of the tendon aponeurosis of the shoulder joint in anterior inferior dislocation. *Acta Chir Scand* (suppl)77:1–184, 1942.

51. Pink M, Perry J, Browne A, et al: The normal shoulder during freestyle swimming. *Am J Sports Med* 19(6):569–576, 1991.

52. Quillen WS, Mohr TM, Reed BV: High voltage pulsed galvanic stimulation as a modifier of sports-induced inflammation, in Leadbetter W (ed): *Sports-Induced Inflammation.* Park Ridge, IL, American Academy of Orthopaedic Surgeons, 1990, pp 493–497.

53. Rabin SI, Post M: A comparative study of clinical muscle testing and cybex evaluation after shoulder operations. *Clin Orthop* 258:147–156, September 1990.

54. Ringel SP, Treihaft M, Carry M, et al: Suprascapular neuropathy in pitchers. *Am J Sports Med* 18(1):80–86, 1990.

55. Rivenburgh DW: Physical modalities in the treatment of tendon injuries. *Clin Sports Med* 11(3):645–659, July 1992.

56. Roy S, Irvin R: *Sports Medicine: Prevention, Evaluation, Management, and Rehabilitation.* Englewood Cliffs, NJ, Prentice-Hall, 1983.

57. Saha AK: The classic mechanism of shoulder movements and a plea for recognition of the "zero position" of the glenohumeral joint. *Clin Orthop* 173:3, 1983.

58. Scovazzo ML, Browne A, Pink M, et al: The painful shoulder during freestyle swimming. *Am J Sports Med* 19(6):577–582, 1991.

59. Sobel J: Shoulder injuries: A rehabilitation perspective, in Knortz K, Lewis C (eds): *Orthopedic Assessment and Rehabilitation of the Geriatric Patient,* St Louis, Mosby, 1993.

60. Stuart MJ, Azevedo AJ, Cofield RH: Anterior acromioplasty for treatment of shoulder impingement syndrome. *Clin Orthop* 260:195–200, November 1990.

61. Townsend H, Jobe FW, Pink M, Perry J: EMG analysis of the glenohumeral muscles during a baseball rehabilitation program. *Am J Sports Med* 19(3):264–272, 1991.

62. Valtonen EJ: Double-acting betamethasone (Celestone Chronodose) in the treatment of supraspinatus tendonitis: A comparison of subacromial and gluteal single injections with placebo. *J Int Med Res* 6:463–467, 1978.

63. Walker SW, Couch WH, Boester GA, Sprowl DW: Isokinetic strength of the shoulder after repair of a torn rotator cuff. *J Bone Joint Surg (Am)* 69A(7):1041–1044, 1987.

64. Warner JJP, Micheli LJ, Arslanian LE, et al: Patterns of flexibility, laxity and strength in normal shoulders and shoulders with instability and impingement. *Am J Sports Med* 18(4):366–375, 1990.

65. Watson K: Impingement and rotator cuff lesions, in Nicholas J, Hershman E (eds): *The Upper Extremity in Sports Medicine.* St Louis, Mosby, 1990, chap 8, pp 213–220.

66. Weiner DS, MacNab I: Superior migration of the humeral head. *J Bone Joint Surg (Am)* 52B:524–527, 1970.

67. Withrington RH, Girgis FL, Seifert MH: A placebo-controlled trial of steroid injections in the treatment of supraspinatus tendonitis. *Scand J Rheumatol* 14:76–78, 1985.

68. Wolf WB III: Shoulder tendinoses. *Clin Sports Med* 11(4):871–890, October 1992.

69. Zuckerman JD, Mirabello SC, Newman D, et al: The painful shoulder, part II, AFP 43(2):497–512, February 1991.

CHAPTER 20

Shoulder Rehabilitation—Instability

Perry S. Esterson

INTRODUCTION

Athletes with shoulder instability fall into two broad categories, those with ligamentous laxity and those whose instability has been induced by trauma. The incidence of recurrent instability in athletics has been well documented. Successful nonoperative rehabilitation following shoulder dislocations has been demonstrated by several authors.[1,3,34] Patients in the first group may initially present not with frank instability but with impingement symptoms because of weakness.[8] When the instability is secondary to trauma, patients will present in the clinic for an initial conservative course of treatment or will have already had surgery. The treatment goals of both groups are to stop the progression of instability through a treatment of exercise and when necessary with surgery. Furthermore, it is through appropriate training. Treatment of shoulder instability is essentially the same whether it is preceding or following surgery. Only the time constraints of tissue healing and pathology sustained in the shoulder will modify the treatment regimen and outcome. A review of the biomechanics of the shoulder as it specifically relates to rehabilitation will be useful, as this will be the foundation of any treatment program.

BIOMECHANICS

The shoulder is a shallow ball and socket joint that maintains static stability through the labrum and shoulder capsule. The glenohumeral ligaments stabilize the shoulder anteriorly and inferiorly.[16] External rotation is more restrained by the anterior superior capsule with the arm in adduction while the inferior glenohumeral ligament provides restraint at 90° of abduction.[7,21] In the horizontal plane there is precise centering of the humeral head in the glenoid fossa. Howell et al.[13] suggest that an intact capsule and labrum maintain this centered position of the humerus rather than the contraction of shoulder musculature. This is significant clinically in that flexibility programs that overstretch the shoulder capsule may contribute to shoulder instability. Furthermore, posterior translation of the humeral head in the horizontal pain was not mediated by the pectoralis major and anterior deltoid, suggesting that strengthening exercises will not provide the necessary dynamic stability to effect this normal gliding motion. Dynamic stabilization is provided through various muscle groups about the shoulder.[9,10] The scapular rotator muscles include the serratus anterior, rhomboids, levator scapulae, and trapezius muscles. Together these muscles stabilize and rotate the scapula on the thorax, providing critical proximal stability for the motion of the more distal arm. The rotator cuff muscles—the supraspinatus, infraspinatus, teres minor, and subscapularis—work in concert to maintain the head of the humerus centralized against the glenoid.[30] The deltoid initiates abduction while the rotator cuff muscles work together to prevent superior migration of the humerus in the glenoid.[16] It is the maintenance of these critical force couples that will reduce shoulder pain in the weak shoulder and provide stability in the loose shoulder with static stabilizers that are no longer effective.

HISTORY AND PHYSICAL EXAMINATION

Prior to embarking on a rehabilitation program, it is important to obtain a thorough history and physical examination.[11,27] A sports-specific history will include the athlete's age, type of sport with particular emphasis on throwing and blocking positions, frequency and level of participation, and target date to return to sports. The complaints of pain and instability should be analyzed to determine what is the offending mechanism of injury and whether this mechanism is from weakness or instability.

The physical examination will include a visual inspection of the shoulders and spine for atrophy or asymmetry. Manual glenohumeral joint laxity tests as previously described in other chapters will assess joint play in the anterior, posterior, and inferior planes. Range of motion measurements should be obtained actively and passively. Impingement tests in flexion, abduction, or external rotation may be performed with and without resistance. Strength testing as advocated by Cyriax[4] to selectively test each shoulder muscle as well as the specific supraspinatus test with the arm internally rotated in the plane of the scapula (scaption)[22] will identify weak muscles. The examiner should take note whether these tests elicit dynamic results that are weak or strong and painful or painless. A strong strength test will signify patency of the musculotendinous structure while a weak strength test indicates the degree of strain or tear. Painful responses are present in acute injuries. Painless tests are present in a noninflamed structure or a totally ruptured musculotendinous unit that is unable to develop any tension. These tests will guide the therapist into developing a rehabilitation program that is appropriate to the level of injury.

THE REHABILITATION PROGRAM

As mentioned earlier, the goal of rehabilitation is to stop the progression of instability that may first present as either pain or frank instability. Burkhead and Rockwood[3] reported different success rates in rehabilitation programs for patients with traumatic vs. atraumatic shoulder instability. Only 15 percent of the traumatic instability group had a good or excellent result compared with an 83 percent success rate in the atraumatic group. Aronen and Regan[1] described a 75 percent success rate in patients with primary anterior shoulder dislocations, using a rehabilitation program with strict adherence to an aggressive exercise regime and rigid restrictions on activity until program goals are met. Yoneda et al.[34] also reported a satisfactory result in 82.7 percent after an exercise program for patients with traumatic anterior dislocation. These studies stand in contrast to the work of Rowe[25] showing a recurrence rate between 79 and 94 percent.

Rehabilitation can be divided into four phases.[31,26] Phase I involves the control of inflammation and the initiation of motion in a protected range. The goals of phase II are to gain pain-free range of motion, allow only minimal tenderness and pain, and begin strengthening of the shoulder rotator and scapular stabilizer muscles. In phase III dynamic exercises are utilized to maximize strength, power, and endurance. Full and pain-free range of motion will be present. Phase IV comprises the return to activity with functional exercises performed in a progressive sequence.

To control inflammation in the acute stage, use modalities of choice that include both physical agents and nonsteroidal anti-inflammatory medication. Applications of ice in the initial stages of injury will reduce pain and inflammation. Electrical modalities using microampere current, interferential current, or high-voltage galvanic stimulation may be used to decrease inflammation. The hallmark of the rehabilitation program consists of strengthening the shoulder musculature. Pink and Jobe[22] have divided these muscles into three groups: the glenohumeral protectors (rotator cuff muscles), the scapulohumeral pivotors (scapular rotator muscles), and the humeral positioners (deltoid, pectoralis major, and latissimus dorsi muscles). The first two groups are initially strengthened while the positioners are subsequently involved. The normal progression of strengthening starts with isometric exercises followed by isotonic exercises in a limited and pain-free range, then full range of motion. Isokinetic exercises are added utilizing various speeds and positions.[31,5] Finally functional activities that mimic the sport are included to prepare the athlete for a successful return to competition. Exercises include both concentric and eccentric contractions performed in both an open and a closed kinetic chain.

Glenohumeral Protectors

This group includes the supraspinatus, infraspinatus, teres minor, and subscapularis. In phase I, strengthening exercises for this group start isometrically with the arm in the neutral position by the trunk. Patients are then progressed using latex tubing to perform isoflex exercises as advocated by Nirschl.[19] Dumbbells can be utilized for these same exercises in the side-lying position (Fig. 20-1). To decrease strain, or "wringing out," across the critical zone of the rotator cuff that Rathbun and MacNab have described,[23] place a small roll in the axilla. Latex tubing or Theraband (Hygenics, Akron, OH) has the advantage of being able to position the upper extremity in many positions against resistance without regard to gravity. Different grades of tubing can be used to increase resistance. These exercises can be started in the side-lying or standing position with the arm by the side.

Different positions have been advocated for strengthening the supraspinatus. Jobe, Moynes, and Pink[15,22] advocate maximum supraspinatus activity in the standing or seated position with the arm positioned in the plane of the scapula at 90° abduction, 30° horizontal flexion, and fully internally rotated. In contrast, Blackburn et al.[2] reported the greatest supraspinatus EMG activity in the prone position with the humerus horizontally abducted 100° and externally rotated with the thumb up (Fig. 20-2). Worrell et al.[33] compared these positions and agreed with Blackburn's findings. Worrell also found significantly greater strength generated in the standing position as compared with the prone. However, this

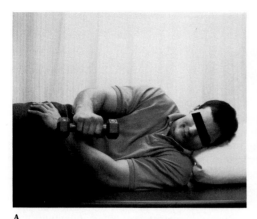
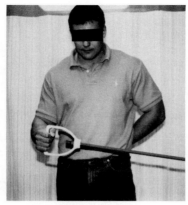

A   B

FIGURE 20-1
A. External rotation with dumbbell. B. External rotation with latex tubing (isoflex technique).

may be related to deltoid activity. When first facilitating supraspinatus strengthening, Blackburn's prone position will cause less impingement and soreness. Additionally, the scapula may be manually stabilized by the therapist. Overhead exercises such as the military press will tend to increase impingement in the shoulder and should therefore be avoided until the final stages of rehabilitation.

Isokinetic activities, both concentrically and eccentrically, can be started with the arm slightly abducted and the patient standing beside the dynamometer with the elbow centered over the axis of motion. Warner et al.[30] proposed isokinetic testing for external and internal shoulder rotation in approximately 25° of scapular plane abduction to avoid impingement or subluxation. When there is a negative impingement sign, the exercises can be progressed with the shoulder in a more elevated position in the plane of the scapula at 90° of flexion and the elbow flexed to 90° (Fig. 20-3). This position is useful for those athletes in throwing activities but is also potentially dangerous because it places the arm in a vulnerable position to dislocate or sublux. When

starting isokinetics, speeds under 100°/s are preferable so the athlete can learn to control the shoulder motion at various speeds. Speeds up to 300°/s on the various dynamometers can be used to mimic sports movements; however, functional shoulder speeds are far in excess of these machines.

The supraspinatus and infraspinatus muscles are critical in preventing superior migration of the humerus. Townsend et al.[29] describe four exercises that are responsible for a high level of EMG activity in the supraspinatus. Scaption with internal rotation, flexion, horizontal abduction in external rotation, and the press-up should be considered as core exercises for the rotator cuff and humeral positioners.

The Scapular Pivotors

This group includes the above-mentioned scapular rotators with the addition of the pectoralis minor. Since the shoulder is primarily a non-weight-bearing joint with an emphasis of mobility and not stability, it is essential to strengthen these muscles in the re-

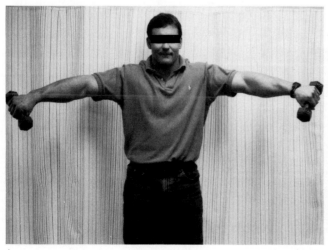

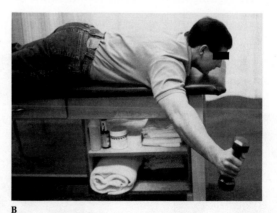

B

FIGURE 20-2
A. Elevation of the arm in the plane of the scapula (scaption) for supraspinatus strengthening. B. Supraspinatus strengthening in the prone position.

A

273

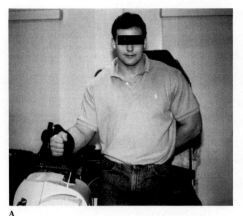

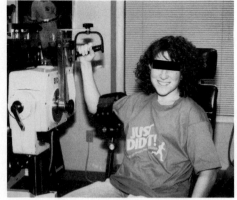

FIGURE 20-3
A. Isokinetic exercises for internal and external rotation in a protected range of motion. B. Isokinetic external and internal rotation in the plane of the scapula at 90° of abduction.

A

B

habilitation program. Strong and effective scapular pivotors will maintain the scapula in an optimum position so that the rotator cuff muscles will perform most effectively. Pink and Jobe, and Moseley[22,18] have found rowing and horizontal shoulder abduction to be excellent exercises for the trapezius, levator scapulae, and rhomboid muscles (Fig. 20-4). Exercises for the serratus anterior and pectoralis minor include the shoulder shrug, press-up, and push-up with a "plus" (Fig. 20-5). The "plus" part of the push-up enhances scapular protraction and may be done as a bench press at the fully extended end range of motion or as push-up. Glousman et al.[9] stress the protraction of the scapula provided by the serratus anterior in throwing. With weakness in this muscle, there will be increased anterior laxity due to the increased stress of the humeral head on the anterior glenoid labrum and capsule. Care must be taken to avoid full lowering of the body to the floor in the push-up or lowering the bar to or below the chest in the bench press because of anterior migration of the humeral head (Fig. 20-6). This will impinge the rotator cuff as well as stress the anterior static stabilizers of the shoulder and may increase instability. This is particularly significant in anterior subluxations or dislocations.

The Humeral Positioners

This group includes all portions of the deltoid, the pectoralis major, and latissimus dorsi muscles. Various authors[18,22,24] have indicated the best exercises for this group include scaption, horizontal abduction with humeral external rotation, and the press-up. Strengthening these muscles will provide the foundation for high-level athletic activities including throwing and tackling.

The exercise program in phase III progresses through the isotonic and isokinetic phase including both concentric and eccentric strengthening at various velocities. Proprioceptive neuromuscular facilitation (PNF)[17] exercises on all fours such as rapid reversals promote closed-chain kinetic stabilization of the shoulder without risk of instability[5] (Fig. 20-7). The final phase of rehabilitation includes returning to functional activities that are found in the patient's sport. Throwing cannot be started until full range of motion has been obtained. Specific throwing programs[11,31] require several months before the athlete can return to hard throwing and pitching. Patients in contact sports may require specialized bracing to restrict the end range of abduction and external rotation. This can be accomplished with the

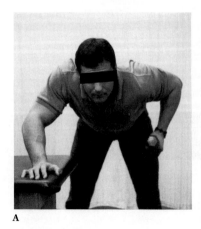

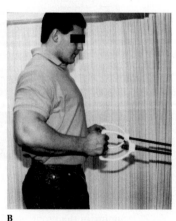

A

B

FIGURE 20-4
A. Rowing with dumbbell. B. Rowing with latex tubing.

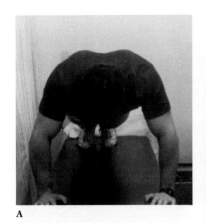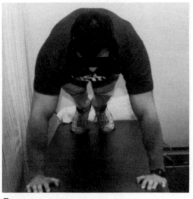

A   **B**

FIGURE 20-5
A. Normal push-up.   *B.* Push-up with a "plus" for scapular protraction.

C. D. Denison-Duke Wyre (Micro Bio-Medics, Inc., 846 Pelham Parkway, Pelham Manor, NY 10803) or SAWA brace (Brace International, P. O. Box 19752, Atlanta, GA 30325). For more details on bracing see Chap. 27.

As the patient progresses through the strengthening program, the therapist must correct range of motion limitations that may exist in the nonsurgical shoulder. Mobilizing the posterior and inferior capsule will help regain full mobility necessary for normal shoulder motion (Fig. 20-8). Prolonged stretching of 15 to 30 s will effectively stretch the capsular tissues. Limitations in pectoralis flexibility will place the scapula in a protracted position and increase the risk of impingement. Care must be taken to stretch this area without overstretching the anterior capsule. Ultrasound to the axilla will help create elasticity in the inferior capsule.[36] Once this mobility and a negative impingement sign are present, the patient starts on a progression of sports-specific exercises as outlined above.

While the majority of the rehabilitation program has been directed toward anterior or anterior-inferior instability, posterior shoulder instability is occasion-

ally seen. Posterior dislocations account for 2 percent of shoulder dislocations.[35] However, Norwood and Terry find recurrent posterior glenohumeral subluxations common in athletics.[20] The athlete will usually fall on an outstretched and internally rotated arm, forcing the humerus posteriorly. Rehabilitation will follow the above outline with particular emphasis on the supraspinatus, infraspinatus, and teres minor to more effectively stabilize the posterior aspect of the shoulder.[6] Generally most nonsurgical candidates will return to their sports within 3 months if they have been faithful with their rehabilitation program. See Appendix C for a rehabilitation protocol for following conservative and surgical treatment.

Surgical Rehabilitation

The advent of arthroscopy has enhanced the return to sports and function with shoulder instability. The main open surgical repairs for anterior or anterior-inferior instability include the Bristow, Putti-Platt, Magnuson-Stack, and Bankart procedures. The cap-

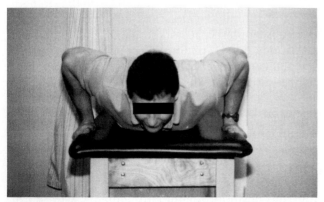

FIGURE 20-6
Full lowering of the body in a push-up can cause anterior migration of the humeral head.

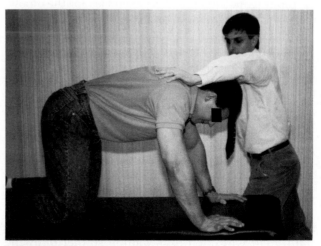

FIGURE 20-7
Closed-chain kinetic shoulder stabilization exercises on hands and knees.

275

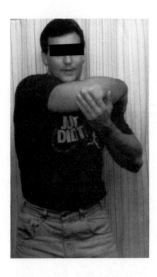

FIGURE 20-8
Stretching of the posterior capsule.

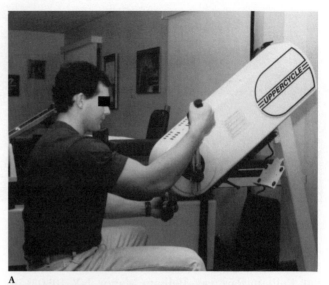

A

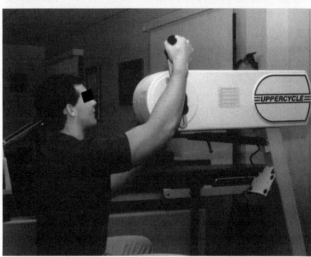

B

FIGURE 20-9
A. Upper body ergometer with shoulder flexion below 90° to avoid impingement.   B. Upper body ergometer with shoulder flexion about 90° in more advanced stage of rehabilitation.

sular shift procedure and Bankart repairs are now being performed with arthroscopic techniques. Shoulder rehabilitation following surgery will generally follow the above conservative program, but with particular modifications for soft tissue and bony healing constraints specific to the surgical procedure performed. (See Appendixes A, B, and C for specific postoperative protocols.) It is common to maintain the arm in a sling and swathe brace for 4 to 6 weeks after open reconstructive procedures. It is essential to use a team approach so that therapist, physician, and patient jointly understand the goals, time frames, and precautions that are inherent in the surgical repair and the subsequent rehabilitation program. The surgical morbidity is less with arthroscopic procedures.[32] When anterior capsule reconstruction is performed via the arthroscope, range of motion and isometric exercises may be started immediately (Nirschl, personal communication). Active or active assisted shoulder range of motion and isometric strengthening exercises may be initiated without pain. Strengthening exercises for the elbow, forearm, and hand are continued throughout the rehabilitative process. Full motion should be obtained within 6 weeks. Strengthening of the nonaffected arm should continue throughout the course of rehabilitation. Aerobic exercise such as stationary biking is encouraged. Upper body ergometer exercises are begun first with the humerus placed below 90° of flexion and progressed to 120 to 150° flexion (Fig. 20-9). This type of cycling may be performed both forward and backward. Sports activities may be started between 4 and 6 months and return to full activity between 6 and 12 months. Reconstructive procedures such as the Putti-Platt and Bristow will limit full external rotation and abduction.[24] The Putti-Platt will often limit motion so that throwing activities are not possible and return to the prior sports level is precluded. When faced with patients

with these surgical procedures, full mobility is sacrificed for stability. Emphasis will be on the strengthening of internal rotators and adductors, including the subscapularis, pectoralis major and minor, and latissimus dorsi. Anatomic reconstructions such as the Bankart procedure or capsular reconstructions may allow full return to sports.[12,14,22]

Posterior Instability Rehabilitation

Stabilization of the shoulder with posterior instability has had less consistent success. Norwood and Terry[20] treated symptomatic posterior subluxation first with exercises to strengthen the posterior deltoid and posterior rotator cuff. Patients who continued to exhibit posterior subluxation with the abducted arm in forward flexion for pulling, pushing,

276

and lifting activities were surgically treated by an opening wedge posterior scapular osteotomy with a bone graft from the angle of the acromion. Soft tissue laxity was also surgically corrected. Postoperatively, abduction and internal rotation were avoided until the osteotomies had healed. The rehabilitation program consisted of regaining range of motion and strengthening the pectoral girdle, posterior deltoid, and rotator cuff. Most athletes in their study returned to their sport. In Tibone et al.'s study,[28] 10 athletes in throwing sports were treated with staple capsulorrhaphy for recurrent posterior dislocation. None of the athletes were able to return to their previous level of throwing owing to a loss of "whip," or velocity. Their conclusion was only patients with significant pain and/or functional impairment should be treated surgically.

Engle and Canner,[6] in one of the few references on rehabilitation of posterior shoulder instability, state most patients return to full activity following labral resection and remain asymptomatic despite the presence of posterior laxity. A 6-week program of rehabilitation was outlined beginning with restoring normal scapulohumeral rhythm using linear and diagonal patterns of scapular facilitation. Isolated internal and external rotation exercises between 10 and 45° abduction are then instituted. Overhead motions are avoided to prevent further damage to the labrum or rotator cuff. After 2 weeks of symptom-free movements, more aggressive diagonal patterns and overhead resistive exercises are included (Fig. 20-10). Engle and Canner have found most patients rarely require therapy beyond 6 weeks. However, if surgical correction is required, this time frame is lengthened to accommodate soft tissue healing.

SUMMARY

A rehabilitation program for the unstable shoulder has been outlined. Symptoms may range from shoulder impingement to frank instability. The basic rehabilitation program remains the same whether it is conservative or postoperative. Careful monitoring of pain, range of motion, impingement signs, and instability will determine the progression and speed of the rehabilitation program. It is essential to strengthen all shoulder musculature to achieve maximum function and stability. Total body fitness will speed the return to sports and help reduce the risk of reinjury. A team effort of the physician, therapist, and athlete will allow for the maximum safe return to activity. A critical understanding of the anatomy, biomechanics, and surgical procedures of the shoulder will help the therapist to design a rehabilitation program to maximize the chances for rapid return to sports and activity.

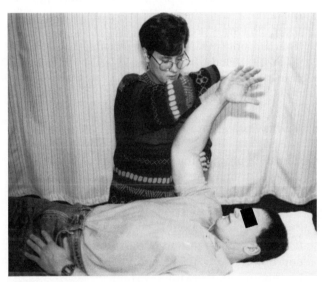

FIGURE 20-10
PNF diagonal exercise patterns.

APPENDIX A: ANTERIOR CAPSULOLABRAL RECONSTRUCTION REHABILITATION PROGRAM*

0 to 2 Weeks Postsurgery:

- Patient is immobilized in an abduction pillow at 80 to 90° of abduction and 45° external rotation for 2 weeks.
- Splint may be removed for gentle passive abduction, flexion, and external rotation two times per day and to allow the shoulder to adduct. Abduction and external rotation are performed in 20 to 30° horizontal adduction. Do not force external rotation.
- Isometric abduction, horizontal abduction and adduction.
- Active elbow flexion and extension strengthening exercises.
- May squeeze a soft ball.

2 to 6 Weeks Postsurgery:

- Patient no longer required to wear splint.
- Continue gentle ROM exercises with emphasis on protecting the anterior capsule.
- Active internal rotation with the arm at the side.
- Active external rotation from full internal rotation to 0° rotation using surgical or rubber tubing as tolerated. Full active external rotation is not allowed in this phase as this will place stress on the anterior capsule.
- Perform ROM exercises and mobilization techniques as needed (i.e., wand exercises, wall climbs, etc.).
- Active shoulder extension in the prone position. Only extend the arm until it is level with the trunk.
- Shoulder shrugs.
- By 4 to 5 weeks postsurgery, progress to side lying external rotation exercises.
- Supraspinatus strengthening exercise.
- Shoulder abduction to 90°.

6 to 8 Weeks Postsurgery:

- Continue strengthening exercises with emphasis on the rotator cuff muscles.

- Shoulder flexion strengthening exercise.
- Horizontal adduction (from 15 to 20° horizontal adduction to 90°).
- Upper body ergometer for endurance training beginning at low resistance.

2 to 4 Months Postsurgery:

- Progress with weights as tolerated (i.e., shoulder flexion, abduction, extension, supraspinatus, etc.).
- By 2 months, patient should have full range of motion.
- At 2 months, continue emphasis on strengthening the rotator cuff musculature.
- May include isokinetic strengthening and endurance exercises at the faster speeds (e.g., 240°/s) for shoulder flexion and abduction.
- At 2 to 2 ½ months, add push-ups lowering the body until arms are level with the trunk. Begin with wall push-ups, progressing to modified (on the knees) and then military push-ups (on the toes). The arms are positioned at 70 to 80° abduction. Do not lower the body causing the arms to go past the body, which would stress the anterior capsule.
- Horizontal abduction.

4 Months Postsurgery:

- Continue progressing weights. May add isokinetic strength training at different speeds with emphasis at the higher speeds. Position the arm by the side for internal and external rotation.
- Perform first isokinetic test over a 3-day period.
- If the isokinetic test indicates adequate strength and endurance (70 percent or above) begin with tossing in the throwing program.

5 Months Postsurgery:

- Chin-ups.
- Continue with throwing program as tolerated.

6 Months Postsurgery:

- Continue strengthening and endurance exercises with emphasis on the muscles needed specifically for their playing position.
- Add total body conditioning.

*From the Kerlan-Jobe Orthopaedic Clinic Department of Physical Therapy: FW Jobe, CE Brewster, and JL Seto.

APPENDIX B: REHABILITATION FOLLOWING ARTHROSCOPIC SHOULDER RECONSTRUCTION*

Guidelines for shoulder rehabilitation following arthroscopic Bankart repair. Treatment should be modified as dictated by signs and symptoms.

PHASE I: The initial phase emphasizes beginning ROM recovery without unduly stressing healing tissue.

1. Sling—encourage use of uninvolved joints and ice three times per day.
   0 to 3 weeks.
2. Gentle Codman exercises in sling.
   Start at 1 to 2 weeks.
3. Gentle pain-free isometric exercises.
   Start at 1 to 2 weeks.
4. Begin mobilization out of sling, passive ROM, mobilization, and supine wand exercises (avoid aggressive anterior and inferior humeral glides; avoid external rotation initially).
   Start at 3 weeks.
5. Active-assistive ROM against gravity (wand, wall climb, pulley, etc.: start into flexion and gradually progress to abduction).
   Start at 3 to 4 weeks.
6. Active ROM against gravity, same considerations as no. 5.
   Start at 4 weeks.
7. Limited-arc dynamic resistive exercises; avoid external rotation beyond 0°; emphasis on anterior shoulder musculature; low resistance, high repetition program initially.
   Start at 4 to 5 weeks.

PHASE II: This phase is directed toward increasing ROM, strength, and neuromuscular control—no end range loading.

1. Progressive ROM—begin working into external rotation with arm at side, as appreciation for end feel is essential; full flexion should be obtained by 10 to 12 weeks.
   Start at 5 to 6 weeks.
2. Increase vigor of strengthening exercises, avoiding combined position of external rotation and abduction. Address both muscle isolation and synergy, emphasizing rotator cuff and scapular muscles. We utilize a lot of manual resistance initially, then progress to isokinetic and finally isotonic exercises, emphasizing concentric-eccentric specifically for sports. Strengthening exercises generally performed 90° or below and utilize principles of submaximal to maximal and controlled arcs of motion.
   Start at 6 weeks.
3. Mobilize into external rotation with arm abducted, 60° external rotation by 12 weeks.
   Start at 8 weeks.

PHASE III: This phase increases the intensity and specificity of exercise and prepares for return to full activities.

1. Vigorous strengthening program—high load, low repetition plus endurance, and isokinetic velocity spectrum as indicated.
   Start at 12 weeks.
2. Full ROM as required for function is usually obtainable. This may require rather vigorous mobilization and stretching.
   Obtain by 12 to 16 weeks.
3. Advanced neuromuscular training, quadruped training, pro fitter, etc.
   Start at 14 to 16 weeks.
4. Functional progression for sports and high demands.

PHASE IV: Discharge

1. Maintenance—exercise program.
2. Counseling—equipment, activities, position.

*TB Fleeter, R Thal, Town Center Orthopaedic Associates, P.C. (adapted from Joe Sutter, Tuckahoe Physical Therapy).

APPENDIX C: SHOULDER REHABILITATION PROTOCOL

	Anterior instability	Posterior instability	Posterior surgery	Multi-instability
Phase 1 (0–6 weeks);				
Sling 2–4 weeks	x	x	x	x
Modalities for pain and swelling	x	x	x	x
Pendulum exercises	x	x	x	x
Submaximal isometrics (no pain)	x	x	x	x
PROM and AAROM:*				
Flexion	90°	0°	0°	90°
Abduction	45–60°	45–60°	45–60°	45–60°
External rotation	45°	45–60°	45–60°	45°
Internal rotation	45–60°	0°	0°	20°
Horizontal abduction	30–45°	90°	90°	30–45°
Horizontal adduction	Full	0°	0°	0–20°
Joint mobilization:				
Scapular	x	x	x	x
Glenohumeral anterior glide		x	x	Midrange
Glenohumeral posterior glide	x			Midrange
Scapular PNF patterns:				
Anterior elevation	x	x	x	x
Posterior elevation	x	x	x	x
Anterior depression	x	x	x	x
Posterior depression	x	x	x	x
PREs for hand and wrist	x	x	x	x
Manual resistance scapular PNF	x	x	x	x
Phase II (6 to 10 weeks):				
AAROM and AROM for:				
Full forward flexion	x	x	x	x
Full external rotation	50–75%	x	x	50–75%
Full internal rotation	x			50–75%
Full horizontal abduction	50–75%	x	x	50–75%
Full horizontal aduction	x	50–75%	50–75%	50–75%
Continue PRE scapular stabilizers	x	x	x	x
Protect anterior capsule	x			x
Protect posterior capsule		x	x	x
Begin PRE glenohumeral protectors	x	x	x	x
Begin PRE scapular pivotors	x	x	x	x
Continue PRE humeral positioners	x	x	x	x
PNF on all fours for kinesthesia	x	x	x	x
UBE or upper cycle with light resistance	x	x	x	x
Isokinetics at 20° scaption for external and internal rotation, submax	x	x	x	x
Phase III (10 to 16 weeks):				
Full ROM all planes of motion and normal G/H rhythm	x	x	x	x
Dynamic strengthening at 90-90 position for external and internal rotation	x	x	x	x
PNF patterns, full ROM	x	x	x	x
Isokinetics concentric and eccentric submaximal:				
Flexion and extension	x	x	x	x
External-internal rotation	x	x	x	x
Abduction and adduction	x	x	x	x
UBE upper cycle for endurance	x	x	x	x

APPENDIX C (continued)

	Anterior instability	Posterior instability	Posterior surgery	Multi-instability
Phase IV (16 weeks +):				
Functional sports-specific training	x	x	x	x
Maximum strength training	x	x	x	x
Plyoball training	x	x	x	x
Maintain overall flexibility	x	x	x	x
Maintain cardiovascular endurance	x	x	x	x
Gradual return to sport with proper technique	x	x	x	x

*Progression of range of motion is determined by the specific surgical procedure, tissue healing constraints, and the philosophy of the operating orthopedic surgeon. The therapist must work in concert with the surgeon to progress the patient at the appropriate pace.

REFERENCES

1. Aronen JG, Regan K: Decreasing the incidence of recurrence of first time anterior shoulder dislocations with rehabilitation. *Am J Sports Med* 12:283–291, 1984.
2. Blackburn TA, McLeod WD, White B, et al: EMG analysis of posterior rotator cuff exercises. *Athl Training* 25:40–45, 1990.
3. Burkhead WZ, Rockwood CA: Treatment of instability of the shoulder with an exercise program. *J Bone Joint Surg (Am)* 74-A:890–896, 1992.
4. Cyriax J: *Textbook of Orthopaedic Medicine*, vol I, 6th ed. London, Bailliere Tindall, 1975.
5. Davies G: APTA National Convention, 1992.
6. Engle RP, Canner GC: Posterior shoulder instability: Approach to rehabilitation. *J Orthop Sports Phys Ther* 13:488–494, 1989.
7. Ferrari DA: Capsular ligaments of the shoulder: Anatomical and functions study of the anterior superior capsule. *Am J Sports Med* 18:20–24, 1990.
8. Garth WP, Allman FL, Armstrong WS: Occult anterior subluxations of the shoulder in non-contact sports. *Am J Sports Med* 15:579–585, 1987.
9. Glousman R, Jobe F, Tibone J, et al: Dynamic electromyographic analysis of the throwing shoulder with glenohumeral instability. *J Bone Joint Surg (Am)* 70a:220–226, 1988.
10. Gowan ID, Jobe FW, Tibone JE, et al: A comparative electromyographic analysis of the shoulder during pitching: professional versus amateur pitchers. *Am J Sports Med* 15:586–590, 1987.
11. Halbach JW, Tank RT: The shoulder, in Gould JA (ed): *Orthopaedic and Sports Physical Therapy*. St Louis, Mosby, 1990, pp 483–521.
12. Hastings DE, Coughlin LP: Recurrent subluxation of the glenohumeral joint. *Am J Sports Med* 9:352–355, 1981.
13. Howell SM, Galinat BJ, Renzi AJ, Marone PJ: Normal and abnormal mechanics of the glenohumeral joint in the horizontal plane. *J Bone Joint Surg (Am)* 70A:227–232, 1988.
14. Jobe FW, Giangarra CE, Kvitne RS, Glousman RE: Anterior capsulolabral reconstruction of the shoulder in athletes in overhand sports. *Am J Sports Med* 19:428–434, 1991.
15. Jobe FW, Moynes DR: Delineation of diagnostic criteria and a rehabilitation program for rotator cuff injuries. *Am J Sports Med* 10:336–339, 1982.
16. Kapandji IA: *The Physiology of the Joints*, 2d ed. Edinburgh, Churchill Livingstone, 1970, vol 1, *Upper Limb*.
17. Knott M, Voss DE: *Proprioceptive Neuromuscular Facilitation*, New York, 1969, Harper and Row.
18. Moseley JB, Jobe FW, Pink M, et al: EMG analysis of the scapular muscles during a shoulder rehabilitation program. *Am J Sports Med* 20:128–134, 1992.
19. Nirschl RP: Prevention and treatment of elbow and shoulder injuries in the tennis player. *Clin Sports Med* 7:289–308, 1988.
20. Norwood LA, Terry GC: Shoulder posterior subluxation. *Am J Sports Med* 12:25–30, 1984.
21. O'Connell PW, Nuber GW, Mileski RA, Lautenschlager E: The contribution of the glenohumeral ligaments to anterior stability of the shoulder joint. *Am J Sports Med* 18:579–584, 1990.
22. Pink M, Jobe FW: Shoulder injuries in athletes. *Clin Management* 11:39–47, 1991.
23. Rathbun J, MacNab I: The microvascular pattern of the rotator cuff. *J Bone Joint Surg (Br)* 52:540–553, 1970.

24. Regan WD, Webster-Boaert S, Hawkins RJ, Fowler PJ: Comparative functional analysis of the Bristow, Magnuson-Stack, and Putti-Platt procedures for recurrent dislocation of the shoulder. *Am J Sports Med* 17:42–48, 1989.

25. Rowe CR: Acute and recurrent anterior dislocation of the shoulder. *Orthop Clin North Am* 11:253–270, 1980.

26. Slaughter D: Shoulder injuries, in Sanders B (ed): *Sports Physical Therapy*, Norwalk, CT, Appleton & Lange, 1990.

27. Tank R, Halbach J: Physical therapy evaluation of the shoulder complex in athletes. *J Orthop Sports Phys Ther* 3:108–119, 1982.

28. Tibone JE, Prietto C, Jobe FW, et al: Staple capsulorrhaphy for recurrent posterior shoulder dislocation. *Am J Sports Med* 9:135–139, 1981.

29. Townsend H, Jobe FW, Pink M, Perry J: Electromyographic analysis of the glenohumeral muscles during a baseball rehabilitation program. *Am J Sports Med* 19:264–272, 1991.

30. Warner JJP, Micheli LJ, Arslanian LE, et al: Patterns of flexibility, laxity, and strength in normal shoulders and shoulders with instability and impingement. *Am J Sports Med* 18:366–375, 1990.

31. Wilk KE, Arrigo C: An integrated approach to upper extremity exercises. *Orthop Phys Ther Clin North Am* 9(2):337–360, 1992.

32. Wolf WB: Shoulder tendinoses. *Clin Sports Med* 11:871–890, 1992.

33. Worrell TW, Corey BJ, York SL, Santiestaban J: An analysis of supraspinatus EMG activity and shoulder isometric force development. *Med Sci Sports Exerc* 24:744–748, 1992.

34. Yoneda B, Welsh RP, MacIntosh DL: Conservative treatment of shoulder dislocation in young males, in proceedings of the Canadian Orthopaedic Association. *J Bone Joint Surg (Am)* 64-B:254–255, 1982.

35. Zarins BZ, Rowe CR: Current concepts in the diagnosis and treatment of shoulder instability in athletes. *Med Sci Sports Exerc* 16:444–448, 1984.

36. Ziskin MC, McDiarmid T, Michlovitz SL: Therapeutic ultrasound, in Michlovitz SL (ed): *Thermal Agents in Rehabilitation*. Philadelphia, FA Davis, 1990, pp 134–169.

SPORT-SPECIFIC PROBLEMS

CHAPTER 21

Golf

John R. McCarroll

The person who never plays golf may imagine that it is a harmless activity less taxing than other sports. However, bad backs, sprained wrists, and aching shoulders lead the list of ailments affecting the golfer.

Unfortunately, golf injuries have received very little attention in the literature. There have been isolated reports of carpal fractures,[1] ulnar and median nerve injuries,[2] tendinitis in various areas,[2] skin rashes,[3] and eye injuries.[4–6]

Two studies[7,8] have reported on injuries in the professional and amateur golfer. In the professional golfer, the most common injury was to the wrist, followed closely by the back, hand, shoulder, and knee. In the amateur golfer, the most common injury was to the lower back, followed by the elbow, wrist, shoulder, and knee (Table 21-1).

Most of these injuries were caused by too much play or practicing causing overuse syndrome. The other causes such as poor swing mechanics, hitting an object other than the ball, or poor warm-up are summarized in Table 21-2.

There are also interesting isolated reports of injury and death, psychologic aspects of golf, and ocular physical problems experienced by the golfers.[5,22–24] One such case is related to injuries involving a gentleman who performed a golf swing and broke his tibia in two places.

Excitement on the golf course has also led to some strange injuries. One woman threw her putter into the air after making a long putt, fell over her golf bag, and broke both of her wrists. Another golfer threw his club into the air and knocked out his playing companion.[25]

Many deaths have occurred on the golf course because of lightning, heart attacks, heat strokes, and electrocution after striking power lines.[26]

Likewise, anger has led to death in many cases. One man broke his club on a tree, and the broken shaft subsequently rebounded off another tree. The jagged end plunged into his body. Recently, a golfer in Silver Springs, MD,[26] was charged with attempted murder after a bloody club-swinging brawl with a faster foursome who tried to overtake his group. Finally, back in 1939,[26] a Philadelphia golfer was convicted of involuntary manslaughter for killing his caddy after swinging his club in anger after missing a shot.

There is a golfing disease known as the twitch or yips[24] that is such a ridiculous disease that nonsufferers can hardly credit it. It attacks the victim almost always on short putts. One becomes totally incapable of moving a putter head to and fro without giving it a convulsive twitch at the critical moment of impact. Some players simply strike the ground whereas others move the ball only a few inches. Bobby Jones, Harry Vardin, Sam Snead, Ben Hogan, and Henry Longhurst have been afflicted with this disease. There has been some basis to the fact that yips could actually be a mental disease. However, many attempts at cure utilizing hypnotism, changing of putters, changing of grips, or putting styles have all been tried but to no avail.

There appears to be a paradox involved that many excellent players have very poor eyesight yet cannot play with glasses. The long game seems to depend on pure physical action rather than ocular physical coordination. On the other hand, the short game depends on ocular physical coordination. This is where high refractive error is common, as astigmatism and muscle imbalance may take their toll.[5]

In order to evaluate, treat, and prevent golf injuries one must understand the biomechanics of the golf swing. For the purpose of this chapter the golf swing will be broken down into three parts: takeaway, impact, and follow-through.

The golf swing occurs in two planes, the plane of the backswing and the plane of the downswing. The swing evolves around three dimensions: (1) vertical, (2) lateral, and (3) rotatory.[9]

Take-away (Fig. 21-1A) consists of the setup and movement to the top of the backswing (Fig. 21-1B).

283

TABLE 21-1
Frequency of Injuries

Body part	Professional (393)	Amateur (908)
Lower back	93 (23.7%)	244 (34.5%)
Wrist	105 (26.7%)	142 (20.1%)
Elbow	26 (6.6%)	234 (33.1%)
Shoulder	37 (9.4%)	84 (11.7%)
Knee	26 (6.6%)	66 (9.3%)
Neck	12 (3.1%)	28 (4%)
Hip	4 (1.0%)	22 (3.1%)
Ribs	12 (3.1%)	22 (3.1%)
Ankle	8 (2.0%)	18 (2.5%)
Foot	13 (3.3%)	12 (1.7%)

TABLE 21-2
Mechanisms of Injury

	Professional's injuries	Amateur's injuries
Too much play or practice	270	204
Poor swing mechanics	0	150
Hit ground (divot)	40	171
Over swing	0	85
Poor warm-up	0	60
Twist during swing	18	22
Grip or swing change	0	26
Fall	2	24
Bending over putt	5	8
Injury secondary to cart	0	18
Hit by ball	3	36

The golfer rotates the knees, hips, lumbar, and cervical spine while the head remains relatively stationary as the weight shifts to the right side. The prime mover at this phase in the right shoulder is the supraspinatus portion of the rotator cuff and not the deltoid.[10,11] In the left shoulder, the rotator cuff muscles (supraspinatus, infraspinatus, and teres minor) fire minimally while the subscapularis is quite active.[10,11] Deceleration to a momentary arrest is accomplished by the right-sided muscles that later will accelerate the downswing. There is a hyperabduction of the left thumb, radial deviation of the left wrist, and dorsiflexion of the right wrist. However, less than 25 percent of all golf injuries occur during this part of the golf swing (Table 21-3).[7,8]

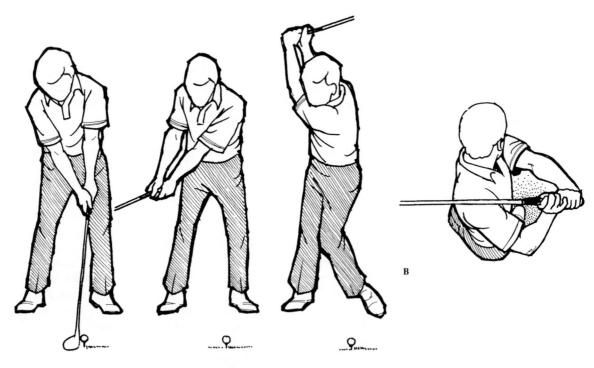

TAKE-AWAY

A

B

FIGURE 21-1
A. Take-away. B. Top of backswing or take-away. Momentary arrest before acceleration into the downswing; the right arm is abducted, externally rotated, and horizontally extended. The left arm is adducted across the anterior chest.

TABLE 21-3
Relationship of Injury to Swing

Swing	Total injuries
Take-away	
Back	28
Wrist	25
Elbow, neck, knee	9
Hand	7
Shoulder	6
	75
Impact	
Wrist	73
Back	50
Elbow	22
Hand	16
Shoulder	9
Knee	7
Upper back	2
	179
Follow-through	
Back	43
Shoulder	18
Ribs	12
Knee	10
Wrist	9
Neck	6
Hand	4
Elbow	4
	106

Impact (Fig. 21-2A) consists of the downswing (Fig. 21-2B) and the impact of the ball (Fig. 21-2D). Table 21-3 shows that there are more injuries during impact than during any other stage of the golf swing.

As the downswing (Fig. 21-2B) begins, golfers shift their weight to the left side by moving their hips toward the target. Good golfers actually begin this hip movement about 0.1 s before the downswing starts.[12,13] In order to develop maximum acceleration in the downswing phase, the golfer applies the stretch reflex principle. When the whole muscle is stretched, the stretch of the muscle spindles causes a reflex contracture of the host muscles. As a result, the contractile force of the muscle increases and facilitates the recoil of elastic tissue. This principle can further be developed by increasing the flexibility of the major muscle groups. Thus the farther a person can rotate the shoulders away from the target, the greater clubhead speed can be generated, thus increasing distance.

This counterclockwise torque in the upper body is generated by the buttocks, quadriceps, hamstrings, and lower back muscles. This torque causes mod-

erate levels of activity[10,11] in the pectoralis major, latissimus dorsi, and rotator cuff muscles in both shoulders. The power phase (Fig. 21-2C) of the downswing is produced by near maximal contractions of the pectoralis major and latissimus dorsi and moderate subscapularis and the other rotator cuff muscles firing on the right, and less so by the subscapularis, pectoralis major, and latissimus dorsi on the left.[10,11] During the downswing, the wrists apply a negative torque by remaining cocked. At this time, the right wrist is in maximum dorsiflexion, the left thumb is hyperabducted, and the left ulnar nerve, elbow, and forearm muscles are under tension. When the club is approximately in the horizontal position (Fig. 21-2C) to the ground, the wrists uncock, and this uncocking of the wrists accelerates the club into the ball (Fig. 21-2D).

In the impact stage of the golf swing (Fig. 21-2D) the maximum clubhead velocity (up to 110 to 130 mph)[14] is reached. From a performance aspect, the purpose of the impact is to hit the ball as far as possible in the proper direction. From the safety aspect, the purpose of the impact stage is to have a smooth transition from acceleration to deceleration.

At impact the weight is shifted to the left side so hat 80 to 95 percent of the weight has been transferred.[15] This is true of both low- and high-handicap golfers. Skilled golfers, however, have their weight supported toward the heel of the foot whereas the less skilled golfers tend to support themselves right in the middle of the foot.[12] This probably implies that a skilled golfer gets more counterclockwise rotation during the swing.

About one-fourth of all golf swing injuries occur during the follow-through (Fig. 21-3A). After impact (Fig. 21-3B) the left forearm supinates, the right forearm pronates, and the lumbar and cervical spines rotate and hyperextend. Hip rotation is also completed. The subscapularis along with reduced levels of the latissimus dorsi and pectoralis muscles of both arms continue to be active in order to decelerate the golf swing[10,11] (Fig. 21-3C). Both knees rotate, the right knee flexes, and the left knee everts. Now all weight should be transferred to the left side (Fig. 21-3D).

The golf swing is the cause of many injuries. The physician can certainly treat many of the medical problems related to the shoulder. However, in order to correct the cause of these injuries, one must correct the faulty swing mechanics. The teaching golf professional, using years of experience with such equipment as video recording, can correct these problems. Also the golf professional should be consulted about the many different types of clubs,

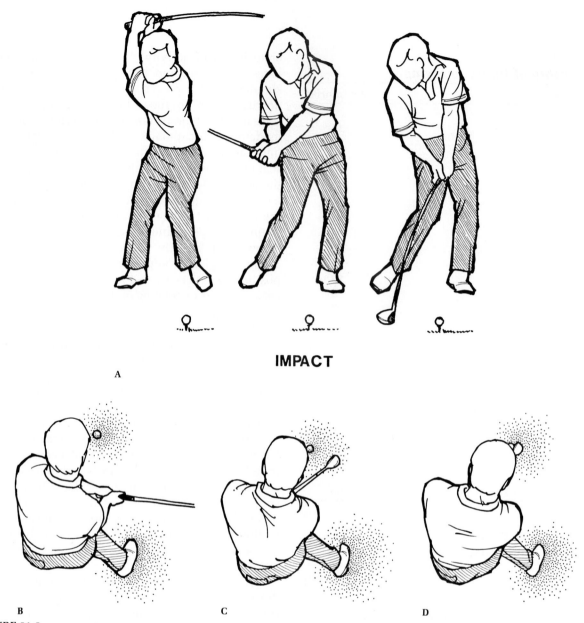

IMPACT

A

B   C   D

FIGURE 21-2
A. Impact. *B.* Beginning of the power phase of the downswing. The right arm is adducted to 0° and still is externally rotated. The left arm is adducted and internally rotated. *C.* Midpower phase. Near maximal internal rotator muscle activity in the right arm and early forceful abductor activity in the left arm. *D.* Near impact. Maximum clubhead velocity. Both arms fully extended (forward flexed) and adducted.

shafts, and other equipment before the golfer makes a final decision.

In considering proper equipment, it is very difficult to find any equipment changes or modifications that really apply to injuries about the shoulder from golf. It has been well shown that equipment changes certainly make a difference in golf injuries, especially to the hand, wrist, forearm, and elbow. For instance, the new graphite shafts have much less torque and therefore cause a lot fewer impact problems in the hand, wrist, and elbow areas during the golf swing. They have been recommended for pa-tients with tennis elbow or wrist problems in the past.

However, equipment is not nearly as important when related to the shoulder because the shoulder is a more rotational type of injury problem and does not get the impact problems that occur in other areas such as the wrist, hand, or elbow. However, I do feel that flexibility of the shaft is very important for someone who has shoulder problems, especially if it is a metal-shafted club. If it is indeed a graphite-shafted club, it is important to work with a golf professional to understand the stiffness and the

286

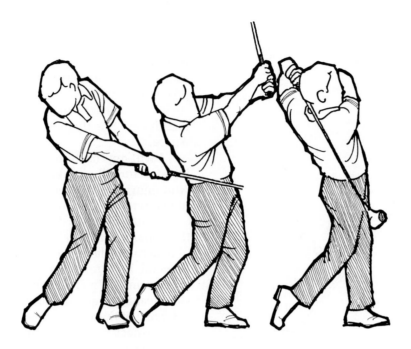

FOLLOW-THROUGH

A

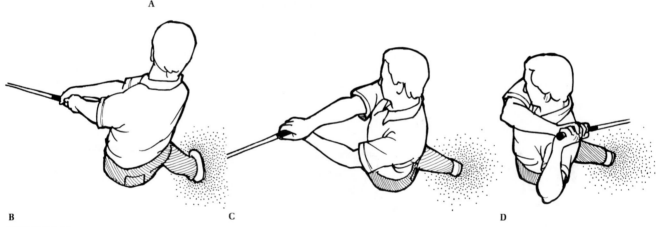

B   C   D

FIGURE 21-3
A. Follow-through.   B. Early deceleration phase of follow-through with left arm abducted and right arm adducted. C. Midway through the follow-through phase. The left arm is forward flexed, and the right arm is adducted across the chest. D. Completion of follow-through. The left arm is abducted and externally rotated, while the right arm is adducted horizontally and forward flexed.

"kick point" of the shaft (Fig. 21-4). This means that the shaft bends at a certain point to give a certain type of trajectory to the ball. For example, some golfers who have a high kick point of a graphite shaft and a very stiff graphite shaft are actually trying to hit the ball with a lower trajectory, causing more roll. A golfer who has this type of club and doesn't know its specifics may try to do some things such as hit the ball higher with that type of shaft and in trying to do this can certainly cause faulty mechanics and thus injure a shoulder or muscles about the shoulder. It is important for golfers, for instance, to know which way they want to hit the ball. For the golfer who wants to have a higher trajectory and less roll, it is

important to have a lower kick point in the graphite shaft; that means it is closer to the club face, which sends the ball on a higher trajectory. It is also important for the golfer who wants to hit a little bit higher shot to have less stiffness in the graphite shaft. When buying a club, have the golf professional look at your golf swing and help you pick the equipment that is proper for your type of swing. I don't see how the type of grips, the weight of the club, and other mechanical aspects of the club will make a difference in either preventing or treating shoulder injuries in golf (Fig. 21-5).

In treating shoulder problems in golf as in any medical problems, a thorough history of predispos-

287

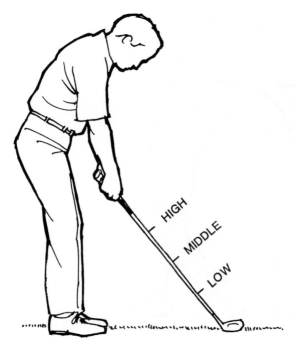

FIGURE 21-4
Club showing different levels of flex, high, mid, low.

ing factors must be taken before a treatment plan is prescribed. Such problems as constitutional acute trauma, insidious trauma, postinflammatory conditions, postinfection, tumors, and congenital defects can all predispose the golfer to injury.

In this chapter, I have elected not to cover the physical examination of the shoulder, surgical treatment of specific problems, or the use of diagnostic tests because they have been well documented in the preceding chapters. The injuries that occur in golf such as impingement, instability, and other abnormalities are exactly the same as those described elsewhere.

I will approach the shoulder and the surrounding structures individually and try to correlate specific injuries with specific structures and their relationship to the golf swing.

Included in the shoulder girdle are the clavicle, the scapula, and four articulations: the sternoclavicular, acromioclavicular, scapulothoracic, and glenohumeral. Each relationship reacts to a repetitive athletic trauma in a characteristic manner. To omit the significance of any underlying pathology or to consider one of these structures without considering the other, especially with the overuse stress of golf, leads to misdiagnosis.

The sternoclavicular joint is subject to medially directed forces on the left at the top of the backswing (Fig. 21-1B) and on the right at the end of the follow-through (Fig. 21-3D). In addition, when the right arm is abducted and fully coiled at the end of the backswing and the beginning of the downswing (Fig. 21-2B) there is posterior retraction of the shoulder that results in anterior sternoclavicular joint stress.

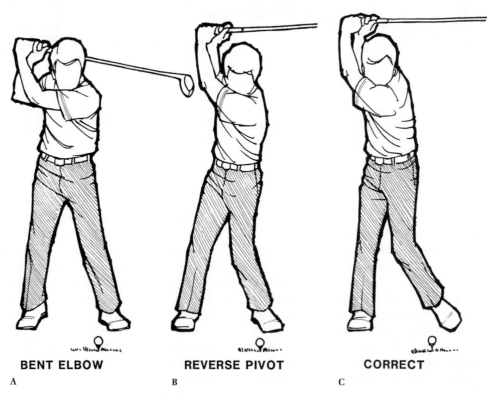

BENT ELBOW

A

REVERSE PIVOT

B

CORRECT

C

FIGURE 21-5
Three golfers: *A.* Bent elbow and poor swing mechanics. *B.* Poor weight shift reverse pivot. *C.* Proper swing positive.

Because less force is involved, similar but less stress is noted on the left sternoclavicular joint at the end of the follow-through. Ordinarily, such sternoclavicular joint stress or sprains produce minimal symptoms and findings, but when the ligamentous supports are sufficiently irritated by the repeated microtrauma of stretching, the sternoclavicular joint can become inflamed and in rare instances unstable to some degree and thus may become degenerative.

The acromioclavicular joint is usually injured by falls on the point of the shoulder resulting in various grades of sprains. It is occasionally the target of arthritis, gout, and more often degeneration due to separation and/or mild repetitive localized trauma. These problems can cause disturbing symptoms of aching after exercising, localized pain after push-ups, chin-ups, throwing, and golf.

In the powerful golf swing of today, the injured or repetitively stressed acromioclavicular (AC) joint can become symptomatic in all segments of the shoulder biomechanics since scapular motion is involved in essentially all components of the golf swing. In the power phase of the golf swing (Fig. 21-2C), the AC joint ligaments are laterally stretched or sprained when the scapula is externally rotated (downward) and the clavicle remains relatively fixed with little rotation on the sternum. A somewhat lesser amount of compression force on the AC joint occurs on the right when the extended right arm crosses the chest just above the horizontal on the follow-through swing (Fig. 21-3C). Lateral stretching and medial compression forces are not as severe on the left AC joint in the right-handed golfer because of a lesser amount of force employed when the left arm crosses the chest on the take-away (Fig. 21-1B) and on the follow-through when the left scapula is elevated (Fig. 21-3D).

With degenerative changes occurring in the acromioclavicular joint secondary to overuse as well as with advancing age, decreased gliding and rotation may occur alone or in concert with sternoclavicular joint pathology. However, should glenohumeral motion be restricted, compensatory increased laxity may develop in the AC joint to aid shoulder motion.

In strict anatomic terms, the scapulothoracic joint would not be recognized as a true articular junction, but for the purpose of this chapter we are describing the scapula and the posterior chest wall. Often neglected as a site of shoulder pathology is the anterior surface of the scapula in relationship to the underlying musculature over the posterior rib cage.[16] In a 2:1 ratio of glenohumeral to scapulothoracic movement, the scapula is intimately related to arm flexion and extension, and abduction and adduction

motion. With repetitive stress as in the repeated golf swings, and at times impeded by inadvertently striking unrelenting turf surfaces and such objects as roots of trees, the costal surface of the scapula may develop osteophyte formation at its inferior medial border. Also a bursa located at this junction may become inflamed owing to chronic irritation and clinically develop into a palpable tender mass.

Insidious weakness of the serratus anterior due to disease of the long thoracic nerve is often difficult to detect but may well be the cause of soaring golf scores. At the top of the backswing (Fig. 21-1B) and continuing into the first phase of the downswing (Fig. 21-2B) the medial border of the right scapula is held tightly to the posterior chest wall. Less or localized force is noted as the swing is accelerated and continued in the follow-through (Fig. 21-3A). On the left side, a similar but less vigorous relationship of the medial scapular edge to the posterior chest wall occurs as the follow-through swing slows to a stop.

The glenohumeral joint is a relatively unstable articulation that is designed to allow a remarkable amount of motion.[17,18] The much larger head of the humerus is held against a variable and shallow concavity on the glenoid of the scapula. This anatomic relationship is somewhat analogous to a golf ball resting on a tee. If the tee is held horizontally, the golf ball falls away from the tee. Such would be the case with the head of the humerus if it were not for the tendinous, ligamentous, and muscular supports that surround this articulation. Anything that weakens or inflames these structures can lead to instability, impingement, or both and affect the golfer's performance. The most common problems we have seen in the golfer are impingement and instability, especially in the rare but many times missed mild multidirectional instability leading to impingement signs and symptoms.

The long game in golf is physically dependent in contradistinction to the short game, which requires hand, arm, and eye coordination. The modern golfer, on today's longer courses, is well aware of the length of the carry and the run of the drive. The typical golfer places less thought on the determinants of the total length of the drive. Disregarding the elasticity and weight of the ball, the clubhead mass and its speed at impact primarily determine the resulting yardage. Distance then can be a measure of efficiently recruiting and applying muscle action about the shoulder that propels the club from a momentary standstill to a maximum velocity at impact and subsequent restitution of forces on the follow-through.

The following paragraphs detail the function of the rotator cuff in different parts of the golf swing to demonstrate how the pathology may occur if weakness or instability is present.

In the backswing, the right supraspinatus abducts the humerus while the left subscapularis internally rotates and adducts the arm across the anterior chest. Other musculature is dynamic, but relatively quiet, and acts as joint stabilizers. When fully coiled at the top of the backswing (Fig. 21-1*B*), the right articular capsule is wound proportionately taut. If the right supraspinatus is weak, the right deltoid overacts to abnormally raise the humeral head. If the left subscapularis is weak, its function of helping to prevent anterior subluxation is decreased. On both the right and left, restraints must be poised to prevent stretching of the soft tissues and abnormal humeral head movement when the forceful downswing begins (Fig. 21-2*B*).

In the initial or acceleration phase of the downswing (Fig. 21-2*B*), more total force is expended on the right than on the left with moderate firing of the right pectoralis major, latissimus dorsi, and subscapularis. These muscles adduct and internally rotate the arm and must be counterbalanced by increased infraspinatus and teres minor activity. Should these external rotators be weak, the unwanted posterior gliding of the humeral head and posterior capsule and infraspinatus stretching are possible. On the left, in the first phase of the downswing (Fig. 21-2*B*) the subscapularis is moderately active as the latissimus dorsi aids in adduction and internal rotation. Also on the left, there must be increased activity of the cuff muscles for checking the primary activators to maintain a proper glenohumeral relationship.

In the power, or second, phase (Fig. 21-2*C*) of the downswing, there is near-maximal force generated on the right by the latissimus dorsi and pectoralis major and somewhat less by the subscapularis. Correspondingly, more activity is also seen in the stabilizers. The long head of the biceps at the elbow counterbalances the full extension activity of the triceps and proximally holds the humeral head up against the glenoid.

On the left in the power phase, there is near-maximal EMG activity noted in the subscapularis and slightly less in the pectoralis major and latissimus dorsi. Maintenance activity of the supporting muscles is again necessary to maintain normal functional glenohumeral activity. Should such support be diminished or overwhelmed by the power activators, soft tissue stretching and then subluxation can follow.

It is to be noted that in the power segment of the downswing (Fig. 21-2*C*) both on the right and on the left, the greatest amount of activity is exerted by the subscapularis, pectoralis major, and latissimus dorsi muscles. The supraspinatus, infraspinatus, teres minor, and deltoid muscles play a lesser role. Additional force is developed in the power segment by a large moment of rotation transmitted from the counterclockwise uncoiling of the hips and trunk to the origins of the pectoralis major and latissimus dorsi on the chest wall. This portion of the downswing is potentially injurious to the glenohumeral joint and surrounding tissues if there is not a balance in total motion, right to left shoulder, and intrinsically on each side because of the considerable magnitude of power (3 to 4 hp) generated.

Just at impact (Fig. 21-2*D*) or at the conclusion of the downswing, the clubhead is traveling at its maximum velocity.[19] Both arms are fully extended and resisting centrifugal force of the clubhead on the hands. At this point, the anterior capsular structures and restraints are fully operational, comparable with throwing a softball underhand on the right side and simultaneously hitting a low backhand with a racket on the left. Should this clubhead strike an immovable object, momentarily the arms would continue their motions before the weaker external rotators and the abductors could decelerate bilateral glenohumeral motion. This would allow each humeral head to ride acutely forward upon and damage the anterior labial rim. A milder, more gradual, and cumulative deleterious effect on anterior capsular and supportive muscular structures would be expected from years of driving practice and from frequent production of fairway divots with woods or bunker holes with high irons.

Fine tuning of the clubhead in the last few inches of the power phase before impact is a delicate function of the intrinsic rotator cuff musculotendinous units and the glenohumeral joint relationship. If muscle imbalance, tendinitis, or improper humeral head seating are present, there will be a disturbance in the critical orientation of the club face to the ball and in the smooth application of the correct speed.

Follow-through, or deceleration, phase (Fig. 21-3*B*) functions, as in other sports, to permit gradual slowing of the club and body movements after impact. On the right, there is slowing by the pectoralis major and latissimus dorsi to a moderate level of activity along with a slightly greater subscapularis contraction while the supraspinatus, infraspinatus, teres minor, and deltoid firing remains at a low level. Should the long head of the bicipital tendon be weakened by inflammation and erosion, the function proximally of holding the humeral head down is diminished when the right elbow is flexed. As the right arm assumes a cross-chest position, further irritation of the anterior labrum can take place, especially if the external rotators are inefficient.

Proper follow-through on the left at the glenohumeral joint is dependent on continued near-maximal subscapularis activity and moderate firing of the pectoralis major, latissimus dorsi, infraspinatus, teres minor, and supraspinatus muscles. If intermuscular synchronism is negated by joint erosion or soft tissue pathology, there is augmentation of any existing glenohumeral joint and rotator cuff lesion. As left-sided recoiling proceeds to a stop, abduction above 90° is produced by increased deltoid activity. Impingement can ensue at this point, especially if superimposed upon tendinitis, wear, and inflexibility due to healed scarring or aging.

The golfing and scientific worlds are knowledgeably enhanced by the accurate research done by Dr. Frank A. Jobe and coworkers in EMG studies of the rotator cuff during a golf swing. The foregoing discussion places much credence in and gives credit to their published works.[10,11] Also much of this information is from an excellent review of shoulder injuries in golf by Dr. James Andrews and Dr. James A. Whiteside in a textbook *Medical Aspects of Golf,* yet to be published by F. A. Davis Publishers.

In the previous paragraphs, I have talked about the mechanics of the golf swing in relationship to the anatomy of the shoulder joint. I have also tried to point out that in certain parts of the golf swing you can see certain stresses put upon certain muscles, ligaments, and tendons. What does this mean when one is facing a golfer who comes into the office with shoulder injuries? For example, let's say that a 45-year-old avid golfer with an 8 to 9 handicap, who plays golf probably 2 to 3 times per week and perhaps hits golf balls while practicing another 2 times per week, has developed shoulder pain. When he* presents to the office, obviously one must take a good complete medical history of his shoulder problems, past medical history, and the history of his golf with its relationship to his shoulder problem. After x-rays, to rule out any obvious changes in the bony structures about the shoulder, the physical examination, of course, is extremely important in a diagnosis. If the golfer has rotator golf signs and symptoms, which are probably the most common problem we see related to the shoulder in golf, and we are sure we have ruled out any neurologic problems in

the neck or elsewhere, and we are sure there are no instability problems, then we put the golfer on a treatment program.

If I saw that type of golfer, I would approach him with a program consisting first of anti-inflammatory medicines, physical therapy, working on range of motion, decreasing the pain, and increasing the strength of the shoulder with various exercises well documented in this textbook. Once the golfer has a pain-free range of motion of his shoulder, relief at nighttime while sleeping, and feels his strength is coming back, I would then start him on a rehabilitation program for golf. The initial treatment can take anywhere from 3 to 6 weeks. During that time, I would definitely limit him from playing golf at all and slowly start him back into hitting balls.[5] I would also recommend strongly for him to consult his teaching professional to make sure that the mechanics of his golf swing are proper and especially to get a video analysis of his golf swing so he and the golf professional can see any faulty mechanics.[5] Once he is gaining strength and has pain relief, I would recommend that he follow the functional progressive type of activity described in Table 21-5. If he can perform these easily over a 3-week period, I would recommend he go back to his golf activity. I think that initial treatment would take about 3 weeks, but to get down the pain and inflammation may take as much as 6 weeks. If he is doing very well, I would accelerate the interval of golf rehabilitation program and progress him even faster back to playing full activity. One must remember, however, that the recreational as well as the professional golfer probably will not be very compliant with this type of prolonged program, and you may be faced with a person who would go back and play golf and not get better as fast as you would like. You must sit down and spend some time trying to counsel the patient, even though he may be feeling a little bit better, that the prolonged course is much better for the healing of his problems than going back to his previous activities without full strength and rehabilitation. If, however, he continues to have pain and problems with his shoulder during the initial conservative treatment, I would strongly recommend further testing, either arthrogram or MRI of his shoulder. Based on those findings, I would then again continue either a conservative treatment plan, or perhaps he would need some type of surgical intervention. Following rotator cuff surgery on his shoulder, be it arthroscopic or open, I feel this changes the amount of time before he can return to golf. I also feel the functional progressive program in Table 21-5 is extremely important following any type of surgery on the shoulder.

*Throughout this text we will follow the traditional English practice of using the pronouns *he, his,* or *him* in the generic sense whenever it is not intended to designate the specific gender of an individual.

This should just lengthen the period of time from the initial treatment to when he begins his activity. In summary, in treating anyone with shoulder problems in golf, it is extremely important to have a good golf history, a good physical examination including all necessary x-rays, and then in treating to follow a very conservative approach at first, gradually increasing functional activity. Most important, the golf swing should be analyzed and faulty mechanics corrected.

Prevention of injury in any sport is difficult. Golf is an activity demanding a high degree of refined motor skills. Many frustrated golfers are trying to play golf when they are not in shape. The weekend golfer and even the professional golfer must condition the body before going to the course or assume a risk of injury. Injuries, sore muscles, and frustrating days on a golf course can be eliminated by preseason, regular season, and off season conditioning programs.

There are four types of exercises that golfers require to maintain their fullest ability to avoid injuries. Stretching exercises[20] are used to maintain complete range of motion of the hamstrings, back, and shoulders. Without complete range of motion and flexibility, the golfer will put abnormal stress on the various body parts during the golf swing.

Golf is not a strength game like other sports. Strength in itself will not enable an individual to hit a ball farther or longer. However, it will allow the skilled player to strike shots with more consistent, explosive power over extended periods. Any golfer with a weak area, especially the knee, back, or shoul-

der, is at risk for a golfing injury. One can use equipment such as Nautilus[1] (Table 21-4), universal gyms, or home devices such as free weights or weighted clubs to increase strength.[21]

These workout programs also develop endurance strength needed to walk long distances, climb hills, and repeat the swing over and over during the game of golf. There are various muscles that must be strengthened in order to improve basic skills. Table 21-4 reviews the Nautilus workout program for golf. For the golfer who does not have specialized exercise equipment available, an excellent reference booklet by Jobe[20] describes home exercises.

Cardiovascular exercise for endurance is another essential part of conditioning. Climbing hills and walking 18 holes is impossible without a cardiovascular system that responds to strenuous exercise. Follow a preseason conditioning program of jogging, riding a bike, walking, or using a Stair Master in order to get into cardiovascular shape for golf.

In many sports such as football, basketball, or baseball, the athlete is put through a functional progression rehabilitation program before returning to the sport. The same should hold true for golf. Table 21-5 shows a type of interval golf rehabilitation program for the injured golfer to return safely to the sport.

Golfers are athletes, for golf is a sport. To play it well, one must have athletic ability, strength, agility, coordination, and endurance. The golf swing is physically demanding and has contributed to various types of injuries. It may be argued that the shoulder is not the most vital link in the stroke produc-

TABLE 21-4
Nautilus Workout Program for Golf

Exercise	Muscles	Skills
1. Hip and back	Buttocks, lower back	Driving power, walking endurance
2. Leg extension	Quadriceps	Driving, walking
3. Leg curl	Hamstrings	Hip turn, driving
4. Double shoulder (lateral press)	Deltoids	Club control, impact
5. Double shoulder (seated press)	Deltoids, triceps	Shoulder turn, club extension
6. Pull over	Latissimus dorsi	Shoulder turn, club extension
7. Wrist curl	Forearm flexors	Club head control, impact, power acceleration
8. Reverse wrist curls	Forearm extensors	Club head control, acceleration

Perform one set of 8 to 12 repetitions of each exercise. Take no more than 60 s to perform each set. Rest no more than 30 s between sets.

TABLE 21-5
Interval Golf Rehabilitation Program

	Monday	Wednesday	Friday
1st week*†	5-min chip and putt 5-min rest 5-min chip	5-min chip and putt 5-min rest 5-min chip 5-min rest 5-min chip	5-min chip and putt 5-min rest 5-min chip 5-min rest 5-min chip
2d week*†	10-min chip 10-min rest 10-min short iron	10-min chip 10-min rest 10-min short iron 10-min rest 10-min short iron	10-min short iron 10-min rest 10-min short iron 10-min rest 10-min short iron
3d week*†	15-min short iron 10-min rest 15-min long iron 10-min rest 15-min long iron	15-min short iron 10-min rest 15-min long iron 10-min rest 15-min long iron	15-min short iron 10-min rest 15-min long iron 10-min rest 15-min long iron
4th week*	Repeat Wednesdays	Play 9 holes	Play 18 holes

*Flexibility exercises before hitting.
†Ice after hitting.

tion, but there is little question that the shoulder pathology and the pain it produces are the chief cause of stopping golf play.

In treating injuries to the shoulder in golf, one must understand the golf swing and its relationship to the injury. Then in conjunction with a thorough physical examination and proper diagnostic proce-

REFERENCES

1. Torisu T: Fracture of the hook of the hamate by a golf swing. *Clin Orthop* 83:91–94, 1972.
2. Stover CN, Wiren G, Topaz SR: The modern golf swing and stress syndromes. *Physician Sports Med* 4:42–47, September 1976.
3. Mattikow MS: The ubiquitous golfer. *Cutis* 19:471, 1977.
4. O'Grady R, Shock P: Golfball granuloma of the eyelids and conjuctivia. *Am J Ophthalmol* 76:148–151, July 1973.
5. Vallottow W: The ocular aspect of golf. *South Med J* 58:44–47, January 1965.
6. Weston PA: Injury from a disrupted golf ball. *Lancet* 1:375, Feb. 12, 1977.
7. McCarroll JR, Gioe TJ: Professional golfers and the price they pay. *Physician Sports Med* 10:64, 1966.
8. McCarroll JR, Shelbourne KD, Rettig AC: Injuries in the amateur golfer. *Physician Sports Med* 18(3): 122, 1990.
9. Maddalozzo GF: An anatomical and biomechanical analysis of the full golf swing. *NSCA J* 9(4): 6, August/September 1987.
10. Jobe FW, Moynes DR, Antonelli DJ: Rotator cuff function during a golf swing. *Am J Sports Med* 14:388–392, 1986.
11. Moynes DR, Perry J, Antonelli DJ, Jobe FW: Electromyography and motion analysis of the upper extremity in sports. *Phys Ther* 66(12): 1905–1911, December 1986.
12. Hay JG: *The Biomechanics of Sports Techniques.* Englewood Cliffs, NJ, Prentice-Hall, 1973, pp 270–287.
13. Cochran A, Stobbs J: *The Search for the Perfect Swing.* Heinemann Educational Books, 1968.
14. Schulenburge CAR: Medical aspects and curiosities of golfing. *Practitioner* 217: 625–628, October 1976.

15. Richards J, Farrell M, Kent P, Kraft R: Weight transfer patterns during the golf swing. *Res Q Exerc Sport* 56(4):361–365, 1985.

16. Sisto DJ, Jobe FW: The operative treatment of scapulothoracic bursitis in professional pitchers. *Am J Sports Med* 14(3):192–194, 1986.

17. Resnick D: Shoulder pain. *Symp Orthop Radiol Orthop Clin North Am* 14(1):81–97, January 1983.

18. Moseley HF: Athletic injuries to the shoulder region. *Am J Surg* 98:401–422, September 1959.

19. Milburn PD: Summation of segmental velocities in the golf swing. *Med Sci Sports Exerc* 14(1):60–64, 1982.

20. Jobe FW, Moynes DR: *30 Exercises for Better Golf*. Champion Press, Inglewood, CA, 1986.

21. Peterson J: *Conditioning for a Purpose the West Point Way*. West Point, NY, Leisure Press, 1971.

22. Mattikow MS: The ubiquitous golfer. *Cutis* 19:71, 1977.

23. Roberts J: Injuries, handicaps, mashes, and cleeks. *Physician Sports Med* 6:121, 1978.

24. Schulenburg CAR: Medical aspects and curiosities of golfing. *Practitioner* 217:625, 1976.

25. Everard A: Golf. *JR Coll Gen Pract* 293:3, 1970.

26. *Indianapolis Star & Newspaper*, 1982.

CHAPTER 22

Swimming

Peter J. Fowler

The repetitive movements performed by the competitive swimmer through years of training are often associated with a variety of characteristic injuries. The shoulder is the primary target of such injuries. The competitive swimmer's ultimate goal is maximum performance. This goal is shared by all those involved in the athlete's care and development, and as training programs are organized and implemented, prevention of injuries must be a primary focus. A basic knowledge of the mechanical details of the sport along with an understanding of the related anatomic and biomechanical considerations helps physician, coach, and swimmer monitor not only performance but danger signs of impending dysfunction as well.

SWIMMING STROKES

The front crawl, backstroke, breaststroke, and butterfly are the four competitive swimming strokes that are swum in various distances alone or in combination. A working knowledge of the main components of each stroke will provide a basis for an understanding of the pathophysiologic entities common in competitive swimmers (Table 22-1).

Four phases are common to all strokes: the reach, catch, pull, and recovery (Table 22-2). The main power of propulsion (75 percent) is provided by arm action during the pull phase in all strokes but the breaststroke, in which arms and legs contribute equally. In front crawl, backstroke, and butterfly, the motion of the arm through the water starts with hand entry and proceeds with continual adduction and internal rotation of the glenohumeral joint. In the out-of-water phase the arm is in abduction and internal rotation so that it is again positioned for hand entry and repetition of the cycle.

Anatomic Features

As the most mobile joint in the human body, the shoulder has little bony support. The stability that allows the arm to function with power and precision is the result of the interaction of the shoulder capsule, the surrounding ligaments, the rotator cuff muscles, and the pectoralis major and serratus anterior muscles. The rotator cuff muscles, supraspinatus, infraspinatus, teres minor, and subscapularis

(Fig. 22-1), work in a force couple combination with the deltoid and the long head of biceps to contain the humeral head in the glenoid fossa. The long head of biceps is important in stabilizing the humeral head and is active in forward flexion, a function that should not be overlooked in shoulder mechanics. The scapular muscles, the serratus anterior, the rhomboids, and the trapezius work constantly in swimming arm action. If they fatigue, a downward tilt of the scapula may occur that in turn alters the mechanics of the glenohumeral joint and may contribute to the onset of excessive subacromial loading.

TENDINOPATHY—SWIMMER'S SHOULDER

Because there is a lack of understanding of many of its causes (Fig. 22-2), shoulder pain has too frequently become synonymous with the term "impingement." Consequently, inappropriate treatment may be selected for some patients. The term "impingement" should be reserved specifically for those cases where rotator cuff pathology is associated with actual mechanical abutment of the rotator cuff. Rotator cuff tendinopathy is a more appropriate term for pain resulting from dysfunction of the rotator cuff. Although tendinitis is often the descriptive term, inflammatory cells are seldom identified at microscopy. The challenge remains to determine the exact cause of rotator cuff tendinopathy in individual patients. The term "swimmer's shoulder" was first used by Kennedy and Hawkins in 1974 and referred to tendinitis of the supraspinatus and/or biceps tendon.[9] This was staged chronologically by Neer and Welsh. In stage I, there is edema and hemorrhage that occurs in athletes under 25 years. In stage II, fibrosis and tendinitis are seen in those between 25 and 40. In stage III, there is the formation of osteophytes and the occurrence of partial or complete tendon rupture in those over 40.[11] In the competitive athlete, however, these stages are not age-specific. In 1974, Hawkins and Kennedy reported a 3 percent incidence of "swimmer's shoulder."[9] The 50 percent occurrence more recently reported may be the result of an increase in the intensity of training schedules combined with such anatomic features as acromial shape and shoulder joint laxity, and bio-

295

TABLE 22-1
Main Components of the Competitive Swimming Strokes

Front Crawl—fastest, most frequently used practice stroke

- Hand enters water, palm faces downward 1 ft in front of shoulder, reaches ahead until arm is fully flexed
- Pull phase initiated by sculling motion
- Torso is rolled about its longitudinal axis; arm is positioned deeper in water
- S-shaped curving pull, palm facing backward produced under torso
- Recovery of one arm simultaneous with pull phase of other arm
- Using body roll, arm is released from water and swept into entry position
- Arm action continuous; two to six vigorous flutter kicks per arm cycle

Backstroke

- Arm entry straight with shoulder in fully elevated position
- Using body roll arm pulls in S-shaped pattern to side
- Legs perform flutter kick

Butterfly—part of competition since 1952

- Arms and legs enter water and move simultaneously during pull and recovery phases
- A dolphin motion with body relieves stress on shoulder
- Legs perform dolphin kick (a flutter kick with legs moving together)

Breaststroke—oldest swimming stroke

- Arms move together in pull and recovery phases
- Arms do not pull below waistline

Whip kick

- Begins with legs extended, feet plantar flexed
- Recovery begins with flexion at hips and knees
- Recovery ends with foot dorsiflexed and tibia in external rotation
- Angle between trunk and thigh, 120°
- Knee extends, foot pushes outward and backward
- Dorsiflexed foot engages water with sole
- Hip extensors drive thigh toward water surface
- Extension continues at hip and knees while legs are brought together
- Knee almost extended and feet a few inches apart
- Finishes with foot in plantar flexion.

TABLE 22-2
Components of the Four Phases of the Competitive Swimming Strokes

Reach
- Arm reaches forward to enter water
- Synonymous with term *entry*

Catch
- Similar for all competitive strokes
- Elbow flexes 100°
- Shoulder extends, horizontally abducts, and medially rotates

Pull
- Varies slightly with each stroke
- Swimmer sculls or pushes water
- The propulsion phase
- Except in breaststroke, arm action starts at maximum elevation and ends in extension

Recovery
- Out-of-the-water phase
- Arm returns to start pull again

mechanical factors such as overwork, impingement, hypovascularity, and stroke mechanics.

Causal Factors

TRAINING

In today's training programs, a national caliber swimmer typically practices in the water in 2-h sessions nine or more times per week. Each session may range from 4000 to 8000 m. This time in the water serves to improve both conditioning and technique. Also part of the routine is dry-land training to build strength and endurance. With these rigorous schedules, training sessions must be planned, monitored, and modified on an ongoing basis to prevent and reduce the incidence of swimmer's shoulder. Often the sport medicine physician becomes involved only after an injury has occurred. Ideally a collaborative effort between the coaching personnel and the physician will exist to establish training programs that are successful in prevention of injuries and do not compromise performance.

OVERWORK

As the least stable joint, the shoulder is the most vulnerable to injury in the overhead position. To keep up with the continuous, repeated demands made by swimming, the muscles of the rotator cuff may be required to work excessively to contain and stabilize the humeral head. With the resulting cuff fatigue, superior migration of the humeral head may occur, and with this an increase in subacromial loading. This may be a factor that triggers the onset of the tendinopathy.

HYPOVASCULARITY

The functional relationship between arm position and blood supply to the supraspinatus and the biceps tendon was studied by Rathbun and Macnab.[13] In adduction and neutral rotation, the tendons are stretched tightly over the head of the humerus, com-

Shoulder and Acromioclavicular Joints (from above)

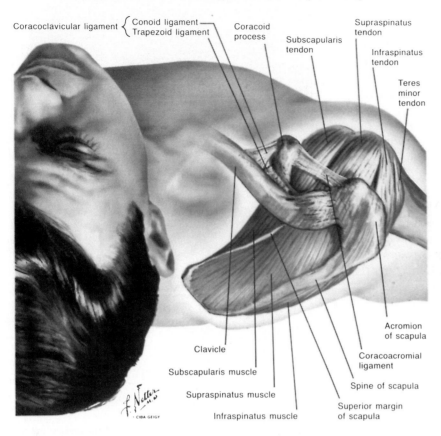

Coracoclavicular ligament { Conoid ligament
Trapezoid ligament

Coracoid process

Subscapularis tendon

Supraspinatus tendon

Infraspinatus tendon

Teres minor tendon

Acromion of scapula

Coracoacromial ligament

Spine of scapula

Superior margin of scapula

Clavicle

Subscapularis muscle

Supraspinatus muscle

Infraspinatus muscle

FIGURE 22-1
Supraspinatus: Inserts on uppermost facet of greater tuberosity; Active during arm abduction; Fulcrum for deltoid during abduction; Helps resist upward displacement of humeral head; during other arm actions. Subscapularis: Primary external rotator; Resists anterior or inferior displacement of humeral; head in glenoid; Stabilizes humeral head. Infraspinatus: External rotator; Extends humerus in horizontal plane; Works with supraspinatus and subscapularis to; depress humeral head. Teres minor: External rotator. (From *The Ciba Collection of Medical Illustration*, 1987, vol 8, part 1, Frank H. Netter: *Anatomy, Physiology, and Metabolic Disorders*, p 33, plate 30. Reprinted with permission.)

promising their blood supply. Circulation is restored in abduction as the vessels fill. This repeated hypovascularity, known as a "wringing out" mechanism, occurs in the area of the tendon most vulnerable to loading and, by compounding the potential for damage by repetitive stress, may contribute to early degenerative changes.

IMPINGEMENT—SOFT TISSUE FACTORS

The supraspinatus and biceps tendons that insert on or across the humerus directly below the coracoacromial arch formed by the coracoid process, the coracoacromial ligament, and the anterior acromion are particularly susceptible to impingement. When the

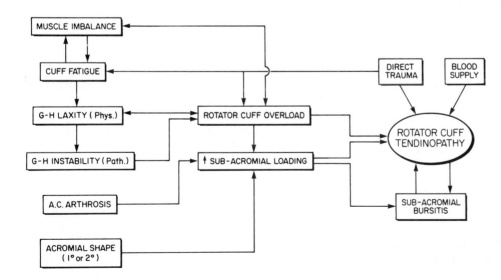

FIGURE 22-2
This algorithm outlines the many pathologic entities that can culminate in rotator cuff tendinitis.

297

arm is in abduction, forward flexion, and internal rotation, a position assumed in the catch phase of all competitive strokes, the humeral head moves under the arch and the tendons may be repeatedly impinged here. A mechanical irritation and subacromial bursa inflammatory response may further compromise the space under the coracoacromial arch.

IMPINGEMENT—OSSEOUS FACTORS

Three acromial shapes have been identified by Bigliani et al.: type I, flat; type II, curved; and type III, hooked.[1] Of these, a type III acromion may be an anatomic factor in refractory tendinitis that does not respond to treatment. Because of the already decreased dimensions of the acromial arch, a competitive swimmer with a hooked (type III) acromion may be predisposed to impingement. Consequently, a tendinopathy that is resistant to treatment may easily develop. Ogata and Uhthoff have suggested that pathologic changes within the rotator cuff substance may be the result of a primary tendinopathy and that the acromial changes observed occur as a secondary phenomenon.[12] In addition, they suggest that the changes seen within the rotator cuff occur initially on the humeral surface of the tendon near the enthesis, as opposed to the bursal side where one would expect to see lesions that are a result of mechanical impingement from the acromion. Theories such as this have precipitated a rethinking of shoulder pathology and its underlying causes.

INCREASED LAXITY

Increased laxity may be a contributing factor in the athlete with resistant shoulder pain. A loose or lax shoulder in the competitive swimmer may cause the rotator cuff muscles to work hard just to contain the humeral head. These fatiguing muscles are further stressed by the rigors of training. A significant observation of the association between rotator cuff tendinitis and shoulder laxity has been made by Fowler and Webster.[5] They assessed 188 competitive swimmers between the ages of 13 and 26 for positive signs of tendinitis and for posterior, inferior, and anterior instability or increased laxity. Fifty recreational athletes without shoulder pain were used as a control group. A formal history was taken of each subject, and episodes of shoulder pain were recorded. The "apprehension test" was used to test *anterior instability*. Any sign of pain or anxiety was recorded as a positive response. *Inferior stability* was assessed using the sulcus sign. The "load and shift" test conducted in both the sitting (Fig. 22-3) and supine (Fig. 22-4) positions was used to evaluate posterior laxity. The excursion of the humeral head relative to the

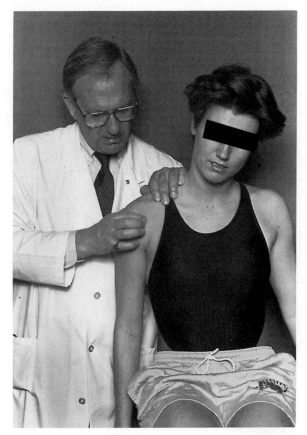

FIGURE 22-3
A second posterior laxity test. Make sure that the patient maintains the correct position and take care when grasping the humeral head, as this area may be tender.

posterior glenoid fossa was used as the index for *posterior laxity*. As in many normal asymptomatic individuals the proximal humerus can be translated posteriorly 50 percent of the glenoid width; any movement greater than this was classified as excessive posterior laxity.

Fifty percent of swimmers had a history of shoulder pain. Some degree of posterior laxity was present in one or both shoulders in approximately 55 percent of the swimmers and in 52 percent of the control group, suggesting that swimming does not predispose an athlete to increased laxity. A history of "tendinitis" and increased posterior laxity was present in 25 percent of the swimmers. In these, "tendinitis" was always present in the lax shoulder, suggesting a relationship between shoulder pain and increased laxity.

SHOULDER STRENGTH IMBALANCE

Manual testing performed on these same swimmers demonstrated external rotator weakness in one or both shoulders in 40, with 33 having both weakness and a history of tendinitis in the same shoulder.

298

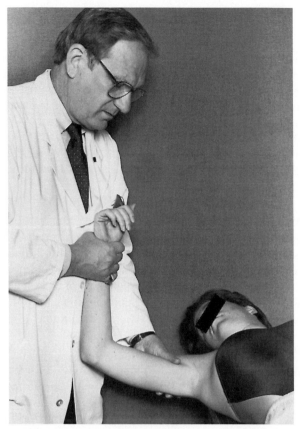

FIGURE 22-4
A clinical test for posterior laxity. The abducted position imitates arm position in variety of activities.

Based on these findings, a second study was conducted to measure rotation strength about the shoulder.[3] One hundred and nineteen swimmers and 51 controls (participants in activities not requiring arm rotation strength primarily) were tested on the Cybex II dynamometer. Internal and external rotation strength were measured in three arm positions: neutral, 90° abduction, and 90° flexion. There was a significant difference in the rotation torque ratio between swimmers and controls in the neutral and 90° abduction positions (Table 22-3). This was attributed to the greater strength of the internal rotators in swimmers. Because the pull-through phase, which involves adduction and internal rotation at the glenohumeral joint, is the "power" portion of the stroke, most swimmers selectively train their internal rotators to improve their power and speed. The resulting imbalance between the internal and external rotators about the shoulder may be a contributing factor in the onset of shoulder pain. It is reasonable to assume that a strong muscle will resist stress better than an unconditioned one. There was no significant difference in external rotation strength between the two groups.

IMPINGEMENT POSITIONS IN SWIMMING STROKES

Positions in swimming strokes during which pain is experienced seem to be associated with the biomechanical factors contributing to tendinitis. This relationship was recognized in a 1981 survey by Webster that reported that 48.4 percent of 155 age 16 and under swimmers had an incidence of past or present shoulder pain.[14] The front crawl was the main practice stroke used by 99 percent of this group. Table 22-4 outlines the occurrence of pain during specific phases of the front crawl. During the entry phase and the beginning of the pull phase (Fig. 22-5) the shoulder is in forward flexion, abduction, and internal rotation, the head of the humerus is forced toward the anterior acromion, and the coracoacromial ligament and the supraspinatus and biceps tendons may be impinged. In the recovery phase, lateral impingement may occur (Fig. 22-6). Here the shoulder is in abduction and internal rotation and the head of the humerus comes up against the lateral border of the acromion. When the shoulder leads the arm through recovery, there is less potential for lateral impingement. The "wringing out" mechanism occurs during the end of the pull phase when the arm is in adduction and internal rotation (Fig. 22-7).

Clinical Evaluation

A thorough history is most important in this assessment. The athlete's pain is characterized in terms of onset, duration, location, quality, and relationship to a specific activity. A systematic physical examination includes inspection, palpation, assessment of range of motion with associated pain, crepitus stability, and motor strength. Tenderness elicited with

TABLE 22-3
Rotation Strength Ratios about the Shoulder: A Comparison of Competitive Swimmers and a Control Group of Athletes

Position	Swimmers	Controls
Neutral	53.7% (SD = 17%)	65% (SD = 15%)
90° abduction	62.1% (SD = 14%)	78.2% (SD = 17%)
90° flexion	Right 46% (SD = 18.4%) Left 42% (SD = 19.7%)	52% (SD = 17%)

TABLE 22-4
Pain during Front Crawl Arm Cycle

Position	Percentage
Entry, first half of pull phase	44.7
End of pull	14.3
Recovery	23.2
Throughout cycle	17.8

palpation of the supraspinatus tendon medial to its insertion on the greater tuberosity is suggestive of tendinopathy. As well, tenderness over the bicipital groove suggests involvement of the long head of biceps. The "painful arc" syndrome that causes pain with active abduction between 60 and 100° is a classic sign of supraspinatus involvement. Biceps tendinitis can be a product of refractory rotator cuff tendinopathy. The straight arm raise with the forearm supinated and the examiner resisting forward shoulder flexion can reproduce symptoms of biceps tendinitis. Infraspinatus or teres minor tenderness may implicate involvement of these tendons.

IMPINGEMENT TESTS

There are various tests in which, by placing the shoulder in an impingement aggravated position, clinical pain is reproduced. An appropriate test for swimmers is one in which the shoulder is forward flexed 90°, elbow is flexed 90°, and the arm is internally rotated by the examiner (Fig. 22-8). This maneuver pushes the head of the humerus against the coracoacromial ligament, aggravating the inflamed tendon and reproducing pain. In a second test described by Neer, the arm is placed in a forward flexed position and forced forward by the examiner (Fig. 22-9). This drives the humerus against the anteroinferior border of the acromion.

MUSCLE WEAKNESS

Resistance (internal rotation force) applied by the examiner when the patient's arm is in adduction and external rotation with the elbow flexed 90° (Fig. 22-10) will determine the presence of muscle weakness. Gross weakness will be conspicuous. Pain may accompany this test.

GENERALIZED LAXITY

Increased laxity or frank instability may contribute to the progression of tendinitis or may be the total cause of the pain. Fowler and Jobe have described tests where the humeral head is levered anteriorly in the abducted externally rotated position. In the presence of anterior glenohumeral instability this maneuver will exacerbate the athlete's discomfort (Fig.

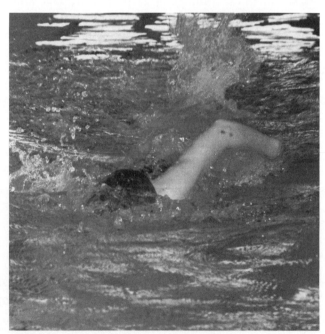

FIGURE 22-6
The recovery phase of the freestyle stroke is demonstrated. In this position the amount of internal rotation of the humerus and the degree of abduction of the arm determine in part the amount of internal rotation. The torso should be turned to recover the arm from the water.

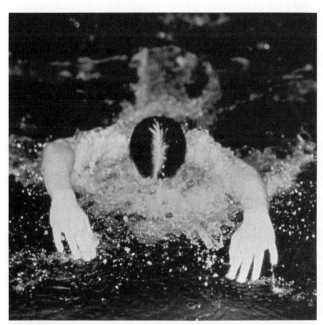

FIGURE 2-5
The reach or entry portion is similar in all strokes. Here it is shown during the butterfly.

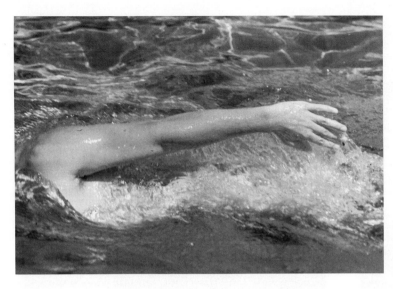

FIGURE 22-7
The "wringing out" mechanism occurs during the end of the pull phase, which is similar for all strokes except the breaststroke.

22-11A). Disappearance of the pain with reduction of the humeral head in the glenoid fossa (positive relocation test) (Fig. 22-11B) is highly suggestive that anterior glenohumeral instability may be the primary underlying pathologic process.

POSTERIOR TRANSLATION

Movement of the humeral head 50 percent of the glenoid width is considered normal. Even though movement in excess of 50 percent is not necessarily abnormal, this would increase the work load of the rotator cuff, thereby influencing shoulder mechanics. To assess posterior translation, the patient is supine and the examiner holds the arm in 90° of abduction and applies posterior pressure to the upper humerus (see Fig. 22-4). If the shoulder is unstable, applying an axial load may reproduce the symptoms the patient experiences during swimming. In a second test for posterior laxity the patient sits while the examiner stabilizes the shoulder girdle with one hand and applies posterior pressure with the other (see Fig. 22-3).

As a tendinopathy progresses, generalized pain about the shoulder is often present at night or at rest. The athlete avoids painful positions and those which aggravate the symptoms. To minimize pain during swimming, subtle changes in stroke mechanics may develop. A gradual loss of shoulder range of motion and muscle weakness may occur over time and supraspinatus and infraspinatus wasting may become apparent. In the mature athlete this may be an indication of gross degeneration of the rotator cuff tendon or a partial tear. Such changes are seldom seen in age-group swimmers and in fact are rare in athletes under 25 years.

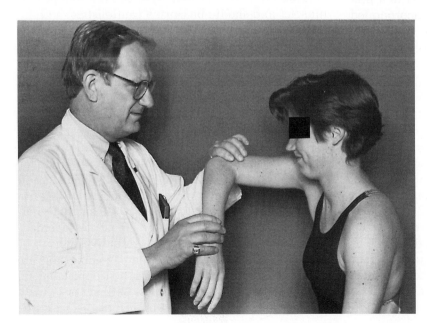

FIGURE 22-8
A clinical test for impingement. Here the tendons are impinged under the coracoacromial arch. Since minimal pressure will cause pain, care must be taken when using this test.

301

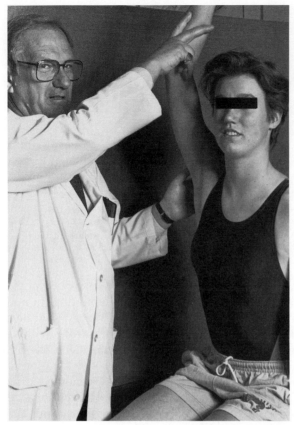

FIGURE 22-9
Here, pressure is applied to the fully forward flexed humerus. Pain may be reproduced if already inflamed tendons are impinged against the anterior acromion.

Prevention

Table 22-5 summarizes a basic preventive program. There are four principles, *balanced muscle strengthening*, *flexibility*, *technique modification*, and *avoidance of overwork*, which are fundamental to a preventive program. These can be readily incorporated into a training schedule as it begins, and any subsequent adjustments to the regimen should be made with these principles in mind.

BALANCED MUSCLE STRENGTHENING

As previously mentioned, in competitive swimming, both pool and dry-land training emphasizes strengthening the internal rotators and extensors important in propulsion. There is little emphasis on strengthening the antagonists, yet they play a significant role in "containment of the shoulder." This can result in an alteration in the balance of muscle strength between internal and external rotation that contributes to tendinopathy. Awareness of an imbalance and early correction play an important part in prevention. An exercise program that includes strengthening the external rotators as well as the biceps and scapular muscles will help avert this im-

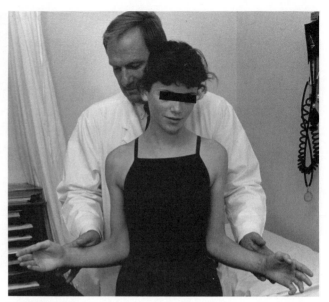

FIGURE 22-10
This manual test determines the gross external rotation muscle strength.

balance. These exercises are simple to perform and require a minimum of readily available equipment such as surgical tubing, pulleys, dental dam, and free weights (Figs. 22-12A and B). They are isotonic and eccentric to improve power and control in both prime mover and antagonist muscle functions. In addition, they are performed in neutral and 90° of abduction to reproduce arm position in the actual sport. Biceps strengthening exercises should incorporate its function as elbow flexor and forearm supinator and should be performed in several positions of shoulder range of motion as well. When doing weight training, painful subacromial loading positions should be avoided. Paddles can produce increased leverage that may overload the rotator cuff muscles and should be caused cautiously.

FLEXIBILITY

In 1985, Griep conducted a study that determined that regardless of sex or stroke most frequently used, those swimmers with restricted flexibility were more likely to develop tendinitis than those who enhanced their flexibility with a stretching program.[7] Stretching should be included in the daily training warm-up routine. Pairs stretching is appropriate for those over 15 years of age (Fig. 22-13). This group should be sufficiently mature to understand that overstretching of the soft tissues can cause irritation to the rotator cuff tendons and must be avoided. Younger swimmers should stretch individually.

The stretching techniques employed by pairs are either passive or proprioceptive neuromuscular facilitated (PNF). In the former, the partner very slowly and gently stretches the swimmer to the pain-free

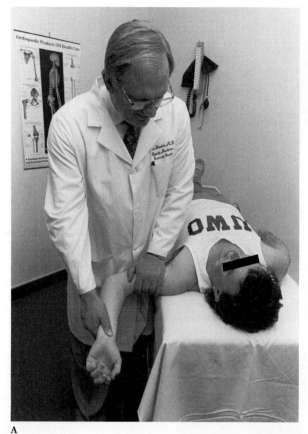

A

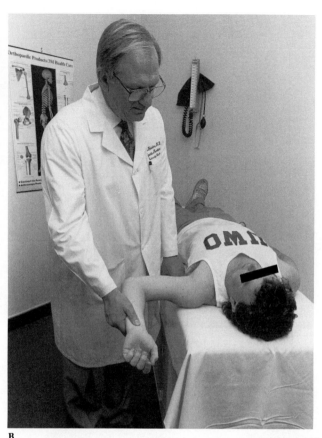

B

FIGURE 22-11
A. The arm is abducted and externally rotated and the humeral head is levered anteriorly. In the presence of anterior glenohumeral instability the athlete will experience apprehension and/ or discomfort. B. Reduction of the humeral head in the glenoid fossa will relieve the symptoms.

limit and then holds this position. In the latter, the swimmer stretches to the pain-free limit. The partner maintains that position while the swimmer contracts against the resistance provided. These are repeated a variable number of times.

TECHNIQUE MODIFICATION

Poor technique not only slows swimmers down but also can be a cause of injury. Again, prevention of overwork and fatigue of the rotator cuff should be foremost in a coach's mind as training programs are planned and the athlete's progress is monitored. Ongoing stroke analysis and recognition of breakdown in stroke mechanics should be part of a routine process that will help the swimmer adjust technique and limit excessive subacromial loading and its stress. Of particular importance is the analysis of stroke mechanics during fatigue. Lateral shoulder impingement can be a result of insufficient body roll in freestyle or backstroke. A high elbow position during the recovery phase of the freestyle stroke must be achieved by body roll. Attempting to force the elbow into a higher position with muscle activity

TABLE 22-5
Prevention of Swimmer's Shoulder

Training regime
- Gradually increase distance
- Gradually increase severity
- Place most vigorous sets at the beginning
- Proper warm-up and warm-down
- Warm-up after kicking sets

Strengthening
- Include external rotators in dry-land sessions
- External rotator strengthening more than 3 times per week
- Include exercises for the muscles surrounding the scapula
- No pain involved

Stretching
- Under 15 years, single stretching
- Over 15 years, pairs stretching
- Passive or PNF stretching only
- No ballistic stretching
- No pain involved

Stroke mechanics
- Proper mechanics, particularly during fatigue situations
- Proper body roll

303

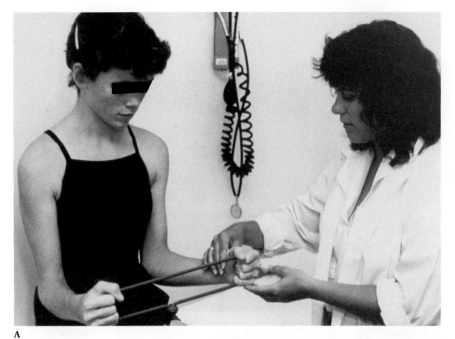

A

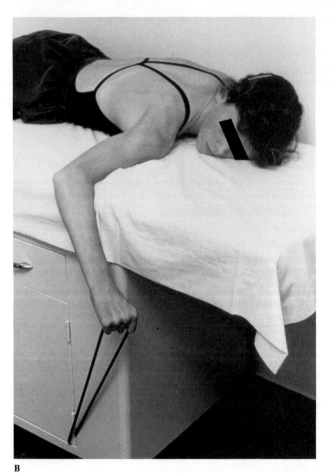

B

FIGURE 22-12
A. Strengthening external rotators in neutral. *B.* Strengthening external rotators in 90° abduction.

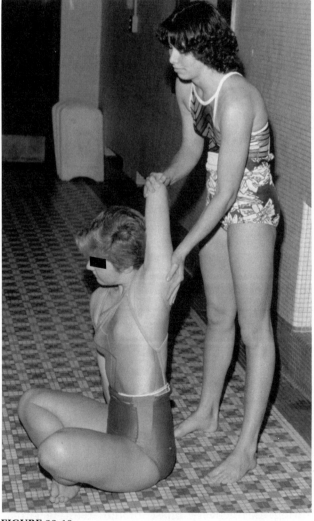

FIGURE 22-13
Pairs stretching requires a knowledge of proper technique and potential pitfalls.

rather than sufficient body roll can induce subacromial impingement.

Overreach with excessive internal rotation during the catch phase of all swimming strokes may cause undue subacromial loading and excessive activity for the cuff muscles to contain the humeral head. Excessive internal rotation may intensify the "wringing out" phenomenon. Changes to body roll, reach, and the degree of shoulder rotation reduce the frequency and the length of time that the shoulder is in a precarious position.

Evidence as to the effect of breathing patterns on the incidence of tendinitis is contradictory.[14] Breathing to alternate sides keeps the swimmer from leaning constantly on the same shoulder.

AVOIDANCE OF OVERWORK

The demands on the swimmer should be increased gradually. Rigorous training sets before the athlete is ready or "extra hard" practices at the beginning of training regimen can trigger the onset of shoulder pain. Training sessions should be designed so that the difficult portion of the workout is completed early in the practice when the swimmer is rested. The workouts should be organized with a focus on providing the swimmer with relative rest to structures at risk. For example, after the difficult work has been completed, the practice can continue with emphasis on stroke drills, alternating stroke and leg work and start and turn techniques. Minimizing the potential for injury is dependent on proper instruction that will teach the swimmer to guard against fatigue and to be aware of the value of good stroke mechanics.

Treatment of Tendinitis (Table 22-6)

CLASSIFICATION OF TENDINOPATHY

Tendinitis is classified in three grades according to the categories for jumper's knee described by Blazina.[2]

Grade I.   Pain is experienced after the activity.
Grade II. There is pain during and after the sport, but it is not disabling.
Grade III. Disabling pain is present during and after activity.

Grade IV describes the group of patients who have stopped swimming but continue to experience pain with activities of daily living.[8]

TABLE 22-6
Treatment of Rotator Cuff Tendinopathy

It is important to identify and treat the primary process in order to initiate sensible treatment.

1. *Rest* from aggravation (not complete rest)
2. *Alter* mechanics if indicated
3. *Anti-inflammatory* medication for a short course
4. *Ice,* first modality, used before and after workouts and therapy
5. *Physiotherapy* modalities—ultrasound, laser, electrical stimulation, friction massage
6. *Restore* motion, strength, power, endurance, stability (individual attention to each depending on deficit)
7. *Steroids:* Occasionally in subacromial bursa; repetitive injections may cause further problems
8. *Functional* sport-specific exercises
9. *Surgical treatment*
   Instability surgery if indicated
   Decompression surgery *only after 9 to 18 months of failed conservative treatment*
   Open or arthroscopic decompression—indications objectives and rehab are same: bursal excision may be sufficient if chronically inflamed and thickened: EUA and explore cuff for tears

Rehabilitation Program
Pain and tenderness
- Mobilizations (grade I + II), transverse frictions, modalities (ice, US, laser, interferential, TNS)

ROM and stiffness
- ROM (pure and combined AROM movements), mobilizations grade IV + V, stretches—later used as prestrengthening warm-up

Muscle imbalance
- Strengthening—always performed in pain-free ROM once shoulder is only mildly irritable
- Emphasis should be placed on internal and external rotator strength balance; high ratio is important to achieve

Isometric
- Work all muscle groups, various ranges, maximal contractions—6 reps, 5 s hold, 3 times per day
  Once isometric work causes minimal treatment soreness, progress to isokinetic training.
- Isokinetic strength evaluation at slow—60°/s and fast—240°/s speeds determines shoulder ratio
- Training commences in the least irritating position—neutral; progresses to 90° as comfort allows
- Concentrates on external rotation
- Tolerance must develop gradually

Isokinetic
- 3 times per week, neutral position
- 240°/s 1 × 20 and 2 × 6 reps
- 180°/s 1 × 15 and 2 × 6 reps
- 120°/s 2 × 10 and 2 × 6 reps

Grade I

Conservative management includes increases in both warm-up and warm-down times, particular attention to prepractice stretching, icing, correction of external rotation weakness, decrease in work load, and temporary elimination of painful strokes. It is important that practice strokes be pain-free. Stretching to increase blood flow, restore range of motion, and decrease potential for impingement should involve all structures about the shoulder including the anterior ones. These are followed by a prolonged, slow-paced warm-up in the pool using pain-free strokes. Additional arm warm-ups are done after kicking sets. The training session is concluded with a warm-

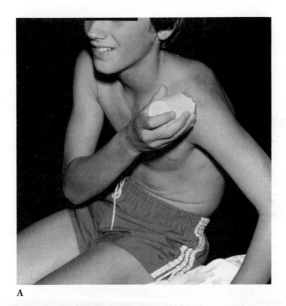

A

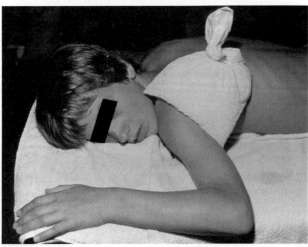

B

FIGURE 22-14
Techniques for icing after practice. *A.* Ice cup. *B.* Ice bag.

down period in the pool. Icing the shoulder for a maximum of 15 min after practice will often reduce pain (Fig. 22-14*A* and *B*). This is conveniently and effectively accomplished using ice cups. Strengthening the external rotators is important to control the glenohumeral joint and increase muscle work efficiency. This is begun by working the external rotators in adduction and progressing to varying degrees of abduction. If symptoms are caused by one stroke only, it should be discontinued until they subside and then gradually reintroduced. Faulty mechanics must be corrected.

Grade II

Management includes the above as well as relative rest, physiotherapy, and medication. Relative rest means using strokes that do not cause pain and emphasis on leg work. Use of kick boards may place the shoulder in pain-provoking positions and should not be used. Running and cycling can augment the limited swimming workouts. Anti-inflammatory medication along with these measures will help provide symptomatic relief. Physiotherapy is indicated at this stage. Treatment is based on the therapist's evaluation, which includes an assessment to determine intensity and duration of pain, range limitations, and strength loss in arm and shoulder girdle muscles. Modalities such as ultrasound, interferential therapy, and transcutaneous nerve stimulation (TENS) are included in the therapy. Passive mobilization techniques and range of motion exercises are used to treat loss of range. Appropriate strengthening programs are organized to correct muscle strength imbalance or weakness. Exercises are isometric, isotonic, or isokinetic depending on the nature and presentation of the pain, joint range, and weakness. Free weights or surgical tubing can be used effectively in treatment programs. It is important that the exercises do not reproduce pain. If pain is felt in certain positions, the exercises should be done around these. Exercise that is painful throughout the range should be discontinued or decreased in repetition or resistance to a level that is pain-free. A successful treatment program will allow the swimmer to gradually return to a full training schedule. However, therapy should not be discontinued until the preinjury activity level is attained.

A steroid injection into the subacromial space should be considered only if there is no response to treatment and if impingement aggravated tests still elicit pain. In situations where its use is warranted, the swimmer's load should be decreased following the injection and return to previous levels should take place over a 4- to 6-week period. Steroid injections should not be used routinely.

Grade III

If the process progresses to grade III and becomes refractory in spite of the measures outlined above, the athlete is faced with options that include a change of sport or surgical intervention. Most young swimmers choose the former, and in most instances this is to be encouraged. If the possibility of a career at the national or international level exists, the athlete should be encouraged to carefully weigh the implications of both alternatives and should be assisted in this process by the coach and physician. Surgery as outlined below should be planned only if the swimmer clearly understands that the postoperative period demands a serious personal commitment to a rehabilitation program and that the success of the procedure is contingent upon cooperation and compliance with this program. Included in this regimen is a progressive exercise program to restore range of motion and balanced muscle strength. Return to the pool should begin with slow swimming that progresses to interval training and guided stroke modification. As well, there should be an overlapping period from formal rehabilitation.

Grade IV

A grade IV process is most often seen in the mature athlete and may indicate a torn rotator cuff. Imaging techniques such as athrography, ultrasonography, and magnetic resonance imaging may help confirm the clinical diagnosis. Lesions such as partial thickness tears and thickened subacromial bursa can be identified by arthroscopy of the shoulder joint and subacromial space. While not a frequent cause of pain in the younger swimmer, anterior and posterior superior quadrant labral tears can cause pain in the swimmer and can be treated successfully with arthroscopic excision.[10] Bursectomy alone followed by appropriate rehabilitation can provide relief in the younger swimmer, but a more radical decompression that includes resection of the anteroinferior acromion and a portion of the coracoacromial ligament is usually recommended. But return to the preinjury level of participation is unlikely, and this should be explicitly understood by the athlete prior to surgery. Postoperatively, range of motion is often low and muscle strength, endurance, and power deteriorate, particularly in the abductors and external rotators. Physiotherapy that rehabilitates all the muscle groups about the shoulder girdle plays a significant postoperative role.

SHOULDER INSTABILITY

Anterior Instability, Prevention, and Treatment

Anterior instability is not often the cause of pain in competitive swimmers and is usually secondary to a traumatic incident in another sport. With the exception of the conventional backstroke turn where the arm is levered anteriorly, the arm is seldom in the provocative position during swimming strokes as compared with throwing activities.

Primary conservative treatment of anterior instability is stroke modification and balancing-strengthening exercises. The traditional turn in the backstroke that reproduces the symptoms of shoulder dislocation can be modified by having the swimmer reach across the body to touch the pool wall and perform a somersault to come out of the turn.

If symptoms do not subside, examination under anaesthesia and/or arthroscopy will assist in diagnosing intraarticular lesions such as a Bankart or Hill-Sachs. An anterior stabilizing procedure can provide relief, and athletes can return to preinjury levels if their motion and strength are regained.

Posterior and Multidirectional Instability, Prevention and Treatment

Swimmers with frank posterior instability may have pain from dislocating their shoulders during the swimming stroke cycle. The at-risk position of forward flexion and internal rotation occurs in all strokes. Pain in swimmers with congenital or acquired multidirectional instability must be differentiated from that experienced by those suffering from painful tendinopathy who have concomitant increased laxity.

In swimmers with prolonged periods of instability, persistence with a nonoperative program is recommended. In most cases, stroke modification, correction of strength deficits, as well as modifying training programs to minimize the magnitude and incidence of abnormal motion, can be successful. Surgical intervention such as an inferior capsular shift, "a reefing procedure" to the posterior cuff and capsule, and a glenoid osteotomy should be considered only when all nonoperative treatments have been exhausted. These procedures, while providing symptomatic relief from pain for daily activities and for recreational participation in swimming and other sports, may because of restricted motion terminate a highly competitive swimming career.[4,6]

REFERENCES

1. Bigliani NU, Morrison DS, April EW: The morphology of the acromion and its relationship to rotator cuff tears. *Orthop Trans* 10(2):216, 1986.

2. Blazina ME: Jumper's knee. *Orthop Clin North Am* 4(3):65, 1980.

3. Fowler PJ: Shoulder injuries in the mature athlete, in Grana WA (ed): *Advances in Sports Medicine and Fitness*, Chicago: Year Book Medical Publishers Inc, 1988, p 225.

4. Fowler PJ: Evaluation, treatment and prevention of upper extremity injuries in swimmers, in Nicholas J, Hershman Elliott B (eds): *Upper Extremity in Sports Medicine*. St Louis: Mosby, 1990, p 891.

5. Fowler PJ, Webster MS: Shoulder pain in highly competitive swimmers. *Orthop Trans* 7(1):170, 1983.

6. Fowler PJ, Webster-Bogaert MS: Swimming, in Reider Bruce (ed): *Sports Medicine—The School-Age Athlete*. Philadelphia, Saunders, 1991, p 429.

7. Griep JF: Swimmer's shoulder: The influence of flexibility and weight training. *Orthop Trans* 10(2):216, 1986.

8. Kennedy JC, Craig A, Schneider RC: *Sports Injuries: Mechanics Prevention and Treatment*. Baltimore, Williams & Wilkins, 1985,

9. Kennedy JC, Hawkins RJ: Swimmer's shoulder. *Phys Sports Med* 2(4):35, 1974.

10. McMaster WC: Anterior glenoid labrum damage: A painful lesion in swimmers. *Am J Sports Med* 14(5):383, 1986.

11. Neer CS, Welsh RP: The shoulder in pain. *Orthop Clin North Am* 8:585, 1977.

12. Ogata S, Uhthoff HK: Acromial enthesopathy and rotator cuff tear. *Clin Orthop* 254:39, 1990.

13. Rathbun JB, Macnab I: The microvascular pattern of the rotator cuff. *J Bone Joint Surg (Am)* 52(B):540, 1970.

14. Webster MS, Bishop P, Fowler PJ: Swimmer's shoulder. Undergraduate thesis, in University of Waterloo (ed): *Waterloo, Ontario, 1981*.

CHAPTER 23

Tennis

Robert E. Leach

INTRODUCTION

As first-year medical students, we remember the anatomy instructor telling the class that the primary role of the shoulder was to put the hand into position to function. Even these many years later, that seems a good functional definition for the shoulder. When it comes to sports, however, the shoulder must add certain other functions to its primary role. Mobility plus stability and even strength are needed for tennis.

In tennis, the racket is held in the hand, and the shoulder, elbow, and wrist must place the hand and racket into position to strike the ball. Mobility is then the primary objective of the shoulder. Conversely, when the racket meets the ball, force will be transmitted through the racket and its strings to the upper extremity, and stability of the upper extremity, particularly of the shoulder, must be present or pain may occur. Also, if there is instability, one may not be able to have the shoulder assume and hold the correct position to position the racket to strike the tennis ball.

The ability to strike the ball hard and thus produce more ball velocity is a function of many parameters, including the speed of the racket head as it contacts the tennis ball. Strength is one physical function that helps to produce power and racket head speed. In particular, the muscles of the shoulder should be strong for the serve and the overhead strokes to increase power, which may increase the velocity of the tennis serve. Some studies have been done to show that increasing the strength of the internal and external rotators of the shoulder will increase the speed of the tennis serve. However, much of the power of the serve is generated by the legs and the trunk. At the beginning of the serve, the knees flex and as they go into extension, power is generated into the body and eventually through the shoulder to the racket. Trunk rotation also accounts for much of the power generated in the serving motion. It is, in fact, a coordinated effect of all these separate factors that combine to make a fast tennis serve.

Shoulder pain can be a major consideration and cause of disability for a tennis player.[9,12] For elite junior tennis players, the shoulder is the most common site of injury. For older players, a number of acute and chronic conditions can interfere with playing tennis. Fortunately, most shoulder disorders can be well managed with conservative treatment and most players will return to full tennis activity.

COMPARISON WITH PITCHING A BASEBALL

Hitting a tennis serve and pitching a baseball have often been compared and, less often, contrasted.[8] Parts of the motion of hitting a tennis serve and pitching a baseball are comparable. However, the mechanics of pitching a baseball are much more violent for the shoulder[11] and its soft tissues than the act of hitting a tennis serve. This is so despite the fact that the fastest tennis serves are between 118 and 130 m/h and the act of throwing a baseball at its fastest is around 92 to 98 m/h. The difference in the speed produced is the mechanical advantage gained by the racket and the increased lever arm that this provides. This also makes it easier on the shoulder to serve than it is to throw a baseball.

Virtually every day during the baseball season, we read about a pitcher who is having new problems with a shoulder or recovering from old problems. Many baseball pitchers' careers end as the result of problems with the shoulder.[12] We do hear of tennis players who have significant problems with the shoulder, but it is unusual to have a career end as the result of a shoulder problem. Generally, even at the top level, a player may sit out several tournaments but does not miss a year.

In baseball, the average starting pitcher may throw 110 to 130 pitches during the course of a game, but that starting pitcher will not pitch again until the fifth day after the previous performance. In tennis, a routine three-set match could easily involve 30 games, 15 of which would be served by each person. At an average of six points per game, with 50 percent first serves in, this would add up to 135 serves during the course of that three-set match. Many collegiate and even professional tennis players will play doubles on the same day, which could add another 60+ serves. All would be expected to be in condition to be able to play the next day and throughout a 5- or 6-day tournament. Clearly, the tennis player is going to serve many more times than the baseball pitcher, and the incidence of significant acute or chronic injury is lower in the tennis player. Since we know at the top levels that the velocity of the tennis serve is higher than the velocity of the baseball pitch, the act of hitting a tennis serve must be easier on the shoulder soft tissues than the act of pitching a baseball.

We have already mentioned that the racket provides an increased lever arm so that more force and speed is generated at the racket head than can be generated at the hand, which is the delivering agent in baseball. Most baseball pitchers have excessive external rotation of the shoulder that allows them to obtain a significant rotatory moment as the pitching arm goes from extreme external rotation to internal rotation. This rotatory moment, with the coordinated help of the legs and body mechanics, helps to increase the velocity of the pitch. This rotatory force also increases the stress on the muscle tendon units and other soft tissues around the shoulder as the arm quickly and powerfully goes from external rotation to internal rotation. There is initially great stress on the anterior glenoid labrum and anterior capsule and later severe eccentric stress on the external rotators during the deceleration phase. Careful examination of the tennis service motion shows that what appears to be a great deal of external rotation of the shoulder

is achieved by arching the dorsal spine backward, laying back the wrist, and some opening of the face of the racket head (Fig. 23-1*A*, *B*, *C*). The total effect is similar to more external rotation of the shoulder, but it is achieved with far less tissue strain. The arc of rotatory motion at the shoulder is thus less, and it would seem that the deceleration phase would be less severe, indicating why less stress is produced on the soft tissues around the shoulder. On the contrary, the racket head goes through a major arc of motion, and that is one reason why the stroke is so powerful.

The rest of the tennis game, ground strokes and volleys, produces relatively few problems for the shoulder, as the usual positioning of the shoulder is well below 90° of forward flexion or abduction, which produces less stress on the soft tissues. It is only when one is forced to extremes, i.e., reaching wide for a high forehand or backhand ground stroke or volley, that we find people complaining of their shoulder in the usual ground stroke or volley sequence. Tennis would be quite easy on the shoulder, except for the serve and overhead.

TREATMENT

The strained muscle needs time to repair itself and regain its functional strength. Palliative treatment

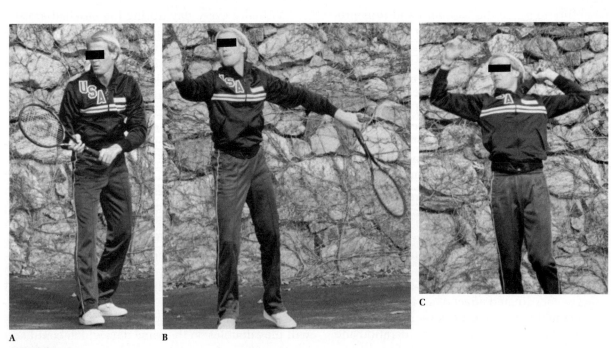

FIGURE 23-1
A. Serve starting position; shoulder is in internal rotation.   *B*. Midway in serve shoulder is still internally rotated.   *C*. Much apparent shoulder external rotation is rotation of torso and laying back of wrist.

such as NSAIDs may cause further damage if this allows the player to again serve without treatment. The player must cease those strokes, usually the serve and overhead, that cause pain in the muscles, but we frequently allow players to continue to hit ground strokes trying to keep the ball waist high or below. A full range of motion must be kept, and if there is loss of elevation or rotation, the player should be started on active and active-assistive exercises. The usual muscle strain needs a rest period of somewhere between 10 and 21 days, and the gradual elimination of pain is a good criterion for how to progress. Once the offending muscle group has been identified, and after a period of rest, exercises should be starting to strengthen this muscle group gradually. The internal rotators of the shoulder are strong, and frequently, as they contract and bring the shoulder into internal rotation, it is the external rotators, the decelerators, that bear the strain. We certainly agree with Chandler that these muscles are frequently underpowered and start the patients on a general program of external rotation exercises against light resistance, with either an elastic cord or light weights. We would start with these low-resistance exercises and gradually increase the number of repetitions. The shoulder elevators and abductors should also be strengthened, but initially the internal rotators seldom need to be worked on. As pain decreases and strength increases, the resistance is gradually increased and the repetitions are increased proportionally.

When the player can go into external rotation against manual resistance without pain, it is time to resume serving and overheads. We do not want the player changing a previous service motion unless there has been a history of chronic shoulder problems or if the service motion, by either history or observation, is obviously awkward. In such an instance, the coach or other related professionals should be brought into the picture. Otherwise we think that there are potential problems if the physician begins to advise players to modify a tennis stroke without the advice of teaching tennis professionals.

ACUTE MUSCLE STRAINS

All the muscle groups of the shoulder girdle have a function while playing tennis, but during the serving and overhead motion, it is the internal and external rotators of the shoulder, particularly the rotator cuff muscles, that are the most subject to acute muscle strain. The usual history of a player suffering an acute strain of the rotator cuff muscles is that of having previously played a long match or practice with a great deal of serving, perhaps playing under conditions where the balls have become wet or heavy on a clay court surface. In some instances, there has been a short warm-up, particularly for the service motion. Generally, the player has noticed something going on in the shoulder during the course of playing, but typically will continue through that practice or the match and wake up the next day with a sore feeling in the shoulder. Elevation of the arm above 80° of abduction or external rotation beyond 70° may be painful. Typically, the player will warm up more slowly the next day and then while hitting serves or overheads may notice that the pain becomes more acute and is present with each shot when the racket is raised above the head. Classically, the muscle strains around the shoulder are felt with the serve, overhead, and sometimes, with a high backhand ground stroke. On physical examination, for an acute muscle strain, observation will disclose no atrophy of the involved muscle groups. The range of shoulder motion is usually complete, but as the player starts to elevate the arm above 80° of forward flexion or abduction, some pain may be produced. The examiner may see asynchrony of scapulothoracic motion as viewed from the back, while the arm is going through the final 100° of elevation. This finding may be similar to that seen in a chronic impingement syndrome, but the history easily differentiates these two entities. There may be some local tenderness of the involved muscles, but this is not common. External rotation or elevation against manual resistance may produce pain in the involved muscle groups. X-rays show no significant findings and we believe that an MRI is not needed at this stage in acute muscle strain.

Chandler et al.,[4] in a study of college tennis players, found both acute and chronic muscle strains relatively common. They found that the more powerful internal rotators around the shoulder seemed to overpower the external rotators, which they believe is the potential cause of injury (Fig. 23-2). They also found that the eccentric contraction of the external rotators that is demanded as it slows the arm down was a likely cause of problems.

Frequently, tennis players with an acute strain of the rotator cuff muscles continue to play because they can hit their ground strokes without difficulty. There is a tendency to modify the motions of the serve and the overhead or to decrease the number of times that the ball is hit with these strokes and thus to not seek assistance early. During the several weeks

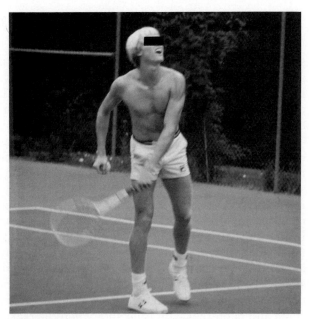

FIGURE 23-2
Internal rotation acts powerfully on finish of serve and overhead.

that can pass, the muscle that has been strained is continuing to be damaged by activity.

CHRONIC MUSCLE STRAINS

Acute strains of the muscles around the shoulder usually respond well to rest and conservative management. Certain chronic muscle conditions are more of a problem. These arise from the overuse of the muscle groups and, to some extent, from the maladaptation of these muscle tendon units around the shoulder.

As the tennis player uses the arm and shoulder more and more for tennis, particularly for serving, there is a gradual hypertrophy of the muscle groups on that dominant side. There is usually some contracture of the posterior capsule of the shoulder and some loss of internal rotation. There also may be some gradual tightening and contracture of the scapula muscles, including levator scapulae, the rhomboids, and the serratus anterior, all of which are used in the action of scapular retraction and protraction while serving and, to a lesser extent, during the ground strokes.

Chronic pain in these muscle groups is not uncommon. In some instances, the pain is in the body of the muscle, particularly with regard to the rhomboids, and in some instances it is closer to where the muscles attach to the scapula, such as where the levator scapulae and serratus anterior attach. Techni-

cally, we should call the process in the muscle body a type of myositis, and the process at the attachment sites would be a tendinosis. In some instances, both the body of the muscle and the attachment sites are involved and are tender. The player has trouble with the service motion. Pain is produced, and it is described as a deep, aching pain. There is a scapula dyskinesia that affects the service motion. Local tenderness is common. Pain in the muscle body or at the attachment sites, while produced with hitting a tennis ball, is also present as a dull ache during ordinary activities. As the scapula muscle groups become gradually painful, there is some contraction of these muscles and some loss of both strength and endurance.

Initial treatment must be directed by resting the shoulder muscles from the strains of playing tennis, particularly in serving. However, the muscles themselves need to be rehabilitated. Exercises must be done to stretch out the levator scapulae, the rhomboids, and the serratus anterior maximally. This means that the patient must elevate and depress, protract and retract this scapula maximally. Very specific instructions have to be given to the patient to achieve these aims. Any internal rotation contractures of the shoulder should be stretched out at the same time (Fig. 23-3).

After several days of rest and the initial stretching exercises, the next move is to gradually strengthen the scapular muscles, paying particular attention to those muscle groups that are the most painful and dysfunctional. These muscle groups are not the ones that most athletes are used to working on, and it usually requires the use of a physical therapist or trainer to devise the exercises to work on these particular muscles. The authors have found that deep massage followed by range of motion and strengthening exercises seems particularly helpful in these muscle groups. Anti-inflammatory agents may decrease pain during the treatment time and be helpful in allowing the exercises to be done. Some people have found that ultrasound applied to the points of maximal tenderness is helpful, and we have used this with some success. The basic concept has been to get rid of all the muscle tenderness and the shoulder dyskinesia before allowing the patient back into normal tennis activities.

In some instances, the pain at the site of the levator scapulae has been more of a problem than certain other muscle groups. If this is at the attachment site to the scapula, occasionally we have used a local steroid injection followed by the same treatment plan that we outlined as a means of alleviating the pain.

It is very easy at a younger age for players to overuse these muscle groups and these syndromes

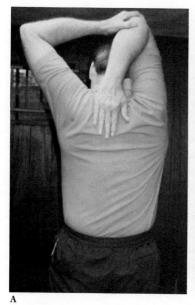
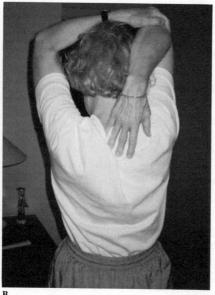

FIGURE 23-3
A. Exercise to stretch shoulder capsule; subject has less contracture than *B.* *B.* Exercise to stretch shoulder capsule; subject cannot bring arm to midline.

are basically an overuse type of problem. Younger players have to be cautioned against too much serving, overheads, and the like, particularly when they begin to experience soreness that lasts overnight.

TENDINITIS, TENDINOSIS, AND IMPINGEMENT SYNDROME OF THE ROTATOR CUFF

During the past decade, tendinitis of the rotator cuff has become seemingly synonymous with the impingement syndrome. Similarly, there has been difficulty in distinguishing between tendinitis and tendinosis of the rotator cuff. Tendinitis implies that there is inflammation of the tendons, whereas tendinosis implies that there is intrinsic damage to the cuff without inflammation. In this section, the authors try to distinguish among these three entities and show how they play a role in problems of the shoulder in tennis players.

We believe that impingement of the rotator cuff against the anterior portion of the acromion and the coracoacromial arch may cause changes in the rotator cuff that lead to inflammation and chronic tendinitis. We also believe that tendinitis of the shoulder may occur de novo without the impingement syndrome acting as the initiating factor. With tendinitis, an inflammation of the tendons of the rotator cuff, there may be a secondary involvement of the overlying bursa. As the rotator cuff becomes weaker, one would expect proximal migration of the humeral head, and the impingement syndrome may then become the more important aspect of this symptom complex.

Andrews and others have hypothesized that the action of throwing a baseball with the tremendous stresses that are placed on the rotator cuff may produce changes in the substance of cuff tendons as the result of the acute action of throwing the baseball. Nirschl[11] has described what he calls a traction or tensile failure of the cuff that occurs on the undersurface of the tendons near the attachment to the greater tuberosity. This fiber failure, which usually occurs on the undersurface of the cuff but can occur within the substance, leads to a loss of integrity of the cuff and since it is not accompanied by inflammation should be called tendinosis. Previously mentioned authorities and others[14] feel that this is caused by an eccentric overload primarily of the supraspinatus and infraspinatus tendons. As the cuff becomes weaker, again, one would expect proximal migration of the humeral head and more impingement against the acromial arch.[6]

A primary impingement syndrome secondary to acromial morphology seems rare in tennis players. The secondary impingement syndrome could result from failure of some of the fibers of the rotator cuff that would allow proximal migration of the humeral head and impingement of the humeral head and intervening rotator cuff against the acromion. This type of impingement syndrome could result from anything that causes weakness of the muscle tendon units of the rotator cuff. This secondary impingement syndrome definitely occurs in tennis players, and particularly is seen in the over-40 age group.[10] Another possible scenario that produces impingement occurs because many tennis players have a very tight posterior capsule with decreased internal rotation. With elevation of the arm, there may be an-

313

terior translation of the humeral head and a tendency to have the head ride up against the anterior aspect of the acromion, producing impingement and more changes in the rotator cuff. One final possible cause for a secondary type of impingement syndrome in tennis players is an altered rhythm of the scapula due to strain of the scapula stabilizers. If the scapula does not protract properly, the acromion may not move so as to be cleared by the humeral head as the arm elevates, and an impingement syndrome could result.

Tendinitis of the shoulder in tennis players usually occurs following episodes of serving or hitting overheads and probably represents the strain of the muscle tendon units. The resulting pain in the shoulder region may be nonspecific, although there is often radiation into the area of the deltoid muscle attachment on the humerus. The pain is intensified with elevation of the arm past 85°, particularly in abduction. There may be local tenderness over the rotator cuff, but it may be difficult to detect on physical examination because of a large deltoid muscle or an inability of the patient to relax well. Early in the disease process, there may be some weakness of the muscles of the rotator cuff, particularly the supraspinatus and the external rotators. This weakness may be initially produced because of pain, but as the condition persists, the weakness becomes more notable.

Players with chronic tendinitis usually have a slight hesitation of the scapulothoracic motion as the arm is abducted between 85 and 120°. This momentary hitch of the scapula can be viewed when standing behind the patient. Frequently, as the arc of motion goes beyond 120°, the pain disappears and full elevation is usually possible, particularly in the early phases of the disease. There is frequently an element of impingement with tendinitis as the condition progresses. At that time, the impingement sign should be positive. The arm is forcibly forward flexed by the examiner to 90° and then put into internal rotation. This brings a greater tuberosity with the attaching tendons against the anterior-inferior surface of the acromion and possibly the coracoacromial ligament. In the over-40 patient, it is best to obtain a supraspinatus outlet view to see if there is any problem with the morphology of the acromion. One other test is similar to a tennis player hitting a high backhand. The involved shoulder and arm are brought across the body and then the patient attempts to push the arm against resistance away from the body. The cross-body excursion of the shoulder and arm is often decreased, and this attempted for-

ward motion of the shoulder usually causes pain. Atrophy of the shoulder girdle muscles is difficult to pick up unless the condition has been long-term or unless there is a rupture of the tendon. Rarely, we have found major tenderness over the biceps tendon, indicating that this tendon is also involved. One should always compare the tenderness over the bicipital groove on the unaffected arm with that of the affected arm. Many patients experience some discomfort with palpation of the tendon in its groove. Loss of elevation, particularly in abduction, and loss of internal rotation are common. One should always measure this accurately, as it may be very helpful in predicting a full return of function and in monitoring the patient's progress.

Treatment

Treatment of these chronic problems of the rotator cuff will vary with the acuteness and intensity of the symptoms, the duration of symptoms, the age of the patient, and to some extent, the tennis desires of the patient. Directed physiotherapy will be the backbone of treatment. We first start range of motion exercises to be sure that the patient has full abduction plus full internal and external rotation. Pendulum exercises can be done by the patient, but increases in internal and external rotation may be difficult to gain and the patient is often dependent upon active-assistive exercises done with a therapist. Generally, there is no particular reason to stretch the anterior capsule, and thus exercises should be directed toward stretching out the posterior capsule and increasing internal rotation.

There is agreement that strengthening the rotator cuff muscles is necessary in dealing with these syndromes, but there has been some change in the thinking as to which muscles need to be worked on and exactly how they should be strengthened. The prevailing view is that eccentric overload is a major cause for many of the problems involving the rotator cuff. We now recommend working on both the internal and external rotators of the shoulder, feeling that they both play a major role. The easiest way to strengthen the external rotators is by working against a rubber bungee cord or surgical tubing, but with the arm held below 60° of abduction (Fig. 23-4*A*, *B*). Resistance can be varied by using various types of tubing and we start with low resistance and high repetitions, gradually working up to higher resistance. We would also perform the same type of exercises for the internal rotators. By using a bungee cord or similar apparatus to work both muscle groups, we

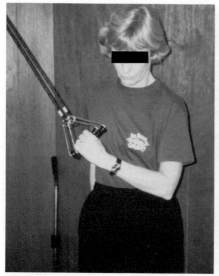
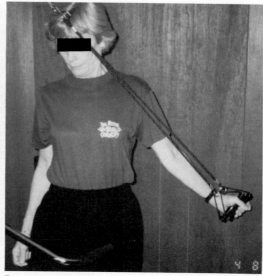

FIGURE 23-4
A. Starting position to strengthen external rotators. *B.* Finishing position; subject would do better to keep elbow against body.

are getting a combination of concentric and eccentric strengthening. We hope that this combination will work to increase both strength and endurance of both muscle groups. The internal rotators are generally quite a bit stronger than the external rotators. However, Chandler[4] found that the endurance of the internal rotators was not as good as would be expected in collegiate tennis players. He and Hawkins[6] both state that the subscapularis is very important and must be strengthened along with the external rotators. The concept is to gradually stress the appropriate muscle-tendon units with the hope that this will cause a repair process as its normal homeostasis is regained.

The role of nonsteroidal anti-inflammatory medications has been debated. They certainly may be used to alleviate pain and are very helpful in allowing people to carry out their exercises. In mild cases of tendinitis of the shoulder, their use may be sufficient to allow people to play some tennis. If, however, the medication is used to mask the pain while playing and the basic problem is not corrected, the ongoing condition gradually will be exacerbated. We do not have a problem with players using a nonsteroidal at moments of pain exacerbation or to relieve mild pain as long as they are working on alleviating the causes of the pain.

During the past 15 years, we have used few steroid injections into the subdeltoid bursa as the treatment of chronic tendinitis. If the pain is thought to be due to chronic tendinitis with a secondary bursitis and the patient was making no progress with other treatment modalities, a subdeltoid bursal injection with a steroid preparation is a possibility. We would recommend that following that, the patient

rest the shoulder for 2 weeks and do nothing more than range of motion exercises. Then the follow-up care must consist of range of motion exercises plus strengthening exercises, as previously outlined.

When impingement seems to be a major part of the painful shoulder, as it often is in the older patient, the supraspinatus outlet view may show a type I, II, or III acromion, as described by Bigliani.[2] If symptoms persist over a 6- to 12-month period despite good conservative care, operative intervention is a possibility. At that time, the surgeon inspects the anterior aspect of the acromion and the undersurface of the acromioclavicular joint. A partial acromionectomy, as previously advocated by Leach et al.,[8] was effective in alleviating pain and allowing athletes, including tennis players, to resume their careers. However, the anterior acromioplasty as described by Neer[10] and modified by others is now the open procedure of choice.[14] Anterior acromioplasty can be done effectively arthroscopically. This allows for an easier rehabilitation for the tennis player. In an athlete in whom impingement has occurred, there is always a question as to what is happening to the undersurface of the cuff, so shoulder arthroscopy should be performed at the time of any arthroscopic decompression of the acromion. If there are areas of deterioration of the cuff on the undersurface, these can be debrided prior to the acromioplasty and the glenoid labrum is also inspected. Labral debridement, however, has not been a good long-term procedure.

The rehabilitation period following arthroscopic decompression has been well outlined by others. Range of motion exercises are instituted quickly. If there are changes on the undersurface of the rotator

315

cuff, one should wait a period of at least 3 weeks before undertaking any vigorous resistance exercises. Following any surgical decompression, we like to decrease the posterior capsular contractures and increase the eccentric and concentric strength of both the internal and external rotators of the shoulder. Realizing that shoulder motion is a complex motion, we recommend work on the scapula muscles to be sure that these are not contracted and have not weakened during the time of relative incapacity.

ACUTE ROTATOR CUFF TEARS

Acute tears of the rotator cuff do occur as a result of playing tennis, but it is not a common occurrence. It is much more likely that a tear will occur as the result of chronic changes in the rotator cuff in the over-45 player. In such an instance, while the tear itself may be acute, the condition arises from chronic changes in the rotator cuff.

We have seen two professional players with tears of the rotator cuff, which occurred acutely. In each instance, the men, who were in their mid to late twenties and playing regularly on the tour, were involved in a long, hard match under adverse circumstances. They sustained small tears of the rotator cuff while serving. The diagnosis was not obvious, primarily because although they lost some strength and it affected their ability to serve, their youth and lack of acute symptoms did not point immediately to an acute rotator cuff tear. Cuff tears in the older player do occur acutely but are superimposed on chronic problems. We discuss rotator cuff tears below.

CHRONIC ROTATOR CUFF TEARS

Acute tears of the rotator cuff are uncommon, particularly in younger tennis players, but tears of the rotator cuff in the over-45 tennis player are seen more often. With aging and repetitive use of the arm overhead, a number of tennis players have chronic shoulder problems. Most of these patients suffer from either chronic tendinitis, tendinosis, or the impingement syndrome (Fig. 23-5). Some of these patients go on to sustain a tear of the rotator cuff, and in this instance, this is basically a continuum of a process starting with tendinitis or tendinosis and/or impingement, which progresses to degeneration and finally, acute dehiscence of the rotator cuff tissues, i.e., a tear. In some players, the rotator cuff tear does occur de novo and players state that they have had no significant shoulder trouble but all of a sudden had pain in the shoulder and the inability to elevate the arm in the normal manner.

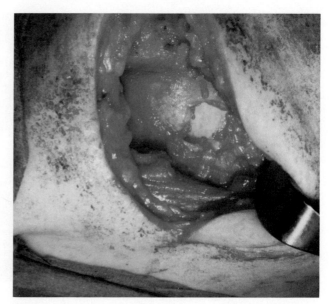

FIGURE 23-5
Chronic cuff tear typical of over-50 tennis player.

The usual history that the patient gives is one of the two instances cited above. More commonly, patients have had chronic shoulder problems for which they may or may not have sought treatment and then have had superimposed upon that a sudden episode with pain and inability to properly elevate the arm. Generally, the pain is not severe, and it is usually this inability to properly elevate or abduct the arm that brings the tennis player to the doctor.

The less common history is that of players playing a lot of tennis and having an episode when pain is felt, usually when hitting the serve. They then realize that they cannot properly use an arm. In both instances, players may not arrive in the doctor's office until several weeks have gone by. Often they assume that the shoulder will get better and may seek help from friends, such as the local tennis professional, or health industry–related people who are often attached to tennis clubs. At times, patients come in more than a few weeks after the initial episode, telling you that they have been on an exercise program that has been prescribed by somebody at the tennis or health club. Pain is a lesser part of this player's complaint.

On physical examination, there will be a problem with elevation of the arm. Patients seem to do better in forward flexion than in true abduction. Sometimes, there is a major loss of elevation, being able to get the arm up to only 65 to 70°. Other times, the patient may gradually elevate the arm, but there is distinct asynchrony of the scapulothoracic muscles as the player attempts full elevation of the arm. The patient may lean to the opposite side, trying to stabilize the humeral head against the glenoid,

316

which would then enable the deltoid to assist in elevation past 90°. There will be weakness of the rotator cuff muscles and it is the supraspinatus primarily and the infraspinatus secondarily that are most commonly torn. Isolating the supraspinatus muscle by elevating the arm to 90°, putting it in 20° of forward flexion, and then internally rotating it will almost invariably show weakness of this muscle by the inability to hold the arm in elevation against minor resistance. External rotation will also be weak.

To verify the diagnosis, the clinician has a number of possibilities. An arthrogram may show a tear if there is leakage of dye from the joint through the rotator cuff into the subdeltoid bursa. If the tear is small or if there is a flap tear, an arthrogram may not show it. An MRI will show tears of the rotator cuff, and as experience increases with this modality, it is likely tha this will be the test of choice. In Europe, ultrasound is an effective way of diagnosing tears of the rotator cuff, but it is less popular in the United States. Finally, arthroscopy should enable one to see the tear, evaluate the tissues, and probably in the very near future, enable us to repair the cuff without an open operation.

How should we treat a rotator cuff tear in a middle-aged tennis player? Generally, the patient will say that the shoulder has improved, but it has reached a point at which it is not continuing to improve. Tennis players may volunteer that they can hit ground strokes but not an overhead serve or a high forehand volley. Few players will be aggressive in seeking surgery since most athletic people think that this is the court of last resort. People are often told that surgery is likely to be less successful as one grows older. Patients 60 and 70 may feel that surgery is unlikely to be helpful. We agree with Bigliani et al.[2] who advise repair and who found that the results were quite good in a group of active people with an average age of 58, who had full-thickness cuff tears that were repaired. Six of their patients who had a traumatic event causing the tear suffered this while playing tennis. Eleven had a gradual onset of pain and what one might call an attritional or chronic tear. In follow-ups of between 3 and 4 years, 83 percent of their patients had good results. Although their patients were doing resistive exercises at 3 months, it took about a year for them to be able to return to their preinjury status in serving. One other fact of interest was that 7 of their 23 players had tenderness over the AC joint and 5 of their 23 players had tears of the biceps tendon, although that was not a cause of major symptoms.

We would agree that there is no particular reason that surgery should not be performed, even in

the older player. The success rate is more likely to be related to the size of the tear, the status of the surrounding tissues, and how long one has waited before repairing the tear. It appears that the late performed surgery is less likely to be successful. We believe that in the tennis player who has sustained a tear, even of a chronically inflamed cuff, the most likely way of helping is to repair the rotator cuff.

At the time of a cuff repair in the middle-aged or older tennis player, we advocate some type of acromioplasty with careful inspection of the AC joint to remove any osteophytes that might cause irritation of the underlying cuff. The methods of rotator cuff repair are well outlined in a variety of previously published articles. The principles are simple. You must have adequate exposure, unhealthy tissue that is not able to hold sutures or does not have a vascular supply must be resected, and the surgeon must do enough dissection to bring healthy tissue to healthy tissue for the repair. If the tendinous tissue has torn away from the bone, it must be advanced to the bone and securely fastened so that after the repair, the arm may be brought down to the side with the repair intact. As a general rule, rotator cuff tears occurring in tennis players are not going to be massive and one is not usually faced with the prospect of doing a complicated procedure to close a major defect.

Postoperatively, we advocate early motion of the shoulder, with gentle pendulum exercises the day after surgery. An exact timetable for when to start active or active-assistant exercises would really depend upon the tissues and the repair that was accomplished. In most instances, it is unlikely that one is going to be able to start on active-assistive exercises until 6 to 8 weeks. At that point, one would want to start on forward flexion and external rotation and then gradually push ahead, probably beginning resistive exercises at about 3 months.

Rehabilitation of a patient with a torn rotator cuff in the middle-aged group is not easy. With chronic shoulder symptoms and with complete disruption of the cuff, strength of these muscle groups decreases rapidly. Rehabilitation has to be long-term and assiduous.

It may be difficult to tell patients exactly when they can get back to hitting tennis balls and particularly hitting overheads and serves. There is no particular reason that with competent physical therapy and a cooperative and aggressive patient we could not have somebody out hitting ground strokes at around 5 to 6 months, and serves will happen some months later. Bigliani[2] and his group found that people were serving at about a year, but we have had some patients who have been able to come back at 6 to 7 months, particularly those with cuff tears that were operated upon early. Most of these patients will probably not return to their normal pre-cuff-tear strength. They will also probably never regain complete range of motion, particularly in external rotation. However, there is the reasonable expectation that they will have good strength and motion to get back to playing tennis well.

SHOULDER INSTABILITY

Shoulder instability rarely arises primarily as the result of playing tennis. However, a person who has sustained a previous shoulder injury, which causes recurrent subluxations or dislocations, could have a problem playing tennis. If such a player came into the office with the chief complaint of instability of the shoulder and pain with hitting the tennis ball, this would present a problem for the treating physician. Based upon our personal experience, it is unusual for the shoulder to dislocate while playing tennis. Subluxation is a more likely occurrence but is still rare. A player who has had chronic episodes of subluxation or dislocation may have pain with the serving or overhead motion as the shoulder goes into external rotation and the humeral head moves forward. The tight posterior capsule often seen in tennis players may contribute to this forward movement of the humeral head. The result could be damage to the glenoid labrum or a subluxation of the humeral head.

With a tennis player with apparent shoulder instability, we would treat the patient with strengthening exercises of both the internal and external shoulder rotators. We would try to stretch the posterior capsule by internal rotation exercises. If these measures did not help, the major diagnostic problem for the physician is whether the pain or momentary instability is caused by actual subluxation of the humeral head over the anterior rim of the glenoid, or perhaps by a small tear of the glenoid labrum being caught between the head and the glenoid.

The physical examination will be helpful but may not always solve the diagnostic problem. An apprehension test, which can be performed with a patient lying on the abdomen and the arm held in neutral rotation, should be performed to show either anterior or posterior laxity. Translation of the humeral head over the glenoid rim indicates a chronic subluxation. It can also be present in a tear of the glenoid labrum, as was demonstrated by Altchek et al.[1] in their study, which showed 24 of 40 patients showing at least 1+ laxity in either the anterior or posterior direction. Hawkins[6] likes to perform his apprehension test with the patient sitting and the arm totally relaxed, and he tries to translate the humeral head anterior or posterior.

If the apprehension test is positive and it is felt that the humeral head is moving over the rim of the glenoid, one might expect the player to have trouble with the serving motion or when hitting an overhead. An operative procedure to stabilize the shoulder would probably be necessary. We do not want to limit external rotation in the tennis player, although it is of less importance than it is in the throwing athlete. The literature leads one to believe that despite some early reports concerning certain operations, there is some loss of external rotation in virtually all shoulder repairs. We believe that a capsular repair of some type, usually listed under the generic term "Bankart," would be the best method for restoring stability and cause the least loss of external rotation for the tennis player. We have had tennis players who have had recurrent subluxations who have had capsular repairs of the shoulder done and had a final result of between 90 and 100° of external rotation. They were able to return to playing recreational tennis without difficulty. We have not had a tennis player who was at a high collegiate or professional level who has had the same problem and been operated upon.

Postoperatively, it is critical to try to start a patient on a resumption of early range of motion exercises, which can be done with a good capsular repair. We do limit external rotation to the neutral position for the first 3 weeks postoperatively, but then gradual resumption of external rotation and other motions of the shoulder is done. Strengthening of the internal rotators should be started at approximately 6 weeks with the progressive resistance exercises, and we would start the external rotators at about 8 weeks. We would like the internal rotators to be stronger in order to be protective for the shoulder against the usual anterior subluxation. It may also help to stretch out the posterior capsule. The external rotators should be strong to prevent any future problems involving the rotator cuff.

GLENOID LABRUM INJURIES

Injuries to the glenoid labrum are common in throwing athletes and seen in certain other activities such as racket sports, swimming, and weight lifting. The symptoms that occur from a tear or detachment of the superior glenoid labrum are not specific just to these labral tears. They may mimic shoulder subluxation and even, to a certain extent, the symptoms of impingement. That makes the diagnosis difficult and formulating a treatment plan equally difficult. Most patients with a labral tear will present with shoulder pain, which occurs during forward flexion and overhead use of the arm, such as occurs in the serve in tennis. The pain is usually anterior and occurs only with activity, gradually disappearing as the activity fades. Altchek et al.,[1] in a study of 40 patients with labral tears, found that 38 had a positive impingement sign but a negative impingement test. A majority of such patients are likely to demonstrate positive shoulder laxity, either anterior or posterior, but many fewer will demonstrate frank subluxation of the glenoid humeral joint.

Routine x-rays are usually negative, and even the West Point view will usually not show changes at the anterior glenoid margin. An arthro-CAT scan would be of real value in determining if there is a lesion of the glenoid labrum and is a reasonable alternative to a diagnostic arthroscopy.

If the diagnosis of a tear or detachment of the glenoid labrum is made, it presents a dilemma for the treating physician. Six of the 40 patients were treated by debridement of the glenoid labral tears and yet only 1 of their 40 patients returned to preinjury sports participation level. Seventy-two percent of their patients noted gradual deterioration of their early postarthroscopic debridement status. Given these disappointing results, which were seen over a 2-year period, there is a real question as to what is the best method of treatment. Pappas had reported earlier on labral excision, but this was done by an open operation and it is possible that there was some capsular scarring that may have made the joint more stable and thus was helpful to his patients. His previously reported good results have not been reported by others. While arthroscopic debridement may give reasonable early results, the later results are not as good. If there is a major element of instability, correcting that instability while excising any labral tear would seem reasonable. If the only diagnosis is a tear of the glenoid labrum, and the patient is symptomatic while playing tennis, arthroscopic debridement can be done, but the prognosis frankly is guarded for a tennis player, as the long-term results seem less satisfactory.

ACROMIOCLAVICULAR ARTHRITIS

Considering the amount of motion that occurs at the acromioclavicular joint with elevation of the arm,

such as that which would occur serving or hitting an overhead in tennis, there are relatively few patients who have symptomatic acromioclavicular arthritis that requires treatment. In some instances, the player may notice pain with elevation of the arm, a relatively generalized pain, which could be confused with chronic rotator cuff tendinitis if a careful examination were not done. In other instances, the patient may say that a grinding sensation is felt in the anterior aspect of the shoulder, which is accompanied by pain with the overhead motion. The physical examination will disclose tenderness over the AC joint and, in many instances, a sensation of grinding or crepitus when the arm is elevated over head. Routine x-rays of the acromioclavicular joint will show changes (Fig. 23-6).

Treatment

Several times we have had patients who have come in complaining of pain in the AC area, and after the diagnosis has been made, they seem to have been satisfied. They required no more than occasional use of NSAIDS and have continued to play tennis. In other instances, the pain is severe enough that something needs to be done. To be sure that there is not another concomitant cause of pain in a patient upon whom we are planning to operate, we inject a few milliliters of Xylocaine into the acromioclavicular joint. If the pain disappears completely with that anesthetic in place, even with elevation of the arm, it is likely that this patient is going to benefit from a distal resection of the clavicle.

Although we have resected the distal end of the clavicle in only a few patients who were tennis players, the results have been excellent. These players have been over the age of 50 and had the classic history and physical exam. The distal end of the clavicle was resected in the usual manner and rehabilitation was relatively quick. In each instance, the

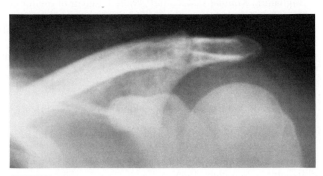

FIGURE 23-6
Acromioclavicular arthritis: An x-ray.

player returned to playing tennis at 6 weeks without apparent difficulty. As the reader knows, in some instances, the undersurface of the distal clavicle may have a large osteophyte that is causing irritation of the rotator cuff, and there are times when resection of the distal end of the clavicle may prove to be efficacious, not only for the AC joint but for the underlying cuff.

COMPRESSION OF THE SUPRASCAPULAR NERVE

Compression of the suprascapular nerve does occur in athletes and thus should occasionally be seen in tennis players, although it is a rare phenomenon overall.[3,5] The authors, however, have seen no tennis players on whom they have made this diagnosis. Pain and scapular dysfunction are caused by compression of the suprascapular nerve as it passes through the suprascapular notch under the transverse suprascapular ligament. Rarely, the nerve can be compressed by an obstruction at the base of the acromion process.

Patients usually complain of a nonspecific pain in the posterior aspect of the shoulder and some weakness of the supraspinatus and infraspinatus muscles. Atrophy and weakness of these muscles may be demonstrated. One would expect that this dysfunction would significantly affect the tennis serve and overhead. The diagnosis can be confirmed by an electromyogram and nerve conduction test.

If the diagnosis is definitive, the usual treatment would be to surgically decompress the nerve. This procedure is well described in other texts.

DOMINANT SIDE HYPERTROPHY

Some tennis players, particularly males, who started playing at an early age will demonstrate in their late teen years and after noticeable dominant side hypertrophy of the muscles of the upper arm and shoulder girdle.[13] This phenomenon would appear to be simply the response of the muscle units that are being used in tennis and that hypertrophy because of the eccentric and concentric strains that are being applied by tennis. It is well recognized in baseball players that the same phenomenon occurs and that the cortical bone of the upper humerus demonstrates increased thickening as compared with the nondominant side. Frequently, there is some depression of the shoulder on the dominant side, and this sagging shoulder may be a cause for having parents bring in the tennis player to be sure that nothing is wrong.

In our experience, this situation is rarely the cause of symptoms. Sometimes patients who present with marked dominant side hypertrophy may complain of weakness or pain, particularly in the posterior scapular muscles. We believe that this is due primarily to the strains of playing tennis as opposed to being caused by the hypertrophy of the upper extremity. Reassurance is usually all that is needed for the parents. If the muscles are strained or fatigued, treatment would be directed at the appropriate muscle groups.

REFERENCES

1. Altchek D, Warren R, Wickiewicz T, Ortiz G: Arthroscopic labral debridement. A three-year follow up study. *Am J Sports Med* 20:702–706, 1992.
2. Bigliani L, Kimmel J, McCann P, Wolfe I: Repair of rotator cuff tears in tennis players. *Am J Sports Med* 20:112–117, 1992.
3. Black K, Lombardo J: Suprascapular nerves injuries with isolated paralysis of the infraspinatus. *Am J Sports Med* 18:225, 1990.
4. Chandler T, Kibler W, Stacener E, et al: Shoulder strength, power, and endurance in college tennis players. *Am J Sports Med* 20:455–458, 1992.
5. Drez D: Suprascapular neuropathy in the different diagnosis of rotator cuff injury. *Am J Sports Med* 4:43, 1976.
6. Hawkins R, Kennedy J: Impingement syndrome in athletes. *Am J Sports Med* 8(3):151–158, 1980.
7. Jobe F: Symposium: Shoulder problems in overhead-overuse sports. *Am J Sports Med* 7(2):139–140, 1979.
8. Leach R: *Tennis Serving Compared with Baseball Pitching. Injuries to the Throwing Arm.* Philadelphia, Saunders, 1985.

9. Lehman R: Shoulder pain in the competitive tennis player. *Clin Sports Med* April 1988: 309.

10. Neer C: Impingement lesions. *Clin Orthop* 173:70–77, 1983.

11. Nirschl R: Prevention and treatment of elbow and shoulder injuries in the tennis player. *Clin Sports Med* April 1988: 289.

12. Priest J: The shoulder of the tennis player. *Clin Sports Med* April 1988: 387.

13. Priest J, Nagel D: Tennis shoulder. *Am J Sports Med* 4:28–40, 1976.

14. Tibone J, Jobe F, Kerlan D, et al: Shoulder impingement syndrome in athletes treated by an anterior acriomoplasty. *Clin Orthop* 198:134–140, 1985.

CHAPTER 24

Baseball

James R. Andrews
Laura A. Timmerman
Kevin E. Wilk

INTRODUCTION

The motions used in baseball, including the pitch, throwing a baseball, and batting, all place tremendous stresses on the soft tissues about the player's shoulder. In order to throw successfully, the shoulder complex must be capable of excessive motion, while maintaining stability of the glenohumeral joint. Injuries to the throwing shoulder can result from acute trauma, such as a fall with a resulting dislocation or fracture; but more commonly disorders about the baseball player's shoulder are the result of overuse injuries from the repetitive throwing act.[1] Imbalance in the muscles and soft tissues about the shoulder can result in an injury secondary to abnormal biomechanics of the glenohumeral complex.

Knowledge of the biomechanics of the throwing motion is crucial to the clinician involved in treating baseball players. Understanding the anatomy of the shoulder complex and the mechanics involved in throwing provides a framework for diagnosis and treatment of shoulder disorders in the baseball player that can be approached in a systematic fashion. This chapter (1) reviews the biomechanics of the throwing motion; (2) discusses the pathomechanics of shoulder injuries as related to the throwing motion; (3) discusses the evaluation of the injured throwing shoulder; (4) reviews specific injuries seen about the shoulder in both the skeletally immature and mature baseball players including diagnosis, treatment, and operative findings; and (5) discusses our approach to the rehabilitation of the throwing shoulder in baseball, including a maintenance program, and the interval before return to a throwing program after conservative and operative treatment of specific shoulder disorders.

BIOMECHANICS OF THROWING

The throwing motion is used in various activities, including racket sports, the javelin toss, and basketball. Analysis of the baseball pitch allows the most comprehensive understanding of throwing mechanics; this information can then be applied to other forms of throwing.[2,3]

Pappas and coworkers analyzed 15 major league pitchers with high-speed cinematography.[4] They divided the pitch into three phases: cocking, acceleration, and follow-through. They found that the shoulder had an average peak angular velocity for internal rotation of 6180° per s just prior to ball release. The movement about the shoulder is impressive. Pappas reported that the entire excursion of the arm through space occurred within a range of 225° with respect to the horizontal plane. This motion is not confined just to the glenohumeral joint; rather it is the result of the composite action of the glenohumeral and scapulothoracic joints, along with trunk extension, flexion, and rotation.

At our Biomechanics Laboratory of the American Sports Medicine Institute, data have been collected using motion analysis of the pitching motion on over 230 baseball pitchers. Based on the analysis of this information, the baseball pitch is divided into five phases of throwing: windup, cocking, acceleration, deceleration, and follow-through.

Windup Phase

The windup phase starts from a two-legged stance to a one-legged stance where the ipsilateral leg is planted with the contralateral leg brought up into a tucked position with the hip and knee flexed to approximately 90°. This phase is complete when the ball is removed from the glove. The pitcher prepares for delivery of the ball by obtaining correct body posture and balance. This is a smooth preparation phase of throwing, and no excessive strain is placed across the pitcher's shoulder or elbow. EMG analysis of the muscles about the shoulder shows minimal activity during this phase, and there is little difference in the activity of muscles in professional as compared with amateur pitchers.[5]

Cocking Phase

The cocking phase involves correct positioning of the body in order to provide the optimum acceleration for ball delivery. The contralateral leg is taken from a tucked position and is planted in front of the body. The pelvis and trunk are internally rotated to face the plate; then the internal rotation of the shoulder follows with maximum external rotation of the humerus while it is in a 90° abducted position. The elbow is flexed approximately 90°, and as the humerus reaches the point of maximum external rotation, the elbow begins to extend. During this position there is very little forward motion of the ball; consequently at the end of this phase the shoulder has advanced, while the hand and ball remain positioned behind the body. This results in an eccentric load applied to the humeral adductors (including the pectoralis major and the subscapularis) and the internal rotators (latissimus dorsi and teres major muscles). This extrinsic muscle tension allows the body to become "coiled" to impart energy to the ball.

With EMG analysis, Gowan and coworkers identified two groups of muscles that are active during the pitching act.[5] The first group included the supraspinatus, infraspinatus, teres minor, deltoid, trapezius, and the biceps brachii. They found that this group was responsible primarily for positioning the shoulder and elbow for delivery of the pitch; while a second group of muscles, including the pectoralis major, serratus anterior, subscapularis, and the latissimus dorsi, displayed stronger activity during the propulsive phase of the pitch. EMG analysis of muscle activity during the early cocking phase showed increased activity of the biceps, with increased activity of the subscapularis and supraspinatus during late cocking.[6,7]

Acceleration Phase

The acceleration phase of the pitch is that time frame between the end of the cocking phase and the point of ball release. The term acceleration refers to the energy imparted to the ball, not to the action of the arm segments during the pitch. Over the course of approximately 50 to 80 ms the ball is accelerated from a stationary position to a speed in excess of 80 mph.[8] The pitcher moves forward and transfers his weight onto the forward-planted contralateral foot and leg. This allows for the transfer of the anterior momentum from the legs to the trunk, and then to the shoulder. As the trunk is rotated anteriorly during the cocking phase, the anterior motion of the shoulder is stopped to allow the transfer of the forward momentum from the trunk to the arm, thereby providing acceleration of the ball. The momentum is carried in a chain reaction from the shoulder to the humerus, elbow, forearm, and eventually the hand, where the energy is imparted to the ball at release.

In addition to this extrinsic load that is applied to the arm, intrinsic acceleration in the horizontal plane results from contraction of the anterior muscles of the shoulder, including the pectoralis and subscapularis. The shoulder internal rotators (subscapularis, latissimus dorsi, and teres major) contract to initiate internal rotation of the humerus. Tremendous forward forces are generated at the shoulder, and during the second half of the acceleration phase the rate of humeral adduction is decreased by the firing of the teres minor, infraspinatus, and supraspinatus muscles. This deceleration of the humerus allows the momentum to be transferred to the forearm and increases the rate of internal rotation, thereby further accelerating the ball. This period of forward hand and ball propulsion is critical for the transfer of energy to the baseball.[5]

Just prior to the point of maximum external rotation of the arm the elbow begins to extend. This rapid elbow extension just prior to ball release is due primarily to the angular velocity of the upper arm and the trunk and not to the elbow extensor muscles.[9,10] The end of the acceleration phase occurs just before ball release. The shoulder external rotators, including the posterior deltoid and the teres minor, begin to contract in order to stop the arm. This allows a transfer of momentum to the hand and the ball, and the ball is released. The phase between stopping the acceleration of the arm and complete extension of the wrist with subsequent ball release is called the release point. From this moment on the relative arm motion is decelerated, and this marks the beginning of the deceleration phase.

Deceleration Phase

The deceleration phase lasts from the point of ball release to the end of humeral internal rotation. This is the most violent phase in the pitching mechanism because the momentum generated during the acceleration phase results in an outward force on the arm of approximately 200 lb,[8] which must be opposed by muscle contraction at the shoulder to maintain stability of the glenohumeral joint and resist the forward motion. The forces during deceleration are much higher but of a much shorter duration than the forces during the acceleration phase. The combination of these compressive forces and the abnormal anterior or posterior subluxation of the humeral head that is seen with glenohumeral joint instability can result in labral tearing.

Follow-through Phase

During the follow-through phase of the pitch the body moves forward with the arm, thereby reducing the distraction forces applied to the shoulder, and allows the pitcher to regain his balance. The follow-through allows for the energy generated during the pitching motion to be dissipated. By utilizing a long follow-through pathway with the arm combined with forward trunk flexion, extension of the front leg, and swing of the back leg forward, the load across the arm can be transferred into the larger body parts, resulting in a reduction of tension to the posterior side of the arm.

PATHOMECHANICS OF SHOULDER INJURIES

The forces generated during the pitch result in adaptive physiologic changes. This includes an alteration in the range of motion with a gain in external rotation of the shoulder at 90° of abduction, and a loss of internal rotation. The humerus may hypertrophy in response to exercise.[11] The repeat stress on the rotator cuff and biceps tendon can result in inflammation with eventual tearing. The labrum is subject to repeat stress and can detach or tear. Repeated stress to the ligamentous capsule can result in instability. More rarely, chondromalacia of the humeral head and glenoid can result.[12] In the skeletally immature a stress reaction or separation of the proximal growth plate may occur.[13]

An alteration in the normal muscular balance about the shoulder can result in distraction and subluxation of the glenohumeral joint, which can lead to injury of the involved soft tissue and bony structures. The types of injury can be related to the phases of throwing: (1) anterior impingement, (2) posterior tension, (3) avulsion, and (4) anterior laxity.

Anterior Impingement Injuries

During the throwing motion the humeral head and the overlying soft tissue sleeve of the rotator cuff and biceps tendon must pass rapidly under the coracoacromial arch. The arch consists of the anterior acromion and the coracoacromial ligament. Impingement of the soft tissues under this arch can result from several different mechanisms. An increase in the bulk of the muscles of the rotator cuff secondary to strengthening or inflammation can cause impingement. The actual space may decrease secondary to osteophyte formation of the acromion and fibrosis of the subacromial space. Actual weakness or incompetence of the rotator cuff may allow the humerus to ride up and impinge against the coracoacromial arch.

Posterior Tension Injuries

The most severe insult to the soft tissues about the shoulder occurs during the deceleration phase of the pitch since the posterior shoulder muscles must contract eccentrically to counteract an outward glenohumeral distraction force equal to the body weight of the thrower. These deceleration torques are nearly twice as great as the acceleration torque on the arm. During deceleration the rotator cuff muscles may fail under tension and result in posterior rotator cuff tears.

Avulsion Injuries

Avulsion of the anterior-superior labrum at the insertion of the biceps tendon is well described in pitchers.[14–17] The biceps contracts during the late cocking phase in order to flex the elbow, and then during the deceleration phase the biceps is actively eccentrically contracting to oppose extension of the elbow.[6] Andrews and coworkers[6] demonstrated that with stimulation of the long head of the biceps muscle the tendinous portion became taut near its attachment to the glenoid labrum, and actually lifted the labrum off the glenoid. As the humerus is rapidly internally rotated, additional forces are placed on the biceps tendon between its position in the bicipital groove and its attachment to the glenoid tubercle. The combination of these two forces can result in avulsion of the anterior-superior labrum at the site of insertion of the tendon of the long head of the biceps.

Anterior Laxity

In order to throw successfully, a pitcher requires laxity in his shoulder to allow for the extreme amount of external rotation of the humerus that is observed in the pitching motion. This external rotation places a tremendous amount of tension on the anterior stabilizing structures of the shoulder, including the anterior capsulolabral complex and the rotator cuff. During the deceleration phase of throwing the muscles about the shoulder contract to oppose the outward distraction and internal rotation of the humerus, resulting in anterior translation of the humerus on the glenoid. Howell and coworkers[18] demonstrated that with anterior instability the humeral head glides anteriorly when the arm is flexed or rotated from the cocking stage of the throwing motion, producing a shearing stress on the glenoid and labrum. In the normal shoulder the center of the humeral head rested approximately 4 mm posterior to the center of the glenoid cavity during the cocked stage of the throwing motion; otherwise the humeral head remained centered in the glenoid. The anterior translation of the humerus on the glenoid results in repetitive microtrauma to the anterior labrum and capsular structures, which over time can result in anterior labral tears and capsular laxity.

EVALUATION OF THE THROWER'S SHOULDER

History

The patient's history is the first and usually the most important step in evaluating an injury. We evaluate our patients initially with four simple questions: (1) what, (2) how, (3) when, and (4) where. In the shoulder the chief complaint is usually pain, but the important determinants include how, when, and where did the pain start. The level and length of time a pitcher has been throwing, type of pitching style (either overhead, three-quarter throw, or sidearm), the speed and types of pitches (fastball, curveball, breaking, slider) usually thrown, any recent changes in throwing style, the length of time since he last threw, and whether he has noticed any change in velocity or accuracy are important pieces of information. It is important to determine the mechanism of injury; for example, was it a sudden onset of pain with one pitch or did the condition develop slowly over time? Ascertaining in what portion of the pitch symptoms occur is useful in localizing the pathology. Whether the pain occurs only with throwing, before warm-up, or after the game, and what relieves or aggravates the pain is helpful knowledge.

The occurrence of other associated injuries, including elbow, back, and lower extremities, that may have altered the biomechanics of the body should be sought out. History of previous treatment, including rehabilitation, medication, injections, and surgery is important. The specific type of previous rehabilitation exercises should be defined in order to determine whether an adequate course of conservative treatment has been followed.

Physical Examination

The physician should perform a consistent exam of the throwing shoulder on every patient. This avoids missing positive findings and allows one to relate the functional phases of throwing to the findings on physical exam. With experience, the physician becomes familiar with normal physical findings in a throwing shoulder. The uninjured shoulder should always be included in the exam for comparison.

Initially one inspects the shoulder. Any signs of atrophy or swelling can be noted. One should carefully assess the scapular motion and contour of the scapular stabilizing muscles, as this is often missed on physical exam. The scapula plays a pivotal role in the stability and motion of the glenohumeral joint.[19] A simple test for this is to have the patient perform a sitting lift off the table, and then to observe the scapula while patients elevate their arms overhead. The posterior musculature of the shoulder is examined to determine the development of the external rotators. The biceps can be easily inspected while standing behind the seated patient with his hands placed on the back of his head.

The shoulder should then be palpated for areas of tenderness or crepitus. This includes not only the glenohumeral joint but also the sternoclavicular and acromioclavicular (AC) joints, the clavicle, the scapulothoracic joint, and the soft tissues about the shoulder. The best position to examine the posterior capsule and external rotators is with the patient prone and the arm relaxed over the side of the table. While in this position the quadrilateral space can be palpated inferior to the teres minor muscle, a rare site of axillary nerve and posterior humeral circumflex artery compression.

Range of motion should be carefully assessed in the sitting, supine, and prone positions. Sitting internal rotation is noted by recording the spinous process the patient can touch with his thumb. In comparing both sides of a throwing athlete, the throwing side will usually lack internal rotation. External rotation at both 0 and 90° of abduction should be noted. The throwing side should have an increase in external rotation at 90° of abduction. Brown and coworkers[20] reported on range of motion findings in 41 professional baseball players. They noted that pitchers demonstrated 9° more external shoulder rotation and 15° less internal rotation with the arm abducted, 5° more forearm pronation, 5° less shoulder flexion, and 9° less shoulder extension on the dominant side. The amount of forward flexion and abduction should be noted; a painful shoulder will often lack the last few degrees in this plane of motion. True glenohumeral external rotation can be evaluated with the patient in the prone position by fixing the scapula and rotating the humerus in 90° of abduction.

A determination of strength of the muscle groups is a critical portion of the exam. Weakness in one portion of the shoulder musculature can result in an imbalance and subsequent injury. The scapular stabilizers, internal and external rotators, deltoid and supraspinatus, triceps, and biceps strength are all compared with the nonthrowing arm.

Stability testing of the shoulder is at times the most difficult portion of the physical examination, especially in large musculatured patients. It is necessary to compare the stability findings with that of the uninjured shoulder in order to determine the amount of baseline laxity present. Initially one can evaluate glenohumeral translation in the sitting position with the arm relaxed. The sulcus sign, or inferior translation of the humeral head, is assessed. The humeral head can be gently pushed in the anterior and posterior planes in this position. With the patient supine, and the shoulder abducted approximately 130° and externally rotated 90°, anterior translation of the shoulder can be performed by grasping the humeral head with one hand while stabilizing the distal humerus with the other and lifting up on the humerus (Fig. 24-1). This is similar to the Lachman test of the knee. Posterior instability can be determined by bringing the arm across the chest in 90° of abduction and then placing a posterior force across the humerus while palpating the humeral head posteriorly. Any apprehension with anterior or posterior translation can be determined. One of the best positions to detect anterior instability is with the patient prone (Fig. 24-2). The arm is externally rotated at 90° of abduction and a forward force is applied to the humerus. If there is any apprehension with anterior translation it will be detected with this test, and the symptoms will be relieved with posterior translation of the humerus.

Special tests in throwing shoulders include a careful assessment of the labrum. Andrews and Gillogly first described this as a "clunk test."[21] The test is performed with the patient in the supine position. The examiner's hand is placed posteriorly on the humeral head, and the opposite hand holds the humeral condyles at the elbow to provide a rotating motion. The patient's arm is brought into full overhead abduction, and the examiner's hand on the humeral head provides an anterior force while the opposite hand rotates the humerus. A "clunk," or grinding, can be felt in the shoulder as the humerus hits or snaps on the labral tear. The location, either superior, anterior, or posterior, of the labral tear is determined by the position of the humeral head at the time the grinding is felt. This "clunk" can also be felt with the patient in the prone position and an-

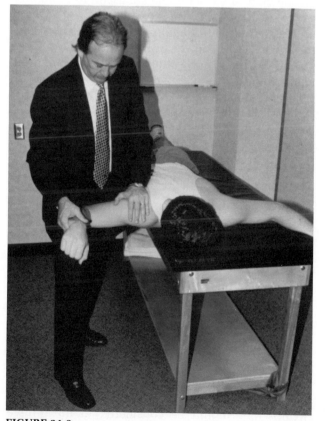

FIGURE 24-2
The prone apprehension test is performed with the patient prone, the arm abducted and externally rotated, with pressure applied to the posterior arm in the anterior direction.

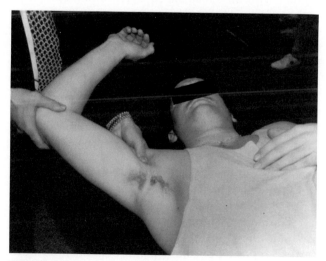

FIGURE 24-1
Test for anterior instability of the glenohumeral joint. The patient is supine; the examiner grasps the humerus and humeral head, and then performs an anterior drawer, akin to the Lachman exam of the knee.

terior force directed on the humeral head as it contacts an anterior labral tear.

It is often difficult to determine whether pain with abduction and external rotation of the humerus is due to shoulder or to rotator cuff tendinitis. Impingement is elicited by internal rotation of the forward flexed arm. This can be done in both the sitting and supine position; in large athletes the latter is easier. Throwers with undersurface rotator cuff tears may not have obvious signs of impingement, and subtle clues indicating irritation of the rotator cuff should be noted. By internally rotating and adducting the arm across the patient's chest the supraspinatus tendon can be palpated just anterior to the acromion process, with the infraspinatus palpated posteriorly.

Ancillary Tests

We obtain a "thrower's series" radiograph of the shoulder on all pitchers, including internal and external rotation A/P views, a modified Stryker (Fig. 24-3; the humerus is abducted 45° to allow visualization of the glenoid rim and AC joint), and an axillary view. A coracoacromial arch, or outlet view, and a profile view of the acromion are useful in evaluation of the subacromial space.[22]

In the past arthrograms were used to evaluate the rotator cuff, and the arthrogram-CT scan of the shoulder allowed for evaluation of the glenoid and labral pathology. We are now using injections of 15 to 20 mL of saline into the shoulder joint followed by an MRI study instead. The saline outlines the labrum and rotator cuff, and tears can easily be seen. This avoids the possibility of a contrast reaction and has no exposure to radiation.

Isokinetic testing of muscle strength is helpful in determining the strength of specific muscle groups. Not only will this at times delineate specific pathologic conditions, but it also assists in developing a rehabilitation program for the injured pitcher.[23,24]

Diagnostic testing with local anesthetic is useful in determining the source of pain. The subacromial space can be injected, as well as the AC joint. This can help to separate intraarticular pathology such as labral tears or anterior laxity from impingement or AC joint pain.

Finally, diagnostic arthroscopy is the last step in evaluating the injured pitcher's shoulder. Every effort is made to reach a diagnosis prior to surgery, with appropriate conservative treatment instituted. Arthroscopy should be considered in the athlete who fails a conservative treatment course. At times, the diagnosis is not confirmed until the shoulder is examined under anesthesia and then systematically inspected arthroscopically.[25–27]

INJURIES IN BASEBALL PLAYERS

History and Epidemiology

In 1941, Bennett[6] first reported on shoulder and elbow lesions of the professional baseball pitcher. He divided the pathologic changes into two groups—the anterior and the posterior group. The anterior group included inflammatory and traumatic lesions of the supraspinatus tendon, subacromial space, and the biceps tendon. The posterior lesions were described as an exostosis that developed on the posterior-inferior margin of the glenoid secondary to the constant strain during the deceleration portion of the pitch.

In 1969, King and coworkers[28] reported over 50 percent of the professional pitchers examined had a flexion contracture in the elbow, 30 percent had a valgus deformity of the elbow, and a rather uniform finding of an increase in external humeral rotation with a concomitant decrease in internal shoulder rotation in the pitching arm.

In 1978, Barnes and Tullos[1] reported on an analysis of 100 symptomatic baseball players. Fifty-six of the 100 players had shoulder problems, with 29 anterior lesions, 24 posterior lesions, and 3 miscellaneous. The anterior lesions included bicipital tendinitis, supraspinatus tendinitis, pectoralis major tendinitis, latissimus dorsi tendinitis, and acromioclavicular joint injuries. All 24 of the posterior lesions were described as posterior capsular syndrome, with an exostosis seen on radiographs in 8 patients.

As arthroscopy has developed over the last two decades, the nature of diagnosis in the throwing shoulder has changed. Initially bicipital tendinitis and bursitis was a common diagnosis.[29,30] This was replaced with the diagnosis of impingement syndrome.[31–33] Despite relief of pain with treatment of impingement syndrome, the actual return to previous level of performance with an acromioplasty alone was poor in some series;[34,35] for example, in one series only 4 of 18 athletes involved in pitching and throwing returned to their preinjury status after acromioplasty.[34]

The concept of recurrent shoulder instability began to develop in the early 1980s. In 1980, Rowe and Zarins[36] reported on the use of a Bankart procedure to treat recurrent transient subluxation of the shoulder; although their series reported 70 percent excellent results, only 4 of 8 pitchers were able to return to throwing. Garth and coworkers[37] reported on a series of patients with occult anterior subluxation in noncontact sports who at arthroscopic exam of the shoulder were noted to have pathology consistent with anterior subluxation. With an increase in shoulder arthroscopy, previously unrecognized lesions of the capsule, undersurface of the rotator cuff, and labrum became important diagnoses.[14,17,27]

A dynamic electromyographic analysis[38] in throwers with anterior instability demonstrated a marked reduction in activity of the pectoralis major, subscapularis, and latissimus dorsi. This in turn added to the anterior instability by decreasing the normal internal rotation force that is required during the late cocking and acceleration phases of the pitch. The activity of the serratus anterior was also decreased in the throwers with anterior instability, which is associated with decreased protraction of the scapula and increased anterior laxity. The neuromuscular imbalance seen in the throwing athletes with anterior shoulder instability was felt to be either part of the primary pathology or a secondary phenomenon.

Current concepts regarding shoulder pain in the throwing athlete are based on early instability of the glenohumeral joint, which can lead to muscular imbalance and abnormal demands on the muscles about the shoulder including the scapular stabilizers and the rotator cuff. Rotator cuff irritation can result because the cuff is attempting to stabilize the humeral head. With persistent instability, labral tears and capsular laxity can develop. With subluxation of the shoulder, secondary impingement can develop.[39]

Rotator Cuff Pathology

Rotator cuff pathology in the thrower is comprised of three main entities: (1) tensile failure, (2) impingement "compressive" disease, and (3) instability. Acute traumatic tears can occur, but these are less common than the injuries due to repetitive activity. In the thrower a common rotator cuff lesion seen is a tensile failure of the undersurface of the rotator cuff, most commonly found in the region of the supraspinatus and infraspinatus tendons. This tensile failure is due to repetitive microtrauma with eccentric overload during deceleration. These lesions can also be found isolated to the infraspinatus tendon and the posterior glenohumeral capsule. Athletes will complain of pain with overhead motion, and they may complain of pain only with throwing. On physical exam they may be tender over the rotator cuff. Obvious weakness or atrophy of the rotator cuff is not usually present. A saline-MRI may demonstrate a partial undersurface tear of the rotator cuff.

Initially the athlete is placed on a rehabilitation program with an emphasis on rotator cuff strengthening. If there is no improvement after 2 to 3 months, arthroscopic debridement of the tear is performed with the rationale that this will stimulate a fibroblastic healing response (Plates 29 and 30). Andrews et al.[40] reported on 34 athletes with partial tears treated with arthroscopic debridement; 85 percent of the patients had good or excellent results and were able to return to their previous athletic activities; 15 percent of the patients had poor results and were not able to return to competitive throwing.

If an undersurface tear is present, underlying instability should be ruled out, since this can lead to secondary impingement, or compressive rotator cuff disease. This requires a careful examination of the shoulder under anesthesia, and a careful arthroscopic examination of the glenohumeral joint for signs of instability, including a Hill-Sachs lesion and anterior labral and capsular detachments.

Compressive, or impingement, rotator cuff disease can also result in primary rotator cuff pathology. The hallmark finding of this mechanism is extraarticular superior surface tears (outside to inside) with evidence of subacromial erosion. This can be caused by a type III hooked acromion, os acromiale,[41] degenerative acromial spurs, or congenital thickening of the coracoacromial ligament.[67]

On physical exam the patient's pain will be relieved with an injection of anesthetic into the subacromial space. Treatment consists of stretching the tight posterior capsule often seen in throwers to help prevent the anterior migration of the humeral head, and strengthening of the rotator cuff musculature. Surgical decompression may be necessary if conservative treatment fails.

Full-thickness rotator cuff tears are not often reported in the young throwing athlete, but they can occur. A repair is warranted, but the return to previous level of play is often not successful. In one large series, only 7 of 22 professional or collegiate-level pitchers and throwers with complete or partial rotator cuff tears were able to return to the same competitive level.[35] In our experience, arthroscopic decompression of the subacromial space and arthroscopic debridement of the tear, followed by repair through a small deltoid splitting incision, early results appear to be superior compared with an open acromioplasty and rotator cuff repair.

Instability

Instability in the throwing shoulder can be in either the anterior or posterior direction. The diagnosis is usually made based on the history and the physical findings. The athlete may complain of apprehension and/or pain and clicking in the shoulder. The most reliable finding on physical exam is pain with stressing of the humeral head in either the anterior or posterior direction, or a "positive apprehension test." The mainstay in treatment of instability is strengthening of the muscles about the shoulder in order to provide a dynamic stability to the glenohumeral joint. If labral pathology is present, surgical intervention may be required. If the athlete fails a conservative rehabilitation program, surgery is considered.

After a careful examination under anesthesia, diagnostic arthroscopy is performed. The glenoid labrum is evaluated for evidence of detachment or tears. Under direct visualization the humeral head is pushed in the anterior, posterior, and inferior direction with the amount of subluxation noted. Once the degree of instability is noted, a decision is made regarding treatment. Mild instability is usually best treated with a conservative strengthening program.

With more severe instability an open procedure may be indicated to repair the labrum and capsular structures. The athlete needs to be aware that return to a previous level of throwing is at times difficult after this procedure. In one series that included 12 pitchers who underwent an open anterior capsulolabral reconstruction, only 6 (50 percent) returned to their former competitive level for at least one season, with an average time of return to competition of 15 months.[42]

Arthroscopic repair of labral detachment has been described.[43] The senior author (J.R.A.) uses this procedure very selectively in athletes with early, true Bankart lesions or early detachment of the anterior capsule and labrum. The technique for repair of anterior lesions involves placement of arthroscopic sutures in the labrum, then passing these sutures posteriorly through a drill hole in the glenoid where they are tied down over the infraspinatus fascia. The new development of biodegradable screws or staples that can be placed arthroscopically through the capsulolabral complex is advantageous in that anterior early detachments can be repaired without the concerns of transglenoid drilling, but no long-term results are yet available in throwing athletes.

Posterior instability can occur in throwers and in batters. Most athletes will improve with a strengthening program, followed by an interval throwing program. As with anterior instability, arthroscopy is considered only after failure with conservative treatment; rehabilitation is the crucial and primary treatment option in these patients. The experience with arthroscopic treatment of posterior instability is limited. Debridement of some labral tears may allow the athlete to return to competition, and reverse Bankart lesions may require arthroscopic or open repair. In case of severe instability open stabilization with a capsular shift employing suture anchors into bone may be necessary. The athletes' return to their previous level of competition after posterior stabilization procedures is very unpredictable, and our enthusiasm for this procedure is minimal.

Labral Tears

Labral tears can occur in the shoulder secondary to the large compressive and shear forces that are seen in the shoulder during throwing (Plates 31, 32, 33). A significant percentage of labral tears involve the anterosuperior portion near the insertion of the biceps tendon (Plate 32) and are not associated with instability;[26] in a recent series labral tears occurred without anatomic instability in 72 percent of the patients treated for labral tears.[17] Posterior labral tears can also occur in the lead arm with batting. The labrum can also become entrapped between the humerus and glenoid during a fall and tear, as is often seen when the player dives to catch a ball.

The thrower usually complains of pain during a certain motion and may also have catching, clicking, or locking in the shoulder. Physical exam may be positive for a clunk test. Labral tears can sometimes be seen with either a CT-arthrogram or saline-MRI study of the shoulder. The tear can be visualized at arthroscopy, and a treatment option selected.

For a degenerative or flap-type tear, arthroscopic debridement with a motorized shaver is usually indicated. Debridement should be done with caution; a stable peripheral rim of labrum is desired, and glenohumeral instability may be aggravated or created with excessive labral debridement. Andrews and Carson[14] reported on the results of arthroscopy in 73 athletes with labral tears. The most common tear was anterosuperior, and after arthroscopic debridement 88 percent had good to excellent results with over 1 year follow-up.

Glasgow et al.[17] recently reported on arthroscopic resection of glenoid labral tears in athletes and found a statistically significant difference in the functional outcome at 2 years between patients with stable and those with unstable joints. In the patients with a stable joint there was 91 percent good or excellent outcome, as opposed to a 75 percent fair or poor functional outcome in the unstable shoulder. No patient with a stable shoulder developed subsequent instability after debridement.

However, it should be noted that when a labral tear is present subtle shoulder instability may exist that is difficult to diagnose. This may develop into occult instability with time, and the diagnosis of instability should be considered in a patient with the recurrence of shoulder symptoms after previous treatment for labral pathology.

Biceps Tendon Injuries

The biceps is active in the cocking and acceleration phase and has its highest level of activity during the follow-through phase.[6] With the eccentric contraction during the follow-through phase biceps tendinitis may develop, although, as mentioned previously, this is not diagnosed as frequently as prior to the advent of shoulder arthroscopy.

The biceps tendon can easily be located on physical examination by placing the patient supine and abducting the shoulder 90° with internal rotation of 30°; then the biceps tendon is located directly in front of the shoulder. At arthroscopy a longitudinal split in the intraarticular portion of the biceps tendon is sometimes observed, and fraying with subsequent rupture can also occur. Rupture in a young throwing athlete is rare; if it occurs, it is usually due to chronic inflammation, attrition, or a mechanical spur in the groove. Treatment of biceps tendinitis is usually conservative, with the same protocol used to treat impingement.

Thrower's Exostosis

The term "thrower's exostosis" was first described in 1941 by Bennett,[44] who described an ossification occurring on the posterior glenoid in professional baseball players. The players complain of persistent posterior shoulder pain, and on a modified Stryker view a bony exostosis is seen off the posterior inferior glenoid (see Fig. 24-3). Lombardo et al. reported on four professional baseball players with symptomatic ossification in the posterior inferior glenoid region treated with open excision; all four players were able to return to satisfactory competitive levels of play.[45]

In the past, the exostosis was thought to be a calcification in the long head of the triceps, but open surgical inspection by the senior author (J.R.A.) has shown that the lesion is not located in the triceps insertion. The exostosis is extracapsular, but by viewing the posterior shoulder from the anterior portal with a 70° arthroscope the posterior-inferior capsule can be reflected with a motorized debrider and the exostosis located. A motorized burr can then be used to remove the bony lesion. Although not previously published, the senior author (J.R.A.) has resected this lesion in several pitchers and allowed them to return to competitive pitching.

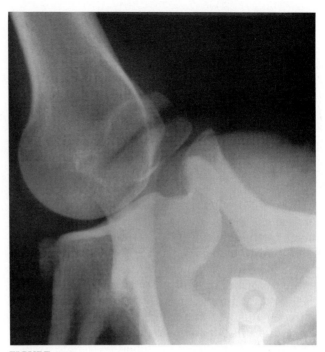

FIGURE 24-3
Modified Stryker view of the shoulder; note the thrower's exostosis off the inferior glenoid rim.

Osteochondritis Dissecans

Osteochondritis dissecans of the glenoid is an uncommon finding in the throwing shoulder. It should not be confused with a common lesion that is seen at arthroscopy in the throwing shoulder, which is an erosion of the center of the glenoid (Plate 34), at times to subchondral bone. We refer to this as a "centering lesion" and consider it a normal finding in the throwing shoulder, as it is seen quite frequently in both young and mature throwers. However, osteochondral defects on the posterior glenoid can occur in throwers (Plate 35) from either direct trauma or insidious onset. This is not a common diagnosis, and unless a loose body is seen on radiographs, it is usually first diagnosed at arthroscopy. Treatment consists of burring or drilling the defect if possible in order to stimulate the formation of fibrocartilage.

Neurovascular Syndromes

Neurovascular disorders about the shoulder are seen rarely, but they may be a source of shoulder pain that is difficult to diagnose. These can include quadrilateral space (through which the axillary nerve and posterior humeral circumflex artery pass) syndrome, suprascapular nerve entrapment, thoracic outlet syndrome, and axillary artery occlusion.[46]

In 1986, Redler et al.[47] reported on a case of quadrilateral space syndrome in a pitcher who complained of an ache in his shoulder with pitching, and the development of weakness and a dead feeling in his shoulder. His EMG and nerve conduction studies were normal, but an arteriogram with the arm in full abduction and external rotation showed occlusion of the posterior humeral circumflex artery. The patient altered his pitching style to a three-quarter overhand throw with relief of his symptoms.

The suprascapular nerve innervates both the supraspinatus and infraspinatus muscles. The nerve can be damaged secondary to stretching from the high speed of pitching, or form compression at several sites, most commonly in the suprascapular notch by the superior transverse scapular ligament.[48] An interesting anatomic and clinical study revealed that otherwise asymptomatic baseball pitchers may exhibit slowing of suprascapular nerve conduction as the season progresses, and that denervation of the infraspinatus and supraspinatus muscles is not always due to entrapment of the nerve at the suprascapular or spinoglenoid notches.[49]

Once diagnosed, this condition should be treated conservatively with emphasis on strengthening the involved muscles and the scapular stabilizers. The authors have observed this pathology on several occasions in professional-level baseball pitchers, and on isokinetic evaluation their strength parameters were within an acceptable range. They were able to pitch without difficulty or evidence of altered body mechanics.

Acromioclavicular Joint

Injuries to the acromioclavicular (AC) joint are often the result of acute trauma from a fall. The type III AC joint sprain, or complete rupture, presents a diagnostic dilemma to the treating physician. The clavicle functions as a strut, which helps to stabilize and position the scapula in order to optimize glenohumeral function. When the strut is damaged, as is seen in a type III AC joint sprain, secondary impingement of the rotator cuff from the acromion can occur from the forward subluxation of the scapula. Although most athletes do well with conservative treatment of type III dislocations,[50] surgical repair of the ligaments should be considered in the throwing athlete.

Degenerative changes in the AC joint are seen more commonly in the baseball thrower. Any athlete who lifts weights or engages in repeated throwing is at risk to develop degenerative changes including bony spurs, osteolysis, and osteophyte formation. Conservative treatment including anti-inflammatory medication, modification of physical activity, and steroid injection into the joint is tried initially. If this fails, arthroscopic debridement of the joint is indicated.

Scapulothoracic Injuries

A stable scapulothoracic articulation is critical in the throwing athlete.[19,38] Bony exostosis under the scapulae can cause a snapping scapula syndrome, and the bony lesion is often seen on radiographs. Sisto and Jobe[51] described resistant scapulothoracic bursitis in four professional pitchers without any bony lesions. All four pitchers returned to professional baseball after excision of the bursa.

Skeletally Immature Thrower

Similar conditions affect the mature and young throwing shoulder, but the presence of epiphyseal plates creates the opportunity for specific predictable injuries.[52] Adams first described Little League shoulder as an osteochondrosis of the proximal humeral epiphysis.[53] This is associated with proximal shoulder pain, and radiographs will show a widening of the proximal humeral epiphysis with demineralization.[52] This heals with rest; however, subsequent proximal growth alterations have been reported.[54] Other reported shoulder injuries in the skeletally immature include a spiral oblique fracture of the proximal humerus and epiphyseal avulsion fractures of the coracoid process with concomitant AC separation.[13]

REHABILITATION

Most injuries to the thrower's shoulder occur from the repetitive microtraumatic stresses that result in adaptive physiologic changes. These adaptive physiologic changes can directly or indirectly lead to shoulder injuries. Most shoulder injuries in the throwing athlete can be treated successfully with appropriate rehabilitation and rarely require surgical intervention. The throwing athlete should perform specific exercises to strengthen the various muscles of the shoulder complex and of the entire body. These exercises should isolate the muscles of the glenohumeral and scapulothoracic joints, and additionally, the muscles of the trunk, arm, and legs. Throwing requires adequate strength of the trunk and legs and the upper extremity. Several investigators[8,55,56] have reported that the trunk and legs are responsible for 52 to 60 percent of the kinetic energy necessary to throw a baseball.

The role of the shoulder musculature is to provide dynamic stability to the glenohumeral joint. The dynamic stabilizers of the glenohumeral joint are the rotator cuff muscles, deltoid, and the long head of the biceps brachii.[57,58] These muscles are responsible for maintaining the congruency of the humeral head within the glenoid fossa. This is accomplished by different mechanisms, including the concept of the muscles acting in force couples. Two of the most important force couples at the glenohumeral joint are the subscapularis counterbalanced by the infraspinatus–teres minor and the anterior deltoid balanced by the contraction of the teres minor–infraspinatus muscles.[57,59] These muscles act together as a force couple to compress the humeral head within the glenoid fossa and thus minimize humeral head displacement.

Additionally, in order to maintain the congruency of the humeral head within the fossa, the musculotendinous units of the rotator cuff blend into the glenohumeral capsule to act as a static and dynamic stabilizing structure. By actively contracting the rotator cuff muscles, the glenohumeral ligamentous capsule tightens and assists in stabilizing the humeral head. This is referred to as dynamic ligament tension.[60,61] Lastly, the muscles provide dynamic stability through proprioceptive input from the capsular neurologic receptors.

The scapulothoracic musculature plays an important role in stabilizing the scapula and maintaining normal scapulohumeral motion. The scapular movement is also controlled through several force couples. The rhomboids and middle trapezius with the serratus anterior form one force couple, while the upper trapezius and lower fibers of the serratus anterior form another force couple. The scapular muscles play a vital role in normal shoulder function,

and the exercise program should include exercises for these muscles.

The musculature of the shoulder complex can be divided into two groups: stabilizing muscles and prime muscles. The prime movers or acceleration muscles for the throwing athlete are the latissimus dorsi, pectoralis major, teres major, and triceps brachii muscles. The rotator cuff muscles, the deltoid, and the biceps brachii muscles are considered the stabilizing muscles. The exercise program for the throwing athlete must address this consideration and should reproduce the muscular action found in throwing.

The last consideration in the rehabilitation program for the throwing athlete is the concept of periodization. This concept refers to the sequences and progression of year-round sport and weight training in the athlete. The baseball player has four specific and different training seasons during the calendar year: competitive season, active rest phase, off-season training, and spring training (Fig. 24-4 and Table 24-1). The exercise prescription for the "healthy" thrower should reflect this concept of periodization. Thus the type of exercises, number of exercise repetitions, and intensity of exercise should vary during the calendar year.

Competitive Season

During the competitive season the uninjured baseball player is involved with conditioning exercises to maintain the strength, power, endurance, and flexibility that were achieved during the off season.

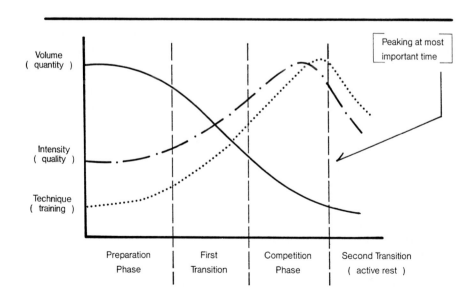

FIGURE 24-4
Matveyev's model of periodization. Volume—the amount of work performed (sets, reps, etc.). Intensity—the quality of effort. Technique—the activity or skill. (*Adapted from Matveyev L: Fundamentals of Sports Training. Moscow, Progress Pub. 1977, pp 167–169.*)

TABLE 24-1
Concept of Periodization in Baseball

Period	Goals	Conditioning Exercises	Skill Training Activities
In-season training "competitive season" (6 months)	• To maintain strength, power, endurance to prevent arm injuries. Prevent the breakdown of tissue	• Low weight, moderate number of repetitions per exercise, throwers' 10 exercise program • Cardiovascular endurance 20–30 min daily to maintain fitness level–stamina training	• Continued throwing activities to maintain proper throwing mechanics and refinement of pitches • Throwing program is designed to emphasize the players' position • Throwing and batting activities (volume) regulated by players' health status
Postseason training "active rest" (2 months)	• Mental and physical recuperation period • Physical activity, but not baseball-type activities • Allows tissues to heal • Relaxation sports participation	• Light conditioning program. Bicycle, swimming, walking, jogging, aerobics • Conditioning, low intensity, long duration	• No baseball-related drills • Relaxation sports, such as golf, tennis, racketball
Preparation phase "off season" (10–12 weeks)	• Gradually and progressively increase exercise demands—throwing exercises and drills • Begin with light isotonic program, progresses to eccentric and plyometric exercises • Skill training is low to start with and throwing begins halfway through this phase • *Ultimate goal* to be *in condition* for spring training reporting date	• Total body exercise program emphasis on large muscle groups • Moderate weight, moderate repetition number to start; isotonic concentric • Progress program to eccentric program, progress to moderate weight—increase repetitions • Cardiovascular training is emphasized 30 min daily to enhance fitness level • Plyometric training drills initiated 2–3 weeks prior to spring training	• Initially no skill training • 4–5 weeks into program, throwing program is initiated, interval long toss program • Batting practice initiated 4–5 weeks into phase
First transitional phase "spring training" (4–6 weeks)	• Enhance conditioning level and skill training (razor shape) • Initially high-volume conditioning, moderate-level skill training • Then moderate-level conditioning, high-level skill training	• Volume of conditioning drills is high at start of phase and sharply down halfway through • Intensity of training and quality of movements are fine-tuned • Plyometrics early phase then discontinued • Thrower's 10 program	• Skill technique training is emphasized • Throwing and batting activities are emphasized, and these skill activities are fine-tuned

These exercises are performed at a moderate intensity level and are intended to retard soft tissue (musculoskeletal) breakdown due to the repetitive stresses during the competitive season. We recommend that the throwing athlete perform a daily conditioning program of cardiovascular fitness through running, bicycling, or stair climbing machines. Additionally, the athlete should perform a daily flexibility program and strengthening exercises. Also recommended for the throwing athlete is performing the thrower's 10-exercise program with a resisted weight that is comfortable. The actual number of repetitions varies based on the health status of that particular player. An uninjured player may perform 40 to 50 repetitions of each exercise while the injured player performs 20 to 30 repetitions of each exercise.

Active Rest Training Phase

The baseball player's season ends when the last game is completed. At this point the athlete should participate in an active rest type of program. This allows the player to disengage himself from baseball and become involved in a recreational sport that he enjoys that will allow the shoulder's soft tissue to heal and will also maintain a general fitness level. Popular sports for the baseball player are golf, tennis, racketball, or basketball. These sports allow the baseball player the opportunity to mentally and physically recuperate from the long competitive season.

First Transitional Training Phase

Eight to 10 weeks prior to the initiation of formal spring training with a team, the baseball player should begin a strength and conditioning program. The goals of this program are to condition and prepare the body for baseball-specific drills and to reestablish muscular and cardiovascular endurance. Exercises including the bench press, shoulder press, biceps curls, triceps extensions, wrist curls, rowing, leg exercises, and a jogging program are instituted to condition the large muscle groups. After several weeks of training the thrower may start specific exercises for the isolated muscles of the shoulder complex. The exercises frequently employed are the "thrower's 10" program (see below). After 6 to 8 weeks of weight training, we initiate plyometric strength training (see below) for the throwing athlete. During this phase the emphasis is placed on a conditioning program that employs high exercise volume and low-skill training volume, such as throwing and hitting. Throwing and hitting activities should be initiated in the middle of this phase. The primary focus of this phase is to condition the athlete to play baseball.

Second Transitional Training Phase

This phase is often referred to as "spring training." The baseball players report to their team and are placed on a conditioning program that the organization's strength and conditioning coach has devel-oped. The early spring training program utilizes a high concentration of conditioning drills such as running, calisthenics, and resisted exercises to strengthen the shoulder musculature. During this time skill training is also performed such as hitting, throwing, catching, and batting. As the spring training period proceeds, the emphasis shifts from conditioning to skill training and by mid to late spring season the baseball player skill level should be near its peak. Additionally, by the end of spring training the player's physical condition should be at a high level, so that he is ready to begin the competitive season.

Thrower's 10

The exercises listed in Table 24-2 have been developed through the collective work of various investigators, who have documented the muscular activity through electromyographic studies during various exercise movements.[23,62–68] These 10 exercises emphasize the muscles primarily responsible for the throwing movement, and utilize various types of muscular contractions. This exercise program is referred to as the "thrower's 10" program. The thrower's 10 program can be used year-round as the core exercises for the shoulder muscles. Additional drills such as plyometrics and eccentrics can be added to enhance the program. The number of repetitions should be altered based on the time of year and the health status of the player. Isokinetic testing of the throwing athlete may assist the clinician in objectively documenting muscular performance of the throwing shoulder. Wilk and Andrews[69] have docu-

TABLE 24-2
Thrower's 10 Program

Scaption (supraspinatus)
ER/IR (90° abduction), with exercise tubing
D2 PNF extension UE, tubing
Shoulder horizontal abduction (prone)
Push-ups
Press-ups
Shoulder abductions to 90°
Elbow flexion and extension
Wrist extension and flexion
Forearm supination and pronation
Daily:
    Stretching of the lower and upper extremity musculature
    Abdominal sit-ups
    Wall squat throws
    Runnning and jogging for endurance

TABLE 24-3
Plyometric Exercise Drills

Warm-up drills:
  Trunk rotation
  Trunk side bends
  Trunk wood chops
  IR/ER exercise tubing 90/90
  Push-ups
Throwing movements:
  Two-hand overhead soccer throw
  Two-hand chest pass
  One-hand step and pass
  Side-to-side throw
  Baseball throwing
  Exercise tubing diagonal plyometrics
  Exercise tubing bicep plyometrics
  Plyometric push-ups
Trunk movements:
  Resisted situps
  Plyometric sit-ups
  Back extensions

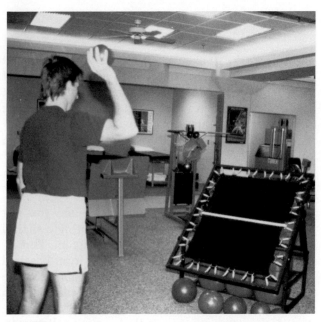

FIGURE 24-5
Stretch-shortening drill (plyometrics) throwing a 2-lb Plyoball (functional integrated technique, Watsonville, CA) into a rebound system plyoback simulating a baseball throw.

mented muscular performance values in healthy professional throwing athletes.

Plyometrics

Plyometric exercise drills are movements that utilize an eccentric muscular contraction prior to a concentric muscular contraction. A weighted ball is used to perform specific stretch-shortening-type exercises for the upper-extremity musculature. Selected plyometric exercises are listed in Table 24-3. This type of muscle contraction activates the stretch-shortening cycle of muscle and employs a stretch prior to the shortening contraction. The prestretch stimulates the muscle spindle and thus facilitates the concentric contraction.[70–72] This type of exercise program has resulted in accelerated strengthening response of various particular muscles. This type of exercise drill is also sport-specific, and all sport movements utilize this stretch-shortening cycle. In baseball, throwing involves a cocking phase prior to the acceleration phase. The cocking phase places a prestretch on the adductor–internal rotator muscles that serves to facilitate the concentric shortening acceleration contractions. The plyometric drill employs a three-phase contraction (see Table 24-4). Figures 24-5 and 24-6 illustrate some examples of plyometric drills for the throwing athlete. Wilk et al. have developed a plyometric training program for

the throwing athlete.[73] Plyometric exercises for the thrower have resulted in an accelerated muscular performance response and serve as an excellent transitional exercise drill prior to resuming activities. This accelerated muscular performance response is probably due to neural adaptions and enhanced neu-

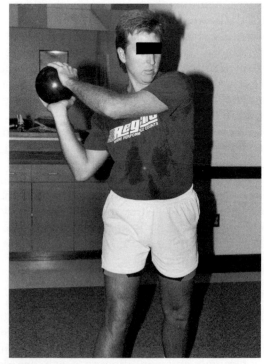

FIGURE 24-6
Two-hand side throw using a 4-lb Plyoball.

TABLE 24-4
Plyometric Exercise, Three Phases

I. Setting phase—eccentric loading (prestretch)
II. Amortization phase (time between phases I and III)
III. Resultant phase—facilitated concentric contraction (response)

336

TABLE 24-5
Interval Throwing Program, Phase I

45-min phase
Step 1:
  A. Warm-up throwing
  B. 45 min (25 throws)
  C. Rest 15 min
  D. Warm-up throwing
  E. 45 min (25 throws)
Step 2:
  A. Warm-up throwing
  B. 45 min (25 throws)
  C. Rest 10 min
  D. Warm-up throwing
  E. 45 min (25 throws)
  F. Rest 10 min
  G. Warm-up throwing
  H. 45 min (25 throws)

60-min phase
Step 3:
  A. Warm-up throwing
  B. 60 min (25 throws)
  C. Rest 15 min
  D. Warm-up throwing
  E. 60 min (25 throws)
Step 4:
  A. Warm-up throwing
  B. 60 min (25 throws)
  C. Rest 10 min
  D. Warm-up throwing
  E. 60 min (25 throws)
  F. Rest 10 min
  G. Warm-up throwing
  H. 60 min (25 throws)

90-min phase
Step 5:
  A. Warm-up throwing
  B. 90 min (25 throws)
  C. Rest 15 min
  D. Warm-up throwing
  E. 90 min (25 throws)
Step 6:
  A. Warm-up throwing
  B. 90 min (25 throws)
  C. Rest 10 min
  D. Warm-up throwing
  E. 90 min (25 throws)
  F. Rest 10 min
  G. Warm-up throwing
  H. 90 min (25 throws)

120-min phase
Step 7:
  A. Warm-up throwing
  B. 120 min (25 throws)
  C. Rest 15 min
  D. Warm-up throwing
  E. 120 min (25 throws)

Step 8:
  A. Warm-up throwing
  B. 120 min (25 throws)
  C. Rest 10 min
  D. Warm-up throwing
  E. 120 min (25 throws)
  F. Rest 10 min
  G. Warm-up throwing
  H. 120 min (25 throws)

150-min phase
Step 9:
  A. Warm-up throwing
  B. 150 min (25 throws)
  C. Rest 15 min
  D. Warm-up throwing
  F. 150 min (25 throws)
Step 10:
  A. Warm-up throwing
  B. 150 min (25 throws)
  C. Rest 10 min
  D. Warm-up throwing
  E. 150 min (25 throws)
  F. Rest 10 min
  G. Warm-up throwing
  H. 150 min (25 throws)

180-min phase
Step 11:
  A. Warm-up throwing
  B. 180 min (25 throws)
  C. Rest 15 min
  D. Warm-up throwing
  E. 180 min (25 throws)
Step 12:
  A. Warm-up throwing
  B. 180 min (25 throws)
  C. Rest 10 min
  D. Warm-up throwing
  E. 180 min (25 throws)
  F. Rest 10 min
  G. Warm-up throwing
  H. 180 min (25 throws)
Step 13:
  A. Warm-up throwing
  B. 180 min (25 throws)
  C. Rest 10 min
  D. Warm-up throwing
  E. 180 min (25 throws)
  F. Rest 10 min
  G. Warm-up throwing
  H. 180 min (25 throws)

Step 14:
Begin throwing off the mound or return to respective position

romuscular control and coordination, not to morphologic muscular changes.[73,74]

Exercise Summary

The exercise program for the throwing athlete should reflect the concepts of periodization and the desired goals and deficiencies of the thrower.[74] Throwing is a full-body activity, where the legs and trunk play a significant role. The exercise program should include exercises for the entire arm, shoulder, scapular region, trunk, and legs. The exercise program for the throwing athlete should change as the calendar year changes. As discussed, the baseball player participates in four different training periods during the calendar year. The exercises and drills should reflect the goals of that particular season. The thrower's 10 exercise program is a core exercise program for the thrower. Plyometric exercise drills appear to enhance strength and dynamic stability for the thrower. Once the injured throwing athlete is allowed to begin throwing, an interval throwing program should be employed (Tables 24-5 and 24-6). The interval throwing program progressively and sequentially increases the distance, number of throws, and types of throws. An internal throwing program facilitates the successful return to throwing. Successful rehabilitation following a shoulder injury in the thrower focuses on the ability of the thrower to dynamically stabilize the glenohumeral joint while performing the throwing activity.

SUMMARY

The act of throwing or pitching a baseball requires coordination of the entire body, including the lower extremities, back, and upper torso. Although common injuries in baseball usually involve the upper extremity, it is important to remember that an alteration in body mechanics can result in a change in pitching style and possible injury. The most critical preventive measure a baseball player can take in order to maintain a healthy throwing shoulder is to participate in a regular shoulder-strengthening program. It is when the muscles about the shoulder become imbalanced, secondary to either injury or relative weakness, that instability and injury can occur. By understanding the pitching motion and the relative contribution of the muscles, the treating physi-

TABLE 24-6

Interval Throwing Program, Phase II

Stage One: Fastball Only
Step 1: Interval throwing
  15 throws off mound 50%
Step 2: Interval throwing
  30 throws off mound 50%
Step 3: Interval throwing
  45 throws off mound 50%
Step 4: Interval throwing
  60 throws off mound 50%
Step 5: Interval throwing
  30 throws off mound 75%
Step 6: 30 throws off mound 75%
  45 throws off mound 50%
Step 7: 45 throws off mound 75%
  15 throws off mound 50%
Step 8: 60 throws off mound 75%
Stage Two: Fastball Only
Step 9: 45 throws off mound 75%
  15 throws in batting practice
Step 10: 45 throws off mound 75%
  30 throws in batting practice
Step 11: 45 throws off mound 75%
  45 throws in batting practice
Stage Three
Step 12: 30 throws off mound 75% warm-up
  15 throws off mound 50% breaking balls
  45–60 throws in batting practice (fastball only)
Step 13: 30 throws off mound 75%
  30 breaking balls 75%
  30 throws in batting practice
Step 14: 30 throws off mound 75%
  60–90 throws in batting practice 25% breaking balls
Step 15: Simulated game: Progressing by 15 throws
  per workout

Use interval throwing to 120-min phase as warm-up.

All throwing off the mound should be done in presence of pitching coach to stress proper throwing mechanics.

Use speed gun to aid in effort control.

cian has a framework on which to build knowledge regarding physical findings and diagnosis of shoulder injuries in baseball players. Once a diagnosis is made, a successful treatment plan may be developed for the player, including both conservative and, at times, surgical means.

REFERENCES

1. Barnes DA, Tullos HS: An analysis of 100 symptomatic baseball players. *Am J Sports Med* 6:2, 1987.

2. Albright JA, Jokl P, Shaw R, Albright JP: Clinical study of baseball pitchers: Correlation of injury to the throwing arm with method of delivery. *Am J Sports Med* 6:1, 1987.

3. Gainor BJ, Piothrowski G, Puhl J, et al: The throw: Biomechanics and acute injury. *Am J Sports Med* 8:2, 1980.

4. Pappas AM, Zawacki RM, Sullivan TJ: Biomechanics of baseball pitching: A preliminary report. *Am J Sports Med* 13:4, 1985.

5. Gowan ID, Jobe FW, Tibone JE, et al: A comparative electromyographic analysis of the shoulder during pitching: Professional versus amateur pitchers. *Am J Sports Med* 15:6, 1987.

6. Jobe FW, Moynes DR, Tibone JE, Perry J: An EMG analysis of the shoulder in pitching: A second report. *Am J Sports Med* 12:3, 1984.

7. Jobe FW, Tibone JE, Perry J, Moynes D: An EMG analysis of the shoulder in throwing and pitching: A preliminary report. *Am J Sports Med* 11:1, 1983.

8. Fleisig GS, Dillman CJ, Andrews JR: Proper mechanics for baseball pitching. *Clin Sports Med* 1:151–170, 1989.

9. Feltner ME: Three-dimensional interactions in a two-segment kinetic chain. Part II: Application to the throwing arm in baseball pitching. *Int J Sports Biomech* 5:420–450, 1989.

10. Feltner ME, Dapena J: Dynamics of the shoulder and elbow joints of the throwing arm during a baseball pitch. *Int J Sports Biomech* 2:235–259, 1986.

11. Jones HH, Priest JD, Hayes WC, et al: Humeral hypertrophy in response to exercise. *J Bone Joint Surg (Am)* 59-A:2, 1977.

12. Warren RF: Instability of shoulder in throwing sports. *Instr Course Lect,* 34, 1985.

13. Ireland ML, Andrews JR: Shoulder and elbow injuries in the young athlete. *Clin Sports Med* 7:3, 1988.

14. Andrews JR, Carson WG: The arthroscopic treatment of glenoid labrum tears in the throwing athlete. *Orthop Trans* 8:44, 1984.

15. Andrews JR, Carson WG, McLeod WD: Glenoid labrum tears related to the long head of the biceps. *Am J Sports Med* 13:6, 1985.

16. Andrews JR, Kupferman SP, Dillman CJ: Labral tears in throwing and racquet sports. *Clin Sports Med* 14:4, 1991.

17. Glasgow SG, Bruce RA, Yacobucci GN, Torg JS: Arthroscopic resection of glenoid labral tears in the athlete: A report of 29 cases. *Arthroscopy* 8(1):48–54, 1992.

18. Howell SM, Galinat BJ, Renzi AJ, Marone PJ: Normal and abnormal mechanics of the glenohumeral joint in the horizontal plan. *J Bone Joint Surg (Am)* 70-A:2, 1988.

19. Kibler WB: Role of the scapula in the overhead throwing motion. *Contemp Orthop* 22:5, 1991.

20. Brown LP, Niehues SL, Harrah A, et al: Upper extremity range of motion and isokinetic strength of the internal and external shoulder rotators in major league baseball players. *Am J Sports Med* 16:6, 1988.

21. Andrews JR, Gillogly S: Physical examination of the shoulder in throwing athletes, in Zarins B, Andrews JR, Carson WG (eds): *Injuries to the Throwing Arm.* Philadelphia, Saunders, 1985.

22. Andrews JR, Byrd JWT, Kupferman SP, Angelo RL: The profile view of the acromion. *Clin Orthop* 263:142–146, 1991.

23. Pappas AM, Zawacki RM, McCarthy CF: Rehabilitation of the pitching shoulder. *Am J Sports Med* 13:4, 1985.

24. Wilk KE, Arrigo CA, Andrews JR: Isokinetic testing of the shoulder abductors and adductors: Windowed vs nonwindowed data collection. *J Orthop Sports Phys Ther* 15:2, 1992.

25. Andrews JR, Carson WG, Ortego K: Arthroscopy of the shoulder: Technique and normal anatomy. *Am J Sports Med* 12:1, 1984.

26. Andrews JR, Gidumal RH: Shoulder arthroscopy in the throwing athlete: Perspectives and Prognosis. *Clin Sports Med* 6:3, 1987.

27. Scarpinato DF, Bramhall JP, Andrews JR: Arthroscopic management of the throwing athlete's shoulder: Indications, techniques, and results. *Clin Sports Med* 10:4, 1991.

28. King JW, Brelsford HJ, Tullos HS: Analysis of the pitching arm of the professional baseball player. *Clin Orthop* 67, 1969.

29. Neviaser RJ: Lesions of the biceps and tendinitis of the shoulder. *Orthop Clin North Am* 11:2, 1980.

30. Norwood LA, Del Pizzo W, Jobe FW, Kerlan RK: Anterior shoulder pain in baseball pitchers. *Am J Sports Med* 6:3, 1978.

31. Jackson DW: Chronic rotator cuff impingement in the throwing athlete. *Am Sports Med* 4:6, 1976.

32. Neer CS: Impingement lesions. *Clin Orthop* 173, 1983.

33. Penny JN, Welsh RP: Shoulder impingement syndromes in athletes and their surgical management. *Am J Sports Med* 9:1, 1981.

34. Tibone JE: Shoulder impingement syndrome in athletes treated with an anterior acromioplasty. *Clin Orthop* 188:134, 1985.

35. Tibone JE, Elrod B, Jobe FW, et al: Surgical treatment of tears of the rotator cuff in athletes. *J Bone Joint Surg (Am)* 68-A:6, 1986.

36. Rowe CR, Zarins B: Recurrent transient subluxation of the shoulder. *J Bone Joint Surg (Am)* 63-A:6, 1981.

37. Garth WP, Allman FL, Armstrong WS: Occult anterior subluxations of the shoulder in non-contact sports. *Am J Sports Med* 15:6, 1987.

38. Glousman R, Jobe F, Tibone J, et al: Dynamic electromyographic analysis of the throwing shoulder with glenohumeral instability. *J Bone Joint Surg (Am)* 70-A:2, 1988.

39. Jobe FW, Kvitne RS: Shoulder pain in the overhand or throwing athlete: The relationship of anterior instability and rotator cuff impingement. *Orthop Rev* 18:9, 1989.

40. Andrews JR, Broussard TS, Carson WG: Arthroscopy of the shoulder in the management of partial tears of the rotator cuff: A preliminary report. *Arthroscopy* 1:117, 1985.

41. Bigliani LU, Morrison DSD, April EW: The morphology of the acromion and its relationship to rotator cuff tears. *Orthop Trans* 10:216, 1986.

42. Jobe FW, Giangarra CE, Kvitne RS, Glousman RE: Anterior capsulolabral reconstruction of the shoulder in athletes in overhand sports. *Am J Sports Med* 19:5, 1991.

43. Caspari RB: Arthroscopic reconstruction for anterior shoulder instability, in Paulos LE, Tibone JE (eds): *Operative Techniques in Shoulder Surgery*. Maryland, Aspen Publishers, 1991.

44. Bennett GE: Shoulder and elbow lesions of the professional baseball pitcher. *JAMA* 117:7, 1941.

45. Lombardo SJ, Jobe FW, Kerlan RK, et al: Posterior shoulder lesions in throwing athletes. *Am J Sports Med* 5:3, 1977.

46. Tullos HS, Erwin WD, Woods GW, et al: Unusual lesions of the pitching arm. *Clin Orthop* 88, 1972.

47. Redler MR, Ruland LJ, McCue FC: Quadrilateral space syndrome in a throwing athlete. *Am J Sports Med* 14:6, 1986.

48. Post M, Mayer J: Suprascapular nerve entrapment. *Clin Orthop* 223, 1987.

49. Ringel SP, Treihaft M, Carry M, et al: Suprascapular neuropathy in pitchers. *Am J Sports Med* 18:1, 1990.

50. Tibone J, Sellers R, Tonino P: Strength testing after third-degree acromioclavicular dislocations. *Am J Sports Med* 20:3, 1992.

51. Sisto DJ, Jobe FW: The operative treatment of scapulothoracic bursitis in professional pitchers. *Am J Sports Med* 14:3, 1986.

52. Tullos HS, King JW: Lesions of the pitching arm in adolescents. *JAMA* 220:2, 1972.

53. Adams JE: Little league shoulder osteochondrosis of the proximal humeral epiphysis in boy baseball pitchers. *Calif Med Assoc J* 105:22, 1966.

54. Cahill BR, Tullos HS, Fain RH: Little league shoulder. *J Sports Med* 2:150, 1974.

55. Atwater AE: Biomechanics of overarm throwing movements and of throwing injuries. *Exerc Sport Sci Rev* 7:43, 1979.

56. Toyoshima S, Hoshikawa T, Miyashita M, et al: Contribution of the body parts to throwing performance, in Nelson RC, Morehouse CA (eds): *Biomechanics IV*. Baltimore, University Park Press, 1974, pp 169–174.

57. Inman VT, Saunders M, Abbott LC: Observations on the function of the shoulder joints. *J Bone Joint Surg (Am)* 26:1–30, 1944.

58. Saha AK: Dynamic stability of the glenohumeral joint. *Acta Orthop Scand* 42:491–497, 1971.

59. Basmajian JV, DeLuca CJ: *Muscles Alive*, 5th ed. Baltimore, Williams & Wilkins, 1985, pp 270–271.

60. Cleland J: On the action of muscles passing over more than one joint. *J Anat Physiol* 1:85–93, 1865.

61. Matsen FA, Harryman DT, Sidler JA: Mechanics of glenohumeral instability. *Clin Sports Med* 10(4):783–786, 1991.

62. Blackburn TA: Off season program for the throwing arm, in Zarins B, Andrews JR, Carson WG (eds): *Injuries to the Throwing Arm*. Philadelphia, Saunders, 1985, pp 277–291.

63. Blackburn TA, McLeod WD, White B: EMG analysis of posterior rotator cuff exercises. *Athl Training* 25:40–45, 1990.

64. Jobe FW, Bradley JP: Rotator cuff injuries in baseball: Prevention and rehabilitation. *Am J Sports Med* 6(6):378–387, 1980.

65. Jobe FW, Moynes DR: Delineation of diagnostic criteria and a rehabilitation program for rotator cuff injuries. *Am J Sports Med* 10:6, 1982.

66. Moseley JB, Jobe FW, Pink M, et al: EMG analysis of the scapular muscles during a shoulder rehabilitation program. *Am J Sports Med* 20(2):128–134, 1992.

67. Townsend H, Jobe FW, Pink M, et al: Electromyographic analysis of the glenohumeral muscles during a baseball rehabilitation program. *Am J Sports Med* 19(3):264–272, 1991.

68. Wilk KE, Arrigo C, Courson R, et al: *Preventive and Rehabilitative Exercises for the Shoulder and Elbow*, 3d ed. Birmingham, American Sports Medicine Institute, 1991.

69. Wilk KE, Andrews JR, Arrigo CA, et al: The strength characteristics of internal and external rotator muscles in professional baseball pitchers. *Am J Sports Med* 21(1):61–66, 1993.

70. Bosco C, Koni P: Potentiation of the mechanical behavior of the human skeletal muscle through pre-stretching. *Acta Physiol Scand* 106:467–472, 1979.

71. Cavagna G, Disman B, Margari R: Positive work done by a previously stretched muscle. *J Appl Physiol* 24(1):21–32, 1968.

72. Chu D: Plyometric exercise. *Natl Strength Conditioning Assoc J* 6(1):56–62, 1984.

73. Wilk KE, Voight ML, Keirns MA, et al: Stretch shortening drills for the upper extremities: Theory and clinical application. *J Orthop Sports Phys Ther* 17(5):225, 1993.

74. Wilk KE, Arrigo CA: Current concepts in the rehabilitation of the athletic shoulder. *J Orthop Sports Phys Ther* 18(1):365, 1993.

CHAPTER 25

Football

Charles Jackson
Bubba Tyer

INTRODUCTION

Football is a violent sport. It is also a very popular sport; 1,500,000 players participate in junior and senior high school football, 75,000 in college football, and 2100 in professional football, with the numbers likely to increase in the years to come. Initially it was a unique American sport like baseball and basketball, with popularity spreading to include teams in Canada and recently in Europe. The violence of the sport combined with its popularity, especially at lower levels where training and skill levels are marginal, make injury a significant problem. Though injuries about the shoulder girdle may not be as threatening as head and neck or knee injuries, they are the most common injuries in football if we include shoulder "burner syndrome."

In no other sport is there quite the contact with compression, distraction, and torque forces about the shoulder defying protective equipment. Whether a player has the ball or not, brute force not so subtly combined with graceful engagement or evasion meet at or about the shoulder. Half the players on the field are dedicated to throwing the player with the ball to the ground in as hurtful a manner as possible with the express desire of disengaging the ball from the hands of that player. The other half of the players risk the structural integrity of their bodies to keep their opponents away from the ball. In most instances furious contact of individuals is quickly followed by plunging, smashing contact with the turf, and then the pile-on of several other players ensues. This violent contact is what impresses everyone the most standing on the sideline of a professional football game for the first time, more than the noise or the size or the speed or the grace of the huge neuromuscular geniuses at work. After years of professional football sideline work on a team that has gone to the Super Bowl four times in the past 10 years, winning three, we still see violence as the most striking feature of the game whether it is a sold-out superdome with deafening noise or an emotionally supercharged Super Bowl.

The shoulder is the primary weapon of those going after the ball while it is the focal point of pro-

tection for those blocking. Blocking and tackling are the mainstay fundamentals even at the professional level where 300-lb stupendous athletes move about on quick feet getting their shoulders in proper position as nimbly as if in a fencing duel. The great coaches tell us that in tackling it all comes together where the head meets the shoulder and in blocking the shoulders are the pivotal points of protection. In fact, since rules changes initiated for the 1976 football season that eliminated the head as a primary and initial contact area for blocking and tackling, the shoulder has been mandated the primary weapon. It should be no surprise to us then that the shoulder girdle, if we include all categories of shoulder "stingers" or "burners" and clavicle injuries, is the most common part of the body injured in football. It may be surprising to those who follow football in the newspaper because the shoulder girdle injuries do not get a lot of press, unless it is a rotator cuff injury of the quarterback or the like. Understanding these injuries in the football setting and how they affect the player and game has given us knowledge in several ways, and we hope to share this in this chapter.

The basic pathology and treatment modalities of shoulder injuries are well covered by anatomic site and type of injury in other chapters of this book, so our discussion concentrates on those aspects of football injuries that differ or stand out substantially from basic pathology and treatment. Because we are emphasizing the differing aspects and because the role of the physician and medical team highlight these differences the best in professional football, we will concentrate on professional football, the aspect of football we know best, and point out pearls that may apply to all of medicine. There are many surprises evaluating and treating such highly motivated neuromuscular geniuses in a sport as high-profile and violent as professional football.

GENERAL COMMENTS

One of the most surprising conclusions of the sports medicine fellows who work with us in the professional football team clinic is that sports injuries about the shoulder seen in everyday office practice are very similar to the injuries treated at the professional football team clinic, provided the age of the individuals compared is the same. Perhaps this is due to the effective role that protective football equipment plays, with shoulder pads second only to the modern helmet as a protective device and modifier of potential injury. We say perhaps because shoulder pads give protection for direct blows and do not protect from torque forces that produce rotator cuff strains and protect poorly from compression of the shoulder girdle on the thorax in line with the clavicle, producing compression and shear at the clavicular articulations. More likely, the power and conditioning work of the player gives sufficient internal stabilization of the scapula on the thorax and with the humerus that more serious injury is avoided. When we compare this similarity of shoulder pathology with the striking difference seen with neck complaints, the importance of this factor of internal protection is even more appreciated.

As surprising as observations about pathology are, the surprises encountered in treatment and rehabilitation are almost beyond surprise to the point of amazement, certainly not explained by rehabilitation techniques in professional football. The only real difference in technique is the speed that progressive motion, coordination, power, and endurance work have advanced. The rationale and speculation about how fast to move derived from years of experience can help us extrapolate from the amazing neuromuscular genius to the more average weekend warrior we see in the office.

Regardless of how similar the pathology is or how different the response to injury the role of the physician changes dramatically depending on the level of play, with the greatest difference coming between the college and professional levels. Even the most simple question, "can he play," coming from the coach has entirely different implications depending on the level. The primary purpose of the physician of promoting optimal long-term health to the whole individual does not change, of course, but interpretation of health to the whole individual does; and who is responsible for determining the risk of not playing to the health of the whole individual, particularly when the neuromuscular gifts are the only extraordinary gifts far beyond the average intellect that may make up a whole person?

It might be more accurate to say age of the individual player rather than the level of play changes the physician's role, for specialization in career and viable options for "making a living" become more and more focused on neuromuscular skills with age

until age restricts ability to perform. With advancing age even in the professional ranks viable options for anything approaching such career success become more and more remote. Risk of not playing becomes more significant in many ways from simple loss of visibility to loss of confidence of the coach, from opportunity afforded younger competing teammates to trades made necessary for more gifted athletes, not to mention the loss of motor skills and experience, as well as psychological loss of teammate respect, which according to many experts is the single most driving force for early return to play. The maturity of the player and his experience with his own injuries and the injuries he has experienced with teammates and friends give the physician greater confidence that the proper course is to allow greater freedom of a player to determine his own destiny, evaluating his own risk-benefit ratio. Rather than determining what is too much risk for a player and being a gatekeeper, the physician's role becomes more a teacher and adviser. The proper diagnosis with degree of structural damage to the anatomic part of cervical root or plexus, acromioclavicular joint, rotator cuff, glenohumeral capsule or labrum, and bone is crucial and the sole responsibility of physician. The player needs to know how bad this hurt shoulder is and why; what could make it worse and what options there are to maximize healing and rehabilitation and the risks of those options; and who is best to carry out the options and what the parameters are for making decisions about play. The final decision to play is made by the player and coach. The risk of playing before full recovery is shared by the player, physician, and team so that all three have input. The team physician in professional football does not have full veto power; though he may be most knowledgeable about the pathology he cannot be the most knowledgeable about position-specific risk on the field, and certainly not all the risks of not playing that the player faces.

The ability to perform continues to weigh more heavily with level of play and age in the risk-benefit balance. In spite of serious risk on the field, especially when a career is in jeopardy on the bench but not necessarily, a professional player may play if he can perform. If you ask the group of 28 orthopedic surgeons responsible for our National Football League teams how they treat a player with a specific injury, they almost always ask you what position does the player play. This is not because the pathology is likely to be different at different positions, nor is it because the relatively predictable stresses are so different at different positions. The critical fact is that ability to perform is affected so differently by similar pathology at different positions. If the injured part is not crucial to optimal performance, decisions about treatment and the timing of treatment become very personal. Rather than being a source of frustration that the physician is not allowed to treat every injury as an isolated event to the optimal benefit of that part, treating the whole patient and helping him keep his long-term career and life in perspective is a source of individual joy and perhaps significant learning for all of medicine. We learn a lot more when we are challenged to treat out of the routine path of conventional wisdom. We must instruct and educate about the short- and long-term risks to the anatomic structural integrity of the parts while we listen and learn as the whole individual puts into the balance his risk of playing and risk of not playing. We can do our best to add weight on one side but we cannot throw the balance out in the professional ranks. Adding weight at the patient's balance rather than taking the role of balance keeper perhaps is something we should attempt more in our office practices.

THE COMBINE EXPERIENCE

We see very few shoulder "burner syndrome" cases in everyday office practice, yet it is the most common injury seen on the sidelines in college football and one of the most common injuries seen in professional football. There are no published statistical analyses to substantiate this, though other observers have recorded this and we have done a survey at the National Football League Combine after looking at our own records. The combine gives us a unique opportunity to review all injuries to the elite college players about to enter the National Football League and examine every player with appropriate laboratory, x-ray, CT scan, and MRI procedures done all at one time. The purpose of the combine is to protect college players from multiple trips to the 28 cities with professional teams and bring team representatives to one city where all draft potential players are gathered to demonstrate their fitness and ability to play professional football. Teams with large scouting organizations that scour the country and every small college must allow their findings to be exposed at the combine, and thus the player may benefit from this exposure in addition to the convenience.

For the past several years the combine has been in Indianapolis, IN, at the Hoosier Dome in February prior to the National Football League draft in April. Physical exams by internists, orthopedists, and trainers are done prior to the physical workouts and time trials observed by the scouts, coaches, and managers. Players are seen initially on the day of their arrival by the sports medicine fellows working with the NFL physicians and histories are taken with appropriate x-rays ordered, and CT scans or MRI tests if they are considered necessary. These tests are done that first day so the players will be available for the complete physicals done the next day at each of six stations with four or five team NFL physicians at each station. The players are cleared for workout and trials the third day. When the players are drafted, all the test results become part of the player's record at his team. Prior to the draft every team has a copy of all medical reports to assist in their choice of players.

This year 340 elite college players were examined at Indianapolis in February in preparation for the 1993 National Football League draft on Apr. 25, 1993. In addition to the history taken by the sports medicine fellows, all records from the training rooms of the colleges were available. Information about any practice missed over a 4-year collegiate career or any game missed was available. The treatment given was supplemented with operative reports and résumés with prognosis given by treating physicians along with all diagnostic tests.

There were 45 players of the 340 with no history of a significant injury during high school or college play. These players had never missed a day of practice or portion of a game in their career. Of the remaining 295 players, 232 players described injuries to their shoulders. By far the most common injury was a shoulder or arm "burner" with 107 players describing such injuries in 109 shoulders; 40 described at least two injuries in one shoulder. Though a shoulder or arm "burner" that the players describe as shoulder injuries may be referred from the neck and cervical nerve roots, they are all classified here as shoulder injuries for none showed root pathology at the disk or foramen level. Injuries with pain in the shoulder associated with disk or foramen pathology were classified as neck injuries. In no case was there transient quadriparesis or were cord symptoms described and the two players who experienced burners in both shoulders never did so simultaneously or even in the same season. Such injuries would be classified as cervical injuries just as other symptoms from proven disk and spinal canal abnormalities. All players with any neurologic symptoms had a complete cervical spine series, and those with specific or persistent neurologic symptoms had an MRI. The next most common injury described was shoulder separation, admitted by 55 players, an incidence slightly greater than half that of burners, with

37 players describing shoulder dislocation. Twenty players had rotator cuff strains or shoulder bruises and 11 players had fractures about the shoulder with 9 clavicle and 2 scapula fractures.

These numbers of injuries are less than injuries in the overall college population of football players. Speer states that the incidence of burners may approach 50 percent among collegiate varsity players over a 4-year career with 5 to 10 percent being serious enough to have prolonged neurologic deficit. The one in three incidence seen at the combine may be explained by the extraordinary ability and strength of the elite candidates of their hesitancy to report transient symptoms with the typical intense burning pain present for a few moments with little residual.

Certainly the scrutiny with which these players are screened and the records available from their care make it unlikely that any significant number of injuries are overlooked, and they may have less injury. The numerous career-threatening injuries that these elite athletes have sustained debunk the misconception that football weeds out players with injury and that the lucky injury-free players are able to advance perhaps even to the professional ranks, while those unlucky ones with serious injury at high school that we had thought should go on cannot advance. It seems that nearly half of the players that we see in the combine have overcome an injury that would sidetrack most any other individual. The desire, drive, and ability to play become more obvious a factor the higher the level of play until at the professional level it may even dwarf injury.

DIAGNOSIS

Advances made in the past 10 years have changed our understanding and approach to injuries of the shoulder, and nowhere is this better appreciated than in the professional team clinic. The MRI and arthroscopy have become mainstays to supplement a good history, physical exam, diagnostic x-rays, and almost routine procedures such as diagnostic therapeutic blocks and arthrograms, allowing us in many instances to achieve what Burkhart describes as "an anatomic specific diagnosis." Our goal is to localize the structures that failed in injury and also assess the degree of failure that may be superimposed on a preexisting incomplete, morbid, or potentially incompetent structure so that our treatment may be specific to both injury and potential reinjury. No matter how we classify the injury for a diagnosis, whether we include or imply etiology, patterns of

pathologic anatomy, patterns of pathologic response, or patterns of necessary treatment, the anatomic specificity made possible by "seeing" the structures with MRI and arthroscopy has helped us not only for treatment but for understanding the function of anatomic structures. Only when we know exactly what structure was injured and how badly, and we know exactly what that structure does and how well it does now after injury compared with preinjury status and ideal status can we call our treatment truly rational. Of course, we have a long way to go on all counts even in the private, quiet solitude of the examination room or the technological majesty of the MRI suite or the excited bustle of the operating room, all far from the field of play. What we have learned in the past 10 years, though, is helping us on the field to become more rational and hopefully better therefore in our treatment.

Symptomatic conditions that we did not know such as the SLAP variation of the labral tear, as well as labral tears in general other than the Bankart, associated or not with ligament stretch or damage and subtle patterns of instability, have become part of our index of suspicion in individuals who bench press several hundred pounds routinely and are involved in such diverse and violent extremes of trauma. In addition to these "new" or recently recognized types of lesions, new understanding of the types and implications of humeral instability, new understanding of the types of trauma, and new understanding of the risk factors go right along with these modern diagnoses. Tried and true diagnoses such as rotator cuff insufficiency can be more precisely evaluated to the point that we are better able to make conclusions based on the degree of damage and the implications for function, repair, and healing and are called on to do so routinely. All this is challenging, exciting, and difficult enough in the clinic. On the field of play clinical evaluation is a different matter, for diagnosis requires a certain definitiveness without the added data that modern technology provides. It also serves a different purpose for those few hours during and after a game. This difference is most dramatic in a professional football game but has implications for all of us, particularly when our access to technology and all the expense it entails may depend on our "sideline diagnosis" not just of football injuries, or even all sports injuries for that matter, but all of our practice. How we make that "sideline diagnosis," or rather what evidence we have to support it, and how we document it must become more important when unlimited physician access to technologic advances for our patient becomes restrained so another "more needy" patient may have access, with the gatekeeper being a bureaucrat who may not be able to spell "glenolabral."

A real-life example gives the best illustration of this difference. A player who has just signed a contract for over $1 million a year, not to mention his nearly $3 million signing bonus, has just come to you on the sideline during the opening minutes of the game with his left arm hanging to his side after a routine-looking tackle at the sideline in front of you: "Something is moving in my shoulder." Mentioning the money is not done to point out the "worth" of this individual but simply to point out that several groups of individuals including scouts with thousands of hours of observation and miles of recording tape, coaches in countless hours of heated discussion, team managers and owners in their collective wisdom have decided that over $1 million will be given in 16 weekly payments to this individual, one payment for each of the 16 games to be played this season, whether he plays or not. Someone is losing more than $75,000 worth of talent for every game he does not play, including the current game that has just begun. A diagnosis is needed immediately, and so much for the subtle and finer points of diagnosis. We are back to history and physical exam with the option of x-ray in the stadium locker using an x-ray machine bought in 1950.

History in our humble opinion is the mainstay of diagnosis, and by that we mean the patient's own account in the vast majority of cases. There are others on the sideline right by us that saw the injury just as we did from perhaps a slightly different perspective. There are two videotapes taken by our team photographers at right angles to each other, one from the end zone and the other from the 50-yard line. There are several other TV cameras recording the injury from various directions, with slow motion and reverse angle. Certainly we have the mechanism of injury on film. While everyone watching TV is viewing the injury over and over from different angles ad nauseam, we are talking to the patient. We have not seen the TV and our videotapes will not be ready for viewing for 6 h. We are not concerned because our diagnosis has never been changed or modified by this additional videotape information.

We listen to the patient because the pathologic condition is always a subjective phenomenon. Pathologic lesions are always objective. The correlation may seem poor and the patient's perception of the anatomic lesion may be entirely wrong, as is so common about the shoulder with referred pain, but the correlation begins with the patient, and in the end when all is said and done any success ends with the patient. The success in rational therapy is entirely related to just how tight the correlation between subjective complaint and objective pathology is, for if a physician corrects an obvious pathologic lesion seen on MRI or with the arthroscope and the patient continues with symptoms and disability the correlation and the success have to be inadequate. Concentrating on the subjective phenomenon is so important, particularly about the shoulder; this initial focus is clearly overlooked and underestimated by nearly all of us as we move from our observation with all the overwhelming technology and precision back to the patient, rather than beginning with the patient and his observations.

Our acutely injured patient is of course anxious about this rude unhinging of his shoulder but has surprisingly little pain until you reach up under his shoulder pad. There is a golden opportunity before reaching and touching, then, to get a history as he begins to calm down from the game battle. If he can tell what position his arm was in when he was hit, what he was trying to do, what he did do, where his arm went, where his head was in relation to his shoulder, what happened with his head and neck, and most important when he felt pain, numbness, or unhinging, you have some of the most useful information you will ever get. In our case at hand the player states that his shoulder gave a "crunch" feeling when he fell on the apex of his shoulder with his arm across his chest and under him. Something felt loose, though he could use his shoulder with pain only when he shrugged his shoulder under the shoulder pad.

If the player's account of the injury is the most important initial focal point, palpation of the neck and shoulder girdle in systematic order going from painless to painful areas with anatomic-specific finger pressure is next most important. Having the patient localize the maximum tender area with one of his fingers at one point on the skin is the initial step at correlating his subjective symptoms with your initial impression of tissue damage or anatomic structural failure. Every spinous process of the neck should be palpated, and if the patient denies neck pain the exam begins there. The spinous processes of C2 and C7 can be easily palpated while C3 through C6 are deep in the ligamentum nuchae and require gentle resistance of your left hand against the forehead with the neck in relaxed posterior translation and gentle flexion while palpating with the right hand deep in the ligamentum. The sternoclavicular and the acromioclavicular joints with the clavicle need special attention, for the bruised rotator cuff will obfuscate injury transmitted proximally from the point of contact at the apex of the shoulder.

Sternoclavicular injury is the most easily missed, though it is so obvious with palpation. It may be hard to convince the player that his neck spasm with torticollis is related to the sternoclavicular injury. Palpation of the scapular spine and scapular fossae may give useful information concerning supraspinatus and infraspinatus compression vs. traction diagnosis of cuff injuries and brachial plexus injuries giving weakness. Anterior neck triangle and infraclavicular palpation is most important with shoulder burners distinguishing root from plexus compression or traction. Palpation of the acromion from the coracoid along the acromioclavicular arch to the deltoid and entire humeral head in all manner of rotation, abduction, and flexion is imperative to localize impact points made more diffuse with shoulder pads.

The golden opportunity for examination of stability immediately after injury is not so golden with the shoulder as it is with the knee, particularly dealing with football injuries. First of all, the two most likely sites of injury when the shoulder is mentioned behind the acromioclavicular joint are the neck and glenohumeral joint, which do not have palpable or demonstrable endpoints of stability like the knee and for that matter nearly all other joints. Second, there is almost always an element of impingement at the shoulder with football injuries due to the violent ground contact with the upper extremity breaking the fall in different positions and the humerus coming in contact with the acromion and coracoacromial arch. This impingement factor obfuscates motion, stability, and power examination from the moment of impact. Apprehension tests, sulcus test, and SLAP grinding test will be painful even with local anesthetic infiltration. Finally, you have to get the shoulder pads off with or without the stretch jersey, putting the shoulder through dramatic contortion unless the jersey is cut and the strings removed. Perhaps this is why we put our hand up under the shoulder pad to feel the acromioclavicular joint, clavicle, and proximal humerus to determine whether the $50 jersey needs cutting as opposed to the $2500 minute (which is $1.2 million per 16 games with 30 min playing time per game). In our case at hand the player had gross laxity both superiorly and posteriorly of the distal clavicle at the acromion without crepitus and with little pain along the clavicle or greater tuberosity.

He will accept your initial impression and outline for definitive diagnosis and treatment with glazed eyes, and then ask: "How long, doc?" Then comes the coach, "How bad, doc?" just before or after the call from the press box for national television:

"Will he go back in?" The coach and team will understand some delay in definitive clinical decisions with discussion of treatment options, second opinions, and player agent input. The press is a different matter. They will not let you off the hook if you profess to know anything, particularly the future, and insist on a "ballpark figure until return" (for the headlines). These extraordinary pressures for immediate answers emphasize once again the importance of history and physical exam regardless of the dramatic difference of clinical setting.

The "burner syndrome" deserves special attention because it is so common in football. A player experiences burning pain in his shoulder and upper arm with contact, followed by paresthesia, dysesthesia, and/or heaviness or numbness. He can usually tell you if his head was compressed to the involved shoulder or away but cannot give an anatomic description of radicular or peripheral nerve involvement. It is never associated with bilateral shoulder pain or lower-extremity symptoms without grave danger of spinal cord contusion or transient cervical quadriparesis, and should not be called a "burner" if these symptoms are described. Weakness passes before paresthesia which may go away, with the dysesthesia leaving more localized paresthesia but still not over a specific radicular or peripheral pattern. If the head comes toward the involved shoulder and the paresthesia is localized to a root pattern, usually C5, there is a possibility that a root is injured as high as the foramen in the neck. This is fairly rare. Even more rare is a localized radiculopathy due to disk herniation, which is the garden variety of radiculopathy seen in the office. Most rare in football is the root avulsion from the cord seen in high-velocity traction injuries; this should be considered if the head moves away from the shoulder and dysesthesia persists for prolonged periods. These lesions of the root at a level of the foramen and above are neck injuries and not properly classified as shoulder "burners." Though neck x-ray, foramen tomograms, CT scans, EMG, and neurologic consultation with MRI and CT myelogram may need to be done to rule out neck and disk pathology, history and a good motor, sensory, and reflex exam generally rule out either specific root or cord involvement pointing to the neck.

The "burner syndrome" is frequently associated with other structural injuries about the shoulder, especially subtle subluxation and impingement. In football there is always some element of impaction or compression force of the humeral head and cuff into the glenoid and under the acromion during the game and almost on every play. The torque forces centered at the humeral head that strain the rotator cuff and sprain the capsular are almost as frequent as the arms are held up against downward blows of opponents. Translation and shear of the humeral head across the glenoid, which plays such a prominent role in throwing injuries, is infrequent except in the quarterback throws and defensive hand or pull-down tackles with the associated distraction and deceleration forces.

Fortunately acute traumatic impingement pain clears relatively quickly so that more definitive physical tests for stability, especially with the added relief of subacromial local anesthetic injection, which may not work well immediately, may be performed. Definitive diagnostic tests can then be done with CT for bony glenoid lesions, MRI and gadolinium MRI for labral and cuff lesions, and ultimately exam under general anesthesia with arthroscopy.

Careful listening to the patient has proved to be more beneficial than videotapes taken by our team as well as the numerous projections taken from the national media. Understanding the mechanism of injury and the relative forces may be highlighted but does not demonstrate and certainly does not delineate the sensation of the player that his "collarbone is loose" or that his "shoulder is loose." This is particularly true for injuries or pains about the shoulder where subtle subluxations of the humerus, or even clavicle for that matter, are so difficult to pin down within the impingement syndrome. We have come a long way in our precision of evaluation of structural change, better able to "see" the anatomy as never before with modern technology. We still have to correlate this anatomic variation with the subjective symptoms and dysfunction of the player patient. It is better to begin with what the patient says because we will always, no matter how far technology goes with PET scans and the like, end with the subjective relief and restored function of the patient.

TREATMENT

Treatment begins before diagnosis when we are responsible for the safety and care of players on a team. Safety begins with prevention and care begins with honesty and caring and the resultant trust in the medical team. Treatment of an injury requires knowledge and experience and is put into effect with good communication and teaching skills, tempered with common sense, especially about where the communication goes. It is our job to know what injuries are common and what potential dangers for the shoulder are specific to our sport and perhaps to

our specific team with variations occurring in the particular age group, the size and skill level of play, and even the position played on that team. We must move beyond simple explanation to teach enough that the player can "see" his problem and understand the treatment. We must check on his understanding and compliance and motivate with tact and hope. Most of us in our office practices do not have the luxury of demonstrating care before injury as the training staff and physicians of a team do, but we can have our office medical team including those who answer the phone demonstrate care before the injury is evaluated, for there is contact with the patient at our offices, even with us, before injury is discussed. As we say so often, we have a long way to go before we can even begin to fulfill the responsibility so reasonably, or unreasonably, expected of us.

It is important to begin to define where our level of expertise begins and ends and honestly portray this to the entire team. Even though teams below the professional level do not have powerful owners concerned about their players in a special way, nor are there agents concerned about their clients in a special way, there are parents concerned about their children (and their sporting careers), making the triangle of responsibility between player, doctor, and team more of a web of interconnecting links. All the linking people need to know what is going on. All these linking people are who we mean when we say the whole team needs to know honestly where we have special expertise and where we are flying by the seat of our pants. The player and his advocates need to make difficult choices with considerable risk and they need to know what other noted and experienced physicians say and do, not just what we know and what we have been trying recently. Portraying the limits of our knowledge, what diagnostic tests and/or consultations are available and appropriate to increase that knowledge, and just how much more information we need to treat the problem rationally is as important as our natural inclination to promote our considerable and even vast experience treating similar problems in the past.

Prevention of shoulder injuries in football begins with education to maintain proper mechanics and point out potential dangers, a strengthening program to internally support structures, and proper equipment to give external support. The tremendous ballistic overload of tissues in football makes it difficult to defend tissues without internal and external support. Preventing overload to vital structures such as the neck requires special rules and changes in the technique of tackling avoiding "spearing," with the helmet striking first. There are no such rules for the shoulder, with its well-recognized shoulder pad supposedly able to stand up to the extra load placed upon it. The shoulder pad does not protect for the two most common injuries of the shoulder, the "burner syndrome" and acromioclavicular separation. The best current prevention device for the "burner" is a good collar that prevents lateral neck bend as well as hyperextension, helping reduce traction across the brachial plexus with the shoulder compressed and the head tilted away. Unfortunately, any restricting device that would truly limit brachial plexus distraction, such as a shoulder pad helmet band, also limits rotation and is unacceptable for play. A firmer body support from the sternoclavicular area to the acromioclavicular joint under the shoulder pad relieving pressure at the apex or deltoid area would help with AC separation, and we use this protection after injury. The classic AC doughnut with the hole centered at the AC joint under the shoulder pad may accentuate pressure at the shoulder apex distal to the joint, which should be unloaded.

Great emphasis has been placed on conditioning and strengthening work to prevent injury, and rightly so, particularly at the shoulder and neck, concentrating on the rotator cuff and scapular stabilizers for the shoulder. The problem is that all players are increasing their power and strength and stamina, making for more forceful contact for longer periods of the game. Also, individuals are beginning at an early age to strengthen their arms, deltoids, and pectoral muscles, making it even more important to teach about the rotator cuff and scapular stabilizers. Learning to isolate the rotator cuff from the deltoid and getting the greater tuberosity of the humerus under the acromioclavicular arch without supraspinatus impingement is more important before rotator cuff injury and impingement syndrome.

The shoulder has peculiar biomechanics made for motion as the most mobile joint in the body with force couple action. Understanding treatment requires some understanding of the anatomy and biomechanics. Use of models is very helpful with treatment of all parts of the body but is particularly helpful, if not indispensable, with the shoulder. The anatomy of the shoulder cannot be understood looking at an atlas, and the patient cannot understand the treatment without this conceptual visualization. Taking the time for teaching is never better rewarded than at the shoulder.

Compliance may be the most significant factor in any rehabilitation program, but there are few programs outside professional sports where supervision is so intense and so well managed that the limits of compliance become obvious quickly. When recovery stalls in our office practice, the variables that we immediately look to concern patient understanding and compliance of the prescribed treatment protocol. On the other hand, when recovery in a professional athlete stalls, proper diagnosis and what we can do to further clarify a possible incomplete or wrong diagnosis get immediate attention. This is best illustrated in treatment of impingement syndrome in professional football players. With impingement syndrome in quarterbacks atraumatic subluxation must be suspected because of the very nature of the forces involved in throwing a heavy football with inconsistent decelerating actions due to impending possible loss of limb or life just before, during, or at the completion of the throw. Inflammation about the rotator cuff and even traumatic subacromial bursal inflammation may result from superimposed routine game compression trauma. With clinical findings including careful history, physical exam, and x-rays limited to recent-onset impingement and dramatic response to a diagnostic therapeutic block of the subacromial bursa with 10 mL of a local anesthetic and short-acting cortisone preparation, treatment might reasonably include a short period of rest and rapid progression to throwing first for accuracy, followed by progressive distance, then increased speed, frequency, and ultimately duration. No isolated time frame for rotator cuff strengthening followed by endurance work with isokinetic machines would be prescribed with routine parascapular and rotator cuff strengthening continued on an ongoing basis. If progression is stalled, we go back immediately to diagnosis and need not wonder about the compliance of the patient or the management of the rehabilitation program. The coracoacromial arch including the acromioclavicular joint, rotator cuff, and labral capsular complex are studied with our most sensitive tools including MRI, exam under general anesthesia, and arthroscopy.

The program is a symptomatic step program, unless there is third-degree damage with loss of stability, with the period of rest dependent on pain and degree of diagnosed structural loss. Ice and nonsteroidal anti-inflammatory medicines are used routinely, with systemic cortisone used for radicular or nerve root neuropraxia almost exclusively, and local cortisone injection used judiciously. No contact or practice is allowed initially, with direct supervision of all motion and strengthening activities by the training staff. When coordination is perfected, the exercise is continued as an endurance exercise, with the next level of exercise done for coordination. Power exercises are done manually, isometrically, and isokinetically with viscoelastic endurance work. When full motion and adequate power and endurance are achieved, the player is released to the weight training coach to work with free weights and nautilus until his preinjury power is achieved. He is allowed back to practice when his coordination field skills have returned to normal.

Special mention is given to treating the shoulder "burner syndrome" so common in football and relatively rare otherwise. As we stated previously, ruling out neck injury including spinal cord injury with or without stenosis and disk herniation is our primary responsibility, for the condition is relatively self-limited if no neck structure is involved. If pain, dysesthesias, and paresthesias resolve within minutes and no neck symptoms or neurologic findings are present, the professional player is allowed back in the game. At the college level with the first "burner" and no previous neck x-rays with the same negative history and physical, the player may be allowed back after neck x-rays with flexion extension views and foramen outlet views. The high school player usually is not allowed back in the game even with transient pain for it is just too difficult to rule out significant neck injury in young immature and poorly conditioned necks.

A localized pattern of persistent neuropraxia with deltoid hypesthesia for C5, thumb and index for C6, and long and index for C7, without reflex or motor changes, can come from foramen compression of the nerve root, as well as plexus traction or even disk herniation, which is so commonly seen in the office but rarely in football. History will help delineate foramen compression with the head going toward the involved shoulder at contact, and physical exam may help with the foramen compression test's being positive. If there is any indication of possible bony injury at the foramen, multiple-angle foramen views with the player's body rotated slightly less and more than 45° with 15° cranial inclination followed by 45° caudad pillar views can be done on the field x-ray machine to be followed by foramen tomograms, which do better than CT or MRI.

If there are motor and reflex changes consistent with a specific root, plexus injury is less likely substantiated by EMG pattern pointing to one root. MRI would be needed to rule out a herniated disk and CT myelogram to evaluate any cord compression may be necessary. The vast majority of "burners" have no persistent symptoms or neurologic findings and if they do they are not radicular in nature but upper plexus in distribution. An EMG may confirm this and if positive may remain so for many years.

Except for root injuries at the foramen, treatment is symptomatic with activity modification, with the ultimate decision being when the player can return to play. The longer the neurologic symptoms and findings persist the more an extensive workup for neck pathology is indicated. If the workup is negative, gradual increase in activity to contact is allowed with full discussion of the probability of persistent findings.

Root injuries at the foramen that are a compression injury are the one type of "burner" that we treat with cortisone after herniated disk is ruled out. Methylprednisolone (Medrol), 8 mg, is given in dose pack form of 22 tablets with two packs used, six the first and second days, five the third and fourth, etc. One dose pack is never enough in our hands. Cortisone is followed by nonsteroidal anti-inflammatory medication, and activity is gradually increased. Neck motion to maintain mobility and reduce spasm and neck strengthening exercises are prescribed immediately as tolerated. A firm cowboy collar is used that encircles the neck, preventing excessive lateral bend and hyperextension as the helmet abuts it at the back and sides.

PROGNOSIS

Nowhere in medicine does the need for prognosis reach such intensity with such immediacy as in professional sports, especially professional football. National television has a direct phone line to the game sideline with two operators in action on the sideline, one to stay in contact with the medical team and the other in contact with the television booth upstairs. If the game is nationally televised, a much publicized prognosis is going to be made the minute the doctor finishes a preliminary history and physical exam and releases findings to the hovering sideline television operators. The initial publicized prognosis comes not from the doctor but from a commentator in the television booth. Because the diagnosis always comes from the doctor, the press is most anxious to substantiate the broadcast prognosis from the doctor. That means that in the give and take with the press immediately following the game, the doctor, who wants to reveal nothing, is in a defensive position with the press, which has a preconceived idea from someone in the press box, usually an exceptionally experienced and gifted retired coach who has suffered the injury himself; not only that, his two best friends and teammates as well as countless star players that played under his direction had the same injury. After the usual remarks from the doctor about how we will have to reevaluate and do further tests, and simply wait and see how recovery progresses, the press sets in, "Can he possibly by any miracle be back by the Dallas game?" The usual reiteration of the doctor about how we will have to wait and see is followed by the press statement that, "Doctor this is much worse than we have been told if there is a possibility that he cannot be back by the Dallas game." The possibilities at both ends of the spectrum are then attacked with feeding frenzy, the earliest he could be back with supernatural intervention, and the latest if every possibility of complication were to occur. Being able to make a diagnosis as anatomically correct as possible and laying out a plan of action for definitive diagnosis with the need for such diagnosis and the treatment plan dependent on that diagnosis is over the head of the press. Telling them we don't know how many anatomic fibers have been stretched or broken and hopefully the player will do so well we will not have to pursue that definition further satisfies them. These press questions are not unlike the questions we have been receiving from cost control health insurance administrators. Our patient may not be reimbursed for an MRI without answers. Our fear is we will not be answering as intelligent an audience as the press.

CONCLUSION

Treating injuries of the shoulder in a sport as violent and high-profile as professional football offers many challenges. Though the player's history frequently elucidates the mechanism of injury better than videotape recording of the injury, television viewers, commentators, and the press have reviewed the films with slow motion and reverse angle playback ad nauseam before the physician does. The physical exam is obscured by blunt compression and contusion of the acromioclavicular joint, trapezius and deltoid musculature, and subacromial structures regardless of the primary structural damage that may be in the neck, clavicular and subclavicular structures, or the glenohumeral joint itself. Though diagnosis and treatment have been dramatically improved in recent years with the advances in diagnostic radiology and arthroscopy, these modalities are far from the field and do not give immediate answers. These very specific challenges are not unlike the general challenge we will face in the near future with strict cost containment and rationing policies forced by government intervention.

In spite of the dramatic advances highlighted throughout this book, nothing will replace a good history and physical exam on the field. As our knowledge about basic pathologic changes improves with better techniques for evaluating anatomic disruption, our index of suspicion will lead us to a better physical exam and even new physical examination tests. Our accuracy on the field is vital whether we choose to disclose our tentative diagnosis or not, or to issue a prognosis with any authority.

What we can all learn from football whether we stand on the sidelines or not is the discipline of an excellent history and physical exam that can form a tentative diagnosis and game plan of definitive clinical evaluation with treatment and a prognosis that can stand up to publicity, which in professional football includes the national press. We are going to be called upon to defend our requests for expensive testing procedures on a national scale in the not too distant future. The publicity may not come from the national press but from national health agencies and insurance companies. We may be forced to publicize by way of form or physician insurance interrogation, or even nurse insurance interrogation, hopefully never government bureaucrat interrogation, our tentative diagnosis with definitive diagnostic and treatment plan.

BIBLIOGRAPHY

Anderson TE, Clolek J: Specific rehabilitation programs for the throwing athlete. *Instr Course Lect* 38:487–491, 1989.

Bateman JE: The diagnosis and treatment of ruptures of the rotator cuff. *Surg Clin North Am* 43:1523, 1963.

Bergfeld JA, Hershman E, Wilbourne A: Brachial plexus injuries in sports: a five year followup. *Orthop Trans* 12:743–744, 1988.

Bigliani LU, D'Alessandro DF, Duralde XA, et al: Anterior acromioplasty for subacromial impingement in patients younger than 40 years of age. *Clin Orthop* (246):111–116, September 1989.

Bigliani LU, Nichoslon GP, Flatow EL: Arthroscopic resection of the distal clavicle. *Orthop Clin North Am* 24(1):133–143, January 1993.

Bjorkenheim JM, Paavolainen P, Ahovuo J, et al: Subacromial impingement decompressed with anterior acromioplasty. *Clin Orthop* (252):150–155, March 1990.

Blasier RB, Burkus JK: Management of posterior fracture-dislocations of the shoulder. *Clin Orthop* (232):197–204, July 1988.

Blasier RB, Bruckner JD, Janda OH: The Bankart repair illustrated in cross-section. Some anatomical considerations. *Am J Sports Med* 17(5):630–637, September–October, 1989.

Bryan WJ, Schauder K, Tullos HS: The axillary nerve and its relationship to common sports medicine shoulder procedures. *Am J Sports Med* 14(2):113–116, March–April, 1986.

Burkhart SS: Arthroscopic debridement and decompression for selected rotator cuff tears: Clinical results, pathomechanics, and patient selection based on biomechanical parameters. *Orthop Clin North Am* 24(1):111–125, January 1993.

Canale ST, Cantler ED, Sisk TD, et al: A chronicle of injuries of an American intercollegiate football team. *Am J Sports Med* 9:384–389, 1981.

Cantu RC, Mueller FO: Catastrophic football injuries in the U.S.A.: 1977–1990. *Clin J Sports Med* 2(3):180–185, 1992.

Cofield RH, Irving JF: Evaluation and classification of shoulder instability. With special reference to examination under anesthesia. *Clin Orthop* (223):32–43, October 1987.

Constant CR, Murley AHG: A clinical method of functional assessment of the shoulder. *Clin Orthop* (214):160–164, January 1987.

Curtis AS, Snyder SJ: Injuries to the glenoid labrum, including SLAP lesions. *Orthop Clin North Am* 24(1):45–54, January 1993.

Detrisac DA, Johnson LL: *Arthroscopic Shoulder Anatomy: Pathologic and Surgical Implications.* Thorofare, NJ, Slack, 1986.

Dines DM, Warren RF, Inglis AE, Pavlov H: The coracoid impingement syndrome. *J Bone Joint Surg (Am)* 72-B:314–316, 1990.

Ellenbecker TS, Davies GJ, Rowinski MJ: Concentric versus eccentric isokinetic strengthening of the rotator cuff. Objective data versus functional test. *Am J Sports Med* 16(2):164–169, March–April, 1988.

Esch JC, Baker CL: *Surgical Arthroscopy: The Shoulder and Elbow.* Philadelphia, Lippincott, 1993, pp 99–186.

Esch JC: Arthroscopic subacromial decompression and postoperative management. *Orthop Clin North Am* 24(1):161–172, January 1993.

Ferenz CC: Review of the brachial plexus. Part II: Reconstruction after chronic upper plexus injuries. *Orthopedics* 11(3):491–495, 1988.

Freund RK, Terzis JK, Jordan L, et al: Modified latissimus dorsi and teres major transfer for external rotation deficit of the shoulder. *Orthopedics* 9(4):505–506, April 1986.

Fronek J, Warren RF, Bowen M: Posterior subluxation of the glenohumeral joint. *J Bone Joint Surg (Am)* 71-A(2):205–216, February 1989.

Fu FH: Symposium: Controversies in reconstruction of the unstable shoulder: Mobility versus instability. *Contemp Orthop* 26(3):301–322, March 1993.

Gerber C, Ganz R, Vinh TS: Glenoplasty for recurrent posterior shoulder instability. An anatomic reappraisal. *Clin Orthop* (216):70–79, March 1987.

Gibb TD, Sidles JA, Harryman DT II, et al: The effect of capsular venting on glenohumeral laxity. *Clin Orthop* (268):120–127, July 1991.

Gonzalez D, Lopez RA: Concurrent rotator cuff tear and brachial palsy associated with anterior dislocation of the shoulder: A report of two cases. *J Bone Joint Surg (Am)* 73-A:620–621, April 1991.

Goss TP et al: Works in progress 3. Recurrent symptomatic posterior glenohumeral subluxation. *Orthop Rev* 17(10):1024–1028, October 1988.

Halbrecht JL, Wolf EM: Office arthroscopy of the shoulder: A diagnostic alternative. *Orthop Clin North Am* 24(1):193–200, January 1993.

Hamada K, Fukuda H, Mikasa M, et al: Roentgenographic findings in massive rotator cuff tears. A long-term observation. *Clin Orthop* (254):92–96, May 1990.

Hawkins RJ, Bilco T, Bonutti P: Cervical spine and shoulder pain. *Clin Orthop* (258):142–146, September 1990.

Hawkins RJ, Abrams JS: Impingement syndrome in the absence of rotator cuff tear (stages 1 and 2). *Orthop Clin North Am* 18(3):373–382, July 1987.

Jobe FW: Impingement problems in the athlete. *Instr Course Lect* 38:205–209, 1989.

Jobe FW: Rehabilitation of shoulder joint instabilities. *Orthop Clin North Am* 18(3):473–482, July 1987.

Kilcoyne RF, Reddy PL, Lyons F, et al: Optimal plain film imaging of the shoulder impingement syndrome. *AJR* 153(4):795–797, October 1987.

McCain GA: Role of physical fitness training in the fibrositis/fibromyalgia syndrome. *Am J Med* 81(suppl 3A):73, 1986.

McIntyre LF, Caspari RB: The rationale and technique for arthroscopic reconstruction of anterior shoulder instability using multiple sutures. *Orthop Clin North Am* 24(1):55–58, January 1993.

McShane RB, Leinberry CF, Fenlin TM Jr: Conservative open anterior acromioplasty. *Clin Orthop* (223):137–144, October 1987.

Magnusson SP, Gleim GW, Nicholas JA: Subject variability of shoulder abduction strength testing. *Am J Sports Med* 18(4):349–353, July–August 1988.

Maki NJ: Cineradiographic studies with shoulder instabilities. *Am J Sports Med* 16(4):362–364, July–August 1988.

Michele AA, Eisenberg J: Scapulocostal syndrome. *Arch Phys Med Rehabil* 49:383, 1968.

Neviaser RJ, Neviaser TJ: Observations on impingement. *Clin Orthop* (254):60–63, May 1990.

Newhouse KE, d-Khoury GY, Nepola JV, et al: The shoulder impingement view: A fluoroscopic technique for the detection of subacromial spurs. *AJR* 151(3):539–541, September 1988.

Nirschl RP: Rotator cuff tendonitis: Basic concepts of pathoetiology. *Instr Course Lect* 38:439–445, 1989.

Nobuhara K, Ikeda H: Rotator interval lesion. *Clin Orthop* (223):44–50, October 1987.

Nuber GW, McCarthy WJ, Yad JST, et al: Arterial abnormalities of the shoulder in athletes. *Am J Sports Med* 18(5):514–519, September–October, 1990.

Ogilvie-Harris DJ, Demaziere A, Fitsialos D, Stevens JK: Arthroscopic acromioplasty: The superiority of the posterior portal over the lateral portal. *Orthop Clin North Am* 24(1):153–160, January 1993.

Ogilvie-Harris DJ, Wiley AM, Satttarian J: Failed acromioplasty for impingement syndrome. *J Bone Joint Surg (Am)* 72-B:1070–1072, 1990.

Paulos LE, Franklin JL: Arthroscopic shoulder decompression development and application: A five year experience. *Am J Sports Med* 18(3):235–244, May–June 1990.

Rafii M et al: Computed tomography (CT) arthrography of shoulder instabilities in athletes. *Am J Sports Med* 16(4):352–361, July–August 1988.

Rames RD, Karzel RP: Injuries to the glenoid labrum, including SLAP lesions. *Orthop Clin North Am* 24(1):45–55, January 1993.

Randelli M, Gambrioli PL: Glenohumeral osteometry by computed tomography in normal and unstable shoulders. *Clin Orthop* (208):151–156, July 1986.

Rowe CR: Recurrent transient anterior subluxation of the shoulder. The "dead arm" syndrome. *Clin Orthop* (223):11–19, October 1987.

Silfverskiold JP, Straehley DJ, Jones WW: Roentgenographic evaluation of suspected shoulder dislocation: A prospective study comparing the axillary view and the scapular "Y" view. *Orthopedics* 13(1):63–69, January 1990.

Snyder SJ: Evaluation and treatment of the rotator cuff. *Orthop Clin North Am* 24(1):173–192, January 1993.

Snyder SJ, Karzel RP, Del Pizzo W, et al: SLAP lesions of the shoulder. *Arthroscopy* 6(4):274–279, 1990.

Snyder SJ, Rames RD, Wolbert E: Labral lesions, in McGinty JB (ed): *Operative Arthroscopy*. New York, Raven Press, 1991, pp 491–496.

Speer KP, Bassett FH III: The prolonged burner syndrome. *Am J Sports Med* 18(6):591–594, November–December 1990.

Speer KP, Warren RF, Wall DJ: Update on football injuries. *Mediguide Orthop* 10(4):2–4, 1991.

Stuart MJ, Axevedo AJ, Cofield RH: Anterior acromioplasty for treatment of shoulder impingement syndrome. *Clin Orthop* 260:195–200, November 1990.

Tolin BS, Snyder SJ: Our technique for the arthroscopic Mumford procedure. *Orthop Clin North Am* 24(1):143–152, January 1993.

Torg JS, Pavlov H, Genvario SE: Neuropraxia of the cervical spinal cord with transient quadriplegia. *J Bone Joint Surg (Am)* 68-A:1354–1370, 1986.

Warner JJ, Micheli LT, Arslanian LE, et al: Patterns of flexibility, laxity, and strength in normal shoulders and shoulders with instability and impingement. *Am J Sports Med* 18(4):366–375, July–August, 1990.

Warren RF: Neurologic injuries in football, in Jordan BD, Tsairs P, Warren RF (eds): *Sports Neurology*. Rockville, MD, Aspen, 1989, pp 235–244.

Williamson JB: A simple shoulder restraint. *Injury* 20(6):339–340, November 1989.

Williford HN, East JB, Smith FH: Evaluation of warm-up for improvement in flexibility. *Am J Sports Med* 14(4):316–319, July–August 1986.

CHAPTER 26

The Shoulder in Gymnastics

Frank A. Pettrone
Francis G. O'Connor

INTRODUCTION

Gymnastics is one of the oldest sports known to modern civilization. Galen, recognized as the first sports medicine physician, defined gymnastics as a sport to maximize the quality of physical and mental life.[6] As the sport has grown in popularity, however, gymnastics has evolved from an emphasis on improving general physical and mental health to one that focuses on competition. The changing emphasis toward sport-oriented competition has led to injury profiles particular to the gymnast.

The shoulder represents a unique challenge to the gymnastic team physician. As will be reviewed, the shoulder is subject to considerable sport-imposed demands that can result in a variety of overuse and traumatic injuries. Swinging and strength dominated events result in substantial compressive, rotatory, and tensile stress to the dynamic and static structures of the shoulder. Knowledge of the inherent requirements for shoulder flexibility and strength is critical to the team physician, as improper interventions can inadvertently end a gymnast's career. This chapter briefly reviews the historical evolution of modern gymnastics and discusses in detail the epidemiology, diagnosis, and management of shoulder injuries in the gymnast.

HISTORICAL PERSPECTIVE

Gymnastics originated in ancient Greece. The term "gymnastics" actually derives from the original word, gymnasion, which refers to a place where physical exercise was done in the nude. The original gymnasiums, or gymnasions, were designed as educational centers for both the mind and body. The area was used for physical exercise as well as debate and discussion. Early philosophers, including Plato and Aristotle, utilized gymnasions as institutions to promote a high level of philosophical thought.

Early exercises, including wrestling, boxing, and track and field, all came to be known as gymnastics as they were practiced in a gymnasium. It was later, with the development of the early Olympic Games, that these sports gained their own separate identity. After the Olympics were abandoned in A.D. 393, gymnastics disappeared with other sports. Tumbling, derived from an earlier form of acrobatics, persisted mainly as a theatrical exercise.

Gymnastics reappeared in Europe with the Renaissance. Modern gymnastics, as we know it today, is generally considered a result of the efforts of the German Friedrich Jahn. Jahn developed the first modern gymnasium in 1811, which came to be known as a turnverein. The concept of the turnverein, or place for physical exercise, spread throughout Germany. Jahn additionally developed early apparatus work, including the parallel bars, still rings, and pommel horse. In Sweden, Peter Ling promoted gymnastics with an emphasis on rhythm and fluidity. Emigration to the United States brought both the concept of the gymnasium and that of physical exercise for total body health.

The first gymnasium in the United States was established at the Military Academy at West Point in 1817. Gymnastics continues to be the foundation for physical training for West Point cadets. In 1881, the International Federation of Gymnastics was formed to supervise international competition. With the inclusion of gymnastics in the first modern Olympic Games in 1896, gymnastics secured its place as a recognized amateur sport. In 1936, the National Collegiate Athletic Association began annual competitions, and by the 1960s almost every state high school athletic association adopted the sport for boys and girls. With the television exposure provided such great gymnasts as Mary Lou Retton, Olga Korbut, and Nadia Comaneci, gymnastics has come to enjoy tremendous worldwide popularity.

MODERN GYMNASTICS

Modern gymnastics is a demanding sport that focuses on maximizing individual performance. Gymnasts often require unparalleled determination and discipline in refining techniques and skills needed for the pursuit of perfection. The quest of the optimal performance has created characteristic profiles for male and female participants, with unique ages of initiation, peak level of performance, and retirement.

The female gymnast has greater opportunities for earlier participation, as club gymnastics is predominantly female. The elite female gymnast typically initiates her sport at approximately age 6, reaching maximal competitive levels at age 16 and retiring by age 18. Male gymnasts, on the other hand, initiate the sport at about age 9, reach peak level at age 22, with subsequent retirement around age 24.[6]

Gymnastics competition involves an elaborate and subjective scoring system. The maximum score that can be achieved by the gymnast is a 10.0. Scoring is computed from four separate categories: difficulty (4.00); execution (4.40); combination (1.0); and ROV (risk, originality, and virtuosity) (0.60).[4]

Difficulty requires that the gymnast have a variety of skills of differing levels in a complete routine. Execution refers to the ability of the gymnast to complete the skills with proper technique. The combination requirement is fulfilled when the gymnast executes patterns of skills unique to each event; i.e., still rings requires both strength and swinging movements. ROV was created to help separate elite gymnastic performances. The pursuit of ROV creates the exciting performances we come to enjoy as spectators, as the gymnasts continue to push "the edge." An example of a movement that would earn the gymnast ROV points would be a triple back somersault dismount off the horizontal bar.

Modern men's gymnastics includes six events: floor exercise, pommel horse, vault, parallel bars, still rings, and high bar. Women's gymnastics includes four events: balance beam, floor exercise, uneven parallel bars, and vault.

Men's floor exercise requires that the gymnast execute a variety of skills including strength, flexibility, and balance elements. The most important skills, however, are the tumbling elements. Female floor exercise is different in its dance requirement, with accompanying music and time limitations. The spring floor is a relatively new addition to modern gymnastics. While the new floor helps to decrease impact loading, the rebound gymnasts can create from the floor has resulted in a new level of skills. The spring floor enables gymnasts to complete "tricks" once thought to be impossible, such as a triple back somersault and a full twisting double back salto.

Floor exercise has a high injury profile secondary to the time required to master skills on this event, as well as multiple opportunities for adverse landings. A number of tumbling skills require the shoulders to either absorb landings or facilitate momentum required for superior skills. However, wrist and ankle injuries still predominate in floor exercise. The roundoff back handspring is a basic skill used by the gymnast to develop power for backward tumbling movements. These skills, however, can result in repetitive compressive overload to the subacromial mechanism, predisposing to a variety of overuse and traumatic injuries. Rotator cuff tendinitis is not uncommon, with acute anterior shoulder dislocation resulting from adverse landings.

Pommel horse (Fig. 26-1) is perhaps the most challenging of the men's events. The apparatus measures 64 in long and is approximately 50 in above the floor, with two wooden handles, or pommels. The horse requires continuous swinging movements, with a predominance of double leg circles. Because the gymnast supports his weight continuously, the shoulders are predisposed to overuse microtrauma, generally in the form of rotator cuff tendinitis. The current trend in pommel horse competition has been to perform more skills without using the pommels, resulting in significant wrist dosiflexion overload.

The still rings (Fig. 26-2) is perhaps the most shoulder demanding of the current events in modern gymnastics. The event requires an inordinate amount of strength, as the still rings are an entirely

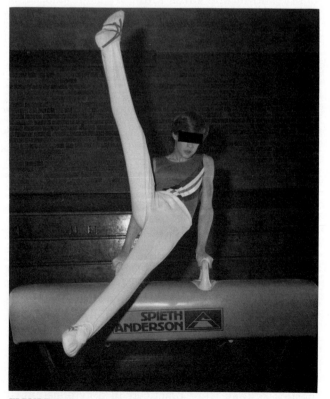

FIGURE 26-1
Pommel horse.

upper extremity apparatus. The gymnast performs on two wooden rings that are suspended from cables 250 cm from the floor. The athlete supports his body as he executes a variety of strength positions and swinging movements. The gymnast tries to keep the rings motionless while performing required elements.

The shoulder is challenged in a variety of ways during still ring competition. Swinging elements require flexibility as the athlete changes his orientation on the rings, by abducting and externally rotating the shoulders in an overhead position. This maneuver clears the surgical head from the acromion, allowing the athlete to move the shoulders from the position of extension to flexion to accommodate giant swings. Gymnasts refer to this action as "dislocating" the shoulders. Accommodating this shoulder movement is the inherent flexibility of the joint capsule. Those athletes with flexible shoulders can accomplish these skills with less strength, and occasionally with less than optimal technique. Accordingly, most gymnasts train shoulder flexibility to facilitate these swinging movements. Shoulder

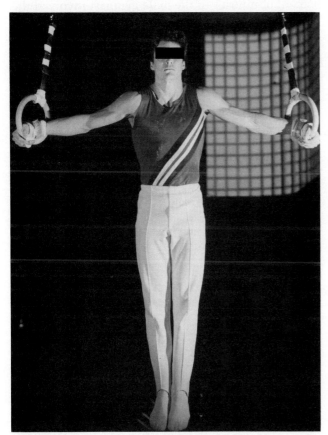

FIGURE 26-2
Still rings.

flexibility, or laxity, is important to the gymnast not only on still rings but also on floor exercise, high bar, parallel bars, and uneven parallel bars. The advantages and disadvantages of shoulder laxity are discussed further in the section on shoulder pathology.

The strength required of still ring competition is extraordinary. Most strength or power elements require "holds" for 2 to 3 s. The forces transmitted to the shoulder are considerable, resulting in a variety of overuse and traumatic injuries to the rotator cuff, acromioclavicular joint, joint capsule, and supporting musculature. As is seen with swinging elements, gymnasts often compromise technique to accomplish skills that they are not prepared to handle. Unfortunately, injury subsequent to improper and abnormal force loading often results. Rehabilitation of shoulder injuries in the gymnast is often plagued by reinjury, because the physician fails to address the role of poor technique and inadequate strength.

The high bar and uneven parallel bars are two of the most exciting events in modern gymnastics. The high bar is a flexible steel bar suspended 250 cm above the floor. The athlete performs swinging or giant movements on the bar, with changes in direction and release-regrasp elements. With the advent of dowel grips, the difficulty of skills performed on the high bar has increased dramatically. It is not uncommon for gymnasts to perform one-arm giant swings, as the dowel grip functions to increase the surface area of the hand on the bar. Grip strength formerly was a limiting factor for the difficulty of tricks performed on the high bar and still rings. With the advent of the use of dowel grips, the limiting factor now is the shoulder. The high bar has a similar injury profile with the still rings, as the event is "swing dominant" and requires "inverted" or "dislocated" giant swings. These swing elements, designated by the inverted giant grip, again require shoulder flexibility to complete successfully.

The women's uneven parallel bars is performed on two wooden bars. One bar is suspended 230 cm above the floor, while the other is 150 cm high. The athlete executes difficult maneuvers while moving from bar to bar. With the advent of the dowel grip, uneven parallel bars has changed dramatically. Female gymnasts now execute male-pattern giant swings on bars that are somewhat farther apart than in prior years. With the complexity of the giant swing comes the shoulder injury pattern that we see in male gymnasts. Once again, the shoulder is subjected to repetitive tensile overload, rotational stress, and the consequences of excessive capsular laxity, particularly in the predisposed female athlete with congenital laxity and weakness.

Vaulting is an event performed by both male and female gymnasts. In men's gymnastics the gymnast vaults over the length of the horse with the use of a springboard. Female gymnasts, on the other hand, vault over the width rather than the length. In most competitions, gymnasts vault twice, with the higher score counting. The absence of shoulder pathology is critical to the gymnast who is attempting to obtain maximum afterflight to accommodate twisting and rotational skills. Gymnasts who have painful shoulders from subacromial pathology are unable to effectively absorb impact and successfully transition quickly from the horse to the afterflight skill, resulting in a poor performance.

The men's parallel bars (Fig. 26-3), like the rings, is an upper extremity event requiring swing and strength elements. The gymnast performs on two wooden bars that are 65 in high. The bars are spaced a variable distance apart, determined generally by the width of the individual gymnast's shoulders. The gymnast has to incorporate release and regrasp movements above and below the bars. Because the weight is suspended for the majority of the routine, the shoulders are subject to both tensile and compressive subacromial overload. A number of overbar release movements, including the back toss and diamadov, require a high degree of flexibility to accommodate shoulder rotation. Gymnasts, once again, train shoulder flexibility to perform these skills. Advantageous flexibility often becomes difficult, if not impossible, to differentiate from detrimental ligamentous laxity.

The balance beam (Fig. 26-4) is an event involving a long wooden beam that is only 4 in wide. The female gymnast uses the full length of the beam to perform acrobatic movements, turns, jumps, and leaps. Recently the difficulty has increased on the balance beam. The beam has transformed from one previously dominated by grace and balance to one that requires power tumbling and strength. The back flip, once thought impossible when popularized by Olga Korbut, is now commonly performed by non-Olympic gymnasts. The shoulder is required for static skills such as the handstand as well as for support during dynamic tumbling movements.

EPIDEMIOLOGY

Despite the enormous popularity of the sport of gymnastics, few epidemiologic studies have been performed to ascertain the frequency and types of injury unique to the gymnast. Those studies that have been done on female gymnasts consistently demonstrate a predominance of injuries in the lower extremity, with ankle sprains representing the most common injury.[3,14] There are fewer reports on men's gymnastics. Weiker, in his review, found that more than 50 percent of injuries in the male gymnast involved the

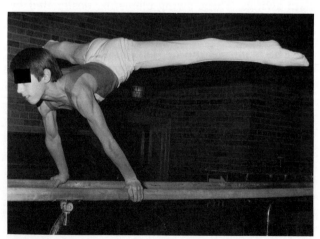

FIGURE 26-3
Men's parallel bars.

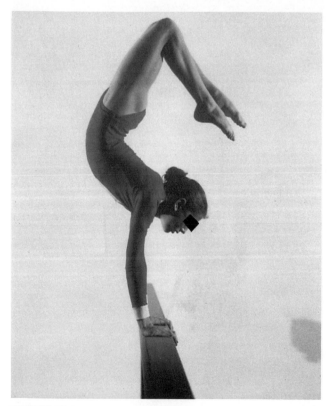

FIGURE 26-4
Balance beam.

upper extremity; however, the study included only 11 injuries.[17]

Pettrone and Ricciardelli performed a prospective analysis of women's club-level gymnastic injuries over a 7-month period.[11] Complete responses from 15 clubs (2550 participants) were obtained. Their results were consistent with prior studies in confirming lower extremity sprains as the most common form of injury and floor exercise as the event with the majority of injuries. They were unable to find any correlation between skill level and type of injury (P + 0.8096) or type of injury and event (P + 0.943). They were, however, able to demonstrate a significant relationship (P < 0.05) between the number of injuries and the duration of the workout. In summary, Pettrone and Ricciardelli were able to define a high-risk gymnast as one who is (1) performing at an advanced competitive level, (2) performing floor or beam exercise, and (3) practicing more than 20 h per week.

Perhaps the most extensive and ongoing review into the epidemiology of gymnastic injuries is performed by the National Collegiate Athletic Association (NCAA).[7] The NCAA developed the NCAA Injury Surveillance System in 1982 to provide current and reliable trends in intercollegiate athletics. The committee's goal is to assess trends in intercollegiate athletics with the intention of reducing injury through suggested changes in rules, protective equipment, and coaching techniques. The committee tracks 16 intercollegiate sports: fall sports (football, men's soccer, women's soccer, field hockey, and women's volleyball); winter sports (men's gymnastics, women's gymnastics, wrestling, ice hockey, men's basketball, and women's basketball); and spring sports (spring football, baseball, softball, men's lacrosse, and women's lacrosse). While club gymnastics is obviously not represented in this report, many useful trends and patterns are identified.

When men's and women's gymnastics are compared against the other 14 intercollegiate sports for injury rates per 1000 athletic exposures, the results are quite enlightening. Women's gymnastics (8.42) trails only spring football (9.64) and wrestling (9.53) in the analysis of combined practices and game injury rates. Men's gymnastics (5.03), on the other hand, ranks twelfth, just behind field hockey. When the committee compared practice injury rates, women's gymnastics (7.22) ranks second only to spring football (9.18); men's gymnastics (4.34) ranked eighth. Men's and women's gymnastics ranks sixth and fourth, respectively, in game injury rates. Football and spring football ranked first and second.

Individual sport data are similar to those reported at the club level. Evaluating women's gymnastics, some interesting trends are noted. When comparing practice vs. game, the injury rate is over three times greater (25.35 vs. 7.95) during competition. A review of the timing of injuries reveals that the majority of injuries occur in the preseason (9.75), with the regular (7.97) and postseason (4.57) following behind. In addition, Division I athletes have consistently greater practice and competition injury rates, when compared with their counterparts in Divisions II and III, these data being consistent with Pettrone's observation that the higher the competitive level of the gymnast, the seemingly higher the risk of injury.

An analysis of individual apparatus injury rates reveals that floor exercise (33.8 percent) and uneven parallel bars (21.1 percent) account for the highest percentage of injuries. Vaulting (13.9 percent), with its inherent trauma during the landing, is surprisingly the least injury-producing of the female events. This observation is probably secondary to the fact that gymnasts spend a relatively small proportion of their time competing and training on this event. A review of the top three body parts injured reveals a striking predominance of lower extremity injuries, with ankle sprain being the most common. From 1985 to 1992, the shoulder has never been identified in the top three body parts injured.

Men's gymnastics has some unique differences from the female injury pattern. In evaluation of injuries throughout division levels, Division III athletes (5.50) had a somewhat higher rate of injury than Division I (4.90) and Division II (5.42), in direct contrast to the women. The timing of injury rates was comparable, with the preseason having the highest rate of injury.

Individual apparatus analysis identifies the floor exercise and high bar as the principal injury-producing events. This is identical with the women, as both these events predispose to landing injuries. Again, like the women, ankle is a consistently predominant injury, occupying 28 percent of the injuries in the 1990–1991 season. The shoulder, in distinction to the women, is almost always identified in the top three body parts injured. The shoulder was the number one (13 percent) body part injured in the 1988–1989 season.

In summary, the epidemiologic data demonstrate that the shoulder is not a commonly injured body part in gymnastics, as lower extremity injuries predominate. The shoulder is more commonly injured in men's gymnastics as opposed to women's gymnastics. As the women's uneven parallel bars continues to evolve to include swinging movements that are traditionally seen in men's gymnastics, we anticipate a higher incidence of shoulder injuries in the female gymnast. Future studies into the epidemiology of shoulder injuries should focus on specific maneuvers during which injuries occur, the timing of injuries into the practice session, the skill level of the athletes, the distribution of overuse vs. traumatic injuries, and the influence of coaching.

SHOULDER INJURIES

Gymnastics differs from other sports in that the shoulder is a weight-bearing joint much of the time.[1,18] The shoulder is subjected to compression loads, torsional and tensile forces, and direct contusive stresses. Conflicting with these forces is the need for the gymnast to maintain a graceful routine and position. As previously described, the sport demands strength, flexibility, and speed, as well as grace. The shoulder is thus subjected to tremendous forces and its function is often compromised. The remainder of this chapter details the concepts of flexibility and training as contributers to injuries unique to the gymnast, as well as management strategies for the successful treatment of these disorders.

TRAINING

It has been noted in several reports that the gymnast trains at least 20 h per week.[3,6,11,16] Injuries have been noted to occur with increased frequency late in the day and week, presumably owing to fatigue. Coaches are advised to allow regular break periods as well as event rotation, not only to rest certain muscle groups and joints but also to keep the athlete mentally refreshed.

An important advance in gymnasts' performance has been the renewed interest in strength training. Where this received lip service before, now it is an integral part of the athlete's weekly training regimen. Strength training will require 1 to 2 h 3 days per week. Obviously in gymnasts, disproportionate attention is given to upper extremities emphasizing the full shoulder circuit as well as biceps, triceps, wrist flexors, extensors, and trunk. Certain strengthening programs are recognized as essential not only to improve performance but to prevent injury. Several coaches interviewed[8,9,10] feel that from ages 10 to 15 technique is as important as strength. With that thinking, body resistance (e.g., pull-ups, handstands, push-ups, and dips) and rubber tubing exercises are best utilized for strengthening—not fixed exercise equipment—with particular emphasis on proper mechanics. Abdominal muscles are needed as in "kip" maneuvers—which also serve to protect the low back. As with throwing sports, the trunk musculature must not be ignored as a base of support for the upper body. Thus the latissimus dorsi and lower trapezius muscles are essential as well. At 16, men are encouraged to add formal weight training for upper extremity strengthening, with the continued use of rubber tubing resistance exercises to protect the rotator cuff. Formal weight training is also most often useful for a specific muscle group or joint when returning from an injury in a rehabilitation mode. Repetition is often emphasized, as anaerobic muscular endurance is frequently required in the gymnast's routine.

FLEXIBILITY

Shoulder flexibility is critical to the performance of many gymnastic movements. Flexibility is a key component of the training program. Stretching exercises to attain maximum shoulder flexibility are essential if the gymnast is to do rotational skills and the newly required release moves on the high bar. A paradox exists, as there is an inherent selection process in female gymnasts that selects lithe hypermobile individuals. These gymnasts' shoulders, when subjected to large forces, particularly at the extremes of motion, develop symptomatic instability. If physiologically hypermobile individuals are allowed to compete without attention to muscle strengthening and proper technique, they run an increased risk of dislocation and subluxation. These individuals, then, in contrast to the inflexible, require comprehensive strengthening of the entire shoulder girdle with particular attention to the adducters, forward flexors, and internal rotators.

Coaches interestingly feel that a unique consequence of shoulder inflexibility is excessive stress to the low back (e.g., poorly executed "back walkovers").[8,10] Thus, particularly in preteens, attention should be given to a shoulder flexibility program (e.g., in the gym and at home).

ACUTE INJURIES

Contusions and Strains

Contusions and strains are the most common acute shoulder injuries seen in gymnastics. Contusions usually result from falls contacting a mat, a piece of apparatus, or another individual (athlete or spotter).

Most of these are due to carelessness or fatigue and can be reduced by improved safety precautions. Break periods allow for release of stress and tension that diminishes the tendency to "fool around" or lose concentration during training drills. As mentioned above, allowing adequate spacing of equipment and athletes running through drills, along with careful spotting, will reduce the frequency of these injuries.

Muscle strains in gymnastics, as in other sports, are related to overtraining to the point of fatigue, inadequate warm-up, improper technique, and premature return to practice after injury, usually to another part of the body. Muscle strains are frequently seen on rings (pectoralis), pommel horse (supraspinatus), and parallel bars (latissimus dorsi). Biceps rupture (long head) has been described in men's gymnastics (rings).[2] Strain of the long head of the biceps is also related to subluxation from its groove.

Treatment of muscle injuries is dependent upon the severity of the strain. Grade I strains involve a small number of muscle fibers, while grade II injuries involve a large number of injured fibers. Grade III strains involve compete rupture of the muscle. Treatment initially consists of ice, compression, and relative rest. Passive range of motion should be started as soon as possible, with progression to active involvement. Strength training is subsequently started when the athlete has full range of motion. Return to sport should be contemplated when there is a return to the preinjury state. Surgical intervention is infrequently warranted. Grade III injuries associated with bony avulsion fracture may require surgical reattachment. The rehabilitating gymnast can be encouraged to work on skills not involving the injured muscle group, as well as enhancing general flexibility. Prevention of future reinjury includes attention to proper strength training, excellent technique, and avoiding excessive training.

Acromioclavicular joint sprains result from falls in a variety of events onto the tip of the shoulder. In general these tend to be mild (grade 1 or 2) and can be treated conservatively.

Fractures

Fractures about the shoulder in gymnastics are relatively infrequent. These injuries are covered in the chapter on fractures and will not be repeated here.

Dislocation

Acute dislocation is readily recognized as a result of a missed movement or a fall from an apparatus. In general the athlete's trunk rotates beyond the fixed hand grip (late release) or the gymnast lands incorrectly on the outstretched arm. In assessing these acute injuries, the physician should first evaluate the athlete for concomitant neurologic injury (usually axillary nerve) or associated injuries (e.g., neck trauma). The examination requires inspection not only of the neck but also of the arm for evidence of brachial plexus injury. Fracture-dislocation in the young athlete is rare in contrast to the elderly adult, but x-ray evaluation of the shoulder is recommended before reduction. After reduction, shoulder immobilization in a sling and swathe is rigidly required for 4 weeks in the initial acute period. Thereafter, rehabilitation first stresses restoration of the range of motion; then comprehensive shoulder strengthening is prescribed. It is our firm belief that gymnasts should be encouraged to stay in the gym during this entire period. It is helpful for them emotionally to still be a part of the team, but also alternative training can be initiated (e.g., stationary bike, stair master, lower extremity strengthening, and flexibility).

Anterior dislocations are statistically the most frequently seen. However, we have also observed posterior dislocations. Today, with an increased recognition of shoulder pathomechanics, the presence of multidirectional instability must be determined. As mentioned above, this usually occurs in the congenitally lax individual. Trauma in the athlete, however, may lead to anterior and inferior instability. Early recognition of the direction or directions of recurrent instability will clarify the treatment regimen selected. Straight anterior dislocation with a traumatic Bankart lesion can be handled by an arthroscopic Bankart procedure. It is our feeling that capsular laxity without traumatic Bankart lesion is best handled by an open capsular shift. Again, comprehensive rehabilitation is necessary after operative correction of instability before the athlete is allowed to return to training and competition.

CHRONIC AND OVERUSE SYNDROMES

Impingement Syndrome

Overuse syndromes can occur in the young gymnast.[1,3,11,12,16] As discussed above, training errors such as overtraining to the point of fatigue, inadequate warm-up, poor technique, and premature return to training after an injury can predispose to overuse injuries. Impingement syndrome is seen in the gymnast. The classic historical complaints are aching subdeltoid pain after workouts and inability to use the arm comfortably in all planes. We have frequently observed these symptoms not only from gymnastics practice, but also in combination with an overly aggressive weight training program. On exam one should look for positive impingement signs (either resisted forward flexion or abduction). The examiner must also check for loss of motion (specifically internal rotation), weakness (usually supraspinatus), and instability. As has been discussed amply by other authors, we concur that the young (under 30) athlete with recurrent rotator cuff tendinitis must be carefully evaluated for concomitant instability. This will clarify the treatment regimen to both the athlete and the coach. In our experience, only early (stage 1 and 2) rotator cuff tendinitis has been seen in gymnasts (no complete rotator cuff ruptures have been recorded). The acute impingement syndrome symptoms respond well to activity modification, rotator cuff exercises (stressing light weights and tubing in repetition), nonsteroidal anti-inflammatories, and ice. This does not mean rest, immobilization, or inactivity, as these all lead to atrophy and deconditioning and are counterproductive. A standard rehabilitation program is presented in Chap. 19. This program is usually successful in 3 to 6 weeks. We stress again that the gymnast is kept in the gym during this rehabilitation program. Strength deficits as noted must be corrected. Routines, as well as training regimens, are modified as necessary. Maintenance of strength training in season, as well as off season, is stressed.

In men's gymnastics the rings, horizontal bar, and pommel horse are all associated with increased shoulder stress, whereas in women's gymnastics the uneven bars are most frequently cited.[1,6,8,10] Again, it must be stated that while the above apparatuses are cited as stressful to the shoulder, the primary culprit is poor technique. It should also be noted that as gymnasts fatigue secondary to prolonged training, they often compensate with poor technique. "Smooth swings" on rings and pommel horse protect from pain and vice versa. Females are now on the higher bar executing giant swings and complex release movements. However, with proper technique there should be no additional stress or pain in the shoulder at the bottom of a "swing-through." Actually, the feeling should be of a pushing away from the bar. Pain occurs with poor technique as the gymnast "drops down" quickly rather than swinging through the movement. The same may be said for men on rings, parallel bars, and high bar.

Instability

Instability has been touched on in the section on dislocation. Gymnasts stress flexibility of the shoulder. The gymnast's shoulder, when confronted with the significant sport-induced force loads, can progress to the point of chronic instability. The natural selection process of the lithe, hyperflexible athlete for gymnastics predisposes the risk of instability. This is frequently accompanied by the symptoms of impingement. Here, accurate assessment of the degree and direction of instability is essential to organizing treatment. Strength deficits must be identified and corrected. Specifically, attention is directed to the shoulder adductors, internal rotators, and forward flexor muscle groups. Strength testing (cybex or biodex) can be helpful in assessment of deficit as well as in guiding rehabilitation. Proper overall conditioning, attention to warm-up, and technique are also needed before return to full training. We have found these programs uniformly successful. One rarely needs to resort to a surgical solution. As with the swimmer's shoulder, surgical intervention in the gymnast to restore stability is problematic. One cannot guarantee gymnasts will be able to return to their previous high level of performance.

As a consequence of the hypermobility of the gymnast's shoulder, chronic subluxation and instability is distinctly more frequent than acute traumatic dislocation. Within this instability we have noted the anterior directional instability most frequently, then multidirectional, then posterior. Men seem to have experienced major difficulties with instability on rings ("dislocated giants") and horizontal bars ("inverted giant swings"), whereas women experience most difficulty on uneven bars.

Acromioclavicular Osteoarthritis or "Gymnast's Shoulder"

Acromioclavicular osteoarthritis following trauma to the distal clavicle and secondary to overload and compression from weight lifting is well recognized. A similar process occurs in gymnasts, termed "gymnast's shoulder." The acromioclavicular osteoarthritis is secondary to the continuous microtraumatic overload from overuse, particularly in overhead activities.[13] The excessive compression effects on the acromioclavicular joints are particularly seen on the rings (e.g., iron cross and shoulder dislocation maneuvers). This process produces local acromioclavicular pain and secondary impingement syndrome. Occasionally surgical intervention is required, and may include arthroscopic decompression or open distal clavicle resection.

CONCLUSION

We have reviewed specific events and their risk of injury, proper training techniques, equipment, acute and chronic injuries, along with appropriate treatment programs. As we have demonstrated, the gymnast's shoulder is caught in the middle of the conflicting demands for flexibility, speed of movement, and grace, as well as power and repetitive overload. We have attempted to shed some light on the particular demands of the sport of gymnastics. The shoulder will be subjected to even greater stress as athletes continue to perform more difficult "tricks" requiring greater speed and strength.

Sports medicine has expanded its scope dramatically in the past decade. As with other sports, the more complete the knowledge of the sport and its particular demands the sports medicine physician has, the better he or she is equipped to treat the athlete. We now have a better understanding of shoulder biomechanics and kinematics. It is our hope to apply this knowledge to gymnastics. This involves injury prevention, accurate pathoanatomic diagnosis, and functional rehabilitation. We must stress this goal to protect and enhance this graceful and artistic sport.

REFERENCES

1. Aronen JG: Problems of the upper extremity in gymnasts, in *Symposium on Gymnastics*, CV Mosby Company (ed). *Clin Sports Med* 4(1):January 1985.

2. delPizzo W, et al: Rupture of the biceps tendon in gymnastics, a case report. *Am J Sports Med* 6(5):283, 1978.

3. Garrick JG, Requa RK: Epidemiology of women's gymnastics injuries. *Am J Sports Med* 8(4):261, July 1980.

4. International Gymnastics Federation. Code of Points/Min, 1989.

5. Kirby RL: Flexibility and musculoskeletal symptomatology in female gymnasts and age-matched controls. *Am J Sports Med* 9(3):180, 1981.

6. Mandelbaum BR: Gymnastics, in Reider B: *Sports Medicine, The School-Age Athlete.* Philadelphia, Saunders, 1991, pp 415–428.

7. National Collegiate Athletic Association: 1991–1992 Men's and women's gymnastics injury surveillance system. Overland Park, KA, NCAA, 1992.

8. Private communication, Gary Anderson, head coach, Marvateens, Rockville, MD.

9. Private communication, Brad Smith, national team trainer. U.S. Gymnastics Federation, Kokomo, IN.

10. Personal communication Milan Stanovich, head coach, K-rons Gymnastics Club, Burke, VA.

11. Pettrone FA, Ricciardelli E: Gymnastic injuries: The Virginia experience 1982–1983. *Am J Sports Med* 15(1):59, 1987.

12. Pettrone FA (ed): Gymnastic injuries, in *Symposium on Upper Extremity Injuries in Athletes.* St Louis, Mosby, 1986.

13. Silvij S, Nolini S: Clinical and radiological aspects of gymnast's shoulder. *J Sports Med Phys Fitness.* 22(1): 1982.

14. Snook GA: Injuries in women's gymnastics. A five year study. *Am J Sports Med* 13:301–308, 1985.

15. Weiker G: Upper extremity gymnastics injuries, in *The Upper Extremity in Sports Medicine.* St Louis, Mosby, 1990.

16. Weiker G: Introduction and history of gymnastics, in *Symposium on Gymnastics*, CV Mosby Company (ed). *Clin Sports Med* 4(1):January 1985.

17. Weiker G: Club gymnastics, in *Symposium on Gymnastics*, CV Mosby Company (ed). *Clin Sports Med* 4(1)39: January 1985.

18. Wetstone E: *The Gymnast's Safety Manual.* University Park, PA, Pennsylvania State University Press, 1977.

CHAPTER 27

Protective Equipment for the Athlete's Shoulder

Frank C. McCue III
Joe Gieck
Susan Foreman
Ethan Saliba

The anatomy of the shoulder joint provides sufficient mobility to allow athletic activities as varied as throwing a javelin, performing gymnastic maneuvers on the rings or high bar, tackling a running back, or dunking a basketball. The same anatomy places the shoulder at risk for injury by direct blows, falls, excess motion, or repeated excursions through a normal range of motion. Injury prevention is an important role of the sports medicine professional. Injury to the shoulder can be minimized by strengthening the muscles surrounding the shoulder, by learning the correct sport-specific technique, and by the development and use of protective equipment.[1]

The shoulder's anatomic complexity, mobility, and poor bony stability make it susceptible to both traumatic and overuse injuries. Athletic participation places great stress on the shoulder, and when problems develop, management is often difficult because of the vulnerability of the joint to reinjury. Protective equipment has been developed and has subsequently been required for some sports to help reduce the incidence of specific injuries.[2] This equipment can have varying styles to accommodate differences in functional needs of the various sports. Additionally, there are subtle differences in equipment even between positions within a sport. For example, lineman shoulder pads typically allow less movement and more protection compared with the shoulder pads for a receiver, which are lighter and allow greater mobility. The materials and types of padding used in shoulder protection are extensive. This chapter addresses the type of protective equipment that is required for specific athletic competition and presents an overview of the various protective equipment that is available for particular injuries.

Protective shoulder equipment is used routinely in sports that place the shoulder at risk of injury. Shoulder pads can restrict the motion of a certain body part, reduce friction between surfaces that come into contact, or absorb energy of a direct blow.[3] The materials allow the force to be dispersed over a greater area so that the force at any one place is minimized. Shoulder pads were originally fabricated out of leather by saddlemakers to disperse forces and reduce shock in football. There are few modifications in the original design, although materials and kinesiologic data have improved the function of protective equipment. Modern equipment is produced from strong, yet lightweight, plastics covering a variety of shock absorbing material. When fitted and used properly, shoulder pads can reduce injury to the upper extremity, the cervical region, and the upper trunk.

Equipment styles in ice hockey and lacrosse have benefited from the original manufacture and design of football shoulder pads. Ice hockey players wear pads to protect their shoulders from impact with opponents, the rink walls, and the ice. Lacrosse players rely on their pads to protect them from their opponent's stick, as well as from direct impact with their opponents, and occasionally the ball. The use of shoulder pads has decreased the incidence of contusion, separations, and fractures in these sports.[4] In addition to football, ice hockey and men's lacrosse require shoulder pads to participate. However, most women's sporting organizations such as lacrosse and field hockey feel that shoulder pads should not be required, as this may change the nature of the game to one with more physical contact.[2]

COMPONENTS OF SHOULDER PADS

Football pads are generally made of a lightweight, hard plastic on the exterior that can deflect a blow, with an inner lining of open-and closed-cell foam padding that absorbs the shock and distributes it over a broad area. There are two main types of football shoulder pads: flat and cantilever.[1] At one time, flat pads were worn by those players such as quarterbacks and wide receivers who were not in constant contact and needed the greater mobility of a lighter pad. However, concern was generated regarding the extent of protection offered by the flat pads. This concern of poor protection resulted in a trend in which flat pads were being replaced by the cantilever pads.[3,5]

Many companies, however, are again producing flat pads, especially for offensive linemen. These pads differ from the earlier generation pads by using the "air management" system.[6] Air management systems use open- or closed-cell foam or combinations of these, specifically located under the protective hard plastic. The padding is encased in a nylon material that restricts the air movement. When contact is made with the shoulder, air is dispersed throughout the padding to create an "air pocket" between the athlete and the shoulder pads. Since offensive linemen principally use their hands while blocking, the less bulky flat pads are felt to allow greater mobility while providing the athlete with protection.

Cantilever pads are named because of the bridge that they make over the superior aspect of the shoulder. This design is to minimize contact with the clavicle and the acromioclavicular joint. They are built to be lightweight, allow maximum range of motion, and distribute the force and pressure of a blow throughout the entire shoulder, chest, and back. Cantilever pads have three types: inside, outside, and the double cantilever. The inside cantilever fits under the arch and rests against the shoulder. It is more common because it is less bulky than the outside cantilever. The outside cantilever sits on top of the pad, outside of the arch. It provides a larger blocking surface and affords more protection to those who are in constant contact such as linemen. The double cantilever, which is a combination of both the inside and the outside cantilever, affords a player with the greatest amount of protection but is not feasible for all positions owing to its bulk.

In addition to the cantilever, the football shoulder pads consist of numerous other structures. The "arch" is the hard outer plastic shell that the padding and other components attach to and is shaped to fit the contour of the upper body. The "epaulets" are padded plastic flaps located on the superior aspect of the shoulder pads and attach to the arch. The shoulder "caps" reach from the edge of the arch down over the arm to cover the deltoid muscle and proximal humerus.

The posterior padding should cover the trapezius and other posterior muscles in addition to covering the scapula and spine. The anterior padding should cover the pectoralis muscles as well as the sternum and clavicle. Anterior padding may be built up for added protection for linebackers and others who routinely receive blows anteriorly or from an upright position.[1] The padding superiorly is designed to create a channel for the clavicle to minimize impact forces. Proper fitting is essential for an appropriate channel to be maintained (Fig. 27-1).

Shoulder pads should be selected for the athlete's position, body type, and history of injury.[7] For example, linemen, especially linebackers and fullbacks, need to have their anterior and posterior padding extend lower in order to protect the sternum and ribs, while defensive ends require the greater protection of larger caps and flaps for tackling. Offensive backs and ends most likely will have smaller caps and flaps to allow them greater mobility when passing and catching. Cantilevers also come in different sizes so that quarterbacks and receivers who need more glenohumeral movement are not restricted while linemen who require little glenohumeral movement but need more protection against constant contact use larger cantilevers (Fig. 27-2).[4]

Ice hockey and lacrosse shoulder pads are less

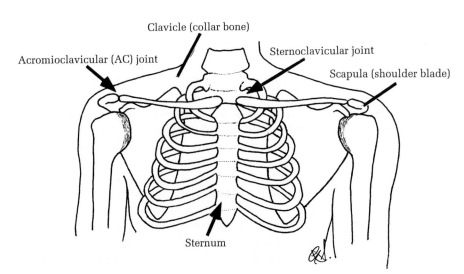

FIGURE 27-1
Shoulder anatomy and football shoulder pad components.

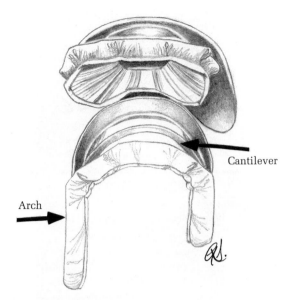

FIGURE 27-2
Cantilever vs. flat pads.

bulky and restrictive than football pads but can have similar characteristics. These sports use equipment with many variations. The shock pads often worn under football shoulder pads may be legal padding for lacrosse. Offensive lacrosse players who must sustain more contact will often wear plastic cups over the acromioclavicular joint encased in canvas. Hockey and lacrosse players tend to wear their

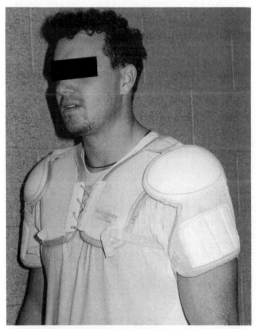

FIGURE 27-3
Standard lacrosse shoulder pads. Foam vest with hard plastic shells to protect AC joints and shoulder tips. Lacrosse pads vary from shock pads to quarterback football pads, depending on the position and a previous injury. Attention should be made to proper fit and wear of lacrosse shoulder pads.

shoulder pads too large or too loose since the pads are more comfortable this way.[4] Coaches, trainers, and equipment personnel should instruct their athletes in the proper fit of the equipment so that the protection that the pads are designed for can be obtained. Additional padding can be added to hockey or lacrosse shoulder pads and the smaller quarterback football pads may be appropriate with these sports if an individual requires more protection (Fig. 27-3).

ADDITIONAL COMMERCIAL EQUIPMENT

Numerous other commercial devices can be added or used in conjunction with shoulder pads to protect specific injuries to the shoulder or cervical region. The following are some of these devices.

Shock pads are worn under football, lacrosse, or hockey shoulder pads. They are felt to improve fit, provide a space to allow better shock absorption, and decrease impact on acromioclavicular joint or on the clavicles.[6] Some equipment personnel feel that this extra pad can be detrimental by removing the air space between the shoulder pads and the player, making them more vulnerable to impact.

The McDavid Cowboy Collar, vinyl neck roll, i.e., longhorn neck roll, or the LaPorta Collar provide additional cervical protection. These devices are used to limit extremes of ranges in the cervical region by limiting the movement of the helmet. Their placement and supplemental padding can be specifically placed to restrict isolated motions. These are particularly helpful with the brachial plexus "burners," which can be very problematic.

Deltoid extensions are extra pads that can be attached to the cap of the shoulder pad. These provide additional protection to the lateral aspect of the arm which is a frequent site of contact with linemen and linebackers. Repeated contusions in this area are a common cause for the development of myositis ossificans, so added protection is periodically necessary.

Rib and back extension pads can also be attached to the shoulder pads. Quarterbacks frequently need rib protection added to their shoulder pads because of the extended position they are in when contact is made. Back extensions are commonly used by running backs (Fig. 27-4).

EQUIPMENT FITTING

Shoulder pads must be correctly fitted and be in good condition to provide optimal protection for the athlete. Prior to the beginning of the athletic season, equipment should be examined by a knowledgeable

367

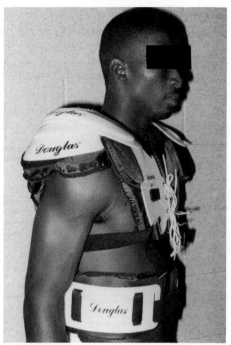

FIGURE 27-4A
Quarterback rib extension combination. Quarterbacks often are hit while their arms are raised. This pad gives additional protection to the ribs and is secured to the existing shoulder pad.

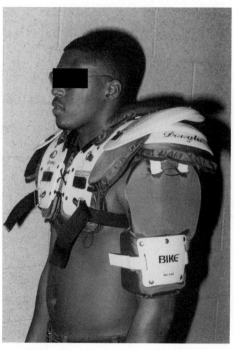

FIGURE 27-4B
Deltoid extension. Elastic band slips over deltoid cap and Velcro secures pad against the arm.

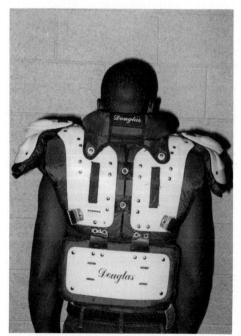

FIGURE 27-4C
Back extension. Flap is attached to shoulder pads with gromets. This type of padding is used routinely for tailbacks or fullbacks who often are hit from behind.

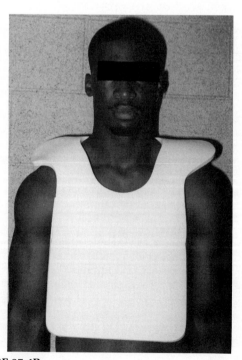

FIGURE 27-4D
Large sternum pad. Worn under shoulder pads to reduce impact on sternum and anterior ribs.

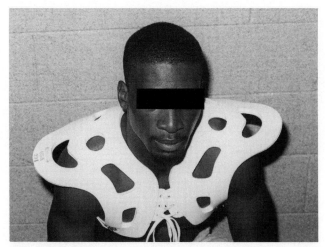

FIGURE 27-4E
Shock pads. Worn under shoulder pads to give added protection to the clavicles and AC joints. Some equipment personnel feel that shock pads reduce the effectiveness of a "channel system" shoulder pad because the fit is altered. Shock pads are often used as lacrosse shoulder pads.

equipment manager. Worn straps, snaps, or buckles should be replaced. If the pads themselves are cracked or otherwise damaged, they should be reconditioned by an equipment company or taken out of service. Used or worn-out pads should not be donated to another team, as this raises a potential liability problem.[6,8]

Each athlete must be fitted with quality equipment by knowledgeable personnel. Many injuries are caused by improper fit of the equipment rather than design flaws.[7] Consultation with the athletic trainer may also be necessary to address unique medical conditions and whether additional padding may be necessary.

Fitting Protocol[5–9]

1. Determine shoulder width and/or chest size and body weight to establish the general size needed. The chest girth measured at the nipple line or the distance between the tips of the acromions may be used depending on the recommendations of the particular shoulder pad companies.

2. Place the shoulder pads on the player and tighten all straps and laces. Check to see if the clavicle is covered completely and that the neck opening is large enough for comfort, but not too large, as this will allow exposure of the clavicles. There should be enough room on either side of the neck roll to allow comfort when the arms are raised fully.

3. Check to determine whether the acromioclavicular joint is covered and bridged by the clavicle

channel. The underneath padding should extend to the lateral aspect of the deltoid. Pads that are not wide enough will not effectively protect the area, while pads that are too wide will not adequately be able to disperse a force across a broad area. The anterior deltoid should be covered by this padding as well.

4. The axillary straps should be secured so that the pads do not shift. The straps should be tight enough to allow only two fingers to be inserted under the strap. The strap is not tight enough if the hand can be slid under the straps or pad. These straps should be as tight as the athlete can functionally tolerate.

5. Check to see if the scapula is adequately covered by the arch and lateral extension of the padding. The plastic shell should extend below the base of the scapula and cover the sternum and pectoralis muscles.

6. Make sure the pads are centered on the player and that the laces are secured with no space between the juncture of the clavicle and sternum.

7. Final inspection: Check the shoulder pads with the helmet and jersey in place to determine the final fit. Have athletes raise their arms to ensure comfort and no impingement in the cervical region.

ADAPTATION TO SHOULDER PADS

Protective equipment is not only available for prevention of an injury but can be available to help protect an already injured area. Protective equipment for specific injuries can be commercially available or can be fabricated by the trainer or therapist. The availability of materials and one's creativity can be the only restricting factors in the fabrication of such a protective piece of equipment. Acute management and rehabilitation must be incorporated when an injury occurs. Proper rehabilitation is essential to help minimize the chronicity of the problem and should be initiated as soon as the injury has stabilized. Once functional criteria have been met to allow the return of the athlete to activity, added protection is considered to help reduce reinjury.[2]

The additional padding should meet the legal requirements for that sport: For example, there should not be exposed metal or hard plastic on the apparatus and it should not have the potential to create harm to other players. Additionally, the modifications of the shoulder pads should not cause stress or cracking of the original material.[7] Drilling holes too closely may weaken or damage the material

369

on impact. Most commercially produced accessory pads fit well on standard shoulder pads and can be secured with the existing brackets or velcro. However, the trainer-therapist may choose to fabricate a customized pad. The customized pads are often smaller and less costly; they perform well but are a challenge to secure in place. For example, foam doughnuts with or without a hard orthoplast or plastic covering can be taped or wrapped on the injured part. Spray adherent on the skin may help prevent slippage of the custom-made pads during competition. The device may be sewn into existing pads.

Specific modifications for various injuries are presented in the following section. These devices are not all-inclusive since most athletic trainers have developed variations that they feel are most effective in certain situations.

CONTUSIONS

Repetitive blows to the football player's arm below the shoulder pad by his opponent's helmet may result in a contusion or hematoma. This injury can evolve into an entity called "blocker's exostosis" since the repetitive contusion can result in the development of myositis ossificans in the deltoid muscle.[6,8] The use of pads that adequately cover the upper lateral arm should prevent this injury. However, if a deep bruise occurs, appropriate treatment should be provided. Subsequently the area should be protected with additional padding. Often pads cut from high-density foam can be more suitably shaped to cover the involved area.[10] A foam doughnut provides pressure around the injured area that minimizes the force on the contusion. The doughnut pad can be covered with an additional layer of foam of a firmer material such as a thermoplastic. The firmer material allows greater dispersion of the force to a broader area, away from the injured site (Fig. 27-5).

ACROMIOCLAVICULAR SPRAINS

Acromioclavicular (AC) injuries can be initially treated with a sling, figure eight brace, or Kenny Howard brace.[6] Following rehabilitative exercises, when the player is ready to return to athletics, a doughnut-type pad may be placed over the AC joint. A thermoplastic material such as orthoplast or hexalite can be placed over the doughnut.[11–14] The pad can be taped to the athlete's shoulder and secured with an elastic wrap or can be sewn into a shock pad to improve consistent positioning. These shock-absorbing cushions may be used effectively beneath football, lacrosse, or hockey shoulder pads. Commercially produced AC pads are also available. A

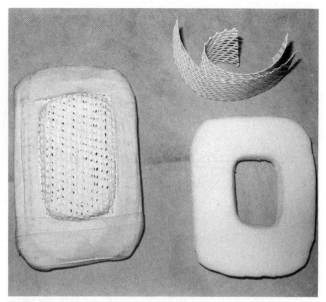

FIGURE 27-5A
Doughnut and thermoplastic material covering. Closed cell foam doughnut disperses force around a contusion. The thermoplastic material increases the amount of protection. These pads are custom made to the size of the injury.

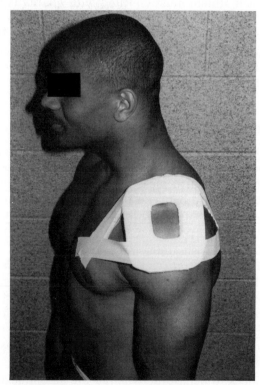

FIGURE 27-5B
Closed cell foam doughnut. Cutout is over contusion to minimize force in that area.

370

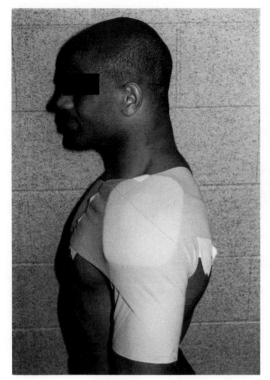

FIGURE 27-5C
Doughnut secured with tape and elastic wrap. Custom pads are more difficult to secure, but can be worn under shoulder pads.

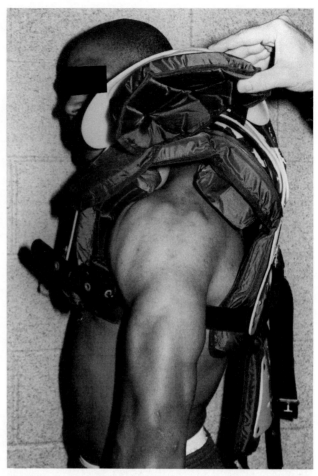

FIGURE 27-6
Channel system. Thick "air management" pads Velcro in place to protect the acromioclavicular joint.

cantilever-type shoulder pad may be appropriate for a football player, if he is not already using one (Figs. 27-6 and 27-7).

BRACHIAL PLEXUS INJURIES

The brachial plexus can be injured in sports with a forceful lateral flexion of the neck or shoulder depression.[8] This injury varies in its severity and is commonly called a "burner" or "stinger" because of the sharp radiating pain along the affected upper extremity. Fit of the shoulder pads is perhaps the most important aspect of preventing brachial plexus injuries.[15] If this injury occurs, the shoulder pads should

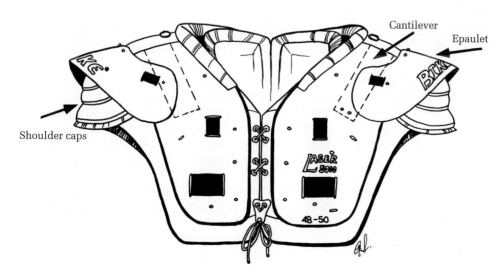

Shoulder caps

Cantilever

Epaulet

FIGURE 27-7
Kenny Howard sling.

371

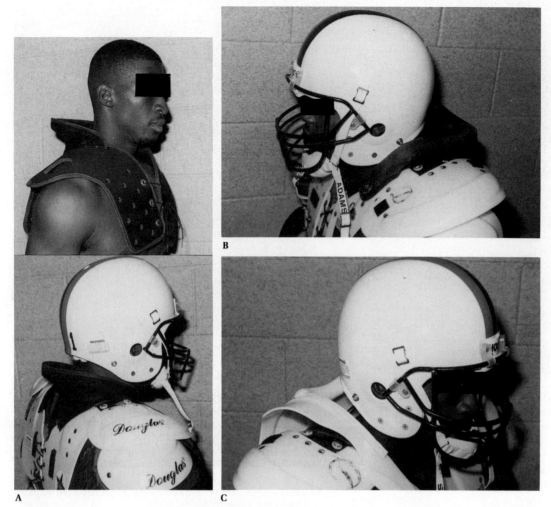

FIGURE 27-8
Cervical protection. Cervical range of motion is restricted as the helmet makes contact with the device on the shoulder pads. **A.** Cowboy collar. Fit under shoulder pads to reduce cervical motion. The device is made from a fairly rigid closed cell foam material. **B.** Longhorn collar. Foam padding is encased in vinyl and secured to the shoulder pads with snaps. Additional padding can be added to any area to further restrict a specific motion. **C.** LaPorta Collar. This raised hard plastic material is secured to the shoulder pads with gromets. The device effectively absorbs shock to the superior aspect of the shoulder and reduces cervical range of motion.

be modified when the athlete is cleared to play so that extremes of cervical motion are restricted. A molded collar around the neck may be used but it must be snug and limit the motion that causes the pain. Commercial products or collars can be added to the shoulder pads to further restrict problematic motions. These include the Cowboy Collar, longhorn neck roll, LaPorta Collar, and numerous others of similar design (Fig. 27-8).

GLENOHUMERAL INSTABILITY

Athletes with glenohumeral instability, shoulder dislocations, or subluxations benefit most from a ro-

tator cuff strengthening program. The incidence of recurrent injury may be reduced sufficiently with exercise to prevent or postpone surgical reconstruction. The high degree of mobility associated with the unstable shoulder may be partially limited by the use of external devices. A strap made out of elastic shoulder strap material encircles the involved arm and attaches to the front of the player's shoulder pads.[16] The strap is adjusted to limit shoulder abduction and external rotation. Success with this type of restraint is limited with hockey and lacrosse padding because these pads actually are less secure on the torso.

Several companies have designed braces to protect the athlete with glenohumeral instabilities.

The SAWA Shoulder Orthosis (Brace International, Scottsdale, AZ) is a reinforced cotton and rubber blend vest with a velcro strap attached to a humeral cuff.[17] The Shoulder Subluxation Inhibitor (Physical Support Systems, Windham, NH) is made of polyethylene and has a strap that limits hyperabduction and external rotation of the shoulder.[18] The CD Denison-Duke Wyre Shoulder Vest (Denison Orthopedic Appliance Company, Baltimore, MD) is made of canvas and leather.[19] Laces attach the biceps cuff to the vest and limit excessive shoulder abduction and extension. No brace or modifications will eliminate all dislocations or subluxations of the shoulder, and certain players may be too functionally restricted to participate with the brace properly in place (Fig. 27-9).

FRACTURES

Scapular fractures are rarely seen in athletes. Sufficient time must be allowed for healing of any fracture. When the player is ready to return, football pads can be reinforced to provide additional protection as the fracture heals. Rib fractures are more common in contact sports. "Flack" jackets or rib extensions can be used to disperse forces around the flank. These pads are usually not routinely worn to prevent rib injuries because they can cause overheating, especially early in the season. However, they should be worn to protect an existing rib or back injury.

ABRASIONS

Although abrasions occur more frequently around the elbow and forearm, they do sometimes occur near the shoulder. The athlete should be instructed to routinely cleanse the area with soap and water in the shower. There are numerous methods to effectively treat skin irritations and abrasions. The abraded area is bandaged for athletic activities and may be covered additionally with a pad if the area is prone to direct impact. Covering the abrasion reduces the possibility of exposing blood or exudate on the padding materials, which can result in contamination. Standardized procedures indicate that exposed areas of plastic padding should be cleaned with a fresh 10 percent solution of bleach. At pres-

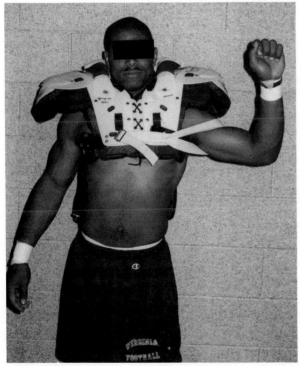

FIGURE 27-9A
Anterior dislocation strap. Elastic strap is secured to the opposite side of the shoulder pads. The strap limits external rotation and abduction.

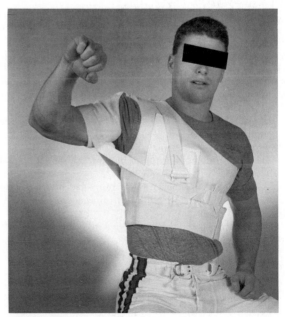

FIGURE 27-9B
SAWA shoulder brace. Harness that restricts excessive glenohumeral motion. Can be worn under shoulder pads or under the jersey. (Photograph courtesy of Brace International, Atlanta, GA.)

ent, there is not a product that is sanctioned as a blood-borne pathogen disinfectant on cloth materials; however, isopropyl alcohol has been suggested.

CONCLUSION

The fabrication, fitting, and use of protective shoulder equipment to prevent or treat shoulder injuries should be coupled with education. Athletes and coaches should be informed that while shoulder equipment is used to decrease the risk of injury or reinjury, prevention cannot be guaranteed. The athlete should be shown how the equipment should be worn and used. He or she should be told to inspect the equipment each day and to replace any damage to the pads, straps, or braces. Additionally the athlete should be asked if the devices fit comfortably and should be told to report any discomfort they cause. Any injury or reinjury should be reported to the athletic trainer and/or team physician. Educating the athlete also includes reinforcing the importance of shoulder conditioning or rehabilitation.

REFERENCES

1. Gieck J, McCue FC III: Fitting of protective football equipment. *Am J Sports Med* 8:3, 192–196, 1980.
2. Kulund D: *The Injured Athlete*. Philadelphia, Lippincott, 1988, pp 301–355.
3. Hodgson VR: Athletic equipment and injury prevention, in Mueller F, Ryan A (eds): *Prevention of Athletic Injuries: The Role of the Sports Medicine Team*. Philadelphia, Davis, 1991, pp 48–62.
4. Gieck J: Protective equipment for sport, in Ryan AJ, Allman FL (eds): *Sports Medicine*. New York, Academic, 1989, pp 211–242.
5. Malacrea R, Protective equipment fit. *Proceedings of the NATA Professional Preparation Conference*, NATA Professional Educational Committee, Nashville, TN, 1978.
6. Arnheim DD: *Modern Principles of Athletic Training*. St Louis, MO, Times Mirror/Mosby College Publishing, 1989, pp 734–775.
7. Fitting shoulder pads. *American Equipment Manager's Certification Manual*, 1992, chap 3, sec 3: pp 1–10.
8. Roy S, Irvin R: *Sports Medicine: Prevention, Evaluation, Management and Rehabilitation*. Englewood Cliffs, NJ, Prentice-Hall, 1983, pp 45–51.
9. Miller R: Presentation on protective padding, in NATA National Convention and Symposium, Columbus, OH, 1987.
10. Rovere GD, Curl WW, Brownig DG: Bracing and taping in an office sports medicine practice, in Collins HR (ed): *Clinics in Sports Medicine: Office Practice of Sports Medicine*. Philadelphia, Saunders, 1989.
11. Silloway KA, McLaughlin RE, Edlich RC, Edlich RF: Clavicular fractures and acromioclavicular joint dislocations in lacrosse: Preventable injuries. *J Emerg Med* 3:2, 1985.
12. Biron SA: Acromioclavicular protection of ice hockey players. *Athl Training* 18:2, 1983.
13. Deitsch MA, Fashover T: Football hip pad protection for hip pointers and AC sprains on ice hockey players. *Athl Training* 16:2, 1981.
14. Wershing CE: A specialized pad for the acromioclavicular joint. *Athl Training* 15:2, 1980.
15. Watkins RG: Neck injuries in football players, in *Clinics in Sports Medicine*. Philadelphia, Saunders, 1986.
16. Gieck J: Shoulder strap to prevent anterior glenohumeral dislocations. *Athl Training* 11:1, 18, 1976.
17. SAWA Shoulder Orthosis. Information Packet. Brace International, Scottsdale, AZ.
18. Shoulder Subluxation Inhibitor: Informative Literature, Physical Supports Systems, Inc, Windham, NH, 1989.
19. CD Denison-Duke Wyre Shoulder Vest: Information Packet. CD Denison Orthopedic Appliance Corp, Baltimore, MD.

CHAPTER 28

Shoulder Problems in the Wheelchair Athlete

Robert S. Burnham
Kathleen A. Curtis
David C. Reid

INTRODUCTION

Sport for athletes who compete in wheelchairs was first introduced by Sir Ludwig Guttmann in 1948 as a means of providing therapeutic exercise for spinal cord injured war veterans. Archery was the first competition and involved only 16 competitors. Since that time wheelchair sport has grown rapidly in popularity and competitiveness, as was demonstrated by the involvement of over 3000 athletes from 96 countries in the 1992 Summer Paralympic Games in Barcelona, Spain. Concurrent with this increase in participation are increases in the quality of competition and athletic excellence. Previously held records are regularly broken by large margins. This may in part be due to increased training intensity and sophistication, availability of adapted training facilities, improved coaching, and advances in sport equipment design. Wheelchair athletes no longer consider sport simply a part of their rehabilitation. For many it is an important and healthy part of their recreational lifestyle. For others, preparing for and participating in high-level national and international competitions is their full-time occupation. Considerable financial rewards and sponsorships are dependent upon their performance. With this evolution it is natural that wheelchair athletes are looking to sport medicine professionals for improved techniques of injury prevention and treatment. Without proper management, aging wheelchair athletes may experience chronic musculoskeletal injury and disability that interferes with all aspects of their daily lives.

WHEELCHAIR SPORT INJURY EPIDEMIOLOGY

The application of sport medicine to athletes with a disability is a relatively new occurrence, and the majority of research to date has been directed toward profiling injury incidence and types. These epidemiologic studies consistently stress the prominence of shoulder injuries.[1–3] When "injury" is defined in terms of time lost from wheelchair sport, the shoulder is the most common injury site.[4,5] Attesting further to its troublesome nature is the observation that shoulder injuries among wheelchair basketball players require professional medical care in 50 percent of cases. By contrast, hand injuries are virtually all self-treated.[6] In Ferrera's survey, 32 percent of the injuries sustained by wheelchair athletes were severe enough to cause the athlete to be off sport for more than 3 weeks.[4] High-injury-risk sports include wheelchair track, basketball, and road racing.[1]

Shoulder pain among wheelchair users is not exclusive to athletes. Wheelchair-dependent nonathletes also suffer from shoulder problems. Nichols found that 266 of 517 (51 percent) of the spinal cord injured patients that responded to his questionnaire previously or currently had shoulder-region pain. The frequency and duration of shoulder pain seemed to increase with time since the onset of disability, and there was a tendency for the pain to be bilateral.[7] Gellman et al. studied 84 paraplegic patients and found that the prevalence of shoulder pain increased with time since injury such that 52 percent had problems within the first 5 years, and shoulder pain was universal by 20 years postinjury.[8] Sie et al. examined 239 spinal cord injured patients, 136 of which were quadriplegics and 103 paraplegics. They found that 33 percent of these patients suffered from "significant" shoulder pain, which was defined as pain severe enough to require medication or limit functional activity or pain experienced with two or more activities of daily living. Again, the prevalence of shoulder pain rose with time since injury in the paraplegic group such that there was a 92 percent prevalence in the group who had sustained their injuries 15 to 19 years previously.[9] It is obvious that shoulder pain is a common and troublesome problem among wheelchair-dependent athletes and nonathletes alike and that the prevalence of this problem increases markedly with long-term wheelchair use.

375

SOURCES OF SHOULDER PAIN IN WHEELCHAIR ATHLETES

It must be remembered that pain in the shoulder can be referred from nonshoulder sources. This is a particularly important consideration in the wheelchair-dependent quadriplegic who has previously sustained neck trauma. Sie et al. determined, on a clinical basis, that 33 percent of shoulder pain among the quadriplegics in their study was referred from the cervical spine.[9] Referred shoulder pain from cervical spine degenerative changes, ligamentous laxity and chronic instability, nerve root entrapment, and posttraumatic syringomyelia should be considered. More commonly, shoulder pain among the wheelchair-dependent comes from pathology intrinsic to the shoulder joint and surrounding soft tissue. In wheelchair-dependent nonathletes, various causes have been described such as adhesive capsulitis and reflex sympathetic dystrophy (usually in the quadriplegic population). Less commonly, undetected fractures of the clavicle, recurrent dislocation, acromioclavicular pathology or suprascapular nerve palsy (which can mimic rotator cuff tears) have also been described.[10] Entrapment and inflammation of the soft tissues of the rotator cuff and subacromial bursa (impingement syndrome) is another potential source of shoulder pain in wheelchair-dependent athletes and nonathletes alike and likely represents the most common cause of shoulder pain in the wheelchair-dependent population.[9,11]

Bayley et al. found that 31 of 97 (33 percent) of wheelchair-dependent paraplegics had chronic persistent shoulder pain, particularly with transferring. Clinical assessment suggested the rotator cuff to be the source of the pain. Twenty-three of these patients underwent shoulder arthrography and 15 (65 percent) had rotator cuff tears. Five had avascular necrosis of the humeral head. The mean onset of shoulder pain in this group was 13 years post spinal cord injury, suggesting the rotator cuff pathology was not sustained at the time of the acute spinal cord injury but was more likely related to subsequent shoulder stresses.[11] Similarly, the rotator cuff was felt to be the most common source of shoulder pain among wheelchair athletes participating in the 1988 Summer Paralympics in Seoul, Korea.[12]

PATHOMECHANICS OF ROTATOR CUFF DISEASE IN WHEELCHAIR ATHLETES

The rotator cuff of the wheelchair athlete is subjected to several unique stresses that may account for its early degeneration. These include:

1. Overuse
2. Impingement related to:
   a. Frequent overhead activity
   b. Arm weightbearing
   c. Shoulder girdle muscle imbalance
3. Inflexibility

Overuse

Repetitive shoulder activity is required for both wheelchair propulsion and to perform most of the activities of daily living. Thus the shoulders of wheelchair athletes are at risk of having inadequate musculoskeletal recovery and regeneration time, putting them at increased risk of overuse injuries. Most athletes spend the majority of their waking hours in a wheelchair. Superimposed on these everyday stresses are the demands of sport training and competition. Many athletes are involved in multiple sports, thus compounding the number of training and competition sessions, as well as shrinking the duration of the off season.[1,2,6] In wheelchair basketball players it was found that they were at a 9 times greater risk of getting injured during the basketball season if they were concurrently involved in sports in addition to basketball. Wheelchair basketball players who trained more than 3 days per week and included weight training as part of their training program had significantly higher rates of injury.[6]

Overhead Arm Activity

Impingement of the rotator cuff, long head of biceps tendon, and subacromial bursa between the coracoacromial arch and the humeral head has been recognized as a major source of rotator cuff trauma—the so-called "impingement syndrome."[13] Furthermore, the multifactorial nature of this problem, particularly the inclusion of passive laxity and functional laxity based on muscle dyssynergy, is gradually becoming more apparent. Traditionally, sports involving repetitive overhead arm positions, such as swimming, baseball pitching, and tennis serving, have been associated with its occurrence. Wheelchair athletes are also frequently required to assume overhead arm positions in sports, such as weightlifting and training, shotput, javelin, tennis, and basketball. It may be for this reason that wheelchair basketball centers were found to have a 4 times greater risk of developing shoulder injuries.[6] Wheelchair basketball players playing the position of center are required to hold their arms in overhead positions frequently and for prolonged periods of time as they rebound and shoot (Fig. 28-1). Overhead arm positions are also frequently required by the wheelchair-dependent,

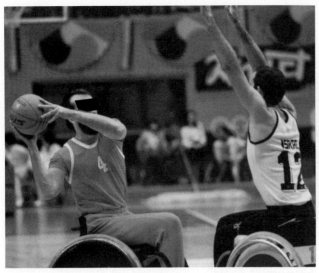

FIGURE 28-1
Wheelchair sport frequently involves assuming positions of shoulder impingement.

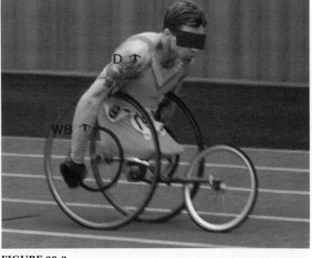

FIGURE 28-2
Deltoid muscle pull (D) and arm weightbearing (WB) result in forces narrowing the acromiohumeral space, causing rotator cuff impingement.

who conduct everyday life activities from the low height of a wheelchair but must reach and operate objects at a height convenient for able-bodied individuals who are standing. Thus requirements of everyday life activities as well as sport frequently place the shoulders of wheelchair athletes in overhead impingement positions.

Arm Weightbearing

The rotator cuff and subacromial bursa can also be impinged in the wheelchair athlete as a result of upper-extremity weightbearing. With each hand strike on the wheel and with each transfer, an axial load is transmitted up the arm, resulting in a force pushing the humeral head cephalad against the coracoacromial arch (Fig. 28-2). If this motion is uncontrolled, the rotator cuff and subacromial bursa within the acromiohumeral space are subjected to high pressures that could result in both mechanical and ischemic injury. Bayley et al. found subacromial pressures rose from 40 to 80 torr in wheelchair-dependent paraplegics during unweighted arm activity, to a mean of 239 torr during arm weightbearing at mid-wheelchair-transfer position.[11]

Muscle Imbalance

Shoulder girdle muscle imbalance is another possible contributor to rotator cuff impingement in wheelchair athletes. The deltoid muscle, when working in isolation, pulls the humeral head cephalad. Normally this force is counterbalanced by the 45 to 55° downward pull provided by the oblique rotator cuff muscles (subscapularis, infraspinatus, and teres minor).[14] Additionally, when the trunk is fixed, the humeral head is pulled downward by the powerful shoulder adductor muscles (latissimus dorsi, teres major, and the lower fibers of pectoralis major). Relative weakness of the shoulder rotator and/or adductor muscles could thus contribute to rotator cuff impingement by providing inadequate counterforce to the cephalad forces acting on the humeral head as a result of both arm weightbearing and deltoid activity (Fig. 28-2).

The role of such a muscle imbalance was recently investigated in 19 paraplegic male wheelchair athletes.[15] Each athlete underwent clinical examination of the shoulders, thus categorizing them as having impingement syndrome or not. It was present in 26 percent of shoulders. Then each shoulder was tested for isokinetic strength (Cybex) in abduction, adduction, and internal and external rotation. The isokinetic torque values were expressed in both absolute terms and as a ratio of strength of abduction to the strength of adduction and internal and external rotation. These values were compared with the values obtained on similar testing of 20 athletic able-bodied men without shoulder problems. Additionally, the isokinetic strength results of the paraplegic shoulders involved with rotator cuff impingement syndrome were compared with those of shoulders that were uninvolved. Not surprisingly, it was found that the paraplegics' shoulders were significantly stronger in all directions than those of the able-bodied athletes. Also, the strength ratio of abduction to adduction was higher for paraplegic athletes (Fig. 28-3). Paraplegics' shoulders with rotator cuff impingement syndrome had significantly higher abduction to adduction and abduction to internal rotation strength ratios than the shoulders of paraplegics without impingement syndrome (Fig. 28-4). This research supports the premise that shoulder

377

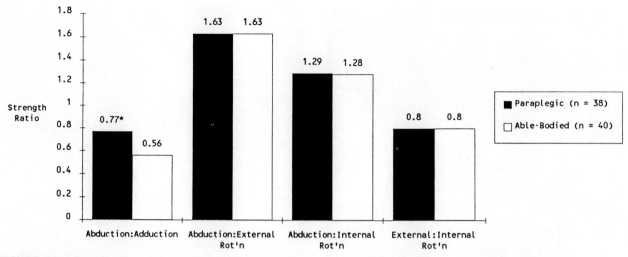

FIGURE 28-3
Isokinetic shoulder strength balance: Paraplegic vs. able-bodied athletes. (*Reproduced with permission from the American Journal of Sports Medicine.*)

muscle imbalance (relative weakness of shoulder rotator and adductor muscles in relation to that of the deltoid) may be a contributor to rotator cuff impingement in wheelchair athletes. Shoulder adductor and rotator insufficiency would also enhance the impingement of the rotator cuff resultant from upper-extremity weightbearing, during wheelchair propulsion and transfers.

Anecdotally, it has been noticed that wheelchair-dependent athletes often assume a position of scapular abduction during sport and at rest (Fig. 28-5). This posture may lead to or result from muscle imbalance, with the scapular adductor group becoming weaker and overstretched as the anterior pectoralis group becomes tighter and stronger. If the scapular adductor muscles (rhomboids and midtrapezii) are

insufficient to control scapular abduction, the scapula will be an unstable anchor for the shoulder rotator muscles that originate from it, thus contributing to the strength insufficiency of the rotator cuff muscles. Additionally, if the scapula remains in an abducted and upwardly rotated position during shoulder weightbearing, the length-tension relationship of the rotator cuff may be altered, further contributing to its weakness and inability to control the upward migration of the humeral head into the acromiohumeral space. The impingement potential of an abducted scapular posture is supported by a recent MRI study that found the size of the subacromial space too narrow as the shoulder moved from an adducted (retracted) to an abducted (protracted) position.[16]

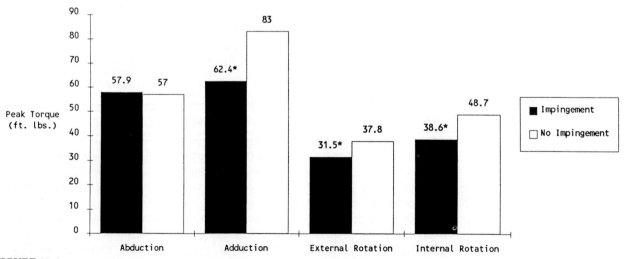

FIGURE 28-4
Isokinetic shoulder strength balance: Paraplegic athletes' shoulders with vs. without impingement syndrome. (*Reproduced with permission from the American Journal of Sports Medicine.*)

378

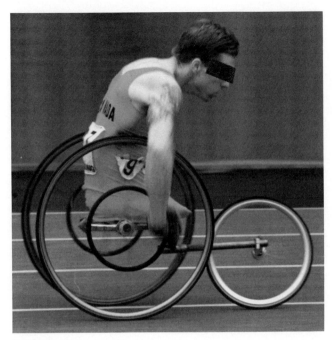

FIGURE 28-5
Internal rotation shoulder impingement position with wheeling. (*Reproduced with permission from the American Journal of Sports Medicine.*)

Wheelchair seat position largely determines the posture the wheelchair user assumes at rest and during activity. Masse et al.[17] studied the relationship of wheelchair seat position to upper-extremity kinematics and EMG activity. It was found that lower seat positions were preferable, as they were associated with lower levels of EMG activity in pectoral and anterior deltoid muscles. Additionally, the kinematics of upper-extremity joints were noted to have a smoother motion, with less abrupt elbow and forearm acceleration.

Inflexibility

Shoulder inflexibility may also be a contributing cause of shoulder pain. Curtis et al.[18] found that spinal-cord-injured wheelchair athletes with shoulder symptoms have less shoulder extension and tendencies to less shoulder abduction range of motion than those without shoulder pain. These tight muscle groups are predominantly those of the anterior shoulder, which is in keeping with the observation of chronic scapular abduction posturing. Insufficient shoulder extension causes the athlete to internally rotate and abduct the shoulder during the recovery and initial contact phases of wheelchair propulsion. This position of shoulder internal rotation and abduction is also a recognized rotator cuff impingement position.[13,16] Overstretching of the scapular adductors may explain the common occurrence of midtrapezius-rhomboid myofascial pain frequently seen in wheelchair athletes.[12]

TREATMENT

Treatment of shoulder problems in wheelchair athletes should be initiated with an appreciation of the magnitude of the disability incurred by shoulder problems and/or iatrogenic immobilization of the shoulder. The several-week period of shoulder rest and immobilization commonly required post rotator cuff decompression and repair renders the wheelchair athlete virtually immobile and dependent. Ideally, prevention of the shoulder problems should be the athlete's, coach's, and sport medicine professional's goal. Preventive measures include:

1. *Allowing adequate rest and recovery time for the athlete.* Training program modifications to allow 24 to 48 h of recovery time between practices and competitions may require rescheduling by the coach or reevaluation by the wheelchair athlete regarding the number of concurrent sporting and recreational activities he or she is involved in.

2. *Minimizing shoulder rotator cuff impingement by minimizing overhead impingement positioning of the arms.* The frequency and duration of shoulder impingement positioning should be minimized by the wheelchair athlete. This could include modifications such as limiting the number of repetitive foul shots performed by a wheelchair basketball player in practice, avoiding extreme forward flexion positions of the shoulders while doing weight training maneuvers such as latissimus pull-downs and military or inclined bench presses. Shorter-arc latissimus pull-downs could be adopted, or a horizontal or declined bench utilized to avoid shoulder impingement positioning. Home or work modifications may be necessary so that the athlete's work space is at a more accessible wheelchair level.

3. *Improving shoulder strength balance.* Strengthening activities of the shoulder rotators, adductors, and scapular adductors should be incorporated into the regular strength training performed by the athlete.[15,19] The wheelchair athlete can easily and inexpensively do these exercises while sitting in the wheelchair utilizing dental dam or surgical tubing (Fig. 28-6). Rowing and backward wheeling are alternative exercises for improving scapular adductor strength and posture[20] (Fig. 28-7). All these exercises should be performed with the arms below the horizontal level of the shoulders to avoid impingement positioning. Resistance and repetition should be modified such that both the strength and endurance components of the muscles are trained.

4. *Posture and flexibility training.* Routine stretching of the anterior shoulder musculature should be included in the training programs of wheelchair athletes by performing exercises that promote mo-

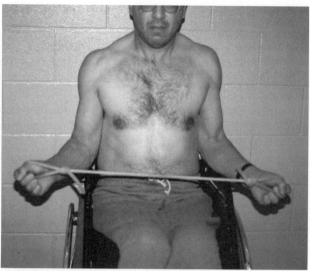

FIGURE 28-6
External rotation shoulder strengthening exercises using surgical tubing.

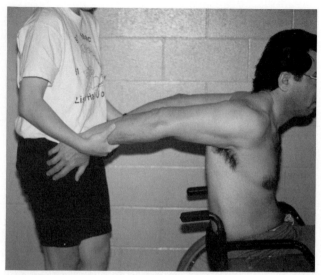

FIGURE 28-8
Assisted stretching into shoulder extension.

tion into shoulder extension, external rotation, and scapular adduction (Fig. 28-8). This may require the assistance of a teammate or trainer to be done adequately.

5. *Wheelchair positioning.* Wheelchair seat position and back height should promote a posture of scapular adduction and provide sufficient pelvic stabilization and lumbar and lower back support. This can be accomplished by using rigid back supports

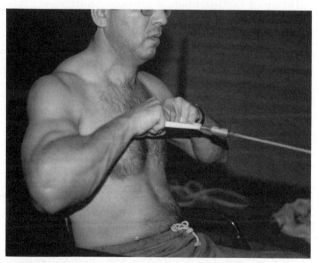

FIGURE 28-7
Rowing is a good scapular retractor strengthening exercise.

and seating systems that encourage an anterior pelvic tilt. Seat height adjustments to lower positions may also help reduce undesirable forces at the shoulders.[17]

It is hoped that with regular adherence to the above program many of the shoulder problems in wheelchair athletes, as well as nonathletes, can be avoided. However, should they occur, early assessment, diagnosis, and appropriate treatment is mandatory to avoid chronic and persistent problems. It has been well documented that wheelchair athletes tend to "self-treat"[1,2,5] and may be reluctant to seek professional medical or paramedical help, as they perceive it as a step backward in their quest for increasing independence. Perhaps they fear being told they can no longer participate in their recreational activities. Many have had negative experiences with physicians, not because of lack of empathy or interest but because medical personnel have had limited opportunities to become familiar with the special stresses, needs, and demands of the wheelchair athlete. Education of the athletes, coaches, and medical-paramedical personnel about proper and effective measures to prevent shoulder injuries, combined with early and effective treatment intervention when warranted, should reduce the morbidity and added disability resultant from shoulder problems in wheelchair athletes.

REFERENCES

1. Curtis KA, Dillon DA: Survey of wheelchair athletic injuries: Common patterns and prevention. *Paraplegia* 23:170–175, 1985.
2. McCormack DAR, Reid DC, Steadward RD, Syrotuik DG: Injury profiles in wheelchair athletes: Results of a retrospective survey. *Clin J Sport Med* 1:35–40, 1991.
3. Bloomquist LE: Injuries to athletes with physical disabilities—Prevention implications. *Phys Sport Med* 4(9):97–105, 1986.
4. Ferrara MS, Davis RW: Injuries to elite wheelchair athletes. *Paraplegia* 28:335–341, 1990.
5. Ferrara MS, Buckley WE, McCann BC, et al: The injury experience of the competitive athlete with a disability: Prevention implications. *Med Sci Sports Exerc* 24:184–188, 1992.
6. Burnham R, Higgins J, Steadward R: Wheelchair basketball injuries. *Palaestra*, in press.
7. Nichols PJR, Norman PA, Ennis JR: Wheelchair users' shoulder? Shoulder pain in patients with spinal cord lesions. *Scand J Rehabil Med* 11:29–32, 1979.
8. Gellman H, Sie I, Waters RL: Late complications of the weight-bearing upper extremity in the paraplegic patient. *Clin Orthop* 233:132–135, 1988.
9. Sie I, Waters RL, Adkins RH, Gellman H: Upper extremity pain in the post rehabilitation spinal cord injured patient. *Arch Phys Med Rehabil* 73:44–48, 1992.
10. Ohry A, Brooks ME, Steinback TV, Rozin R: Shoulder complications as a cause of delay in rehabilitation of spinal cord injured patients. *Paraplegia* 16:310–316, 1978.
11. Bayley JC, Cochran TP, Sledge CB: The weight bearing shoulder. *J Bone Joint Surg (Am)* 69A(5):676–678, 1987.
12. Burnham R, Newell E, Steadward R: Sports medicine for the physically disabled: The Canadian team experience at the 1988 Seoul Paralympic Games. *Clin J Sport Med* 1:193–196, 1991.
13. Hawkins RJ, Hobeika PE: Impingement syndrome in the athletic shoulder. *Clin Sports Med* 2:184–188, 1983.
14. Perry J: Shoulder anatomy and biomechanics. *Clin Sports Med* 2:247–270, 1983.
15. Burnham RS, May L, Nelson E, Steadward R: Shoulder pain in wheelchair athletes—The role of muscle imbalance. *Am J Sports Med* 21(2):238–242, 1993.
16. Solem-Bertoft E, Thuomas K, Westerberg C: The influence of scapular retraction and protraction on the width of the subacromial space—on MRI study. *Clin Orthop* 252:99–103, 1993.
17. Masse LC, Lamontagne M, O'Riain MD: Biomechanical analysis of wheelchair propulsion for various seating positions. *J Rehabil Res Dev* 29(3):12–28, 1992.
18. Curtis KA, Brown K, Gisen T, et al: Shoulder inflexibility and strength in wheelchair athletes: Implications for preventing shoulder injuries. Presented at the 8th International Symposium, International Federation of Adapted Physical Activity, Miami, FL, Nov. 18, 1991.
19. Milliken T, Morse M, Hedrick B: Prevention of shoulder injuries. *Sports 'n Spokes* 17(2):35–38, 1991.
20. Olenik L, Laskin J, Burnham R, et al: Efficacy of rowing, backward wheeling and isolated scapular exercises as remedial strength activities for wheelchair users: Application of electromyography. Presented at Vista '93, Jasper, Alberta, May 15, 1993.

INDEX

Abrasions, protective bandages for, 373–374
Acromial hook, radiographic evaluation, 177
Acromioclavicular joint:
  anatomy, 1, 13, 167, 168
  arthritis, 240
    arthroscopy in, 66
    clinical evaluation, 319
    in gymnasts, 362
    in tennis player, 319–320
    treatment, 319–320
  arthroscopy: anatomy defined by, 13
    in arthritis, 66
    evaluation and debridement in impingement syndrome, 178
  compression test, 252
  degenerative changes in baseball thrower, 332
  examination, 40
  hypomobility, 251
  injuries, 167–174
    in baseball players, 332
    classification, 167–169
    diagnosis, 170–171
    fractures, 169–170
    golf-related, 289
    in gymnast, 361
    mechanisms, 167
    osteolysis of distal clavicle, 173–174
    physical examination in, 170
    radiographic examination, 170, 171
    surgical repair, 172–173
    treatment, 170–174
    type I, 168, 171
    type II, 168, 171–172
    type III, 168–169, 172
    type IV, 169, 172
    type V, 169, 172
    type VI, 169, 172
  shock pad protection, 367, 369, 370–371
  in shoulder biomechanics, 22–23
  sprain, 361
    shoulder pads for, 370–371
  surface anatomy, 1
Acromioclavicular ligament:
  anatomy, 167, 168
  and shoulder stability, 23
  (See also Acromioclavicular joint)

Acromion:
  arch view in impingement syndrome, 147
  arthroscopy, 12–13
  fracture, 169–170
  impingement on rotator cuff tendons, 143–152, 298
    (See also Impingement syndrome)
  shape and slope related to impingement syndrome, 143, 175
  in SLIP lesion, 158
  in tennis-related impingement syndrome, 315
    (See also Acromioclavicular joint)
Acromionizer burr, in arthroscopic subacromial decompression, 150, 151
Acromioplasty:
  arthroscopic subacromial decompression, 149–151
    advantages, 175
    indications, 176, 177
    technique, 177–178, 181
    (See also Subacromial space, arthroscopic decompression)
  for chronic rotator cuff tear, 317
  in full thickness rotator cuff tear repair, 163
Adhesive capsulitis (see Shoulder, frozen)
Adson's maneuver, 40–41, 238
Adson's sign, 231
Age, rotator cuff effects, 247
Air management system, 366
Allen's test, 238–239
ALPSA lesion, 9
Anatomy:
  of acromioclavicular joint, 167, 168
  arthroscopic, 1–14
    (See also Arthroscopy, anatomy visualized by)
Anesthesia:
  for arthroscopy, 67–68
  examination under, in multidirectional instability, 131
Angiofibroblastic tendinosis:
  pathologic changes, 159
  in rotator cuff disease, 156

Angiography (see Arteriography; Magnetic resonance imaging, angiography)
Anterior drawer test (see Drawer test)
Anterior labroligamentous periosteal sleeve avulsion lesion, 9
Anterior slide test, 39
Apical oblique view, 44, 80
Apprehension relocation test, 146
Apprehension sign, absence in recurrent posterior subluxation, 108
Apprehension-suppression test, 146
Apprehension test, 79
  in instability, 39
    multidirectional, 130–131
  in tennis player, 318
  in throwing injury, 327
Arch view:
  in impingement, 147
  after subacromial decompression, 151
Arm elevation:
  biomechanics, 18–20
  clavicular motion during, 23
  external rotation in, 19–20
  scapulohumeral rhythm in, 18–19
Arterial compression syndrome, 238–239
  diagnosis, 238–239
  treatment, 239
Arteriography:
  of shoulder, 51–52
  for tumors, 52
Arthritis:
  acromioclavicular, 240
    arthroscopy in, 66
    clinical evaluation, 319
    in gymnasts, 362
    in tennis player, 319–320
    treatment, 319–320
  crystal-induced, 238, 240
  glenohumeral, 240
    arthroscopy in, 67
  in hemoglobinopathy, 241
  infectious, 237–238
  in inflammatory bowel disease, 241
  in Lyme disease, 241
  in malignancies, 241
  MRI in, 58
  psoriatic, 241

383

external rotation ratio, 256
in locked posterior dislocation, 106
Intramedullary fixation:
of clavicle fracture, 218, 219
in open reduction of humerus surgical neck fracture, 193–194
in three-part tuberosity fracture, 208
Iontophoresis, in rotator cuff disease, 258–259
Isoflex technique, 273
Isokinetic exercises, 259
for external and internal rotation, 273, 274
Isometric exercises, 259
Isotonic exercises, 259

Kehr's sign, 242
Kenny-Howard shoulder brace, in acromioclavicular joint injury, 172
Knot cutter, in arthroscopic stabilization for anterior instability, 92
Knot pusher:
in arthroscopic stabilization for anterior instability, 92
in nontransglenoid arthroscopic stabilization, 97
in transglenoid horizontal mattress technique, 96, 97
in SLAP lesion repair, 123
Knowles pin, for clavicle fixation, 218
distal fracture, 219
Kocher maneuver, modified, in anterior dislocation, 80
Kyphosis, shoulder effects, 249

Labrum:
anatomy, 4–6
anterior wedge, 6
arthroscopy, 4–6, 67, 71
detachment repair, 330
biceps tendon attachment to, 2
classification of variations in anatomy, 6
configuration changes with arm position, 6
degenerative, arthroscopic stabilization influenced by, 90

evaluation in throwing injury, 327–328
flap debridement in recurrent anterior instability, 82
GLAD lesion, 4
and glenohumeral stability, 21
impingement syndrome similar to injury involving, 319
injuries in tennis players, 318–319
in instability, 55, 67
multidirectional, 129
meniscoid, 117, 118
and superior labral injury, 117
MRI for abnormalities involving, 55–56
posterior wedge, 6
SLAP lesion, 2–3
(See also SLAP lesion)
and stability of shoulder, 76–77
superior injuries, 117–124
anterior instability related to, 117–118
avulsion and fraying, 118
biceps tendon role in mechanism, 117, 120
examination for, 39, 40
mechanisms for, 117–118, 120
pathology, 117
SLAP lesion, 118–124
classification, 118–120
diagnosis, 120–121
postoperative rehabilitation, 124
surgical treatment, 121–124
(See also SLAP lesion)
types, 118–120
tears in baseball players, 330–331
vascularity, 117
Lacrosse, shoulder pad in, 366–367, 369
LaPorta Collar, 367, 372
Lateral pull-down, 263, 264
Latissimus dorsi:
exercises in rotator cuff disease, 260
function, 246
in golf swing, 290–291
in pitching, 25
strengthening exercises, 274, 275
Leffert's test, 252–253
Levator scapulae:
exercises for, 274
function, 246
Ligaments:
arthroscopic evaluation, 70–71
glenohumeral, 6–8
(See also Glenohumeral ligaments)

laxity, 79
examination, 131
overuse causing shoulder dysfunction, 248
and shoulder stability, 21–23
Liver, shoulder pain referred from, 242
Load and shift test, 109, 298, 299
Long thoracic nerve:
entrapment neuropathy, 233, 234–235
paralysis causing serratus anterior palsy, 249
Longhorn neck roll, 367, 372
Loose bodies, arthroscopy for, 67
Ludington's test, 252, 253
Lyme disease:
arthritis in, 241
clinical features, 241

Magnetic resonance imaging, 52–60
advantages, 52
over arthrogram, 147
angiography, 52
arthrography: contrast agents with, 56–57
disadvantages, 57
in SLAP lesion, 120–121
in biceps tendon abnormalities, 57
in cervical radiculopathy, 228–229
double-line sign, 58
for ganglion cyst, 58
in humerus fracture, 188
in impingement syndrome, 53–54, 147–148
in instability of shoulder, 55–56, 80
anterior, 55–56
multidirectional, 56, 131
posterior, 56
limitations, 52
in osteoarthritis, 58
in osteonecrosis, 57–58
of rotator cuff, 52–53, 147–148
complete tear, 54
partial tear, 54
in synovial disorders, 58–59
technique, 52
for tumors, 59–60
Malunion, of greater tuberosity fracture, 203–206
Massage, transverse friction, in rotator cuff disease, 258
Mesenchymal syndrome, 248

DATE DUE